30天就會瘦，1天1頁跟著做，
養成易瘦體質不復胖！

最強瘦身教科書

The most effective textbook for losing weight

監修
Sport&Science 負責人
坂詰真二

晨星出版

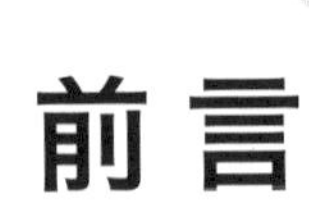

前言

聽到「你覺得為了瘦下來，首先該做的事是什麼？」這個問題時，我想很多人第一個想到的答案是節食與腹肌運動，但很可惜這是錯誤的答案。就真正的意義而言，為了成功減輕體重，第一步該做好的基本功是「準備」！

現在已經是只要利用網路，不論是想得到的資訊還是物品，都能輕易到手的時代。我很明白許多人看了在網路或電視節目中介紹的各種「看起來很有效」的節食方法和運動，馬上躍躍欲試的心情，但是，急著付諸行動，往往只會帶來失敗、挫折，甚至是復胖的惡夢。

準備工作的重要性放諸四海皆準；不論是參加考試還是找工作，甚至是買房子，做好事先準備都很重要。如果在準備不夠充分的情況下貿然行動，就會等到進了新學校或新公司才發現不適合自己，或者是因為買到有缺陷的房子而後悔莫及。

瘦身也是一樣的道理。在毫無準備的情況下，只因看到或聽到一句廣告標語就起心動念，投入必須忍受空腹之苦、有如斷食般嚴格的飲食計畫，或者展開忍不住讓人咬緊牙關的高強度運動，那麼即將降臨在你身上的，除了身心俱疲，還有隨之而來的挫折感，有時甚至連身心健康都因此遭殃。即使靠著強大的意志力勉強自己苦撐，最後看到的轉變不是「精瘦結實的身體」，而是「瘦弱不堪的身體」，與自己原先預期的肌肉變得緊實的健美姿態相差十萬八千里，但是後悔也來不及了。

我要傳授給各位的，不是讓人瘦得看起來一臉憔悴，而是確實能降低體脂肪、仍可保持肌肉結實，而且終身維持的方法。因此，不論是節食還是運動，本書並不建議各位馬上行動。我希望各位首先要具備有關瘦身的正確知識，並掌握自己目前的身體狀況，做好壓力調適，杜絕導致暴飲暴食的可能性。簡單來說，在正式投入之前請先做好身心準備。

接著請開始進行為期30天的瘦身計畫。只要確實完成1日1項的課題，相信各位應該能逐漸感受到身體的變化。30天在我們的一生僅占了１／１０００，但只要各位在這１／１０００的時間付出努力，從此就不必再為體型或體重煩惱。

接下來，請各位開始翻頁，開始閱讀序章吧。

２０２０年12月吉日

Ｓｐｏｒｔ＆Ｓｃｉｅｎｃｅ負責人

坂詰真二

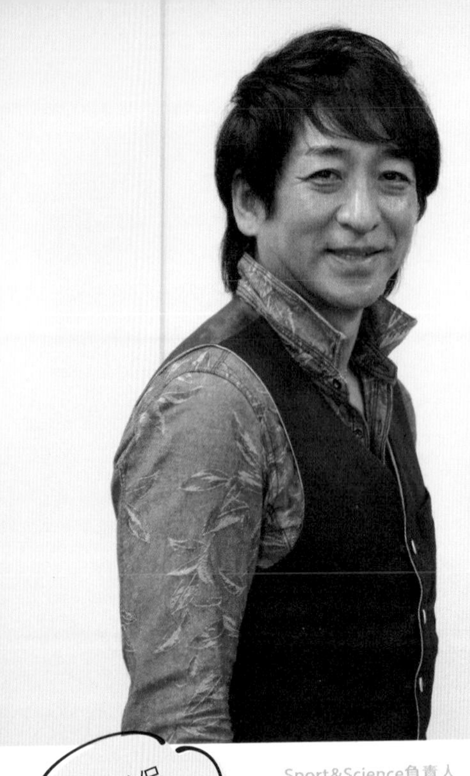
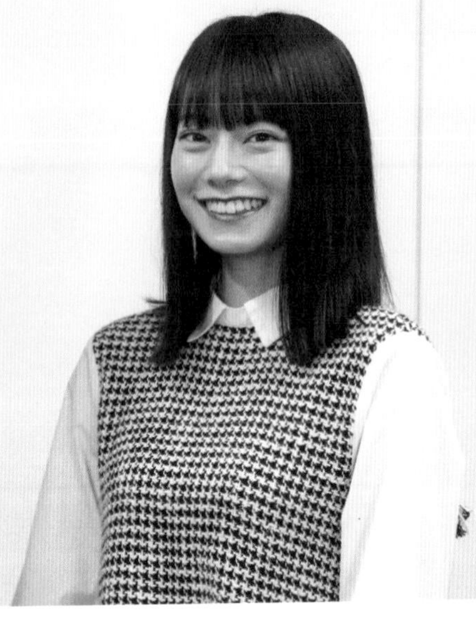

讓你常保
青春美麗

Sport&Science負責人
YouTuber・影片創作者

坂詰真二 × nagomi［對談］

到底什麼才是正確的瘦身方法!?

nagomi是知名的美妝YouTuber，除了透過影片分享美容、健身方式，
本身也靠著好身材獲得同年齡層的壓倒性支持。
藉由這次的對談，她向坂詰老師請教了連粉絲也曾向她諮詢的有關瘦身的煩惱。

第一步是重建減重知識

nagomi（以下簡稱n） 我要把我想問的通通趁今天這個機會請教您。

坂詰（以下簡稱坂） 當然沒問題，想問什麼都可以，不要客氣！

n 經常有粉絲向我尋求有關瘦身的意見，請問第一步該從哪裡做起呢？

坂 說到這個問題嘛，我覺得想要成功瘦下來的人，最好把眼光放遠，抱著長期抗戰的心理準備。不是只有20幾歲的年輕人才希望自己變美吧……應該吧。即使到了30歲、40歲，女性還是希望自己的狀態能維持得很好，就連男性，也希望自己永遠看起來很帥氣。你周圍有沒有人用簡直在虐待自己的方式瘦身呢？

n　有耶，我知道有些人採用很激烈的節食方式。

坂　是啊。從網路等媒體看到什麼好像很有效的減重方法，就馬上跟著做的人還真不少。如果遇到這類的年輕朋友，我第一句想告訴他們的是：請重建減重知識。

n　重建知識是什麼意思啊……？

坂　減重的結果是不可逆的，有些東西一旦失去了，就沒辦法再找回來。為了在短時間瘦下來，身體和精神都要付出很大的代價。

n　很快瘦下來，但馬上就復胖的例子我聽過很多。

坂　剛開始減重時，表現出強大的衝勁雖然不是壞事，但忍耐1個星期、2個星期以後，很多人就因為過度壓抑而反彈，結果食慾爆發，而且一發不可收拾。你不覺得飲食限制愈是嚴格，人就愈容易滿腦子都是食物嗎？

n　真的是這樣。如果忍耐過頭，最後一定會反彈嘛。

坂　選擇錯誤的減重方式，減掉的不只有脂肪，還有肌肉和骨質密度，除了貧血，也會造成免疫力下降。如果是女性，甚至還可能出現無月經症狀。想到將來對身體的各種影響，真的是很可怕的事。所以我希望大家在減重之前，先掌握減重的正確知識。

n　原來如此。為了避免失敗，首先重建原有的認知很重要呢！

強健的心理素質是減重成功的捷徑

坂　重建好有關減重的正確知識以後，我建議大家下一步要做的不是節食也不是拉筋運動，而是想辦法紓解壓力。

n　要先消除壓力嗎？

坂　有過食傾向的人，或是一次吃很多甜食的人，基本上都是為了某些原因而覺得壓力很大。「吃」是生活中的一大樂事，但如果在無法掌控壓力的情況下，受到「限醣」「禁止吃甜食」等各種飲食限制，心理壓力就會不斷升高，造成內心受挫，瘦下來又復胖也是這樣造成的。有些情況嚴重的人，甚至會演變成進食障礙。

n　原來如此啊！

坂　這本書第一個談到有關飲食的部分是「喝水」。食物超過一半的成分是水，所以很多人把想喝水的生理需求和食慾混為一談。明明不是正餐時間，卻老是吃個不停的人，即使只是喝水，就能抑制食慾。

n　沒錯。難怪常聽到人家說減重的時候，一天要喝2公升的水。

坂　你很有概念喔！1天的喝水量，最好是體重的4～5％。建議大家最好一次喝一杯的量。喝完一杯水的時間大約是1分鐘，而且記得慢慢地呼吸。光是這麼做就有紓壓的效果。

n　難道消除壓力後，飲食生活也會跟著改變嗎？

坂　是的。根據我的指導經驗，我可以很肯定地說一定會改變。

n　要不是聽您說，我好像從沒意識到這個問題耶。沒想到暴飲暴飲的原因居然是壓力太大。

坂　我自己還是菜鳥教練的時候也沒發現。因此吃了很多苦頭，也一再犯錯。

n　總之，好好處理自己的壓力，對減重而言是不可欠缺的一環吧。不過，如果想瘦下來，均衡的飲食是不是才是關鍵呢？

坂　沒錯。醣類、脂質、蛋白質、礦物質、維生素、膳食纖維都是很重要的營養素。做到飲食的營養均衡，才能打造不容易發胖的健康身體。

矯正姿勢，把「自我效能」當作獎勵

坂　你是不是有在做什麼運動？

n　我打過硬式網球很長一段時間。

坂　nagomi你的姿勢很端正漂亮，我猜你的網球應該打得很好吧？運動是減重的一環，而運動的第一步是矯正錯誤的姿勢。只要在做拉筋運動的時候，矯正腹肌、屁股、胸部等不應該變硬的地方，姿勢就會變得很漂亮。姿勢如果不正確，不論做什麼運動都做不好。同樣的道理，如果用錯誤的姿勢鍛鍊肌肉，不但效果不佳，還可能會受傷。所以請在進行拉筋運動之前，先矯正自己的姿勢。

n 我以前每個星期會健身2～3次，但現在只會在有重要的攝影工作前臨時抱佛腳，這樣的運動頻率OK嗎？

坂 一開始每星期健身2～3次，慢慢地鍛鍊出肌肉，等到你覺得這些動作都做得很熟練了，就養成每週固定做一次的習慣。1種做3分鐘，總共4種或5種，全部做完大概只要15分鐘。

n 覺得健身訓練好累的時候，有沒有什麼方法可以提高自己的動力呢？

坂 做到讓自己大喊吃不消的程度是NG行為。如果發現自己咬緊牙關，一臉「面目猙獰」的樣子，表示做過頭了。如果只差兩次就達標，但已經覺得很累，就不要勉強自己一定要做完。因為就算差這兩次，效果也不會有什麼改變。

n 您的這番話真的讓我受益良多！因為我常常會勉強自己做到做不下去為止。

坂 我把這本書的重點放在心理問題、認知的問題與如何掌控壓力。有關減重的內容寫在每一頁，讓大家每翻一頁就看一點。希望大家不要急慢慢來，最後都能減重成功，而且永不復胖。

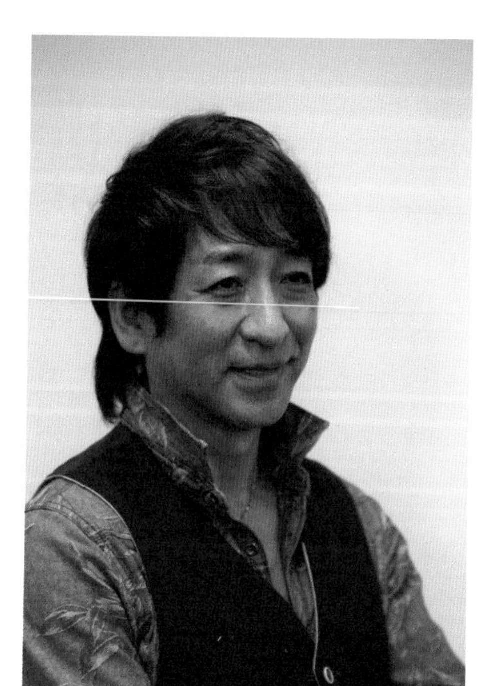

Profile

YouTuber／影片創作者

nagomi

1997年生。與男友Koki共同經營的頻道「Nokonoko Chanel」，訂閱人數已達144萬。在2020年6月開設的個人頻道。在拍攝健身訓練過程的影片中，本人展現的姣好身材也備受矚目。

nagomi的頻道在這裡

Prologue
〔序章〕

減重成功的關鍵在於事前準備!!

在展開節食計畫、健身訓練之前，先搞定壓力問題

如果希望成功減重，最重要的關鍵在於做好充分的事前準備。因為準備工作要是做得不夠充分，減重就可能無法順利進行，容易遇到挫折。

具體而言，應該事先做好的準備有3項。**第1項是拋開有關瘦身的錯誤認知，建立正確的觀念。**有關這部分將從P10開始詳細說明。**第2項是掌握現狀，設定有可能實現的目標。**有關這部分則從P14開始解說。**第3項是做好壓力管理。**原因很簡單，人會胖的主要原因就是飲食過量，而人之所以飲食沒有節制，為了紓壓是其中主要原因之一。

一旦承受壓力，就會大量分泌讓人身心轉向亢奮狀態、進入戰鬥模式的荷爾蒙「腎上腺素」。其實，腎上腺素會隨著身體劇烈的活動而被消耗，壓力也就此消除是身體原有的機制，但是，有過重的心理壓力已經成為現代人的宿命。即使已經解決眼前的問題，但腎上腺

減重的事前準備

1 拋開有關瘦身的錯誤認知，建立正確的觀念

2 掌握現狀，設定有可能實現的目標

3 做好壓力管理

素卻未被消耗，不安與焦躁的心情依舊存在。因此，**人很容易透過暴飲暴食或飲酒等「補償行為」以減緩壓力**。了解這點以後，相信大家都會同意，做好壓力管理確實是減重的必備要件。本書也會仔細說明紓緩、消除壓力的方法，把如何避免因壓力過大而暴食視為優先事項。

即使乍看是繞遠路，但確實做好上述的準備事項，再搭配「適當的飲食控制＋鍛鍊全身肌肉」，就最終結果而言，才是成功減重的最佳捷徑。

有如苦行僧的飲食限制只會造成反效果！

即使在減重期間也要正常享受飲食的樂趣

搞定壓力之後，下一步就是飲食限制。

說到飲食限制，我猜很多人馬上想到的是類似「每天都吃雞胸肉＋青花菜」那種極端低醣、低脂、高蛋白的菜單。如果一直實踐這樣的飲食法，體脂肪確實有可能降低，但「吃的樂趣」很肯定也蕩然無存了。有些人為了徹底執行這樣的飲食計畫，甚至不惜犧牲與家人同桌用餐的機會，另外，有些以營養代餐為主食的人，當然也很難與家人相聚吃飯了。

如果是健美運動員，有時候在減量期會採用上述低醣、低脂、高蛋白的菜單，但只要減量期一過，對拉麵、炸物、甜點也是來者不拒。長期執行極度嚴格的飲食計畫，對身體和心理狀態都會造成負面影響，嚴重者甚至會演變成進食障礙。

每天的三餐是打造健康身心的基礎。最後提醒大家一點，別忘了「吃」對人類而言是最大的樂趣之一。有如苦行僧的飲食限制會讓人

身體必要的營養素

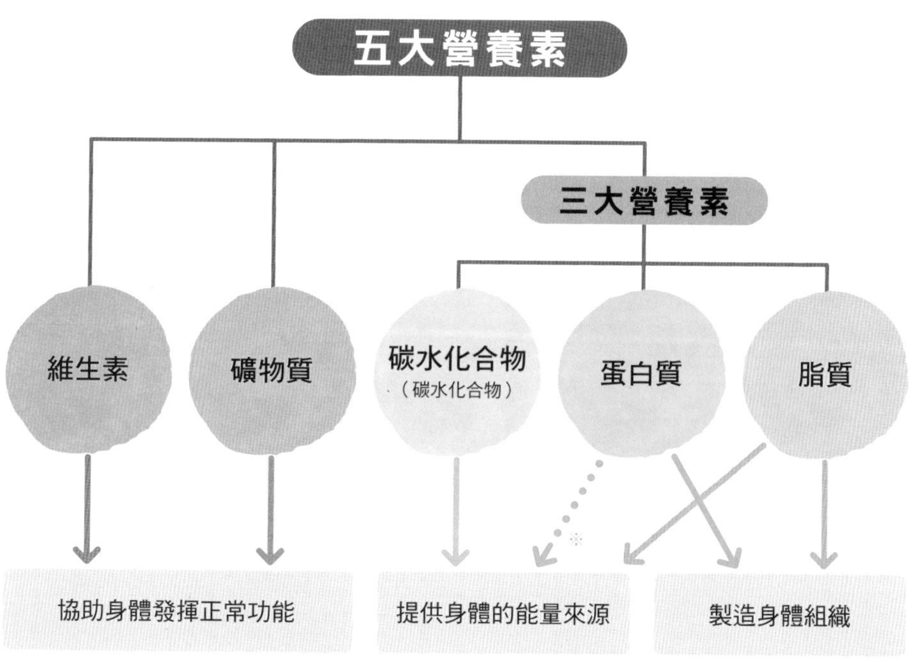

※飢餓狀態及接近飢餓狀態時

不斷累積壓力，最後為了宣洩壓力而暴飲暴食。

有關飲食限制的具體方法容待後述；**在此我要向大家強調的是，最重要的是擁有正確的知識，均衡攝取各類食品以維持營養均衡。**尤其重要的是要均衡攝取碳水化合物（醣類＋膳食纖維）、蛋白質和脂質。因為我們從食物攝取的這些營養素，會轉化成身體活動所需的能量，以及製造肌肉等各種細胞的原料。三大營養素與維生素、礦物質合稱為五大營養素。每一種營養素在體內各司其職，缺一不可。

「鍛鍊肌肉」不僅能夠降低體脂肪，還能維持肌肉量

增加肌肉量、提高基礎代謝，就能打造易瘦體質

飲食限制之後的下一個目標是鍛鍊肌肉。

一旦認真執行節食計畫，體脂肪確實會降低沒錯，但肌肉量無法避免地也會跟著減少。為了彌補流失的肌肉，鍛鍊肌肉是百分之百必要的訓練。

為了讓人體的腦部、心臟、肺部等器官能夠正常運作，維持生命原本就需要消耗大量的能量。為了維持生命所需消耗的最低限度之能量稱為「基礎代謝」。人所消耗的能量可大分為基礎代謝量、運動代謝量、隨著飲食產生的代謝量（DIT），其中消耗量最大的是基礎代謝量，占了整體的60～70％。

基礎代謝量的20～40％，由肌肉所消耗。肌肉是製造體溫的發熱裝置，即使人保持安靜不動，每1kg的肌肉也會消耗15～30大卡的熱量。

簡單來說，**肌肉量愈多的人，即使生活方式與一般人無異，但因消耗的熱量較多，自然**

1日所消耗的熱量比例與基礎代謝的明細

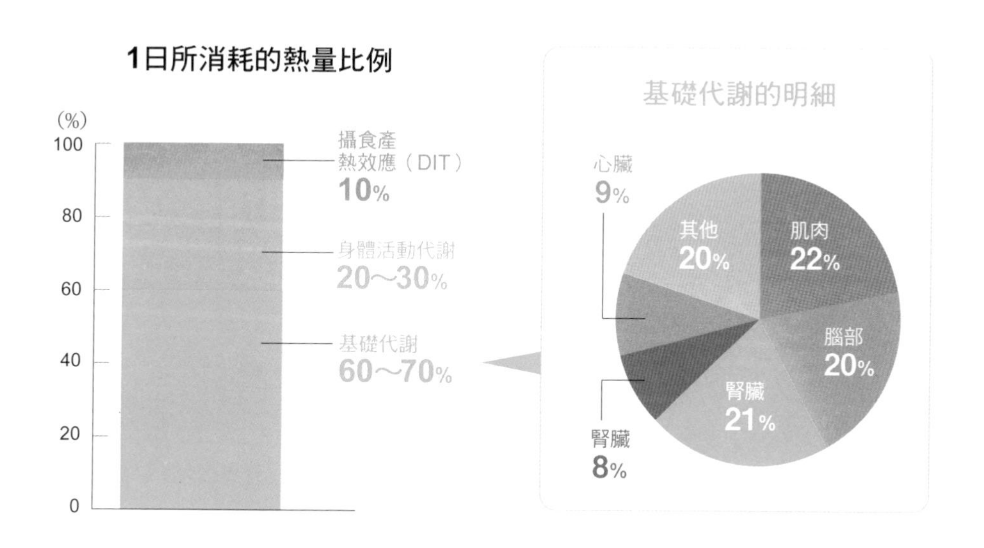

出處：改編自厚生勞動省「身體活動與能量代謝」／厚生勞動省e-健康網「人的器官．組織的靜息代謝率」（糸川嘉則等 編 營養學總論 改訂第3版 南江堂,141-164,2006.）

就比較容易瘦下來。相反地，如果只靠飲食限制以降低體脂肪，那麼連肌肉量也會跟著減少；如此一來，因基礎代謝量下降，使體內囤積多餘的熱量，自然也就成為易胖體質了。除此之外，過於嚴格的飲食限制也會造成復胖。雪上加霜的是，復胖時增加的全是體脂肪。

適度地鍛鍊肌肉，可以讓姿勢更挺拔，達到減齡效果。除此之外，也有幫助細胞修復、促進生長荷爾蒙分泌等功效，另外，預防骨密度降低與貧血的效果也頗值得期待。

客觀地檢視現在的自己屬於哪一種體型

只要有體重計和捲尺，就能掌握自己的體型

為了成功減重，首先必須誠實面對自己目前的體型。從「身高與腰圍、ＢＭＩ（身體質量指數）」就能在某種程度上判斷自己的身體組成，**首先請各位以客觀的眼光檢視自己的體型吧。**

首先請依照左圖算出自己的ＢＭＩ。❶ＢＭＩ的算法是「體重（kg）÷身高（m）÷身高（m）」。❷是測量腰圍，算出「腰圍（cm）÷身高（cm）」是多少。這個數值愈高，表示有可能腹部周圍囤積了內臟脂肪與皮下脂肪，造成體脂肪率過高。

將計算出來的數值與❸的圖比對，就可以大略掌握自己屬於哪一種體型了。

經過比對之後，我想大多數的人都屬於「壯碩體型」「代謝症候群體型」「隱形肥胖體型」「重度肥胖體型」的其中之一。不過，執行30天減重計畫之後，我相信這些人的體型都會轉變為「標準體型」或「結實體型」。

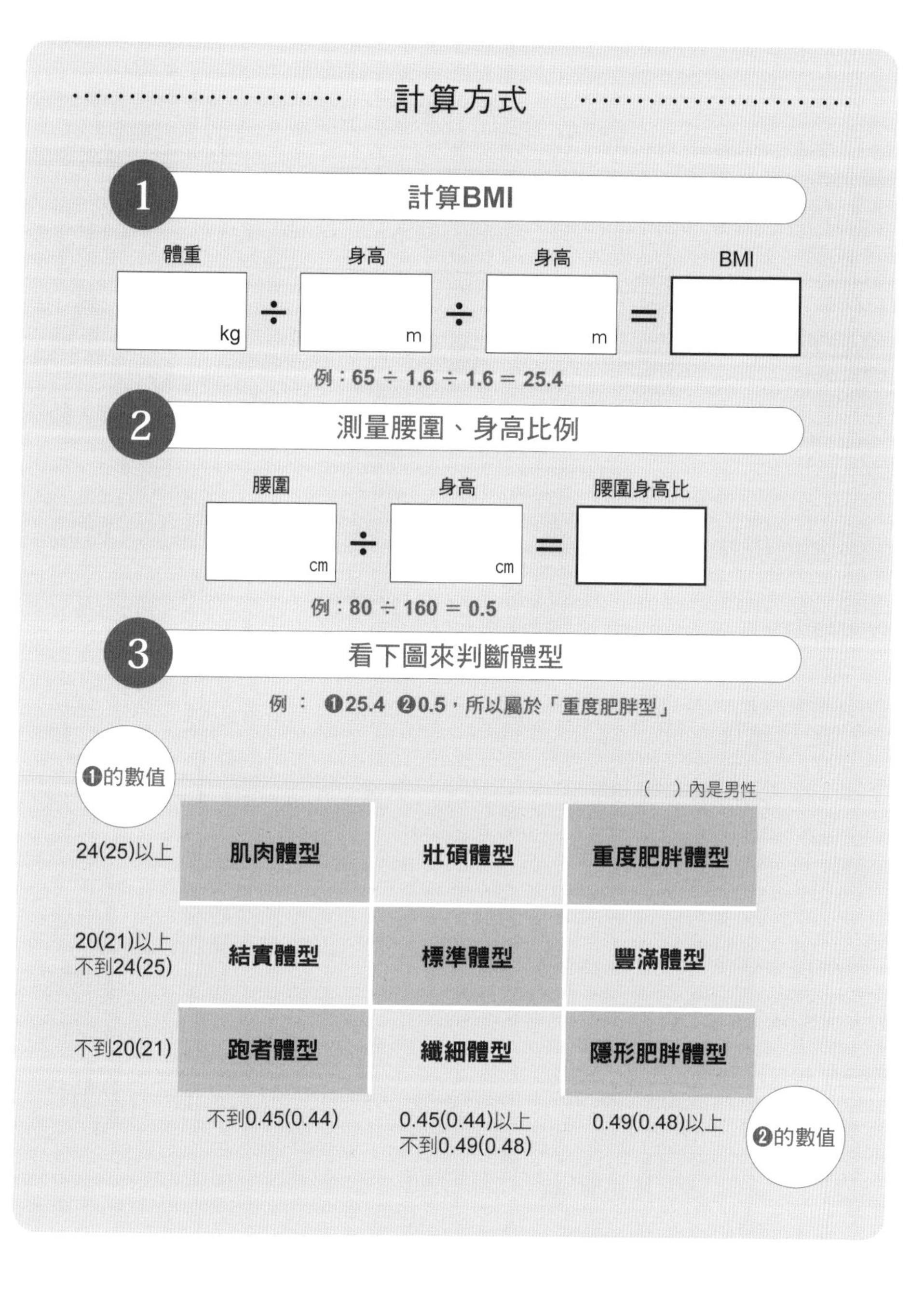

計算方式

1 計算BMI

體重 ＿＿ kg ÷ 身高 ＿＿ m ÷ 身高 ＿＿ m ＝ BMI ＿＿

例：65 ÷ 1.6 ÷ 1.6 ＝ 25.4

2 測量腰圍、身高比例

腰圍 ＿＿ cm ÷ 身高 ＿＿ cm ＝ 腰圍身高比 ＿＿

例：80 ÷ 160 ＝ 0.5

3 看下圖來判斷體型

例 ： ❶25.4 ❷0.5，所以屬於「重度肥胖型」

（　）內是男性

❶的數值 \ ❷的數值	不到0.45(0.44)	0.45(0.44)以上 不到0.49(0.48)	0.49(0.48)以上
24(25)以上	肌肉體型	壯碩體型	重度肥胖體型
20(21)以上 不到24(25)	結實體型	標準體型	豐滿體型
不到20(21)	跑者體型	纖細體型	隱形肥胖體型

坂詰式 設定正確的目標與制定不會受挫的計畫方法

制定具體的計畫，設定到何時為止要瘦下幾kg

確認自己現在的體型後，請先設定「在什麼時候之前要把體重降到○○kg」的目標。這時，為了方便自己掌握更準確的現況，建議大家先準備一台可測體脂率的體脂計。

前提是不能減少肌肉與骨骼、血液的量（除脂體重），只能減去脂肪。另外，考慮到體脂肪也有保護身體免於因衝擊受到傷害、維持體溫等重要功能，所以減少太多也不行。**女性16％、男性8％是維持健康的最低體脂肪量。**

在這個前提下，以女性來說，「體重的下限」的計算方式是現在的除脂體重除以0．84，男性是除以0．92（左表Step❶）。

接著，請自行在自己的體重下限與現在體重之間設定「目標體重」（左表Step❷）。

最後從目標體重反推回去，即可算出「應該減去的體脂肪量」「1星期應減去的脂肪量」，以及「達成目標的所需時間」（左表Step❷❸）。

設定目標的計畫方法

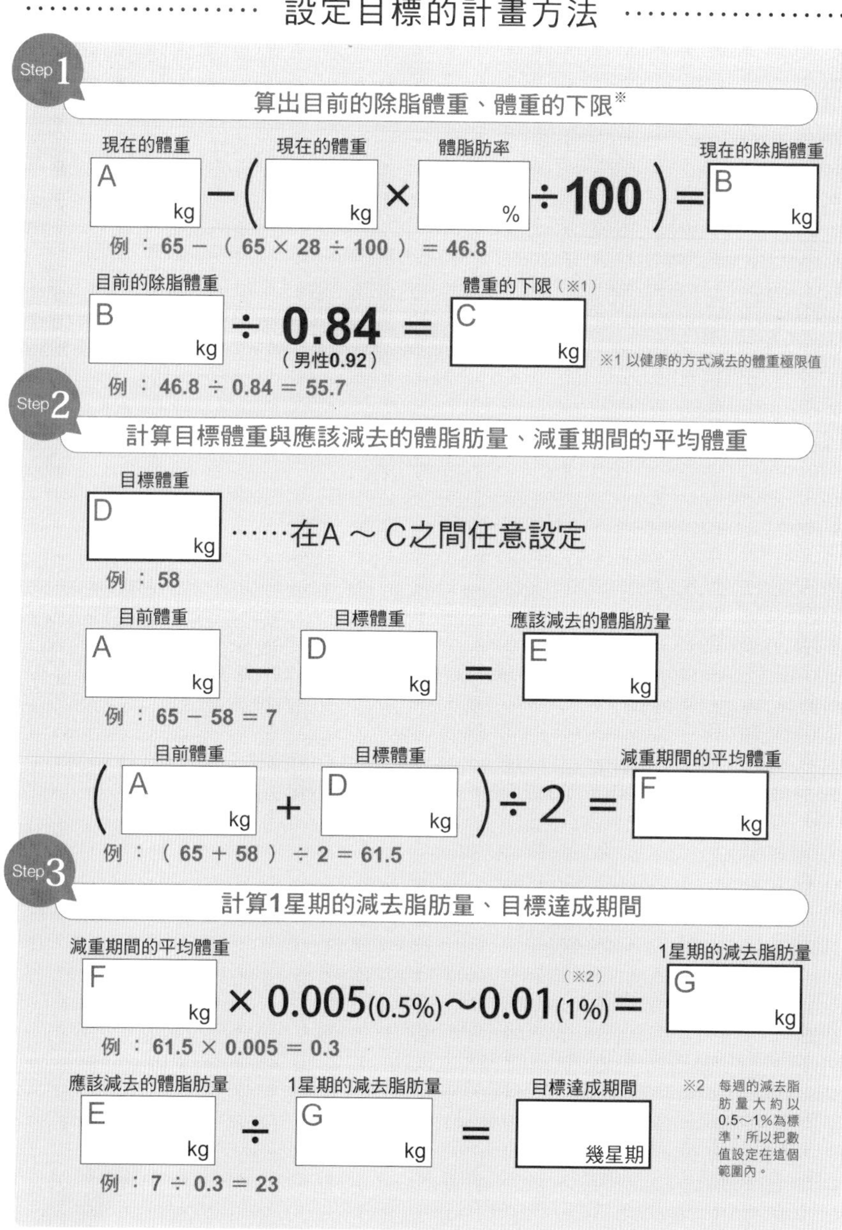
Step 1
算出目前的除脂體重、體重的下限※
現在的體重 A kg －（ 現在的體重 kg × 體脂肪率 % ÷100 ）＝ 現在的除脂體重 B kg
例：65 －（65 × 28 ÷ 100）＝ 46.8
目前的除脂體重 B kg ÷ 0.84（男性0.92）＝ 體重的下限（※1） C kg
※1 以健康的方式減去的體重極限值
例：46.8 ÷ 0.84 ＝ 55.7
Step 2
計算目標體重與應該減去的體脂肪量、減重期間的平均體重
目標體重 D kg ……在A ～ C之間任意設定
例：58
目前體重 A kg － 目標體重 D kg ＝ 應該減去的體脂肪量 E kg
例：65 － 58 ＝ 7
（目前體重 A kg ＋ 目標體重 D kg）÷ 2 ＝ 減重期間的平均體重 F kg
例：（65 ＋ 58）÷ 2 ＝ 61.5
Step 3
計算1星期的減去脂肪量、目標達成期間
減重期間的平均體重 F kg × 0.005(0.5%)～0.01(1%)（※2）＝ 1星期的減去脂肪量 G kg
例：61.5 × 0.005 ＝ 0.3
應該減去的體脂肪量 E kg ÷ 1星期的減去脂肪量 G kg ＝ 目標達成期間 幾星期
例：7 ÷ 0.3 ＝ 23
※2 每週的減去脂肪量大約以0.5～1%為標準，所以把數值設定在這個範圍內。

利用減重清單，挑戰30日減重計畫

每達成1項就打勾確認，體驗滿滿的成就感

請各位善用在卷末附贈的減重清單，充分體驗成就感與充實感吧。本書的3大主軸分別是營養、心態與大腦、運動。**只要每天讀1篇，不斷地增加自己的知識，或者透過身體力行，30天後就能養成容易瘦身的心態，進而自然轉變為易瘦體質。**

這些項目有些是從開始當天之後，每天都要持續進行，也有些只需當天執行。請依照這份清單，閱讀當天的內容，完成後打勾。除此之外，記得每天站上體脂肪體重計，正確掌握現況也很重要。

切記千萬不要因為想快點看到效果而趕進度。偷吃步只會導致復胖與挫折感。正如俗話所說：聚沙成塔。點滴的努力終究會帶來甜美的成果，養出再也不必擔心復胖的體質。

如果執行了30天後覺得意猶未盡，請繼續下去。如果只想維持體型，運動的頻率只需原本的一半就可以了。

P126-127 減重清單的使用方法

DAY	內容	Daily Checks
DAY 1 □	重建有關減重的知識	
DAY 2 □	每餐與兩餐之間一定要喝水	
DAY 3 □	記錄飲食的內容（自我檢核）	□每餐與兩餐之間喝水
DAY 4 □	紓緩壓力	□每餐與兩餐之間喝水 □記錄飲食內容
DAY 5 □	1天吃4餐	□每餐與兩餐之間喝水 □記錄飲食內容
DAY 6 □	做伸展運動	□每餐與兩餐之間喝水 □記錄飲食內容
DAY 7 □	知道瘦得健康的重要性	□每餐與兩餐之間喝水 □記錄飲食內容 □伸展運動（腹部）
DAY 8 □	將減重「可視化」	□每餐與兩餐之間喝水 □記錄飲食內容 □伸展運動（腹部）
DAY 9 □	臀部伸展運動	□每餐與兩餐之間喝水 □記錄飲食內容 □伸展運動（腹部） □將減重「可視化」
DAY 10 □	每餐都有肉類或魚肉當作主食	□每餐與兩餐之間喝水 □記錄飲食內容 □伸展運動（腹部、臀部） □將減重「可視化」
DAY 11 □	對外發表減重宣言	□每餐與兩餐之間喝水 □記錄飲食內容 □伸展運動（腹部、臀部） □將減重「可視化」 □每餐都有肉類或魚肉當作主食
DAY 12 □	擁有品質良好的睡眠	□每餐與兩餐之間喝水 □記錄飲食內容 □伸展運動（腹部、臀部） □將減重「可視化」 □每餐都有肉類或魚肉當作主食
DAY 13 □	減少糖類的攝取	□每餐與兩餐之間喝水 □記錄飲食內容 □伸展運動（腹部、臀部） □將減重「可視化」 □每餐都有肉類或魚肉當作主食
DAY 14 □	利用拱背伸展運動美姿	□每餐與兩餐之間喝水 □記錄飲食內容 □伸展運動（腹部、臀部） □將減重「可視化」 □每餐都有肉類或魚肉當作主食
DAY 15 □	將泡澡的效果發揮到極致	□每餐與兩餐之間喝水 □記錄飲食內容 □伸展運動（腹部、臀部、拱背） □將減重「可視化」 □每餐都有肉類或魚肉當作主食
DAY 16 □	把酒精當作主食看待	□每餐與兩餐之間喝水 □記錄飲食內容 □伸展運動（腹部、臀部、拱背） □將減重「可視化」 □每餐都有肉類或魚肉當作主食
DAY 17 □	慢慢地坐在椅子上	□每餐與兩餐之間喝水 □記錄飲食內容 □伸展運動（腹部、臀部、拱背） □將減重「可視化」 □每餐都有肉類或魚肉當作主食
DAY 18 □	不是替結果，而是為過程打分數	□每餐與兩餐之間喝水 □記錄飲食內容 □伸展運動（腹部、臀部、拱背） □將減重「可視化」 □每餐都有肉類或魚肉當作主食
DAY 19 □	停止傷身的情緒性進食	□每餐與兩餐之間喝水 □記錄飲食內容 □伸展運動（腹部、臀部、拱背） □將減重「可視化」 □每餐都有肉類或魚肉當作主食
DAY 20 □	對自己心懷期待	□每餐與兩餐之間喝水 □記錄飲食內容 □伸展運動（腹部、臀部、拱背） □將減重「可視化」 □每餐都有肉類或魚肉當作主食
DAY 21 □	把樓梯化為訓練裝備	□每餐與兩餐之間喝水 □記錄飲食內容 □伸展運動（腹部、臀部、拱背） □將減重「可視化」 □每餐都有肉類或魚肉當作主食
DAY 22 □	即使外食，也要實踐三菜一湯	□每餐與兩餐之間喝水 □記錄飲食內容 □伸展運動（腹部、臀部、拱背） □將減重「可視化」 □每餐都有肉類或魚肉當作主食
DAY 23 □	養成更添魅力的站姿、走路方式	□每餐與兩餐之間喝水 □記錄飲食內容 □伸展運動（腹部、臀部、拱背） □將減重「可視化」 □每餐都有肉類或魚肉當作主食
DAY 24 □	攝取3K食材	□每餐與兩餐之間喝水 □記錄飲食內容 □伸展運動（腹部、臀部、拱背） □將減重「可視化」 □每餐都有肉類或魚肉當作主食
DAY 25 □	挑戰爬樓梯	□每餐與兩餐之間喝水 □記錄飲食內容 □伸展運動（腹部、臀部、拱背） □將減重「可視化」 □每餐都有肉類或魚肉當作主食
DAY 26 □	鍛鍊背肌以提升代謝	□每餐與兩餐之間喝水 □記錄飲食內容 □伸展運動（腹部、臀部、拱背） □將減重「可視化」 □每餐都有肉類或魚肉當作主食
DAY 27 □	增加NEAT	□每餐與兩餐之間喝水 □記錄飲食內容 □伸展運動（腹部、臀部、拱背） □將減重「可視化」 □每餐都有肉類或魚肉當作主食
DAY 28 □	點心聰明選，安心吃	□每餐與兩餐之間喝水 □記錄飲食內容 □伸展運動（腹部、臀部、拱背） □將減重「可視化」 □每餐都有肉類或魚肉當作主食 □增加NEAT
DAY 29 □	加入腹肌運動	□每餐與兩餐之間喝水 □記錄飲食內容 □伸展運動（腹部、臀部、拱背） □將減重「可視化」 □每餐都有肉類或魚肉當作主食 □增加NEAT
DAY 30 □	為了避免三分鐘熱度的心理建設	□每餐與兩餐之間喝水 □記錄飲食內容 □伸展運動（腹部、臀部、拱背） □將減重「可視化」 □每餐都有肉類或魚肉當作主食 □增加NEAT

DAY 25 ☑

挑戰
爬樓梯

閱讀當天的內容，
完成後打勾

Daily Checks

☑每餐與兩餐之間都有喝水

☑記錄飲食內容

□伸展運動（腹部、臀部、拱背）

□將減重可視化

□每餐都有肉類或
魚類當作主菜

最重要的是記得
每天持續進行

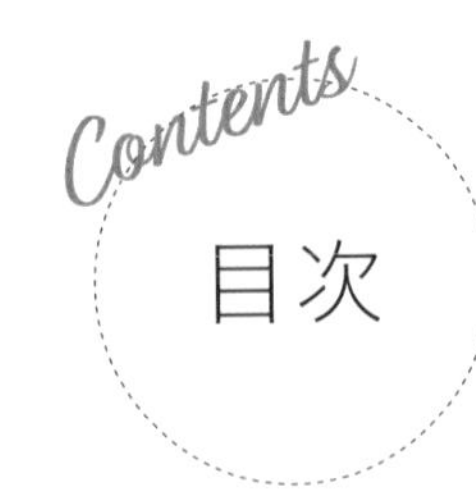

目次

30天就會瘦！1天1頁跟著做，養成易瘦體質不復胖！最強瘦身教科書

2 前言

4 坂詰真二×nagomi〈對談〉讓你常保青春美麗 到底什麼才是正確的瘦身方法!?

Prologue

序章

8 減重成功的關鍵在於事前準備!!

10 有如苦行僧的飲食限制只會造成反效果！

12 「鍛鍊肌肉」不僅能夠降低體脂肪，還能維持肌肉量

14 客觀地檢視現在的自己屬於哪一種體型

16 坂詰式 設定正確的目標與制定不會受挫的計畫方法

18 利用減重清單，挑戰30日減重計畫

Part 1

實踐！30日減重

Day 1 心態與大腦 請重建有關減重的知識 26
Day 2 營養 每餐與兩餐之間一定要喝水 28
Day 3 營養 記錄飲食的內容，以客觀的角度分析 30
Day 4 心態與大腦 紓緩壓力，以免過食 32
Day 5 營養 養成1天4餐的習慣 34
Day 6 運動 首先該做的運動是腹部伸展運動 腹部伸展運動 36
Day 7 心態與大腦 知道「健康瘦身法」與「傷身瘦身法」的差異 40
Day 8 心態與大腦 將減重「可視化」 42
Day 9 運動 利用臀部伸展動作雕塑體態 臀部伸展動作 44
Day 10 營養 每餐一定要吃肉類或魚肉當主食 48
Day 11 心態與大腦 向眾人高調地發表減重宣言 50
Day 12 心態與大腦 「品質良好的睡眠」可預防過食 52

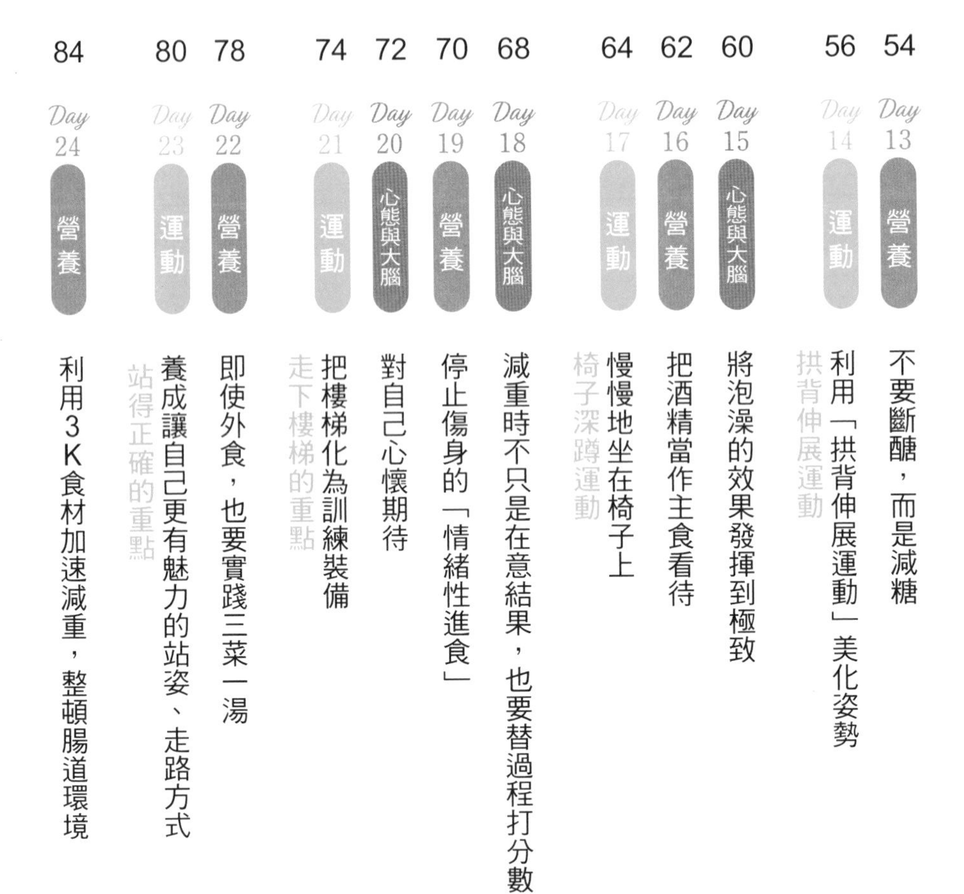

Day 13 營養 不要斷醣，而是減糖 54

Day 14 運動 利用「拱背伸展運動」美化姿勢 56
拱背伸展運動

Day 15 心態與大腦 將泡澡的效果發揮到極致 60

Day 16 營養 把酒精當作主食看待 62

Day 17 運動 慢慢地坐在椅子上 64
椅子深蹲運動

Day 18 心態與大腦 減重時不只是在意結果，也要替過程打分數 68

Day 19 營養 停止傷身的「情緒性進食」 70

Day 20 心態與大腦 對自己心懷期待 72

Day 21 運動 把樓梯化為訓練裝備 74
走下樓梯的重點

Day 22 營養 即使外食，也要實踐三菜一湯 78

Day 23 運動 養成讓自己更有魅力的站姿、走路方式 80
站得正確的重點

Day 24 營養 利用3K食材加速減重，整頓腸道環境 84

目次 *Contents*

86 Day 25 運動 等到身體變得輕盈就挑戰爬樓梯
爬樓梯的重點

90 Day 26 運動 鍛鍊背肌可以進一步提升代謝
背部伸展

94 Day 27 運動 儘量增加日常生活運動量
1天總消耗熱量的明細

98 Day 28 營養 點心聰明選，安心吃

100 Day 29 運動 加入腹肌運動
腹肌運動的正確方式

104 Day 30 心態與大腦 為了避免對減重只有三分鐘熱度的心理建設

106 專欄 建議在超商購買的食品

Part 2 減重的真相與謊言

知識篇

108 只要搓搓揉揉就能瘦是真的嗎？

110 只要矯正身體的歪斜就能降低脂肪是真的嗎？
112 輕斷食、斷食……斷食真的有絕佳的減重效果嗎？

飲食篇

114 只要少吃一餐就能快速瘦下來是真的嗎？
116 最好減少醣類的攝取，改成攝取大量的蛋白質是真的嗎？
118 最好不要吃油是真的嗎？

運動篇

120 肌力訓練最好每天都做是真的嗎？
122 一定要做有氧運動是真的嗎？

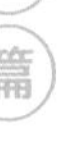
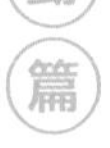

附錄

124 檢視全身的肌肉
125 自我檢核量表
126 減重清單

Part 1
實踐！30日減重

Day 1

心態與大腦

請重建有關減重的知識

Point

- 挑戰了各式減重法，最後、**迷航在減重大海之中**
- 鍛鍊肌肉＝**誤以為**就是練出一身有如健美先生的壯碩肌肉
- 發胖、變瘦的機制其實都**非常簡單**

重新檢討減重方式

全世界有各式各樣的減重方法，從很多年前曾經流行的呼拉圈減重法、紅茶菇減重法，到最近的體幹訓練、減醣飲食等，種類多到不計其數，而且效果參差不齊。有些方法的效果微乎其微，有些則是雖然有效，但是復胖的機率很高，或者會對健康造成危害。必須注意的是，**嘗試這類減重方法的次數愈多，就愈容易累積更多錯誤的知識與經驗，變得很難接受真正有效又安全的減重方法。**

舉例而言，為了抑制食量，雖然有必要積極攝取水分，但曾經嘗試過必須限制飲水量減重法的人，有可能會不自覺地不想喝水。另外，為了只減掉體脂肪，一定要鍛鍊全身的肌肉，但是心裡如果已經產生鍛鍊肌肉就是要練得像猛男一樣的既定印象，就可能只鍛鍊自己在意的部分。

掌握發胖的原因，對症下藥，自然瘦得下來

所謂正確的減重方法，基本上就是「掌握發胖原因加以解決」。如果不從源頭下手，不論怎麼做都看不到效果。

發胖的原因非常簡單，單純是因為體脂肪增加所致。如果換種說法，就是長期從飲食「攝取的熱量」，超過為了維持生命與活動的「消耗熱量」。因此，如果想瘦下來，方法也非常簡單，只要消耗的熱量超過攝取的熱量，當作儲備能量的體脂肪就會被消耗，體重也自然減輕了。

Day 2

營養

每餐與兩餐之間一定要喝水

Point

- 飯前先喝**一杯水**
- 感覺肚子餓的時候，首先**喝杯水**
- 建議喝**氣泡水、礦泉水、麥茶、花草茶**

掌握喝水的祕密

- 餐前先喝250ml左右
- 正在執行飲食限制的人，記得每天的喝水量至少要比平常多1公升

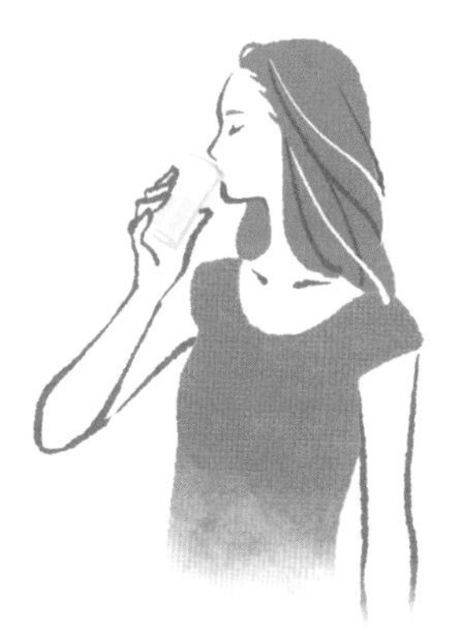

適合喝的水

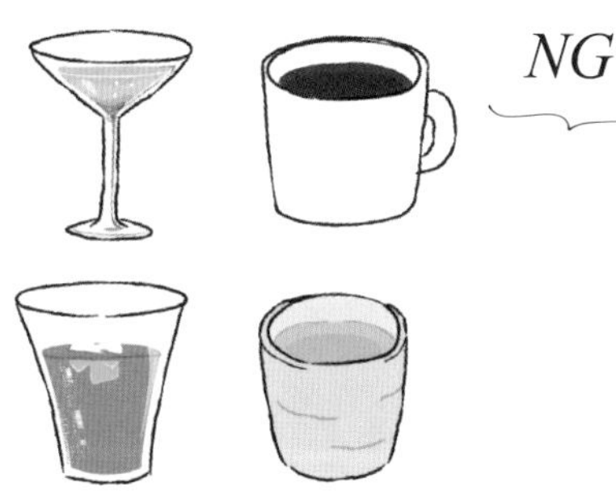

含酒精與含糖飲料。含有咖啡因的咖啡、紅茶、綠茶、烏龍茶等，只能淺嘗則止。

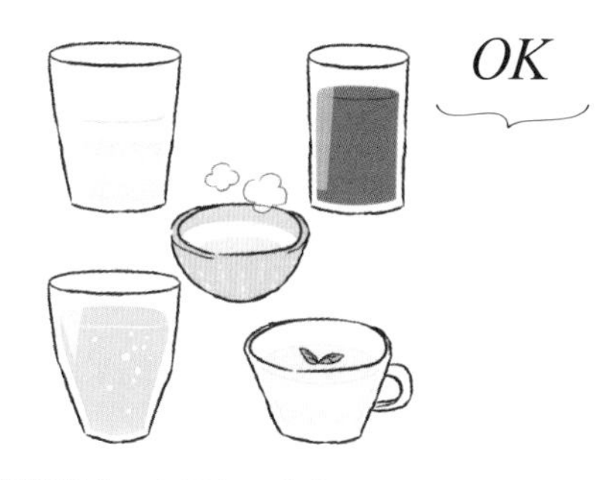

建議選擇水、白開水、麥茶、花草茶等無熱量、無咖啡因、無酒精飲料。特別推薦氣泡水，可以增加飽足感。

只要攝取充足的水分，食量自然會減少

請記得在用餐前，先喝一杯水，吃飯期間也要喝。但不要大口灌水，以免食物未經咀嚼就跟著水吞進去。總之，請記得攝取充足的水分。

食物的成分有一半以上是水，所以只要水喝得夠，食量自然跟著減少。

利用零卡的氣泡水以增加飽足感

特別推薦用餐時選擇無糖零熱量的氣泡水以增加飽足感。另外也可以依照個人喜好，搭配零熱量的礦泉水、麥茶、花草茶等飲料。

Day 3

營養

記錄飲食的內容，以客觀的角度分析

Point

- 進行自我監控，以客觀的眼光**審視自己的飲食生活**
- 回顧1整天的飲食內容，**以達到改善飲食習慣的目的**

透過自我監控，以客觀的眼光審視自己的飲食生活，可以讓我們養成有助於減重的良好生活習慣。也可以利用APP管理，記錄攝取的熱量，掌握是否做到營養均衡。

自我監控的使用範例

10月2日（五）　體重：60kg　體脂肪率：27%

	開始時間	所需時間	主食	主菜	副菜	湯品
早餐	08：05	10分鐘	○	○	×	×
午餐	12：20	30分鐘	○	○	×	○
晚餐	20：30	50分鐘	△	○	○	○
點心	16：00	5分鐘	—	—	—	—

一併記錄體重與體脂肪率，對飲食生活的改善也能派上用場。請利用P125的表格進行自我監控。

利用自我檢核以掌握飲食生活

用餐時當然不用說，只要是把東西送進口中，包括喝水、吃點心等，都要一一記錄下來。如果覺得使用紙本記錄太麻煩，也可以改成拍照記錄，或以手機的APP管理。

回顧1整天的飲食內容，朝想要努力改善的方向前進

光是記錄「吃了什麼」還不夠，最好連同「進食時間」「用餐所花時間」「主食、主菜、副菜、湯品（水分）」的份量也記錄下來。

利用晚上睡前回顧1整天的飲食紀錄，進行檢討，例如「今天副菜吃得太少，明天要記得多吃點蔬菜補回來」，**就能逐漸改善自己的飲食生活**。

Day 4

心態與大腦

紓緩壓力，以免過食

Point

- 大部分瘦不下來的人，**原因出在「過食」**
- **做好壓力控管**能夠防止過食
- **知道讓自己放鬆的方法**很重要

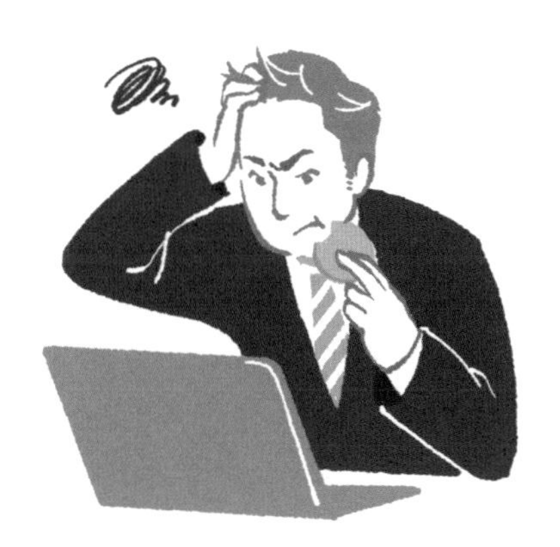

當人承受壓力時，會使交感神經變得活躍，除了心跳次數增加、血壓上升，身體也會處於緊張狀態。

放鬆的方法示範

- 擁有品質良好的睡眠（詳情請參照Day12）
- 悠哉地泡個澡（詳情請參照Day15）
- 覺得壓力很大時改用腹式呼吸（從鼻子深深吸氣，讓腹部鼓起來，再慢慢吐氣）
- 培養正常的休閒嗜好，例如聽音樂、露營等。
- 做拉筋運動（詳情請參照Day6、9、14）

瘦不下來的原因出在「過食」

隱藏在過食背後的原因是壓力。選擇以飲食排遣工作或人際關係造成的壓力的人不在少數。**如果能找回壓力主控權，就不會攝取過多的熱量，體重就會自然下降了。**

嘗試各種放鬆的方法以調適壓力

為了調適壓力，在日常生活中積極利用腹式呼吸與悠哉泡澡等方式（上圖）放鬆自己，讓副交感神經保持優勢很重要。副交感神經是負責啟動放鬆狀態的神經，時常覺得壓力很大的人，尤其應該想辦法鎮定交感神經，讓自己放鬆下來。

Day 5

營養

養成1天4餐的習慣

Point

● **省略某一餐不吃**容易發胖

● 在午餐和晚餐之間**吃點心不容易囤積體脂肪**

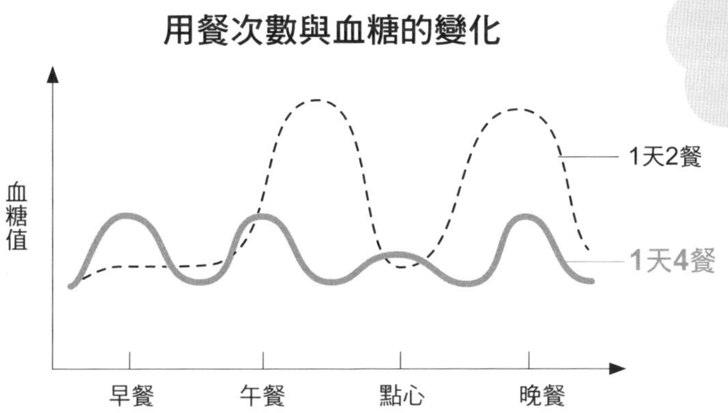

少量多餐可以避免血糖急速上升與急速下降

血糖在飯後上升，胰臟也會分泌胰島素。胰島素會將血液中的營養素帶進體內使用，未消耗完畢的部分主要以體脂肪的形式囤積在體內。

理想的1日飲食

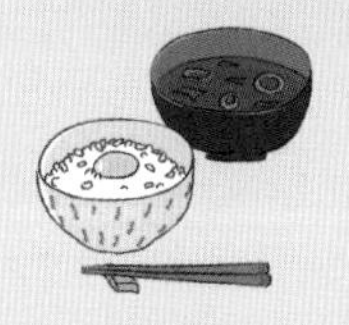
早餐

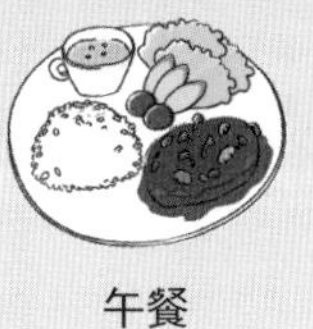
午餐

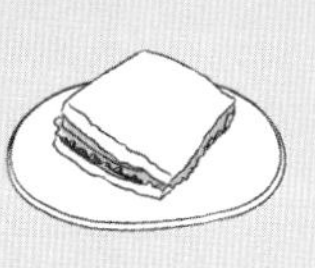
點心

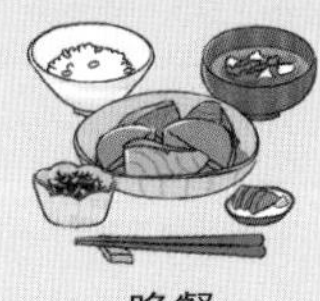
晚餐

建議在下午4點左右吃一個飯糰或小份三明治當作點心。相對地，晚餐的主食份量最好減半。

Day 5 營養

利用少量多餐的方式打造易瘦體質

有些人為了減少一整天的進食量，故意省略某一餐不吃，但這是錯誤的作法。**正確的作法是1天吃4餐**。早餐和午餐要吃得豐盛一點，到了下午4點左右吃個點心，接著晚餐就少吃一點。

大吃大喝的飲食方式容易囤積體脂肪

每次少量進食能夠讓血糖變得緩慢上升，而且攝取的營養大多能當作能量消耗，所以不容易囤積體脂肪。相反地，如果在空腹的狀態下大量進食，血糖會急速上升，這時，身體就不得不分泌大量的胰島素，最後導致沒有完全消耗的營養以體脂肪的形式貯藏在體內。

Day 6

運動

首先該做的運動是腹部伸展運動

Point

- 提升柔軟度，**增加日常的運動量**
- 利用伸展運動**放鬆身心**
- **即使只矯正了姿勢**，馬上有看起來變瘦的效果

透過正確的拉筋運動以提升柔軟度

拉筋運動沒有直接燃燒體脂肪的效果，也沒有增加肌肉、提升代謝的效果。即使如此，**運動時首先該做的就是拉筋**。

我之所以建議大家做拉筋運動有好幾個理由。第一，放鬆肌肉可以提高身體的柔軟度，讓身體活動起來更輕鬆，也不容易疲勞。如此一來，人也會變得更有活動的意願，藉由換衣服、沐浴、買東西和通勤等在日常生活中的活動，可以消耗更多的熱量——NEAT（非運動性活動產熱）。另外，如果身體的柔軟度變得更好，也會提高鍛鍊肌肉的效果。

第二個理由是拉筋運動可以放鬆身心，達到消除壓力的效果。如Day4所言，人在壓力過大，或長期處於被壓力纏身的狀態下，很容易藉由暴飲暴食以排解壓力。

伸展腹部肌肉，調整姿勢

最後，放鬆肌肉還有矯正姿勢，有讓體態顯得年輕的效果。**其中特別重要的是腹部的肌肉。我們在日常生活中伸展腹部肌肉的機會不多，所以肌肉容易僵硬，但長期置之不理，會造成下腹部突出、駝背，甚至使外表看起來超過實際年齡。**拉筋是有速效性的運動，做了很快能矯正姿勢、增加自信。請各位利用下一頁介紹的拉筋運動，找回身體的柔軟度。如此一來，就能消除惱人的小腹，挺直背脊展現迷人的體態。

Day 6

腹部的伸展運動

伸展容易變得僵硬的腹部肌肉（腹直肌），
有助於改善駝背和消除突出的下腹部。
請從今天開始養成伸展腹肌的習慣吧。

10秒 × 1～3組

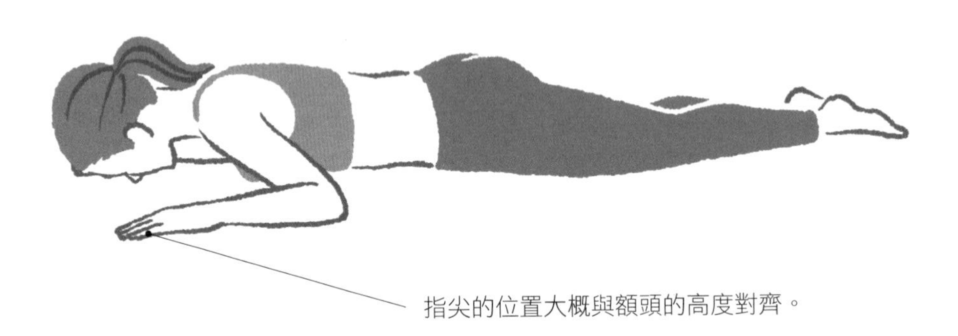

1

臉朝下趴在地板上。夾緊腋下，彎曲手肘，
把手放在臉旁邊。

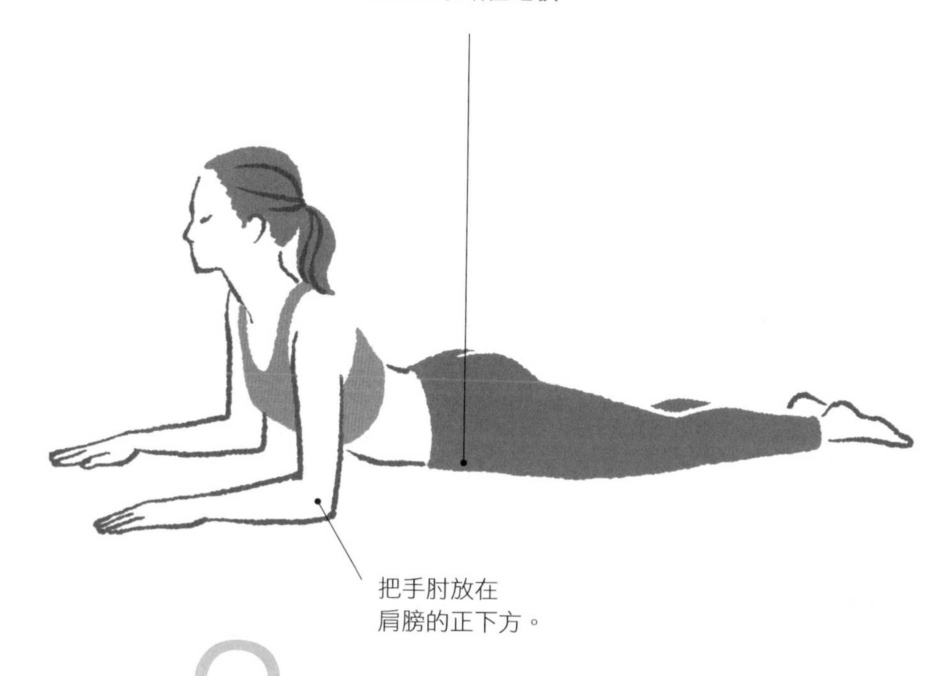

2

慢慢挺起上半身，看正面。正常呼吸，維持這個姿勢10秒鐘。

Day 7

心態與大腦

知道「健康瘦身法」與「傷身瘦身法」的差異

Point

- 在短時間內只減去體重的「**傷身瘦身法**」不可行
- 即使不是馬上見效，但**能夠只減掉體脂肪**
- 理想的減重速度是**1個月瘦2kg**

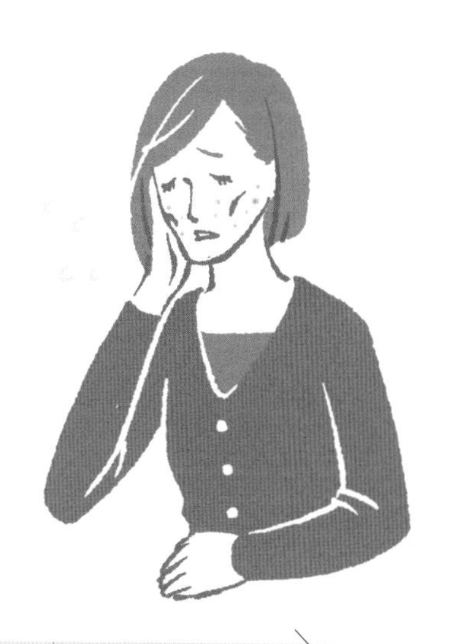

急速瘦身的害處

- 肌肉量減少，人顯得憔悴
- 失去肌肉線條
- 水分流失，皮膚變得粗糙
- 出現貧血等各種身體不適症狀
- 成為復胖與引起飲食障礙的原因

設定正確的減重目標

1週減去體重的
0.5～1%
※以體重60kg的女性為例，大約減去0.3～0.6kg左右。

換算成一個月相當於減去
-1.2～2.4kg

追求急速減重會演變成「傷身減重」

採用讓體重在短時間下降的減重法，會一併減去身體所需的水分、肌肉、骨質，除了引起貧血等各種身體不適症狀，也會導致體力下降。

急速減重對心理也會造成強大的壓力，甚至引起復胖、進食障礙。若是演變至此，便足以證明這不是健康的瘦身法，而是「傷身」的減重法。

請各位選擇即使不能馬上見效，卻能健康減重的方法

正確的減重方法要能做到「保留身體所需的水分與肌肉，只適度減去體脂肪」。**安全的減重進度是1週減去體重的0．5～1％。**以體重60kg的女性為例，大約減去0．3～0．6kg是合理的範圍。

Day 8

心態與大腦

將減重「可視化」

Point

- 把自己現在的照片與擁有理想體型的人進行對照，**提高減重的動機**
- 每天花3分鐘**想像自己變美後的模樣**

充分利用可視化的技巧

為了讓自己對減重持之以恆、成功瘦身，善用各種心理學技巧以增加動力是很有效的作法。**以下為各位介紹其中的一項，也就是正視自己目前的樣貌，將「自己瘦下來後變美的模樣」的意念加以可視化，達到增加動力的方法。**

可視化最簡單的方法就是利用照片。具體而言，如果希望自己恢復以前的體型，就先拍一張與舊照同樣姿勢的照片，接著比較以前的自己和現在的自己有何不同。如果能夠正視現狀，相信一定會提升「我想變瘦」的鬥志。另外，對著鏡子仔細端詳自己最不滿意的腹部、臀部、手臂等部位，或者把自己比較看不到的部位拍下來，以便掌握最真實的現狀，也能發揮同樣的效果。

為了激勵自己，把擁有自己嚮往身材的藝人或模特兒的照片貼在牆上，或設定為待機畫面也是絕招。當然，請儘量挑選身高體格、年齡與自己差距不大的對象，這樣才是可行的目標。

具體描繪出自我的理想形象

另外一個方法是想像自己透過努力改變後的模樣，想得愈具體愈好。例如：「我終於把這件衣服穿得很好看」「自己變得很有異性緣」「連小孩也開口稱讚自己」。養成這個習慣很簡單，每天只需要3分鐘。只要在就寢前或沐浴等可以放鬆的時候，閉上眼想像自己變身後的模樣就可以了。

Day 9

運動

利用臀部伸展動作雕塑體態

Point

- 臀部的肌肉僵硬也是**老態畢現的元凶**
- 持續拉筋會**使肌肉恢復、矯正姿勢**

改善駝背，使臀部恢復緊實挺翹

如同我在Day6所提到的，拉筋具備種種有益減重的效果，包括「提高身體的柔軟度，讓身體活動起來更輕鬆」「可以放鬆身心，消除壓力」。不過，持續拉筋最重要的意義在於放鬆肌肉、矯正姿勢，即使體重不變，體態卻變得挺拔有型，除了增加自信，也能提升繼續減重的動機。

除了腹部的伸展運動，請各位一定要做的還有「臀部」的伸展動作。組成臀部的大臀肌屬於大片肌肉，和腹部一樣，同樣是容易因缺乏運動與年齡增長而變得僵硬的肌肉。**大臀肌若變得僵硬，骨盆就會往後傾，而我們的身體為了保持平衡，就會不自主地拱起背部，形成駝背。**不僅如此，後傾的骨盆會使臀部的位置往下降，讓人的外表看起來超過實際年齡。把大臀肌當作伸展的重點，鍛鍊一段時間之後，自然能找回挺拔的姿勢與緊實的臀部。

在自己能夠輕鬆應付的範圍內進行有效率的拉筋運動

細節留待下一頁說明，但這裡介紹的臀部伸展運動，做起來輕鬆簡單，只要躺在床上就能進行。請搭配在Day6介紹的腹部伸展運動一起進行。

拉筋運動的魅力所在是很快就能見效。做的次數愈多效果愈好，而且還有緩和疲勞與壓力的作用，建議大家養成每天都做的習慣。

Day 9

臀部的伸展動作

組成臀部的大臀肌若變得僵硬，骨盆就會往後傾，造成臀部下垂。
不但顯得腿較短，也是造成駝背的原因之一。
請藉由運動找回臀部肌肉的柔軟度，打造緊實的臀部吧。

左右各**10**秒 × **1～3**組

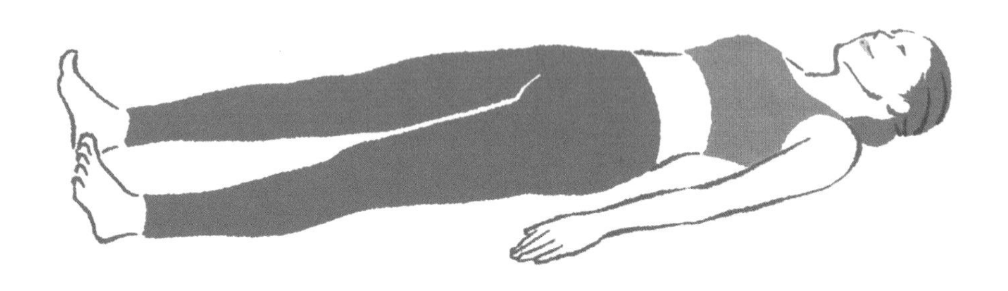

1

仰躺在地板上。雙腳稍微張開，放鬆全身的肌肉。

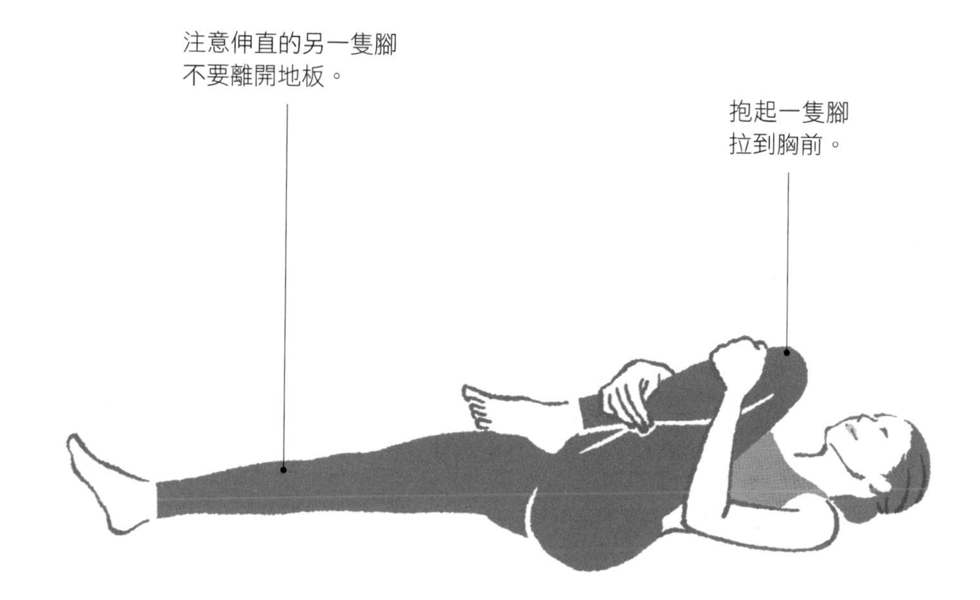
注意伸直的另一隻腳
不要離開地板。
抱起一隻腳
拉到胸前。

2

彎起一隻腳，用兩手抱住，把膝蓋拉至胸前。正常呼吸，維持這個姿勢10秒鐘。

Day 10

營養

每餐一定要吃肉類或魚肉當主食

Point

- 積極攝取蛋白質，增加肌肉量以提升基礎代謝
- 攝取肉類或魚肉也是預防飲食過量的關鍵

三大營養素的功能

碳水化合物	蛋白質	脂質
	成為製造身體的成分	
成為能量來源		

蛋白質的建議攝取量

〔標準〕

體重×1.0g

〔減重中〕

體重×1.2～1.4 g

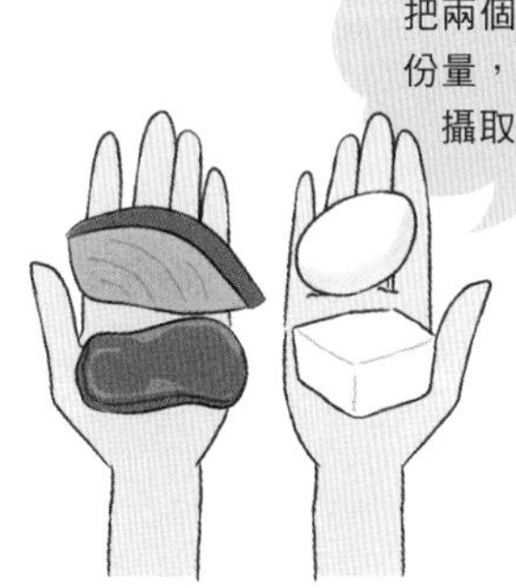

把兩個手掌大小的
份量，當作一天應
攝取的蛋白質

優質蛋白質能發揮持久的飽足感

請各位每餐一定要吃肉類或魚肉當作主食。因為肉類和魚肉是三大營養素之一，富含製造肌肉時不可欠缺的蛋白質。**攝取蛋白質還可以防止肌肉量在減重期間減少。**

透過飲食勤加補充，打造健康的身體

肉類和魚肉另一項值得稱許的功能是能帶來持久的飽足感，避免飲食過量。

蛋白質約占人體組成成分的20％，是製造肌肉時不可或缺的重要營養素。同時也是三大營養素中唯一無法儲存於體內的營養素，所以請務必每餐都要攝取。

Day 11

心態與大腦

向眾人高調地發表減重宣言

Point

- 透過減重宣言，**讓「別人的眼光」成為得力助手**
- 消除「無法忌口」的刺激，**把減重轉換為可長期持續的生活習慣**

公開發表減重宣言，更容易獲得周圍的支持。如果透過SNS公開，就能夠讓更多人知道，對自己形成一種良性壓力。

請向周圍的人宣布「我正在減重！」

為了瘦得健康、美麗，腳踏實地做好壓力控管、飲食改善、拉筋運動等都是掌握成功的關鍵。

不難想見在成功改造體態之前，各位也會有遇到挫折的時候，殊不知能夠在此時發揮鼓舞與支持力量的就是「減重宣言」。舉例而言，只要你告訴周圍的人「其實我正在減重」，那麼就不必擔心到了休息時間會有人拿著零食向自己「推銷」，和朋友一起吃飯時，也能夠毫無顧忌地選擇較無負擔的餐點。

另外，**發表「減重宣言」還有一大好處，就是讓「別人的眼光」成為減重的得力助手**。因為在無法克制想吃甜食的慾望而打算破戒時、再吃下去飲食計畫就要破功的時候，「別人的眼光」將成為讓你懸崖勒馬的救命繩。

改變環境，消除「忍不住想吃東西」的誘因

另外，為了達到成功減重的目的，讓自己不要受到喚醒食慾的刺激也很重要。

「總是在晚餐後又吃點零食」的人，請戒掉「只要零食櫃空了就補貨」的習慣。只要外食，習慣選擇油膩料理的人，也請儘量自己下廚。

總之，打算改變原有的生活習慣時，若先告知家人等身邊的人，他們就會發揮助攻的力量，讓你的減重之路走得更順利。

Day 12

心態與大腦

「品質良好的睡眠」可預防過食

Point

- 良好的睡眠**可預防因壓力過大造成過食**
- 每天至少睡滿6小時，**以7．5個小時為終極目標**
- **保持固定的就寢時間與起床時間**

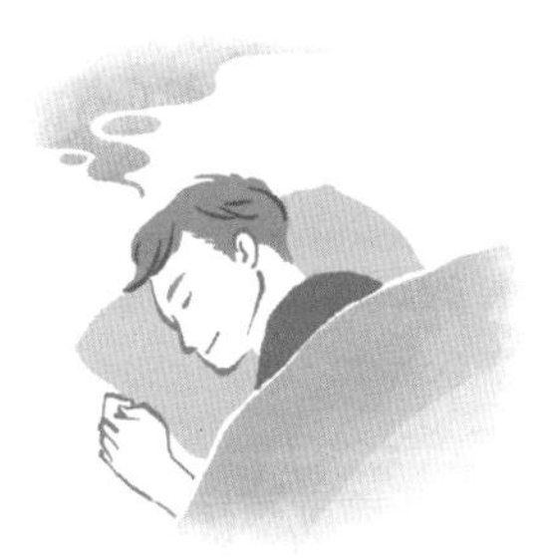

睡眠品質愈好，愈容易忘記負面情緒、不愉快的體驗等不必要的記憶。

如何擁有優質睡眠

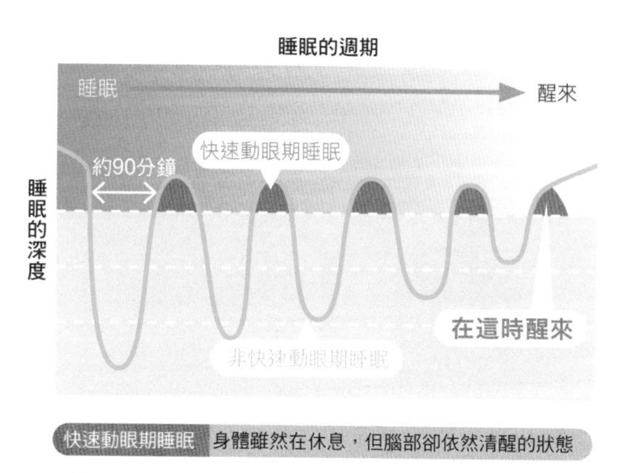

90分鐘×5次＝7.5個小時

為了讓身體充分獲得休息，達到紓緩壓力的目的，至少要讓快速動眼期睡眠、非快速動眼期睡眠完成4個循環，也就是6個小時。理想是5個循環，總共7.5個小時。

為了擁有優質睡眠，請重視睡眠的「時間」

擁有充足且良好的睡眠，是有效減重不可或缺的關鍵。為了確保睡眠品質的良好，養成在固定時間就寢與起床的習慣、**至少睡滿6個小時（理想是7．5個小時）很重要。**

藉由紓緩壓力達到抑制食慾的效果

睡眠所產生的忘卻作用可以消除壓力，間接避免過食。

相反地，目前已經證實如果睡眠時間過短，會使促進食慾增加的荷爾蒙（飢餓素）的分泌量增加，而抑制食慾的荷爾蒙（瘦蛋白）的分泌量減少。

Day 13

營養

不要斷醣，而是減糖

Point

- 了解「醣類」和「糖類」的差異，**打造不會囤積體脂肪的身體**
- 要確實攝取**三大營養素之一的「醣類」**

碳水化合物的組成

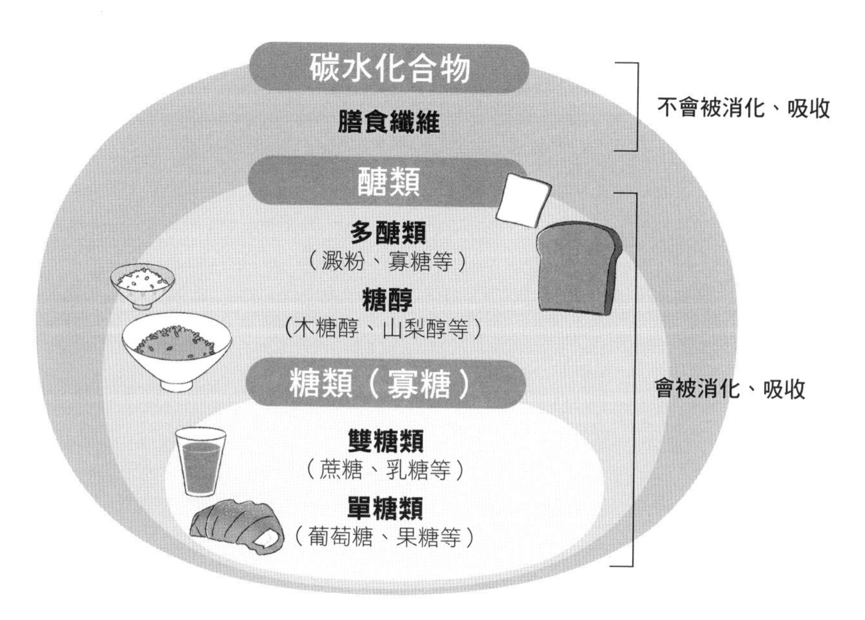

所謂的糖類，就是含於水果中的果糖和葡萄糖等「單糖類」，與由果糖與葡萄糖結合而成的砂糖，也就是「雙糖類」。另一方面，醣類屬於多醣類，含於穀物、薯芋類、蔬菜等。

攝取過多糖類，容易使體內囤積體脂肪

節食時不吃「醣類」是錯誤的觀念，要減少「糖類」的攝取才是正確的作法。

糖類以外的醣類，消化、吸收的速度緩慢，**唯獨糖類會使血糖急速上升，還會促使脂肪合成，囤積於體內**。此外，血糖急速上升後會快速下降，所以會引發空腹感。

對調味料也不可掉以輕心 說不定隱含著糖類

被稱為「高果糖糖漿」的甜味劑含有大量糖類，主要用於添加在軟性飲料、醬料、調味料等，可增添甜味和甘醇味。儘量避免攝取才是聰明的選擇。

Day 14

運動

利用「拱背伸展運動」美化姿勢

Point

- 姿勢就是身體的表情，**只要加以調整就會顯得更有魅力**
- 藉由**拉筋伸展腹部肌肉，調整姿勢**
- 放鬆僵硬的腹直肌，**改善突出的小腹**

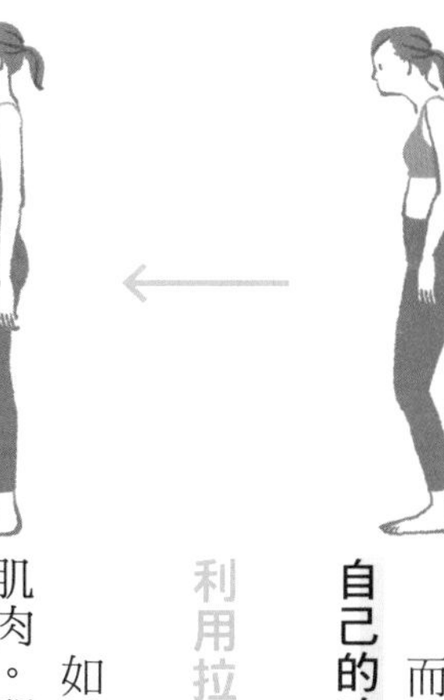

為了改變身體，首先該從「姿勢」下手

維持正確的姿勢能讓體型看起來更有吸引力。所謂理想的體型，就是肌肉和體脂肪都維持適量的狀態，但即使好不容易才獲得這樣的體型，如果姿勢不良，魅力也會跟著大打折扣。相反地，一個人即使體脂肪的比例偏高，肌肉略嫌不足，但只要保持良好的姿勢，體態看起來還是不錯。

而且姿勢可以馬上修正。**調整姿勢會讓體型看起來更有魅力，從鏡中、照片確認自己的改變，除了提升減重的動力，從他人口中聽到的讚美也會成為自己的獎勵。**

利用拉筋運動與意識改變姿勢

如果想要藉由姿勢調整以提升自己的魅力指數，當務之急就是伸展腹部和臀部的肌肉。即使只做在Day6和Day9介紹的兩項拉筋運動，對改善姿勢應該也有相當的幫助。我想，執行一段時間之後，各位都能明顯感受到腰圍縮小，胸部和臀部的位置也改變了。

比較麻煩的是，這兩種拉筋運動都是躺著做，無法利用空檔在辦公室等場地進行。

下一頁將為各位介紹站著就可以鍛鍊腹部和臀部，而且連容易僵硬的胸部和脖子等肌肉也能很快放鬆的「拱背伸展運動」。

為了養成正確的姿勢，隨時提醒自己要保持讓腹部伸展的姿勢也很重要。

Day 14

拱背伸展

拱背伸展運動可以同時伸展脖子正面、胸部、腹部、臀部、大腿內側這5處的肌肉。
請利用工作和家事的空檔等時間，想到就做。

10秒 ×
1~3組

1

雙腳打開，與肩同寬，腳尖稍微朝外。交叉雙手放在臀部後方，同時將臀部往後推，讓骨盆往前傾。

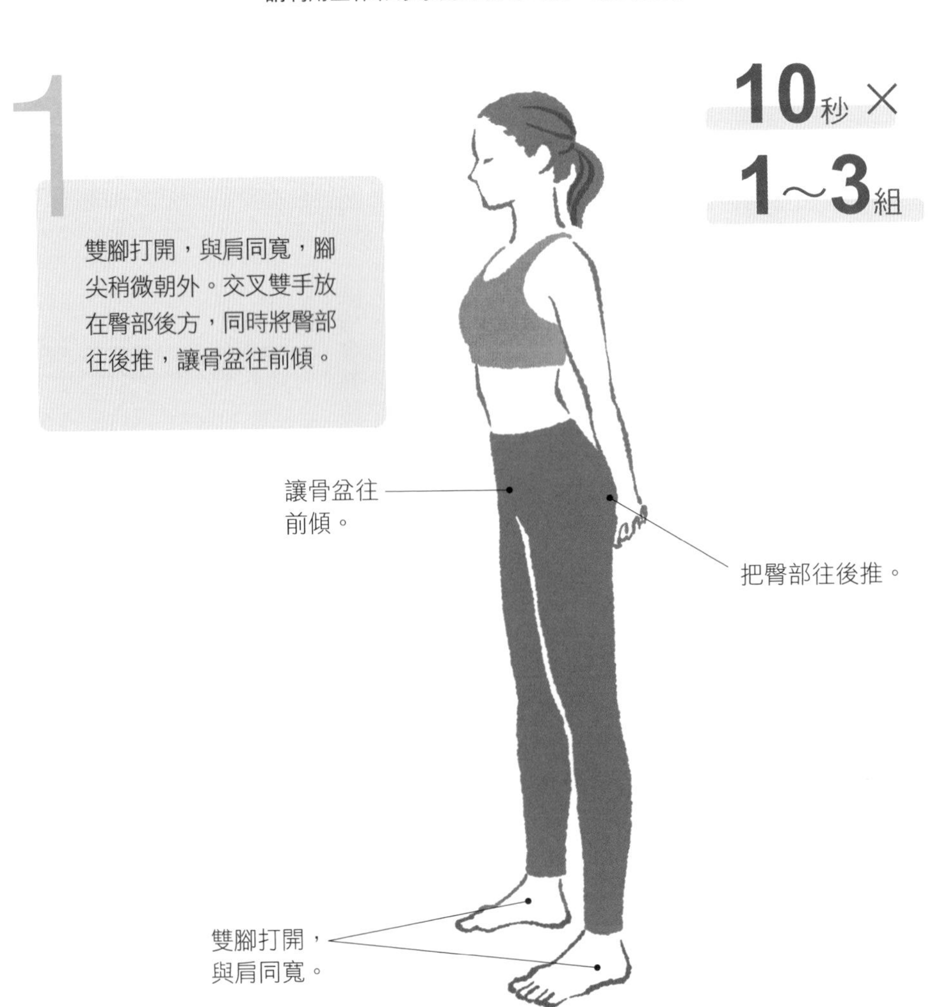
讓骨盆往前傾。
把臀部往後推。
雙腳打開，與肩同寬。

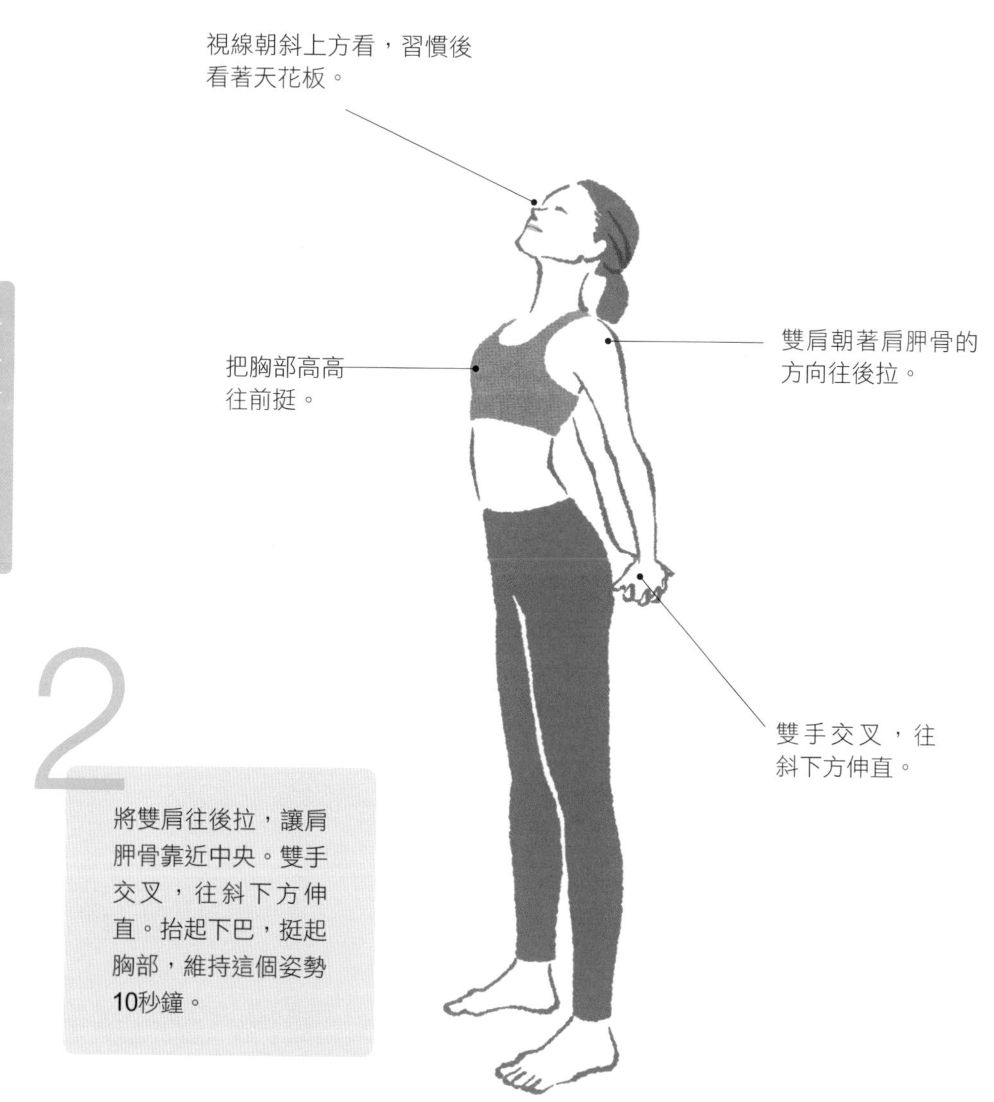
視線朝斜上方看，習慣後
看著天花板。
把胸部高高
往前挺。
雙肩朝著肩胛骨的
方向往後拉。
雙手交叉，往
斜下方伸直。

2

將雙肩往後拉，讓肩胛骨靠近中央。雙手交叉，往斜下方伸直。抬起下巴，挺起胸部，維持這個姿勢10秒鐘。

Day 15

心態與大腦

將泡澡的效果發揮到極致

Point

- 泡澡是**極為有效的放鬆方法**
- 把**水溫設定在38～40度**，悠閒地泡澡
- 透過浮力與水壓，**消除肌肉疲勞**

藉由泡澡使副交感神經保持活躍

如先前所述，壓力是減重的頭號敵人。為了紓緩壓力，**想辦法鎮定會促使身心變得緊張的交感神經，讓有助放鬆的副交感神經保持活躍也很重要。**

Day4也有提到，為了提高副交感神經的作用，悠哉地泡澡是很好的方法。我相信不少獨居的人，或是日子每天都過得很忙碌的人，都只有沖澡而沒有泡澡的習慣。沖澡可以洗去身體的髒污，但無法發揮鎮定交感神經的效果。愈是感覺壓力很大的人，愈應該多留點時間泡澡。

以適當的溫度進行全身浴

以下為各位介紹能夠更有效放鬆的泡澡方法。

第一個重點是溫度。水溫過冷或過熱，都會使交感神經的作用變得更強。適當的水溫是38～40度，不過還是以「讓自己覺得很舒服」的溫度為優先。至少泡澡5分鐘，才能達到紓緩身心緊張的效果。

雖然半身浴號稱有益健康，但如果要消除疲勞，還是全身浴的效果更佳（※）。全身浴的優點除了可藉由浮力讓肌肉從重力得到解放，水壓也有促進血液循環的作用，對消除肌肉疲勞的效果更好。

如果泡全身浴覺得有壓迫感，可以與半身浴交替進行。

※血壓偏高、有心臟疾病的人，為了避免對心臟造成負擔，適合選擇半身浴。

Day 16

營養

把酒精當作主食看待

Point

- **酒喝多**了真的**容易發胖**
- 挑選下酒菜時**以低脂高蛋白為原則**

注意酒精和下酒菜要保持適當的比例

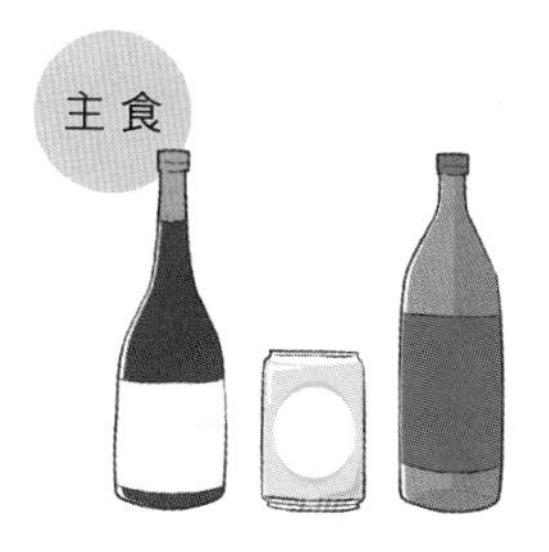

日本酒、啤酒、燒酒等

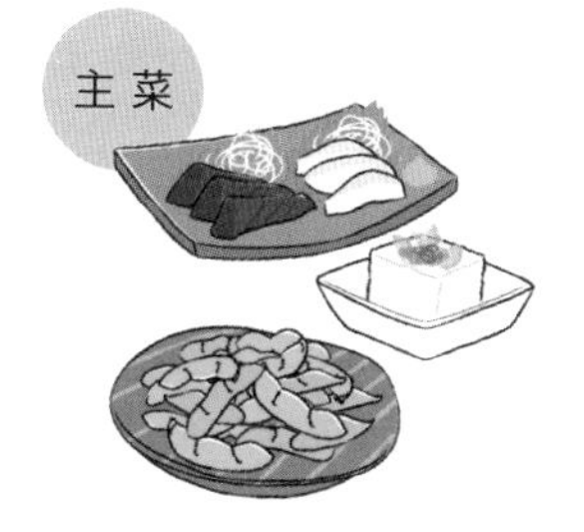

生魚片、涼拌豆腐、毛豆等

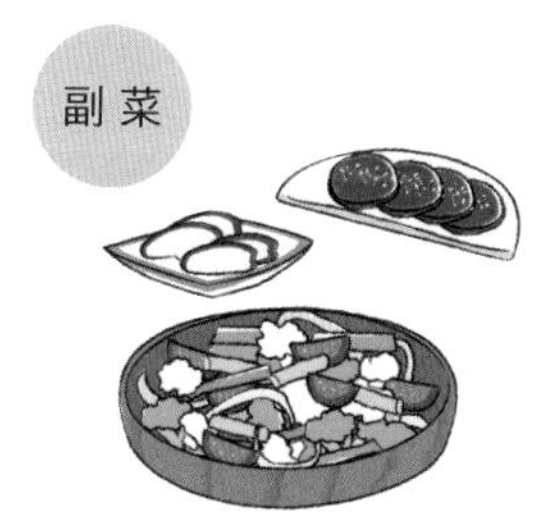

涼拌番茄、淺漬泡菜、生菜沙拉等

適度的飲酒量

根據日本厚生勞動省推動的打造國民健康運動「健康日本21」政策，1日純酒精的適度攝取量大約是20g。

相當於純酒精20g的酒量

酒的種類	量
啤酒（5%）	高罐1瓶（500ml）
日本酒	一合（180ml）
威士忌	威士忌雙份一杯（60ml）
燒酒（25度）	半杯（100ml）
葡萄酒	接近2杯（200ml）
燒酒調酒（7%）	罐裝1瓶（350ml）

喝酒務必適可而止，以免妨礙減重

喝酒會使體脂肪增加的原因是酒精會使血糖急速增加。另外一個問題是，**酒精還有開胃作用，會降低掌管理性的新皮質的功能，使食慾容易變得一發不可收拾**。所以在減重期間，喝酒的頻率和份量都最好減半。

把酒精當作主食，依照三菜一湯的原則選擇下酒菜

如果要喝酒，請把酒精當作主食。選擇下酒菜時，請按照平常用餐時攝取三菜一湯的原則，選擇低脂高蛋白的料理。除此之外，請記得至少加點兩道以蔬菜為主的菜餚。

Day 17

運動

慢慢地坐在椅子上

Point

- 慢慢地放低身體或把重心往下降，有助肌肉的鍛鍊
- 首先鍛鍊**臀部與大腿**
- **花2～5秒的時間完成坐下的動作**

有效鍛鍊肌肉的「離心運動」

近年來，「離心運動」因能有效鍛鍊肌肉而備受矚目。離心運動是一種「慢慢地放低身體或把重心往下降，在負荷過程中伸展肌肉」的運動。若以鍛鍊大胸肌的仰臥推舉當作比喻，離心運動相當於把舉起的槓鈴放在上胸的動作。若以更貼近日常的動作比喻，相當於慢慢往下坐在椅子上或下樓梯時，還有登山下坡時的肌肉動作。

離心運動的特色是相較於傳統的肌肉訓練，做起來較不吃力，而且已經證實在短時間內就能得到效果。只要在短時間內迅速提起重物，再慢慢放下，就能把普通的肌肉訓練轉變為離心運動。

利用椅子深蹲運動，把身體改造為不容易發胖的體質

請各位從今天起開始進行「椅子深蹲運動」，方法很簡單，只要慢慢地坐在椅子上，即可完成這項離心運動。

這項運動不僅便於在日常生活中進行，而且還能完整鍛鍊臀部、大腿等整個下半身。全身有6～7成的肌肉集中在下半身，所以只要好好鍛鍊下半身的肌肉，就能提升代謝，把身體改造為不容易發胖的體質。

進行這項運動時只需要一張不會搖搖晃晃的椅子。細節在下一頁說明，總之，不論在家、辦公室或其他地方，1天做10次左右，每次花2～5秒慢慢地坐下來，即可達到鍛鍊的效果。

Day 17

椅子深蹲運動

利用日常生活中坐在椅子上的時候，花2～5秒慢慢地坐下來。

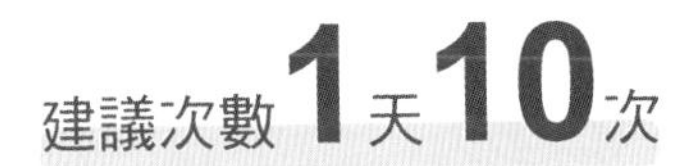

建議次數1天10次

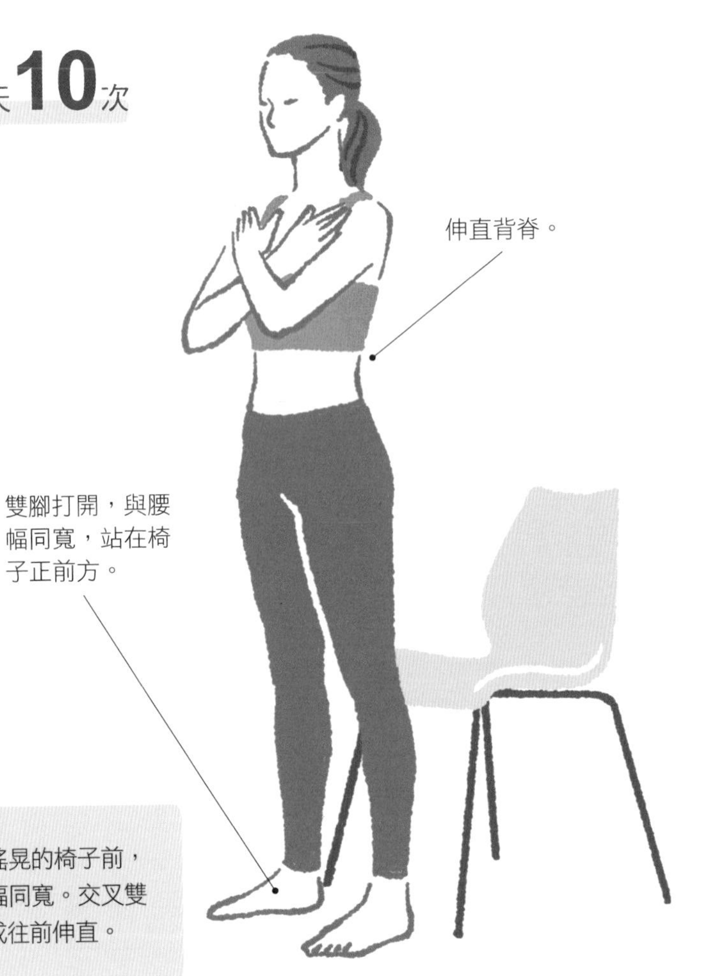

伸直背脊。
雙腳打開，與腰幅同寬，站在椅子正前方。

1

站在一張不會搖晃的椅子前，雙腳打開與腰幅同寬。交叉雙手放在胸前，或往前伸直。

2

吸氣，花2～5秒慢慢地坐在椅子上，接著吐氣，在1秒內站起來。

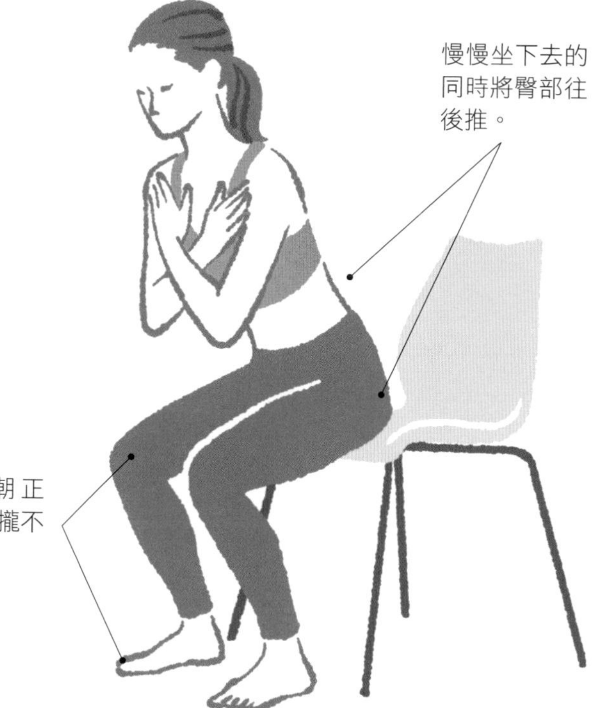
慢慢坐下去的同時將臀部往後推。
記得腳尖朝正面，雙膝併攏不要張開。

Day 18

心態與大腦

減重時不只是在意結果，也要替過程打分數

Point

- 即使看起來不明顯，但**只要付出正確的努力，一定會得到成果**
- **透過自我獎勵**以維持減重的動機

雖然「過程」無法透過數字呈現，但只要完成了就自我獎勵

過程

- 提醒自己喝水
- 睡前做拉筋運動
- 節制砂糖的攝取量
- 不搭電梯，改爬樓梯

雖然要花1個月才會有結果，但來自他人的讚美對自己也是很大的獎勵

成果

- 減去3kg的體脂肪，腰圍縮小5cm

採用正確的減重方式，需要一段時間才能看到成效

人一天只能減掉50～100g的體脂肪，所以要減去1kg脂肪需要10天。而且減掉的是全身每一處的體脂肪，所以要聽到別人讚美自己「你變瘦了耶」「氣色變得很好喔」，至少需要1個月。換句話說，即使透過正確的努力獲得確實的成果，但是需要一段時間才能反映在實質的體重數字和聽到他人的稱讚。

進行自我獎勵以維持動力

因此，**持之以恆地正確填寫卷末的「減重清單」很重要。同時也必須在減重的過程中適度地自我獎勵。**請把一些只有自己知道的變化，例如爬樓梯變得輕鬆了、血液循環變好了，也視為努力的成果。

Day 19

營養

停止傷身的「情緒性進食」

Point

- 「為了抒發情緒而吃」是頭號敵人
- 做好壓力控管以防止情緒性進食
- 「衝動性暴食」「清剩菜剩飯」「禮貌性進食」也是NG行為

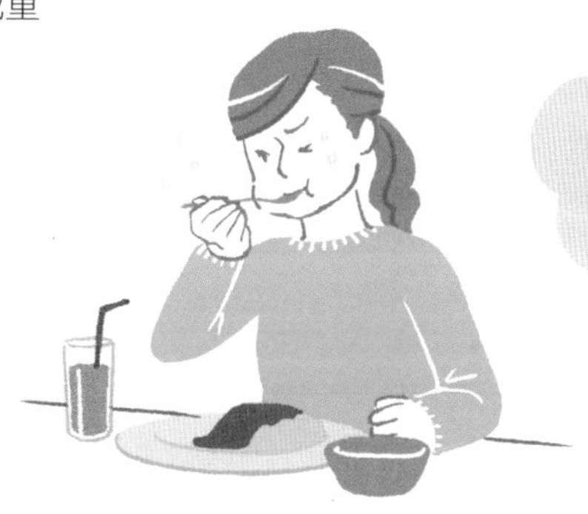

肥胖的原因
源自於飲食習慣

確認自己有沒有符合的項目

☑ 為了發洩情緒而吃東西	因人際關係或工作等方面累積很多壓力時，把吃東西當作宣洩壓力的管道。
☑ 在衝動下暴飲暴食	雖然沒有特別想吃，但只要看到零食就忍不住伸手。
☑ 在家負責吃剩菜剩飯	基於不想浪費的心理，孩子吃剩的飯菜、快到期的食品通通都下肚。
☑ 無法拒絕勸食	對親友送的伴手禮、別人的勸食無法拒絕。

消除壓力可避免情緒性進食

容易發胖的飲食習慣之一是明明不餓，卻忍不住向食物伸手的「情緒性進食」。其中最典型的例子就是為了消除壓力吃甜食的「發洩性進食」。**請保持適當的睡眠與泡澡等習慣，做好壓力的控管以達到預防的目的。**

回顧自己的生活模式，矯正常犯的錯誤飲食習慣

除了情緒性進食，常見的不良飲食習慣還有只要看到點心或試吃活動就無法抗拒的「衝動性進食」、在家負責清空剩菜剩飯和即期食物的「剩菜擔當」、難以拒絕別人提供的點心或伴手禮的「禮貌性進食」等。

Day 20

心態與大腦

對自己心懷期待

Point

● **正向思考**，相信「我一定會減重成功」

● 從各種日常生活的小事肯定自己，**增加自信**

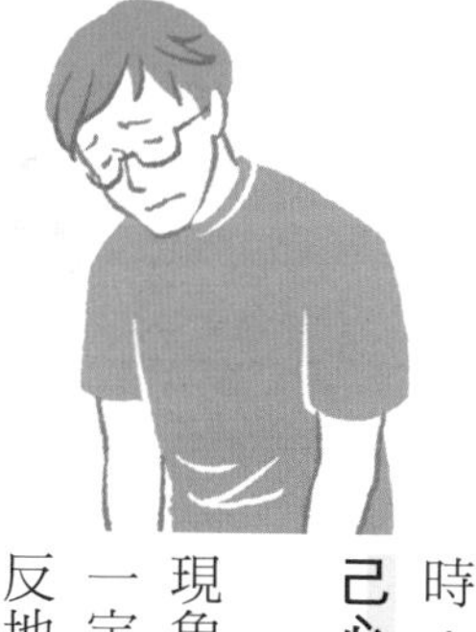

對自己心懷期待是成功減重的助力

不知大家是否看過，在比賽贏得佳績的運動選手接受訪問時，面對鏡頭發表感言時，幾乎都會說「我相信自己一定辦得到」？**正因為他們深信自己能獲得成功，對自己心懷期待，才能馬到成功，享受甜美的果實**。這種思維也可以應用在減重的時候。

人具備的特質之一是很容易按照自己說過的話或想法行動，使其化為現實。這種現象在心理學上稱為「自我實現預言」。簡單來說，只要說出口，或是心裡想著「我一定會減重成功」，就能夠為了達到這個目的而付諸行動，進而提高成功的機率。相反地，如果抱著「我的意志力很薄弱，不可能減重成功」的想法，成功的機率真的就會變得很渺茫。事實上，從減重者的比例來看，想法愈是積極正面、充滿自信的人，減重愈容易成功；而自我評價愈低的人，則傾向於失敗。

提醒自己不要說出負面的話

思考容易趨向負面的人，請不吝於給自己打高分，例如「我本來吃的就不多」「減重對我來說是小事一樁！」，並經常把內心的期待說出口。如此一來，想法也會逐漸從負面轉為正面。

另外，透過「今天很悠閒地泡澡，感覺好紓壓喔」「今天整天沒吃零食」等日常的作為肯定並獎勵自己也很重要。這麼做能逐漸提高自信心，同時提高減重成功的機率。

Day 21

運動

把樓梯化為訓練裝備

Point

- 樓梯就是**「免費的健身房」**
- **只要下樓梯**就足夠
- **只要鍛鍊腰腿，就能提升基礎代謝**，養出易瘦體質

※請務必在觸碰到樓梯的扶手之後洗手或消毒

樓梯就是免費的健身房

本篇為各位介紹在日常生活中，能夠有效鍛鍊下半身的「樓梯的使用方法」。如我在Day17已經說明，下樓梯屬於離心運動，所以樓梯可說是隨處都有設點的健身房，而且完全免費。大家可以使用電梯或手扶梯上樓，只有在下樓時記得走樓梯。下樓梯對身體的負擔較小，相信要各位在日常生活中養成這個習慣並不困難，原則是一天走4層樓。

有關靠下樓梯減重的重點將於下頁說明，**關鍵在於要提醒自己保持挺直背脊的良好姿勢。其次是不要急，一次下一階慢慢走。**一手自然擺動，另一手的指尖則靠著扶手，確保安全。

到了80歲，與20歲時相比，肌肉量只剩下一半

人大部分的肌肉都集中在下半身，而且會隨著年齡增長而逐漸衰退。伴隨而來的變化還有代謝下降，變得不容易瘦下來，所以我們必須積極鍛鍊下半身的肌肉。除了前面介紹的慢慢地坐下來的「椅子深蹲運動」，再加入走下樓梯，可以達到更明顯的效果。

鍛鍊下半身肌肉的另一項好處是可促進IGF－1（類胰島素生長因子）的分泌。IGF－1是一種可促進全身肌肉發達的荷爾蒙，不論從幾歲開始都不會太晚，請各位務必養成走下樓梯的習慣。

Day 21

走下樓梯的重點

只要在日常生活中保持走下樓梯的習慣，就能有效鍛鍊集中了大部分肌肉的下半身。
為了安全與效率著想，請養成正確的姿勢。

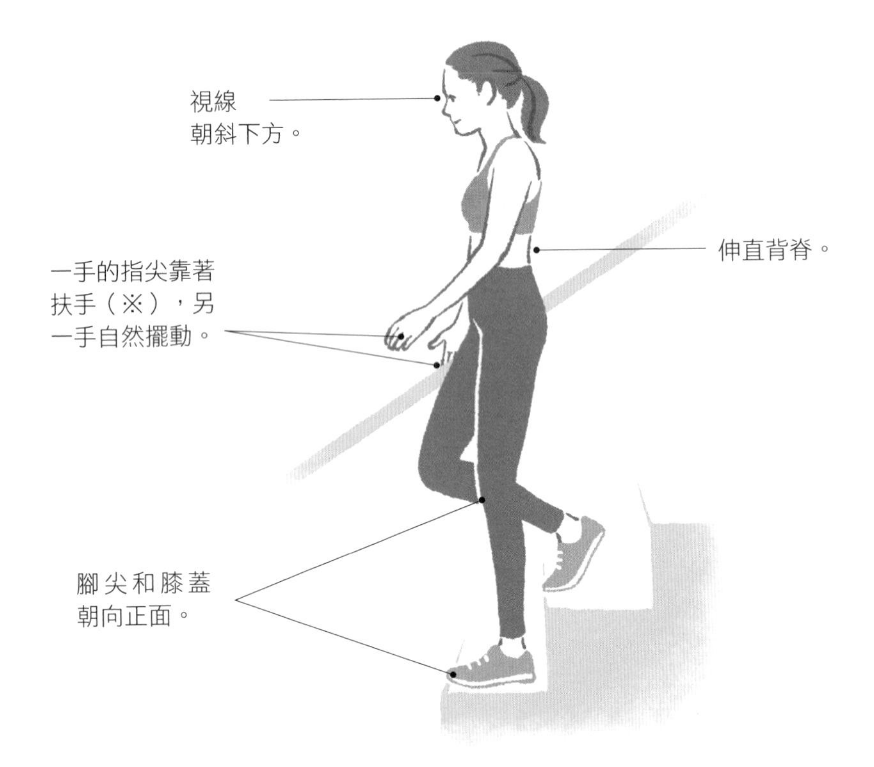
視線
朝斜下方。
伸直背脊。
一手的指尖靠著
扶手（※），另
一手自然擺動。
腳尖和膝蓋
朝向正面。

收下巴，看著斜下方，同時腳尖和膝蓋朝向正面一步一步往下走。挺直背脊，使上半身與地板保持垂直。

※請務必在觸碰到樓梯的扶手之後洗手或消毒。

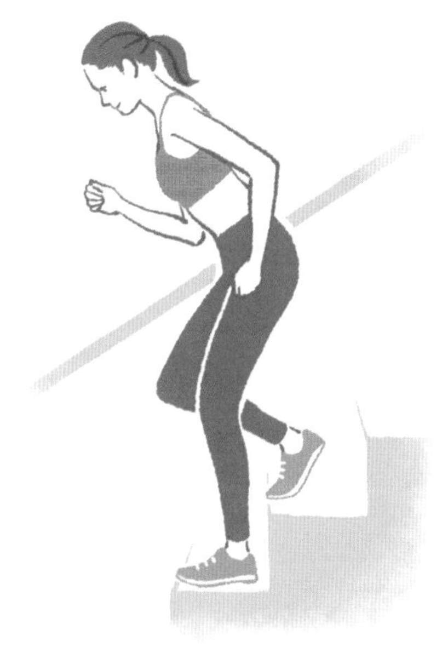

NG

視線朝正下方，背脊彎曲。

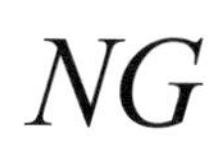

如果腳尖和膝蓋朝外，除了降低鍛鍊肌肉的效果，也會增加膝蓋的負擔。

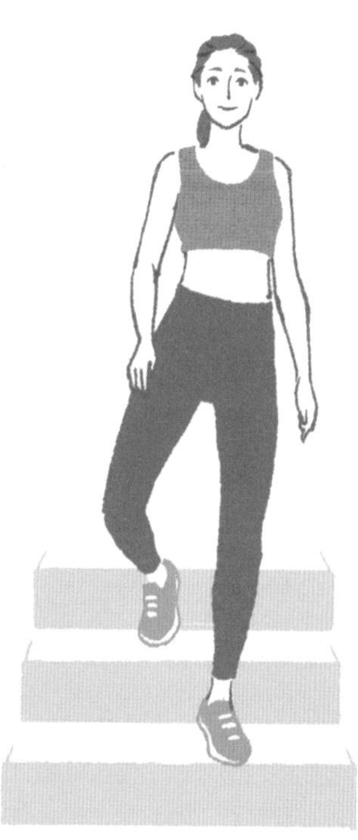

Day 22

營養

即使外食，也要實踐三菜一湯

Point

- 即使外食，也要**遵守三菜一湯的原則**
- 選擇套餐和**單點選項豐富的餐廳**
- **靠配料彌補**主菜與副菜不足的麵類

建議外食時選擇的料理

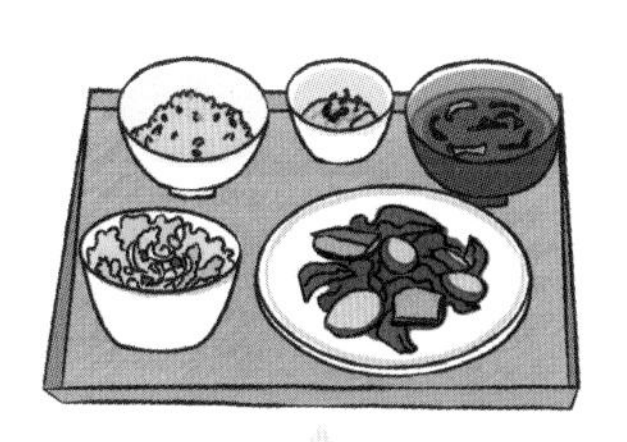

有小缽料理和雜穀米
可供選擇的家庭餐廳◎

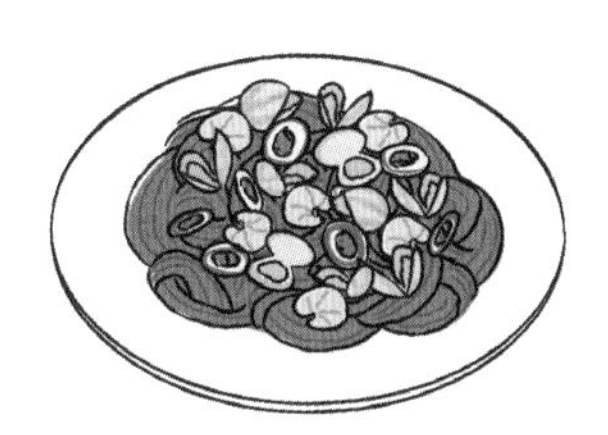

如果要點義大利麵，
就點配料豐富的種類

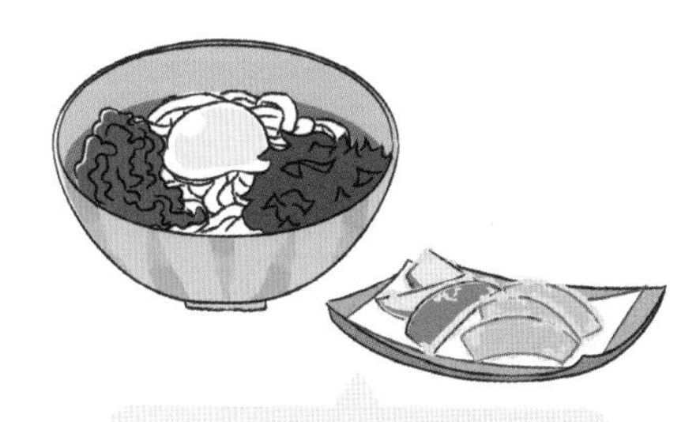

如果點烏龍麵，就靠
配料和小菜調整

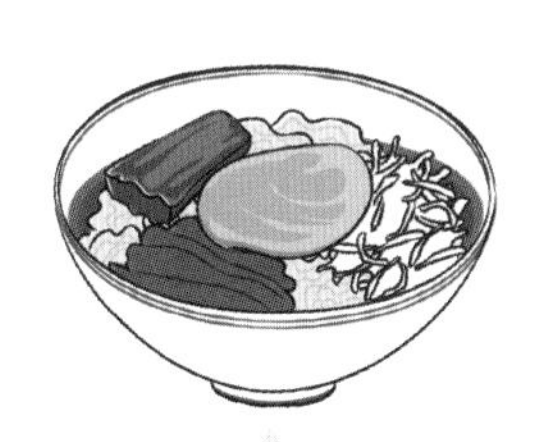

如果點拉麵，可加點
叉燒、蔬菜等配料

選擇家庭餐廳和簡餐店，盡可能遵守三菜一湯的原則

請各位即使外食，也要顧及營養均衡，盡可能做到三菜一湯。挑選外食的餐廳時，首選是家庭餐廳和簡餐店。因為這類餐廳的選擇很彈性，從飯量、米飯的種類等都可以自由選擇，方便顧客兼顧熱量、營養均衡等自身需求。而且也提供許多可單點的主餐，讓顧客能夠享受更多的口味。

點麵食的原則是選擇配料多的品項，以達到營養均衡

麵食類的缺點是幾乎沒有主菜和副菜，難以達到營養均衡。為了改善這一點，建議加點配料和小菜，以攝取充分的肉類、魚肉、蔬菜。

Day 23

運動

養成讓自己更有魅力的站姿、走路方式

Point

- 藉由正確的站姿與走路方式**改善體態**
- 正確的站姿**可預防肩膀僵硬與腰痛**
- 走路時**腳尖和膝蓋要朝向正面**

只要站得正，體態看起來就顯得優美

如同前述，**藉由伸展腹部與臀部的肌肉，隨時提醒自己要挺直背脊，保持正確姿勢，站姿看起來就挺拔美麗。**不僅如此，站得正能夠讓身體不容易疲勞、活動自如，如此一來，日常生活運動量也跟著增加，對減重自然會成為一大助力。

為了養成正確的姿勢，最重要的關鍵在於「腳」。人體所有的肌肉都會連動，只要一個部位產生變化，為了找回平衡，整個身體便會不自覺地發生變化。這種情形稱為「動力鏈」。簡單來說，只要將腳調整到正確的狀態，全身也會跟著調整。

意識到腳部內側的存在，伸直背脊

站著的時候，首先稍微張開雙腳。請把腳尖和膝蓋朝向正前方，大腿內側稍微出點力，讓腳底內側承受體重。如此一來，骨盆自然會挺起來，背脊應該也會伸直。而且肩膀也會往後拉，讓頭部的位置剛好在背骨上方。這種站姿可減輕脖子、肩膀、膝蓋、腰部等對身體的負擔，所以對預防與改善身體各處疼痛也有幫助。

走路時也必須意識到腳的存在很重要。**因為步行是站姿的延長，所以請在走路之前，一樣提醒自己要稍微張開雙腳，把腳尖和膝蓋朝向正前方。**這麼做可以加長步距，讓自己走得更順暢。當然，除了走路方式顯得更有美感，外表看起來也會更加年輕。

Day 23

站得正確的重點

以下為各位介紹保持正確站姿時的幾個重點。站得正不只有美化體態的效果，因為提升身體的活動度，對減重也能發揮正面助益。

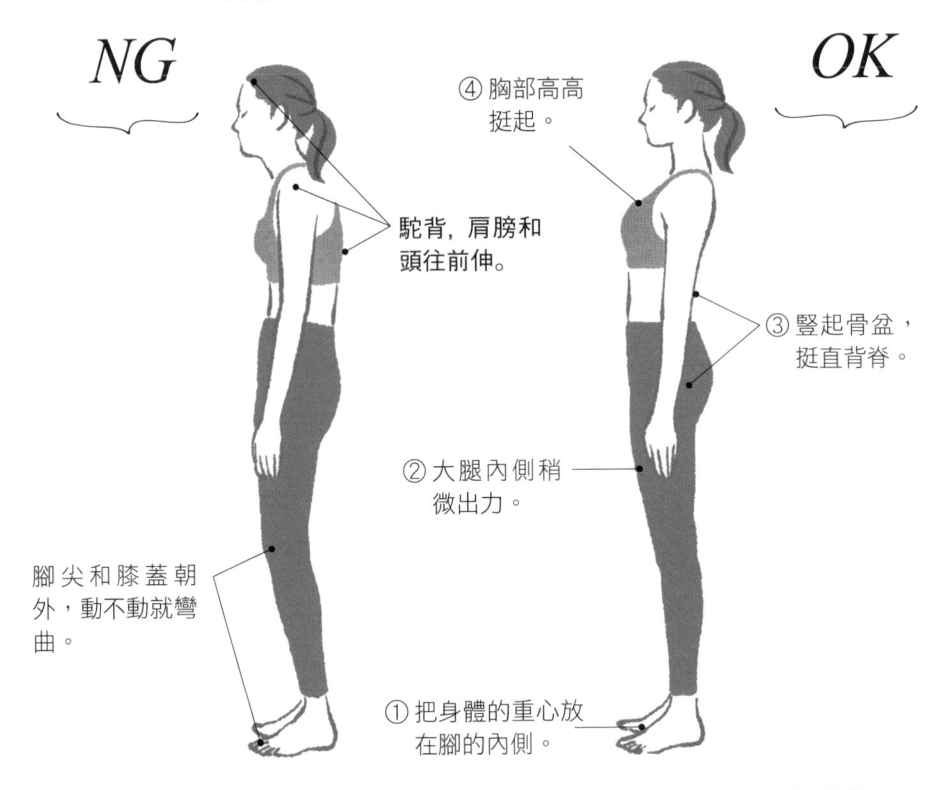

NG
OK
④ 胸部高高挺起。
駝背，肩膀和頭往前伸。
③ 豎起骨盆，挺直背脊。
② 大腿內側稍微出力。
腳尖和膝蓋朝外，動不動就彎曲。
① 把身體的重心放在腳的內側。

如果把身體的重心放在腳的外側，不但容易駝背，肩膀和頭部也會不自覺地往前方移動。

稍微張開雙腳，把腳尖和膝蓋朝向正前方，依照①～④的順序由下往上調整姿勢。

正確的走路方式的重點

右頁介紹的「正確的站姿」為正確的走路方式之本。
提醒自己先保持基本的正確站姿再跨步走出去，想必走路時的姿態看起來會更有魅力。

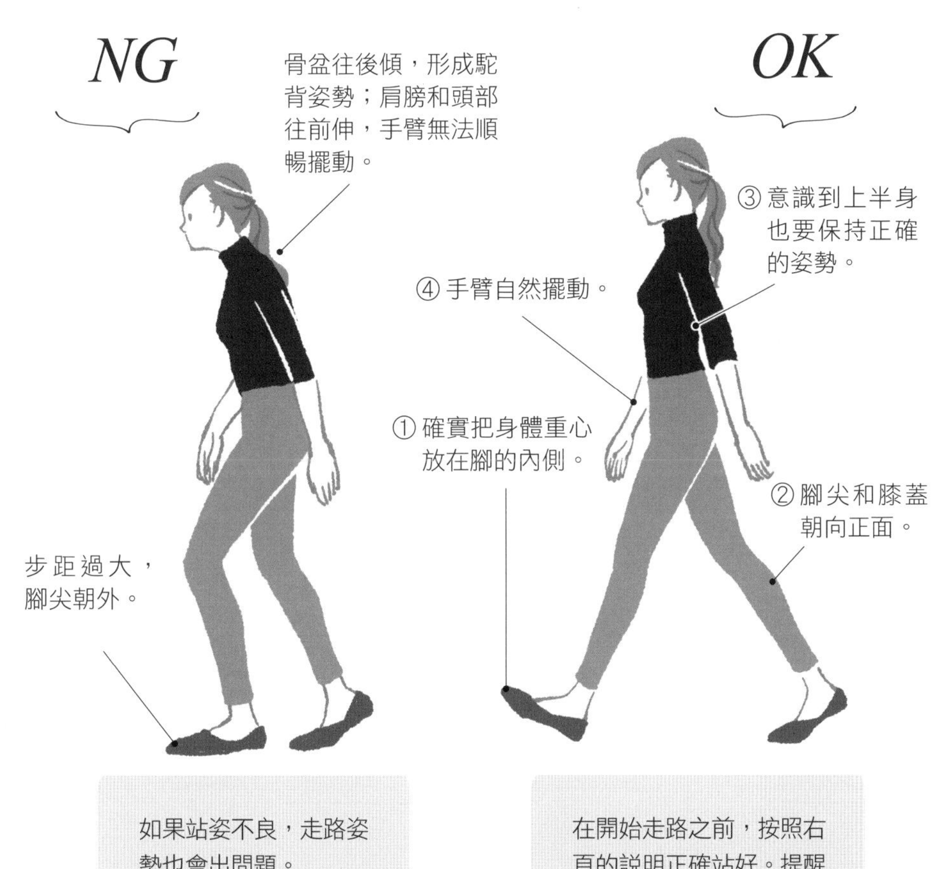
NG
骨盆往後傾，形成駝背姿勢；肩膀和頭部往前伸，手臂無法順暢擺動。
步距過大，腳尖朝外。
OK
③意識到上半身也要保持正確的姿勢。
④手臂自然擺動。
①確實把身體重心放在腳的內側。
②腳尖和膝蓋朝向正面。

如果站姿不良，走路姿勢也會出問題。

在開始走路之前，按照右頁的說明正確站好。提醒自己依照①～④的順序跨步走。

Day 24

營養

利用3K食材加速減重，整頓腸道環境

Point

- 利用**膳食纖維**增加飽足感，調整腸道環境
- 利用富含水溶性膳食纖維的**海藻類維持血糖平緩上升**
- 利用富含不溶性膳食纖維的**菇類與蒟蒻改善便祕**

3K食材

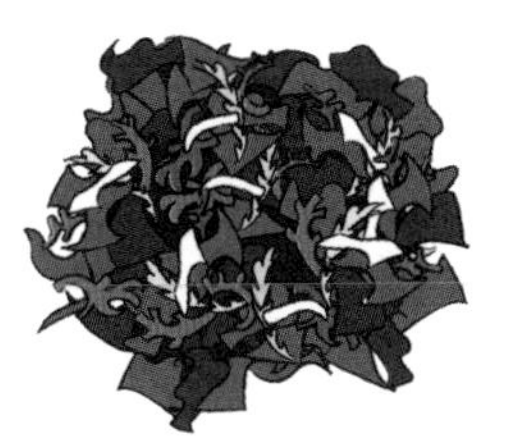

海藻

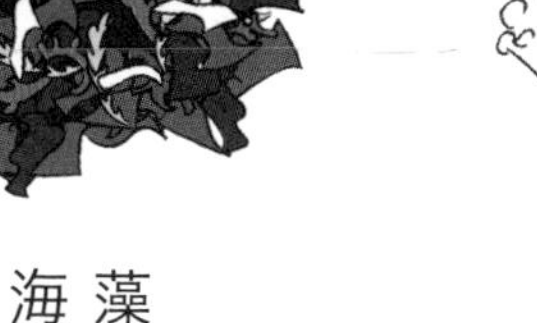

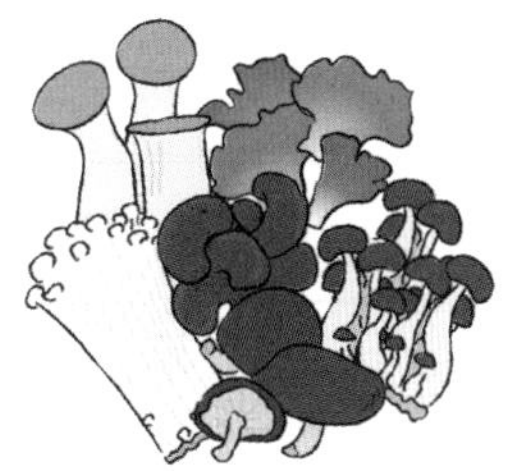

菇類

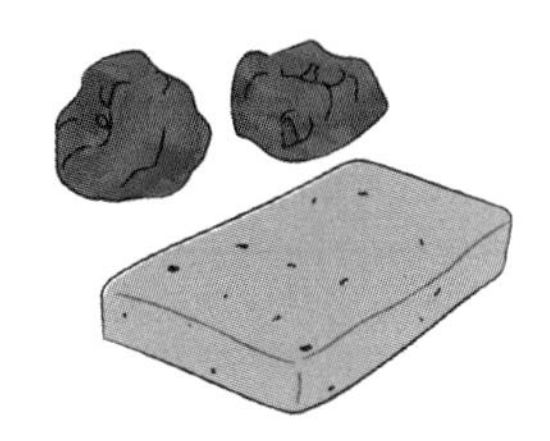

蒟蒻

3K食材的優點

- 幾乎零熱量
- 含有豐富的膳食纖維
- 可增加飽足感
- 整頓腸道環境，預防便祕、腹瀉、皮膚粗糙

高含量的膳食纖維是減重時的強力幫手

所謂的3K食材＝「海藻、菇類、蒟蒻（這3項食材的羅馬拼音都是K開頭）」皆含有豐富的膳食纖維；雖然幾乎不含熱量，卻能增添飽足感。**大量含於海藻類的水溶性膳食纖維，可發揮抑制膽固醇的吸收與血糖急速上升的功能。**大量含於菇類和蒟蒻的不溶性膳食纖維，能夠在腸胃吸收水分，增加糞便體積，有效改善便祕。

整頓腸道環境是保持身體健康的關鍵

膳食纖維到了腸道會成為好菌的食物，可發揮整頓腸道的作用。**積極攝取3K食材，不僅加速減重，對維持健康更是好處多多。**

Day 25

運動

等到身體變得輕盈就挑戰爬樓梯

Point

● 一次兩階，爬兩層樓「往上爬樓梯」會帶來明顯的深蹲效果

● 每增加3kg的肌肉，可多消耗50kcal

※請務必在觸碰到樓梯的扶手之後洗手或消毒

透過爬樓梯提升肌力

1個月的減重計畫轉眼間只剩下6天。目前為止，我已經從各種角度說明如何打造易瘦體質的作法，包括拉筋與矯正姿勢的方法、鍛鍊下半身的方法。我相信到了第26天，應該已經有不少人確實感覺到「身體好像變輕盈了一點」。接下來從今天起，請各位挑戰能加速鍛鍊下半身肌肉的「上樓梯」。

光靠爬樓梯也能得到和深蹲同樣的效果

作法非常簡單。**首先以正確的姿勢站在樓梯前，再一階一階慢慢爬上去。**請從今天開始，以爬樓梯取代搭電梯吧。1天的目標是2層樓。

1天爬滿2層樓持續一段時間後，接下來請試著一次爬兩階。一次爬兩階等同於單腳進行大幅度深蹲，是效果絕佳的肌肉鍛鍊方法（參照次頁）。

重點在於只靠跨上階梯的單腳力量抬起身體。這麼做可以使前腳的臀部與大腿內側的肌肉得到更多鍛鍊。一次爬兩階的訓練頻率以2天1次為宜。

只要增加3kg的肌肉，每天就可多消耗50kcal。為了養成易瘦體質，同時為了彌補在減重過程中分解的肌肉，請務必多加利用樓梯這個免費的健身房。

Day 25

爬樓梯的重點

強力推薦各位在穿著活動方便的褲裝時，務必挑戰的訓練。
若能做到一次爬兩階，肌肉應該可以得到很紮實的鍛鍊。

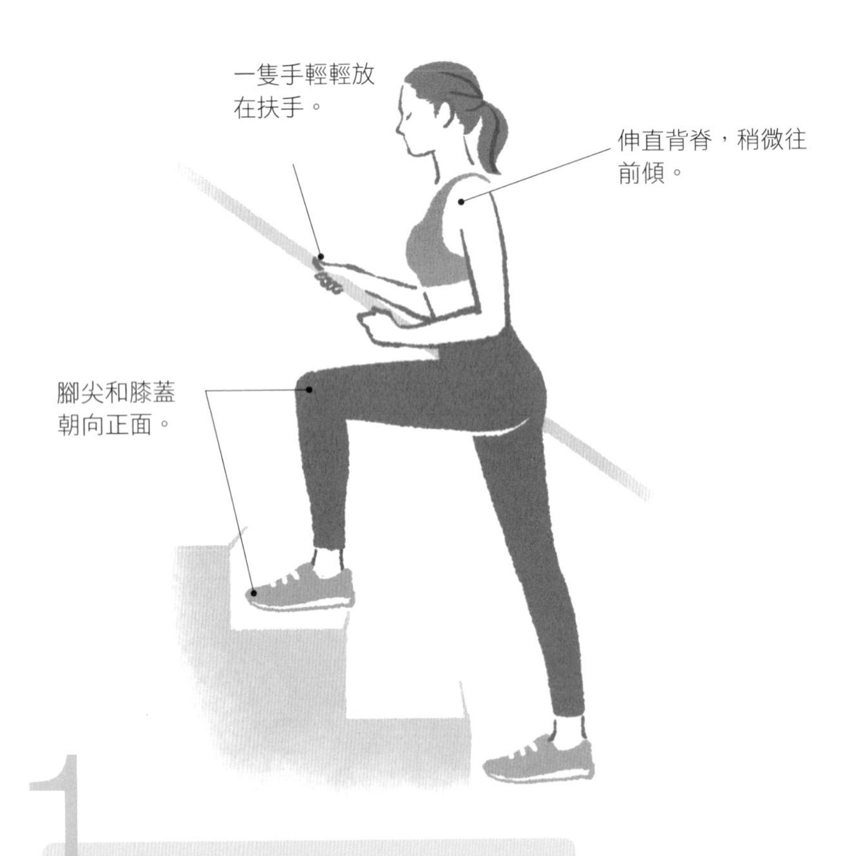
一隻手輕輕放
在扶手。
伸直背脊，稍微往
前傾。
腳尖和膝蓋
朝向正面。

1

以正確的姿勢站在樓梯前，把左腳放在第二階。

※請務必在觸碰到樓梯的扶手之後洗手或消毒

2

儘量只靠左腳（放在前面階梯的腳）的臀部和大腿的力量把身體抬起來。

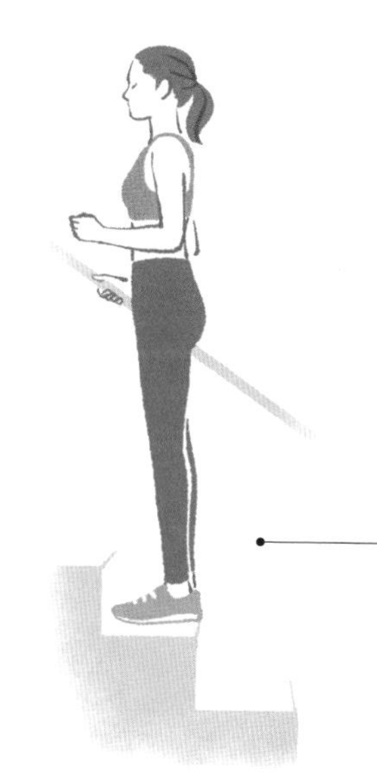

為了避免一開始衝太快，先將兩腳併攏。

3

雙腳靠攏，接著換右腳一次跨兩階。

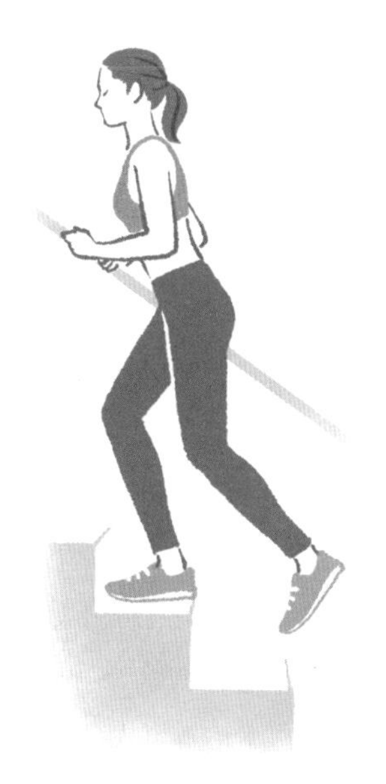

Day 26

運動

鍛鍊背肌可以進一步提升代謝

Point

- 繼下半身之後，下一個應該鍛鍊的是**「核心」**
- **背肌其實比腹肌更重要**
- 只要鍛鍊下半身＋背肌，**就能加強近80％全身的肌肉**

繼下半身之後，接下來鍛鍊背肌

基於美容與健康目的，先前已經說明應該最優先鍛鍊的是下半身的肌肉，因為下半身是支撐身體的根基。等到各位持續鍛鍊下半身的肌肉一段時間，覺得行有餘力之後，接下來應該鍛鍊的就是相當於身體的柱子與牆壁的「核心」。

說到核心，不知道各位第一個想到的是不是腹肌運動？不過，我想告訴各位的是，**其實鍛鍊腰部的背肌比腹部的腹肌更重要**。

理由有兩項。第一，因為脊柱起立肌等背部肌群比腹直肌等腹部肌群更大也更強。反重力，作用是支撐身體的肌肉稱為抗重力肌，而負責將背骨直立撐起，支撐上半身的抗重力肌是背肌而非腹肌。既然要負責撐起背骨，這也意味著不論我們站著還是坐著，背肌隨時都處於上工狀態，所以容易疲勞也是理所當然。因為這個關係，有腰痛困擾的人不在少數，但幾乎沒聽過有人說自己腹肌痛。

鍛鍊下半身＋背肌就能強化全身肌肉的8成

另一個理由是隨著年齡增長，說得精準一點，應該是隨著長期以來的運動不足，更容易衰退的是背肌而不是腹肌。

不論是出於美容目的還是健康目的，只要鍛鍊下半身加上背部肌肉，就能強化全身近80％的肌肉。鍛鍊背肌不但能夠延緩代謝的下降，對挺直背脊，維持年輕體態也功不可沒。另外，強化背肌也能減輕和預防腰痛。

Day 26 運動

Day 26

背部伸展

這套訓練動作是為了鍛鍊背骨周圍的脊柱起立肌等背部肌群。
只要持之以恆地鍛鍊，不但可提升代謝，姿勢也會變得更加挺拔好看。
也很適合想要預防腰痛的人。

10秒 × 1～3組 每週2～3次

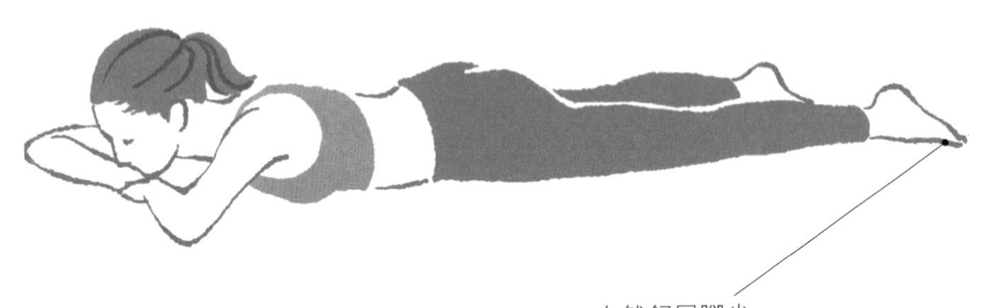

自然舒展腳尖。

1

趴下，雙腳張開與腰幅同寬。雙手相疊，放在下巴下方。

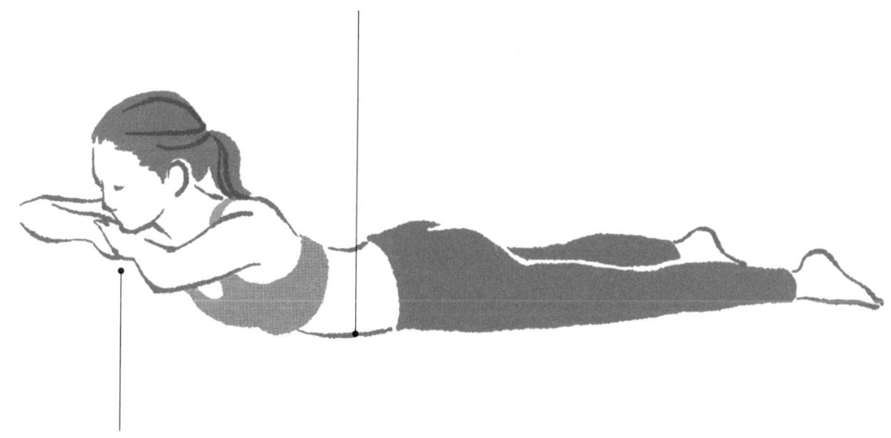
挺起上半身時不可用力過猛，
下腹部以下要全程貼在地板。
上半身挺起的高度大約是手抬
起，距離地板15～20cm的位置。

2

吐氣的同時，花1～2秒挺起上半身，再吸氣，
花2～3秒回到原來的姿勢。

Day 27

運動

儘量增加日常生活運動量

Point

- 在日常生活中有意識地增加運動量
- 以一般的速度步行，取代搭捷運或公車，消耗的卡路里會增加4倍
- 只要增加NEAT，疲勞也能得到舒緩

透過NEAT消耗熱量的方式也受到矚目

如果有人想提高減去體脂肪的進度，請考慮透過全身運動以消耗更多熱量。這裡說的全身運動，並不是游泳和跑步之類的運動。可行性高，又容易持之以恆的反而是藉由移動、做家事等日常生活運動。以下為大家介紹增加NEAT的方法。

在我們一天消耗的所有熱量當中，因身體活動所消耗的熱量約占了20～30%；只要沒有特別運動，那麼大部分都屬於NEAT。事實上，體重過重的人與瘦的人相比，NEAT也有較少的傾向。

在不勉強自己的範圍內增加活動量◎

為了增加NEAT，我希望各位從今天立刻開始實踐的是，減少坐下來的時間。因為和坐著做事相比，站著做事可多消耗2成的熱量。大家可以自訂規則，例如用筆電的時候坐著，滑手機的時候就站起來。做到這點之後，下一步就是儘量找機會走路。因為即使只是按照一般速度走路，消耗的熱量是搭公車4倍。所以我建議大家減少網購和叫外送的頻率，改成自己到實體店面購物。另外，也請多走點路到超市採買，而不是就近到超商購物。如果體力允許，請提早1～2站下車，走路回家。總之，請在不勉強自己的範圍內儘量增加活動量。

現代人的疲勞，有大半是以同樣的姿勢久坐，造成血液循環不良，肌肉不斷累積疲勞。但是，即使放空休息也無法改善這樣的疲勞狀態，唯有藉由活動才能消除。基於這點，增加NEAT也算是能夠一箭雙鵰的好主意。

Day 27

1天總消耗熱量的明細

1天總消耗熱量的60～70%是為了維持生命所需的基礎代謝，
包含NEAT在內的身體活動代謝占了20～30%、攝食產熱效應占了10%。

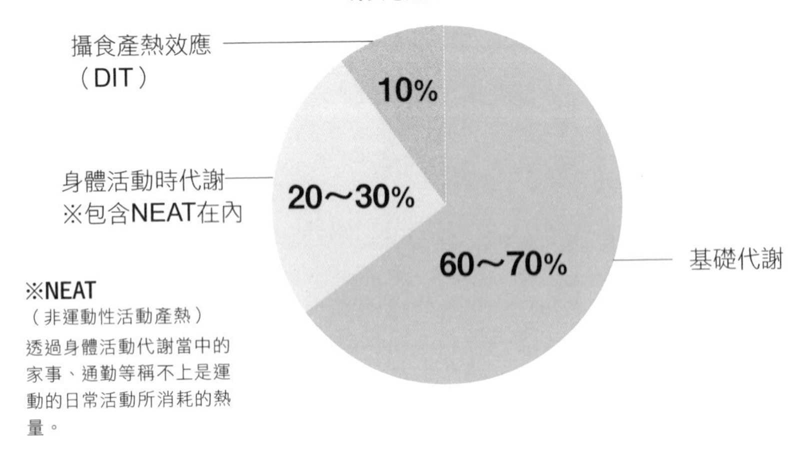

※NEAT
（非運動性活動產熱）
透過身體活動代謝當中的家事、通勤等稱不上是運動的日常活動所消耗的熱量。

可增加NEAT的行動

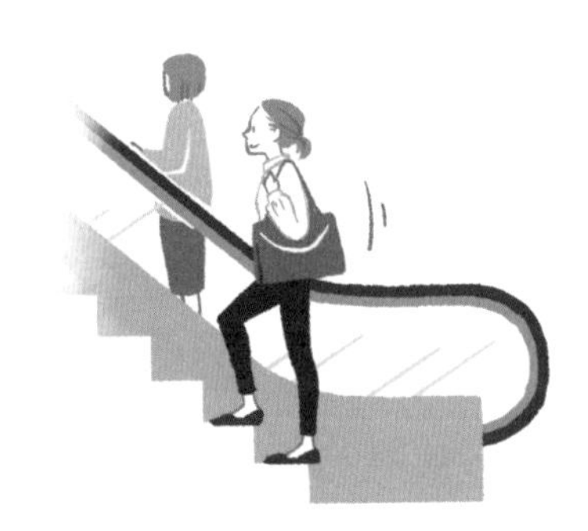

有機會就爬樓梯

移動時儘量步行，以爬樓梯取代搭電梯等。

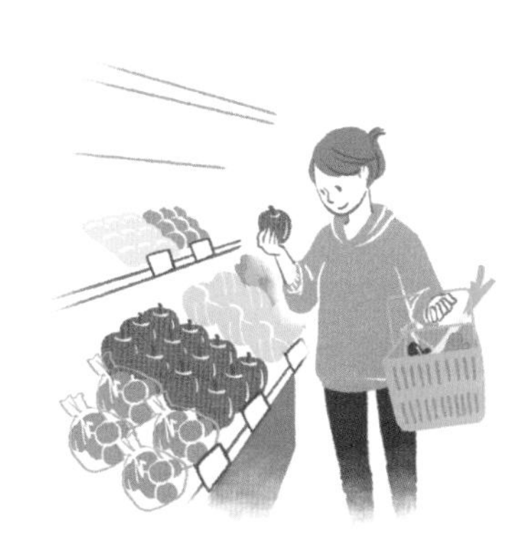

出門採買

減少網購和叫外送的次數，寧願多走點路去超市購物，而不是就近在超商解決。

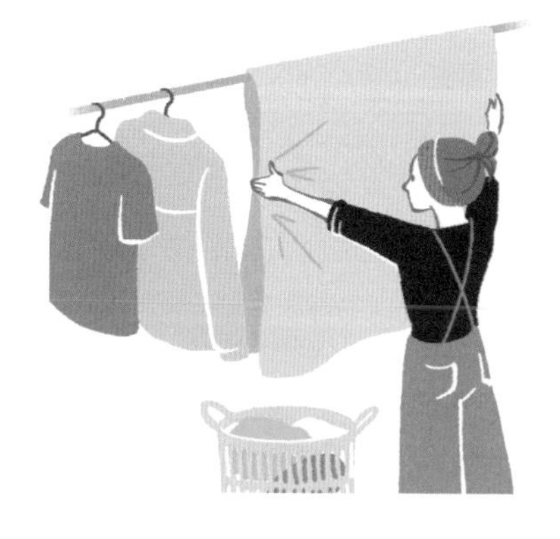

晾衣服

不要仰賴烘衣機，把衣服改成自己晾自己收。

遛狗

延長帶狗出去散步的時間等，在能力所及的範圍內儘量增加步行的距離。

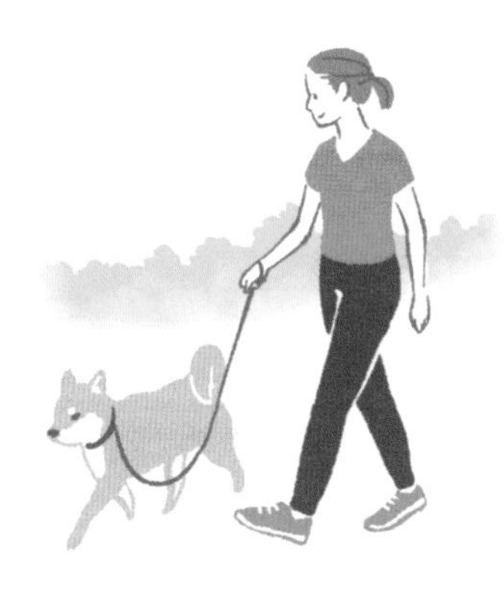

Day 28

營養

點心聰明選，安心吃

Point

- 點心**可防止肌肉的分解**
- 如果要吃點心，最好的時間是**下午4點左右**
- 理想的點心是**接近正餐的輕食，或者含有豐富蛋白質的營養補給品**

吃點心的好處

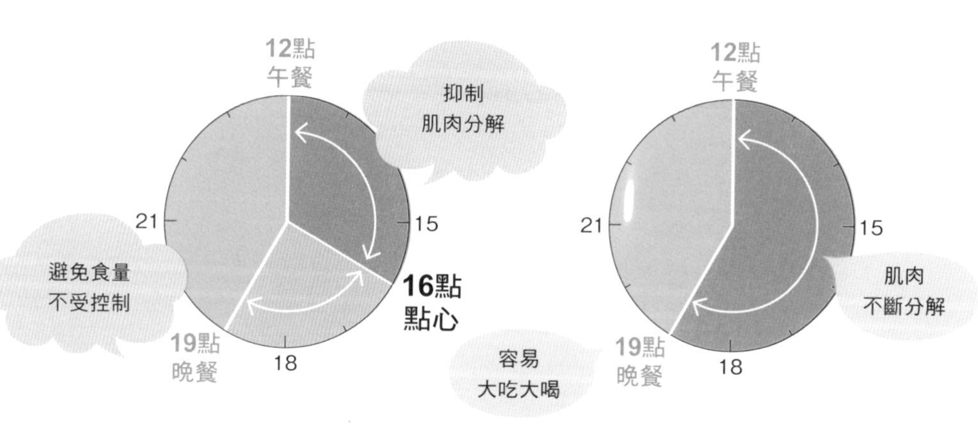

含有蛋白質的輕食是最佳選擇

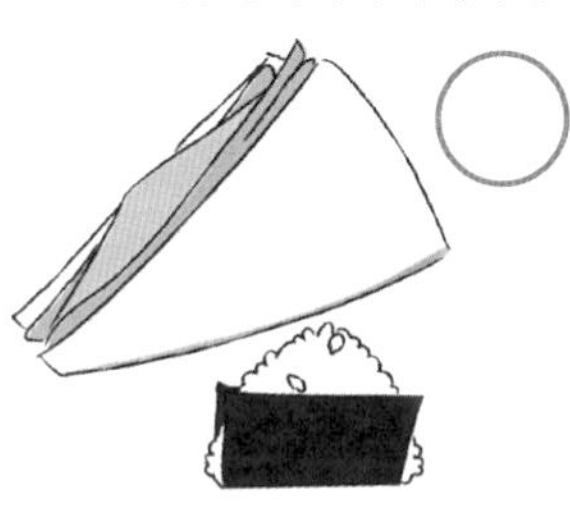

輕食（接近主食+主菜的餐點）如果搭配蛋白質，可以增加飽足感。

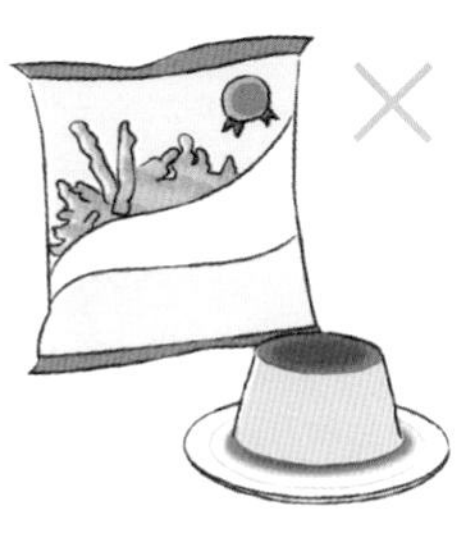

甜食、甜麵包、休閒零嘴會使血糖急速上升再急速下降，反而帶來更強烈的空腹感。

下午4點左右的點心是打造易瘦體質的一大助力

前面已經向各位說明**最聰明的飲食法是「3餐+點心」**。最適合吃點心的時段是下午4點左右，在這個時間攝取150～200大卡的點心，不但能有效抑制肌肉分解，也可以避免晚餐過量。

最理想的點心是「主食+主菜」的輕食

理想的點心包括鮭魚飯糰、火腿起士三明治等由「主食+主菜」組成的輕食。最近幾年，從超商、超市等處也買得到含有豐富蛋白質的營養補助食品，這類產品也是很好的選擇（參照P106）。

Day 29

運動

加入腹肌運動

Point

- 背肌訓練的下一個是腹肌訓練
- 養成正確的姿勢，執行只針對腹部肌群進行強化的鍛鍊

行有餘力之後，請一併挑戰腹肌運動

等到背肌的訓練已經駕輕就熟，接著請加入腹肌運動。腹肌運動分為兩種，一種是將上半身完全抬起的「仰臥起坐」，另一種是只彎曲背部的「捲腹」。大家熟悉的仰臥起坐，除了運用到腹直肌等腹部肌群使背部彎曲，也會運用腸腰肌等肌肉使髖關節彎曲，由兩個地方承受負重。把仰臥起坐做得很熟練以後，做捲腹運動的時候，髖關節很容易不由自主地彎曲，這種現象稱為運動代償。**而為了提升腹肌運動的效率，關鍵便掌握於如何抑制代償，只針對腹部肌群進行鍛鍊**。

養成正確的姿勢，才能得到確實的效果

第一步從確認姿勢開始（P103右上）。首先坐在椅子上，將骨盆貼住椅背，確認自己的背能彎曲到什麼程度，以及眼睛對到大腿的位置在哪裡。切記如果超過這個範圍，髖關節會彎曲，那就NG了。確認完成後躺下來，把膝蓋下方放在椅面上。這時要把髖關節與膝蓋的角度調成為90度。如果身體離開椅子，腰部與地板之間的空隙會變大，換句話說，就是腰椎如果過度朝後方彎曲，背骨就無法順利彎曲。只要背骨能夠從這個姿勢一直前彎到坐在椅子上確認的狀態，而且來到視線正對腳部的位置，自然可針對腹部肌群進行局部鍛鍊。另外，為了進一步提升腹肌運動的效果，請各位也別忘了確認手和手臂的姿勢。

Day 29

腹肌運動的正確方式

等到下半身與背肌的訓練已經駕輕就熟，接下來請加入腹肌的訓練。
只要熟悉以下為大家介紹的正確姿勢，鍛鍊起來就更有效率。

1

讓髖關節與膝蓋呈90度，把腳放在椅子上。把手放在側頭部，指尖深入後頭部的下方，並夾緊手肘。

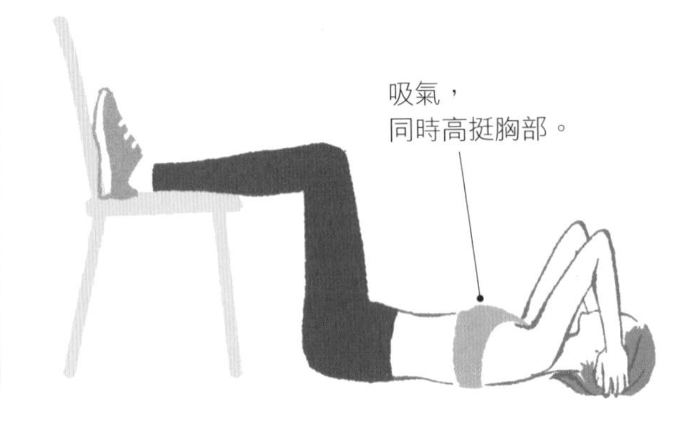
吸氣，
同時高挺胸部。

2

吐氣，同時花1～2秒將背往前彎。接著吸氣，花2～3秒慢慢地恢復原來的姿勢。

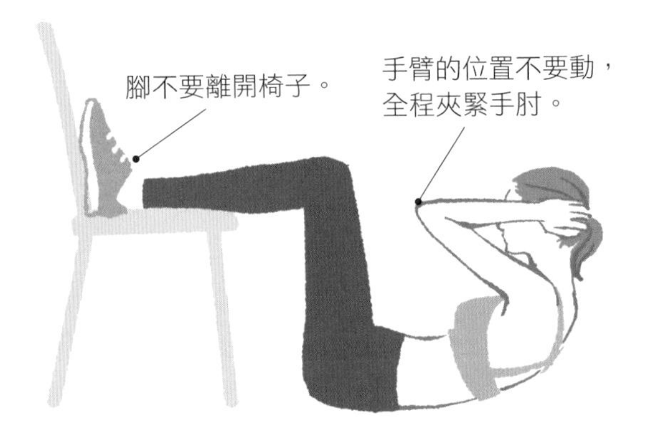
腳不要離開椅子。
手臂的位置不要動，
全程夾緊手肘。

確認腹肌運動的姿勢是否正確

☑ 腳的形狀

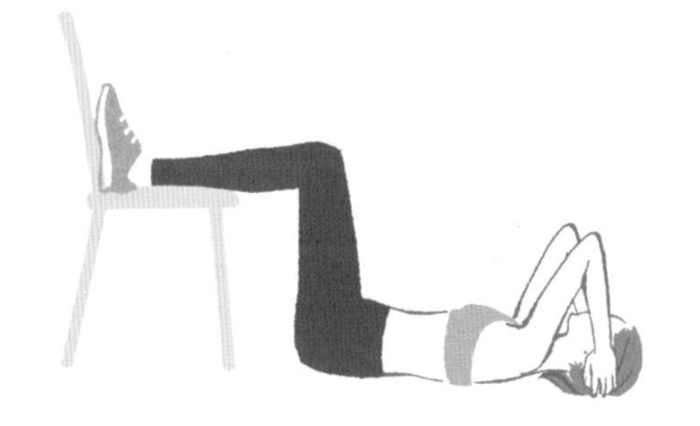

讓髖關節與膝蓋呈90度。如果把椅子放得太遠，腰部與地板會產生過大的空隙。

☑ 確認動作

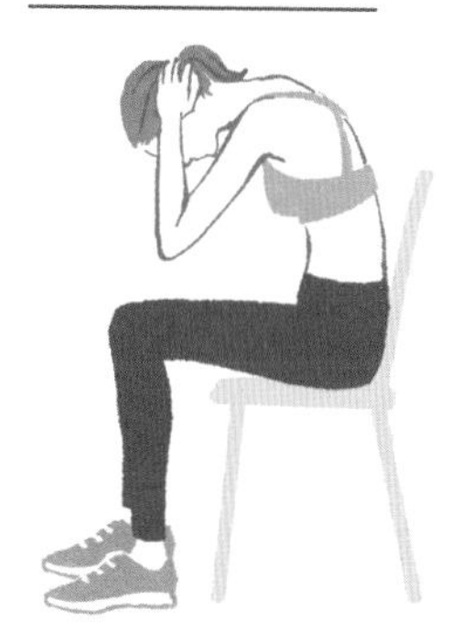

確認坐在椅子上的姿勢是否正確，骨盆如果離開椅背就NG。

☑ 手的形狀

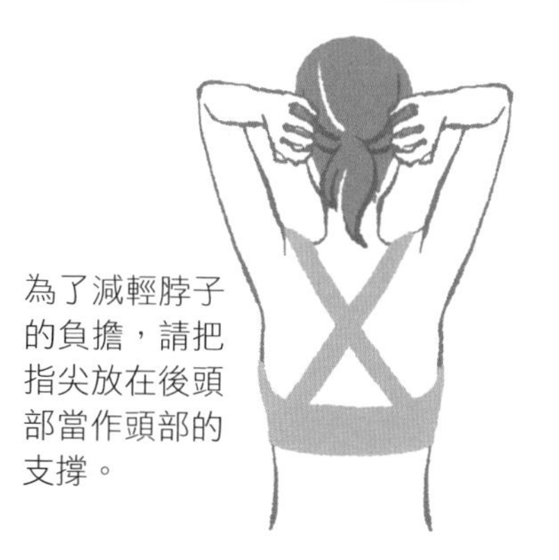

為了減輕脖子的負擔，請把指尖放在後頭部當作頭部的支撐。

☑ 手臂的形狀

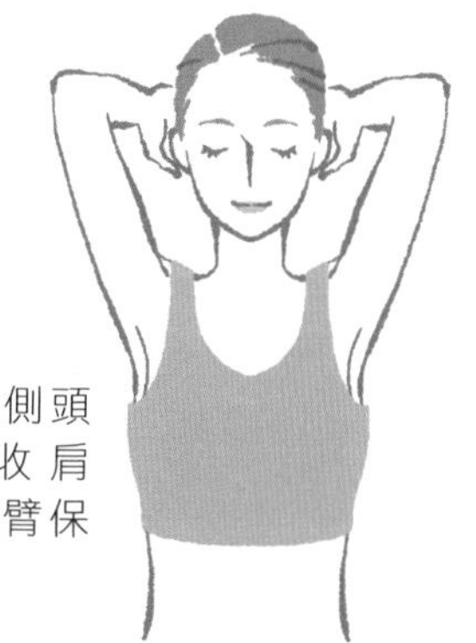

把手放在側頭部，後收肩胛，讓雙臂保持平行。

Day 30

心態與大腦

為了避免對減重只有三分鐘熱度的心理建設

Point

- **努力過頭**是造成挫折的原因
- **懂得見好就收，讓自己意猶未盡**很重要
- **讓身心多幾分從容**，是保持動機不墜的祕訣

總是在減重路上受挫的人

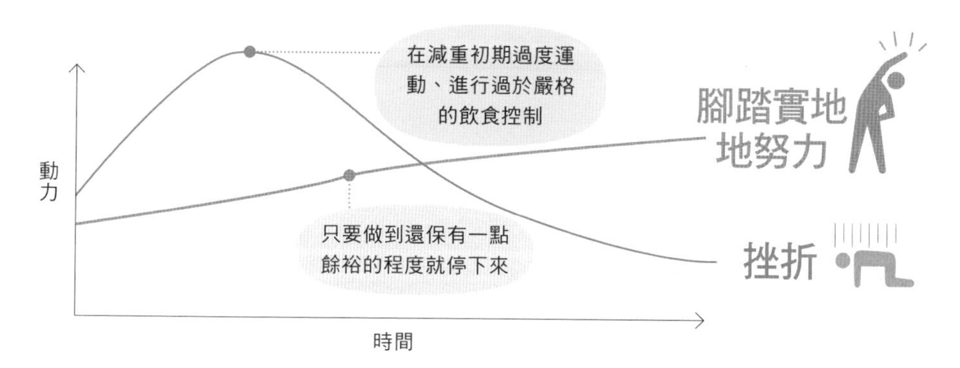

無法持之以恆，減重以失敗告終

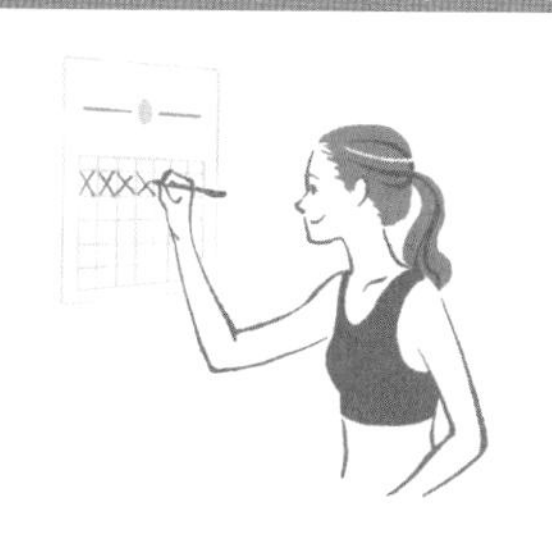

該做的不是一下子給自己太多課題，最理想的狀況是每天腳踏實地地努力，按部就班增加要執行的項目。

初期的「努力過頭」是造成挫折的原因

造成對減重只有三分鐘熱度的最大原因是：一開始衝太快，努力過頭。有些人在鬥志高昂，一心只想著「我要瘦」「我要變美」的減重初期，過度運動或進行過於嚴格的飲食限制，結果在不知不覺中變得身心俱疲，內心受挫。

讓自己保有幾分餘力，減重才可能持之以恆

為了避免受挫，最重要的關鍵在於不論是飲食控制還是運動，在初期階段都要保留幾分實力，不要一下子全力衝刺。這份從容、餘裕可以避免壓力與疲勞上身，是保持動力不墜的祕訣。

建議在超商購買的食品

即使在超商選購正餐和點心，也要顧慮營養均衡與熱量。

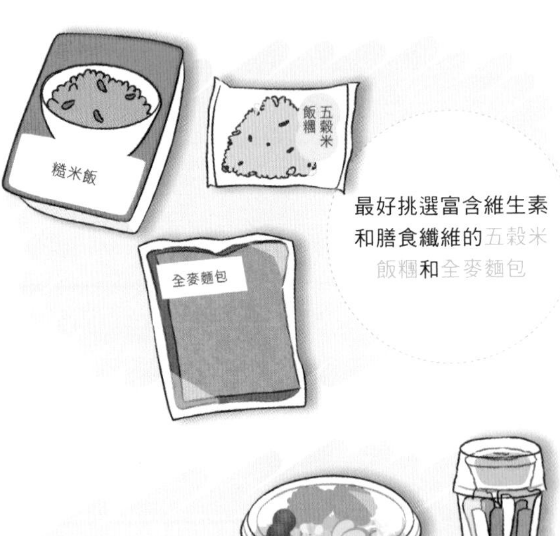

最好挑選富含維生素和膳食纖維的五穀米飯糰和全麥麵包

主菜和蛋白質來源以油脂含量不高的品項為宜

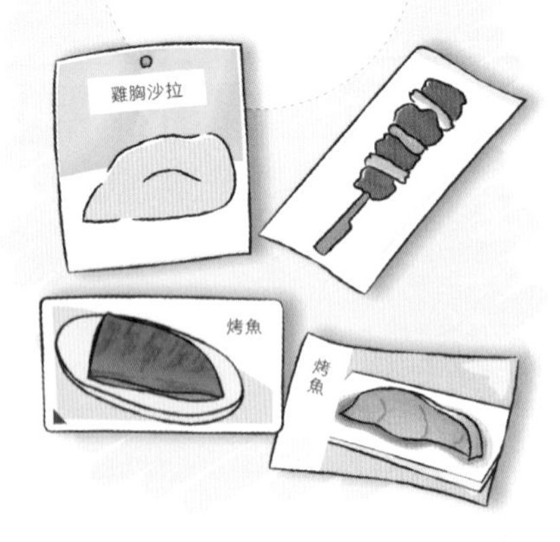

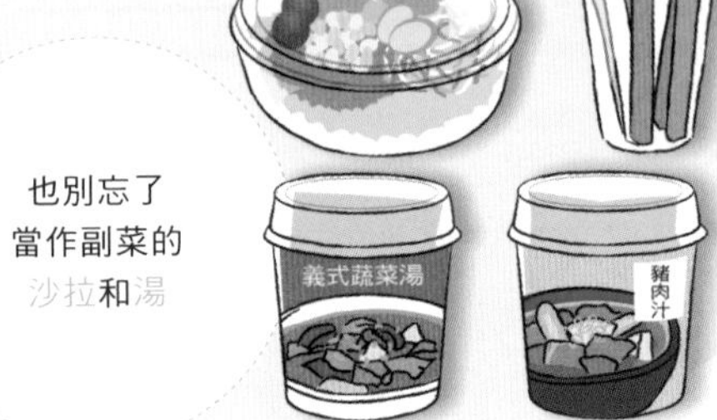

也別忘了當作副菜的沙拉和湯

最適合當作點心的蛋白質補給品

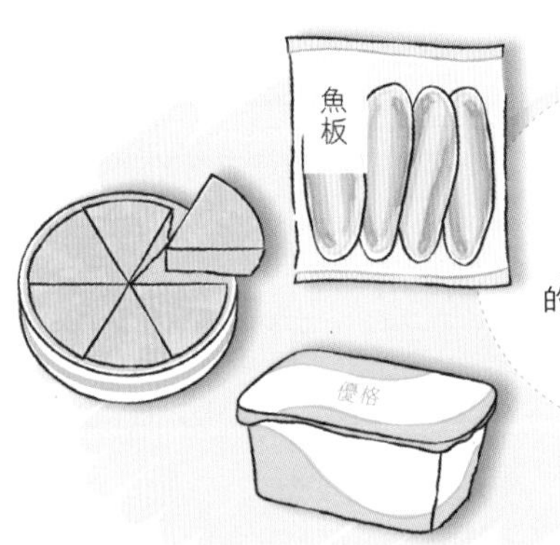

起司和優格可當作主菜的替代品、點心

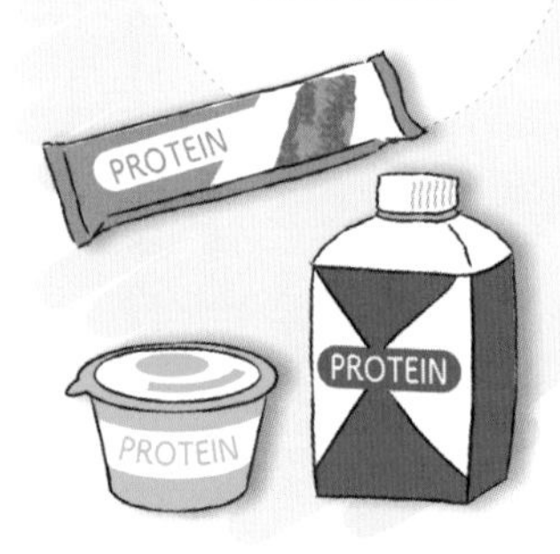

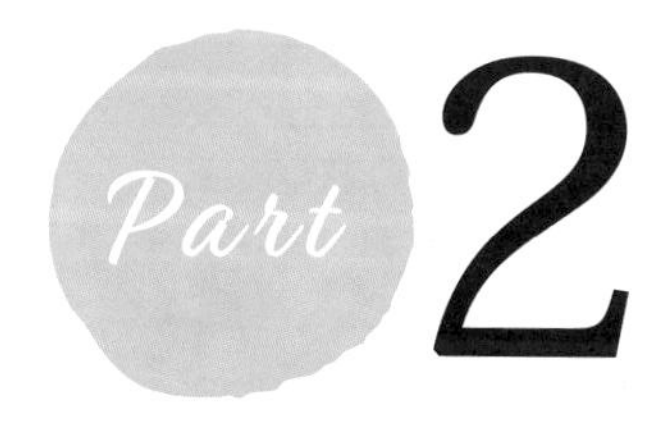

減重的真相與謊言

知識篇

只要搓搓揉揉就能瘦是真的嗎？

只是使水分移動，而不是真正減掉脂肪

我相信不少人都看過類似這樣的廣告台詞，像是「讓脂肪細胞移動」「只要促進淋巴的循環，代謝老舊廢物，身材就會變得苗條」。對此類按摩瘦身法的效果深信不疑的人還真不少，但是我必須告訴大家一個殘酷的事實：**來自外部的物理性刺激，無法分解也無法消耗體脂肪**。

首先，脂肪細胞的周圍有血管和神經通過，而且脂肪細胞之間緊密相連，所以不會移動。透過按摩確實能夠暫時讓腰圍等尺寸縮小，但原因是水分，也就是填滿細胞間隙的組織液移動。尤其是小腿肚，會受到重力的影響，導致水量增加而變得水腫，所以**按摩之後，確實看起來不再浮腫，明顯變細，但大概只能維持1個小時就恢復原狀**。當然也對脂肪的增減毫無影響。

脂肪細胞的化學分解，取決於體內荷爾蒙的指令。例如腎上腺素是一種會作用於全身脂肪細胞的荷爾蒙，並分解儲存於體內的部分中性脂肪，轉換為游離脂肪酸，最後再釋放

到血液中。進入血液的游離脂肪酸會到達肌肉、心臟等處，成為能量來源。當然，這類荷爾蒙的作用，和來自體外的物理性刺激也毫無關係。

不過話說回來，如果能夠讓身心獲得深層的放鬆，那麼按摩就非常值得推薦。因為藉由紓壓以抑制過食，也是有助減去體脂肪的重要一環。

利用按摩消除水腫

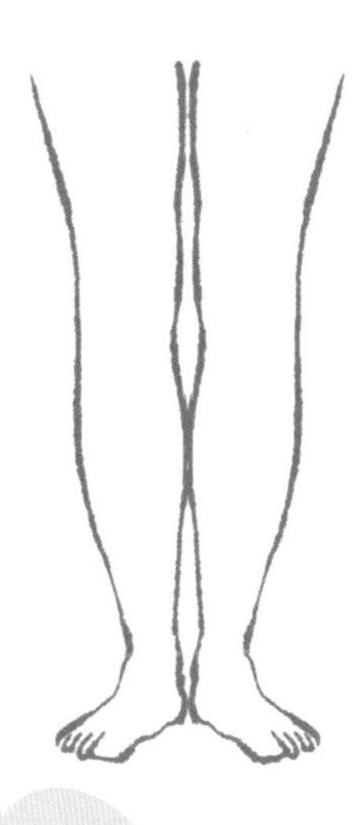

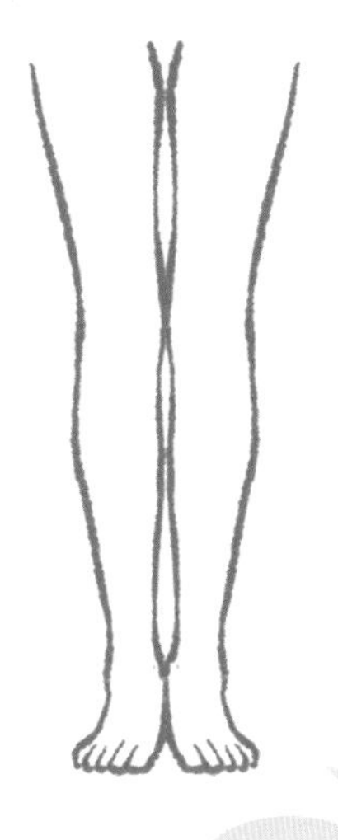

暫時消除水腫，
小腿肚也看起來變細了，
但過了1小時又恢復原
來的樣子！

只要矯正身體的歪斜就能降低脂肪是真的嗎？

誠實面對發胖的真正原因

坊間有不少以整骨為理論基礎的減重法，他們的訴求包括「發胖的原因在於骨盤歪斜」「只要矯正身體的歪斜就能夠瘦下來」。但是，**即使矯正骨骼的歪斜，對降低體脂肪還是無法發揮任何效果。**

身體的姿勢如果出現重大偏差，像是明顯向前後或左右傾斜，確實會影響站立、跑步等日常生活的動作。不良的姿勢會加重腰部、髖關節、膝蓋等處的負擔，也會提高疼痛產生的風險。從這個層面而言，**藉由矯正身體的歪斜，消除疼痛，恢復日常動作的順暢，或許能夠間接發揮降低體重和體脂肪的效果。**

另外，**矯正身體的歪斜還有一個好處，就是改善體態。**如同我在Ｄａｙ14的說明，骨盆過於後傾的人，在骨盆回正後，臀部會變得挺翹。只要矯正駝背，下腹部就會凹進去，胸部變得更堅挺，達到美化體態的效果。但是，僅有矯正身體的歪斜，並無法發揮減輕體重、降低體脂肪的效果。

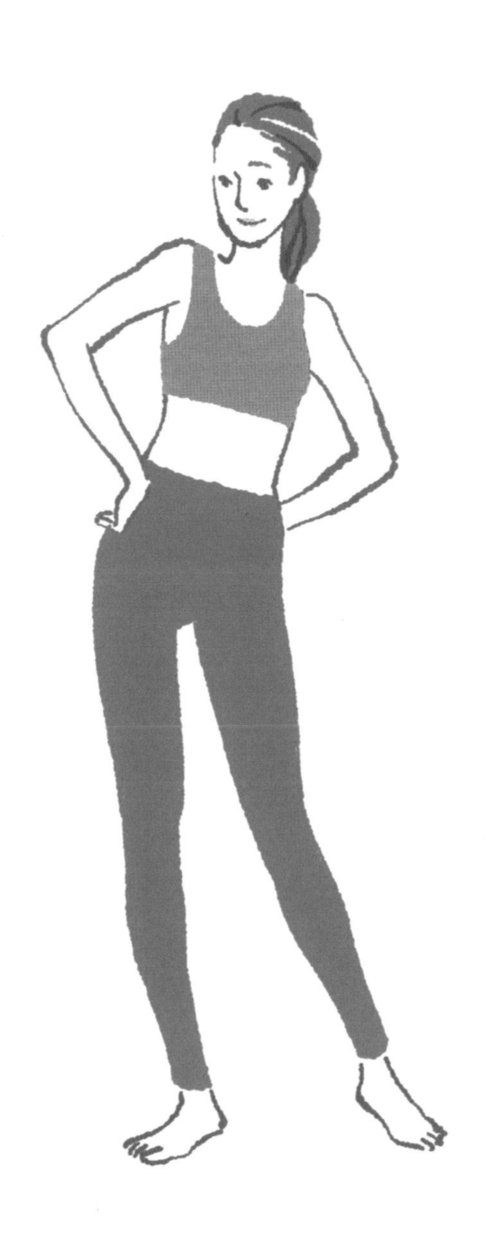

容我再次提醒各位，體脂肪增加的最大原因是飲食過量。而飲食失控源自於每天面對的壓力。其次是運動不足所導致的肌肉減少。如果有心減重，首先請誠實面對自己發胖的原因，改善飲食過量與運動不足的問題，並做好壓力控管，才是成功的不二法門。

輕斷食、斷食……斷食真的有絕佳的減重效果嗎？

之後的復胖很可怕

「輕斷食」「斷食」等禁食性減重法，是一種很危險的減重法，因為若遇到最嚴重的情況，甚至有可能喪命。如果是為過食問題所苦的人，基於改善自己的飲食生活，或者把胃袋縮小等目的，在專家的管理下進行2～3天的斷食，當然另當別論，至於其他人，實在不應該輕易嘗試。

第一個理由是，斷食會造成大量肌肉流失。因為幾乎沒有進食，體重和體脂肪理所當然都會減少，但肌肉也會被分解，當作能量使用，導致肌肉量不斷愈少。肌肉本身就會消耗熱量，所以當肌肉量減少，消耗的熱量也會跟著減少。簡單來說，**難以消耗熱量的身體＝易胖體質**。斷食後，身體已經轉換為「節能」體質，**所以只要恢復到平時的食量，體重又會一點一點增加。不僅如此，體脂肪和斷食之前相比，更是不減反增，體態也走樣了**（左圖）。

此外，斷食也是造成身體出現各種不適症狀的原因。其中必須特別當心的是有致命危險的脫水症狀、低血糖，還有心律不整、骨質密度降低、免疫力下降等。

另外，當食慾受到極度的壓抑也會導致壓力產生。嚴重者，甚至會引起掉髮、失眠，還有過食症、拒食症等飲食障礙。

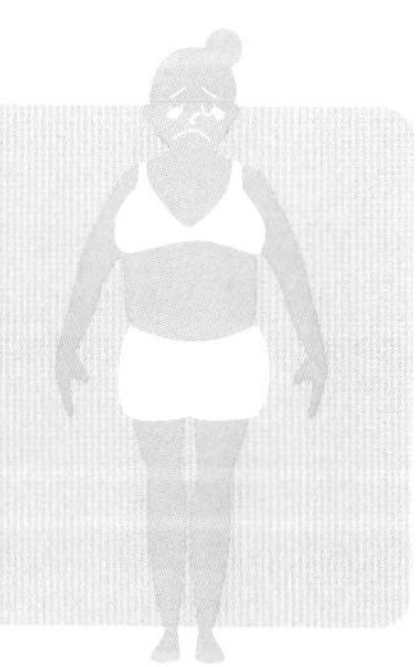

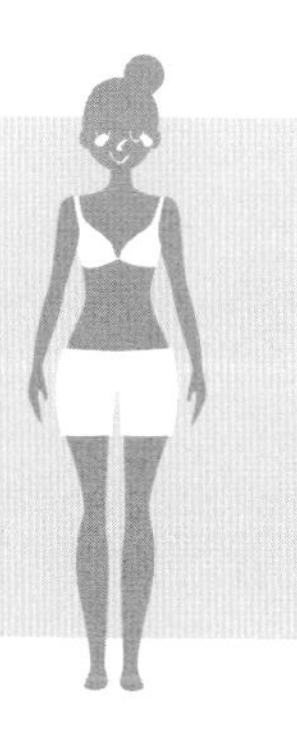

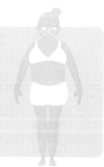

復胖後
60kg
脂肪……33.7% (20.2kg)
除脂肪……66.3% (39.8kg)

減重後，脂肪與肌肉（以除脂肪率計算）會同時減少。一旦復胖，增加的只有體脂肪，換言之，即使體重相同，卻轉變成肌肉少、體脂肪多的體態。

飲食篇

只要少吃一餐就能快速瘦下來是真的嗎？

絕對不要跳過早餐不吃

有些減重的人，因為希望自己吃得少一點，乾脆跳過某一餐不吃，其實這麼做並不正確。**尤其是早餐，如果不吃對減重非常不利。**

千萬不可跳過早餐不吃的理由很簡單。人在睡眠中不吃也不喝，所以**早上起床後，如果不補充熱量，血糖就會降低。如此一來，不僅腦部和身體無法順利運作，連肌肉也會被分解。**其次是，吃早餐有助建立生活的規律。俗話說一日之計在於晨，從一天的開始養成規律作息可提升睡眠品質，身體在白天也能夠充分活動，對減重自然有益無害。

順帶一提，如果想要藉由一件每天早上的例行公事以建立規律的作息，不妨一早出去，曬曬清晨的太陽。我們的生理時鐘把1天設定為大約25個小時，而每天負責重置的是清晨的太陽。生理時鐘一旦重新啟動，大約14～16個小時之後，身體會開始分泌有「睡眠荷爾蒙」之稱的褪黑激素，引導我們進入夢鄉。

請在曬過清晨的太陽後吃早餐。這樣的刺激有助於重置內臟的生理時鐘，讓腦部和內臟保持同樣的步調。為了促進生理時鐘的重置，早餐一定要包括米飯、麵包等含有醣類的食物。

至於晚餐，掌握正確時間點很重要。因為愈晚吃，抑制食慾的荷爾蒙——瘦體素就會分泌得愈少，反倒是促進食慾的飢餓素，分泌量會逐漸增加。所以請儘量在就寢前3～4個小時吃晚餐，最晚不要超過8點。

跳過早餐不吃的比例

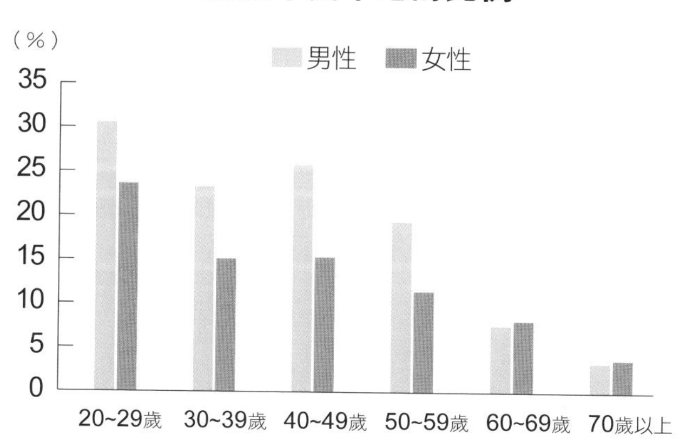

出處：平成29年國民健康、營養調查

一頓理想的早餐
必須具備足夠的份量

最好減少醣類的攝取，改成攝取大量的蛋白質是真的嗎？

減醣雖然可行，但千萬不可減過頭

最近幾年，像是專為健美運動愛好者設計的低醣、高蛋白飲食愈來愈受到矚目，但它絕對不是值得推薦的飲食法。為了打造易瘦體質，均衡攝取蛋白質、脂質、醣類這三大營養素非常重要。另外，要總稱這三項營養素時，蛋白質的英文是Protein、脂質是Fat、醣類是Carbohydrate，各取其開頭的英文字母，稱為PFC。

1日總攝取熱量的比例分別是蛋白質15～20％、脂質20～30％、醣類55～60％是一般公認的看法。另外，如果要按照本書介紹的方法，**透過肌力訓練以降低體脂肪，那麼攝取的比例以蛋白質25％、脂質20％、醣類55％為宜。**

坊間也有非常嚴格限制醣類攝取量的減重法，但醣類攝取量只要減少到平常的一半以下，肌肉就會開始分解，轉變成不易瘦下來的體質。當然，醣類攝取過量會造成肥胖，但吃得太少也不好。另外，大幅減少醣類的攝取，除了造成思考力與判斷力下降，也會引起心律不整發作的機率提高等健康上的問題，以及無法攝取充足的膳食纖維。

蛋白質是構成肌肉等所有身體成分的重要營養素，但如果攝取過量，剩餘的蛋白質會成為壞菌的食物來源，造成腸道環境失衡。同時也會提高肝臟和腎臟的負擔。不論是哪一種營養素，最重要的共通原則是均衡攝取。

一般的PFC比例

蛋白質
15～20%
脂質
20～30%
醣類
55～60%

減重時期的PFC比例

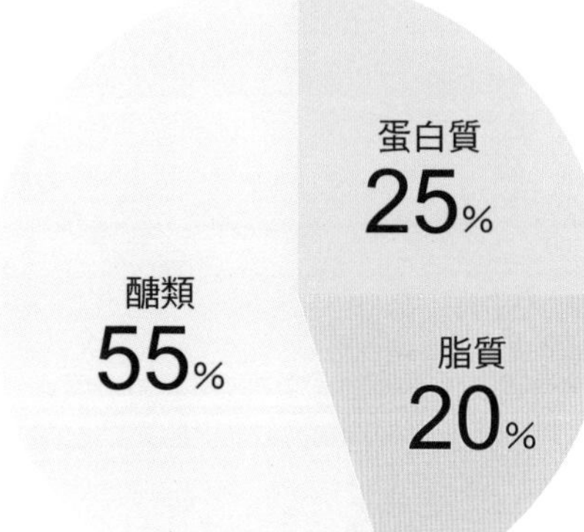

最好不要吃油是真的嗎？

從食品攝取的油也要留意

脂質是製造細胞、膽汁酸、荷爾蒙的材料，是很重要的營養素。更重要的是，如果將油脂從飲食中剔除，會縮短消化和吸收的時間，所以很快就會產生飢餓感，反而更容易飲食過量。因此，如同我在P116已經說明，一天總攝取熱量的約20％，必須從脂質攝取。

脂質的種類很多，首先可大分為飽和脂肪酸與不飽和脂肪酸。肉類的肥肉部分和奶油等在常溫下呈固體狀的油脂屬於飽和脂肪酸。如果食用過量，可能會導致血中膽固醇增加、攝取熱量超標，所以請不要把肉類料理都當作每餐的主菜。

不飽和脂肪酸在常溫之下是液態。不飽和脂肪酸又可分類成Omega-3、Omega-6、Omega-9這3種。Omega-3的代表性種類包括大量含於魚油的DHA、含於亞麻仁油與紫蘇油的α-亞麻油酸。Omega-6的代表性種類包括大量含於葵花油、玉米胚芽油、麻油的亞麻油酸。**Omega-3、Omega-6無法在體**

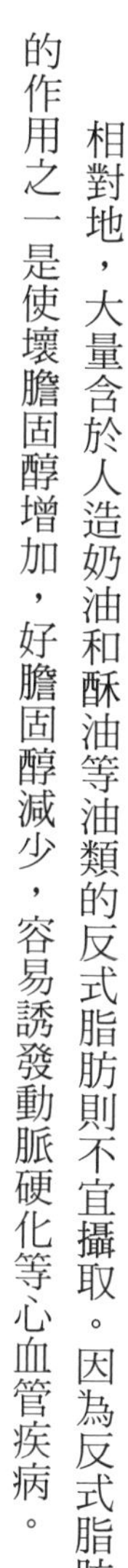
內合成，為了充足攝取，除了1天吃1次魚類料理，也要記得把玉米胚芽油和麻油用於烹調。

相對地，大量含於人造奶油和酥油等油類的反式脂肪則不宜攝取。因為反式脂肪的作用之一是使壞膽固醇增加，好膽固醇減少，容易誘發動脈硬化等心血管疾病。

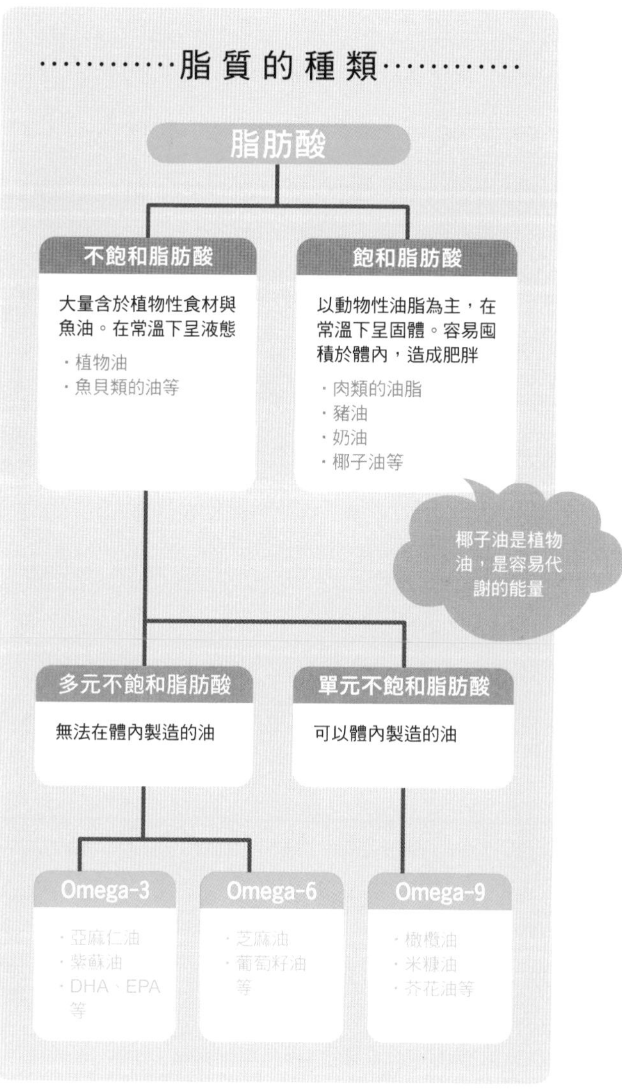

運動篇

肌力訓練最好每天都做是真的嗎？

肌肉在沒有進行訓練的時候成長

認為「肌力訓練一定要每天做」的人不在少數，但這是一個完全錯誤的觀念。**平常幾乎完全沒有運動習慣的人，一旦開始鍛鍊肌肉，即使1星期只做1次也有效果。**等到身體漸漸習慣，再慢慢將次數增加到每週2～3次比較好。至於已經透過肌力訓練，成功把身體鍛鍊成自己想要的樣子的人，如果想繼續維持現狀，即使把鍛鍊的次數減少到1週1次也無妨。

話說回來，所謂的肌力訓練，就是藉由將負荷加於身體，讓肌肉受到些許損傷，並期待肌肉可以從疲勞中獲得升級。換言之，疲勞的肌肉在攝取充足的營養，並獲得完整的修復之後會不斷成長，成長到即使承受同樣的負荷也不容易疲勞的程度。相反地，如果每天都進行肌力訓練，等於讓尚未從疲勞中恢復的肌肉持續受到刺激，那麼只會造成反效果，不但無法提升鍛鍊的效果，肌肉也容易受傷。

復原後的肌肉會變得比原來更粗壯的機制稱為超回復，據說所需時間是48～72個小時。因此，肌力訓練一週只要進行2～3次便已足夠；如果只想繼續維持現狀的人，把頻率降低到1週1次也ＯＫ。

另外，有些人很自豪自己可以一次做１００個伏立挺身、１５０個腹肌運動等，但容我提醒各位一點，能夠一口氣重複做15次以上的訓練，意味著加諸於肌肉的負荷太輕，即使做得再多也沒有意義。為了使肌肉變粗、變得強壯，必須持續施予大約能夠反覆10次左右的負荷。可以連續做１００次的訓練雖然可望增加肌肉的持久力，但無法期待會讓肌肉變得肥大。

休息會讓肌肉成長

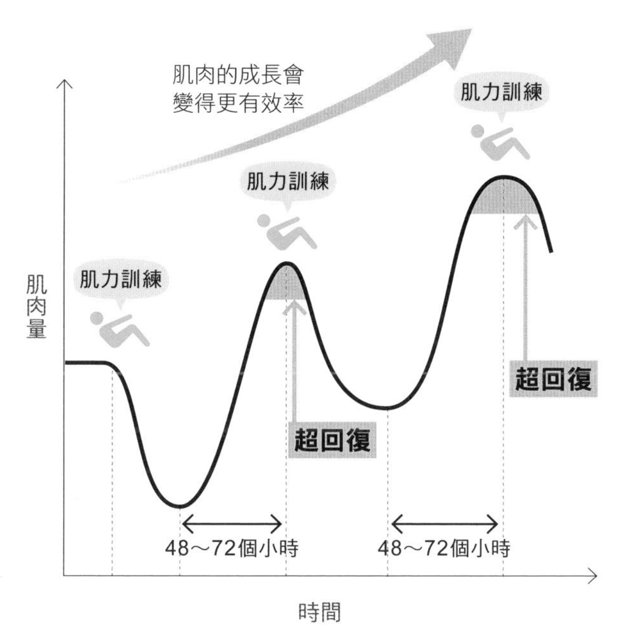

一定要做有氧運動是真的嗎？

如果覺得有壓力，不要繼續勉強方為上策

似乎有很多人認為和進行肌力訓練相比，走路、游泳等有氧運動對減重的效果更好。但正如本書已向各位說明，**只要以正確的方式執行「飲食控制＋肌力訓練」，就不是一定非做有氧運動不可。**

透過飲食控制以減少攝取的熱量，或是進行有氧運動等運動增加消耗的熱量，是減重成功僅有的兩個方法。如果選擇後者，以一個體重為70kg的一般男性為例，如果要消耗400大卡的熱量，必須以時速4公里的速度走路近2個小時，或者以時速8km的速度跑步40分鐘。相對地，如果採取減少食量的方式，那麼假設原本一天攝取的熱量是2800大卡，就必須減少約15%。**從這個例子我們可以清楚知道，要減少同樣的熱量，減少食量明顯會比運動輕鬆，而且更有效率。**

飲食控制＋肌力訓練雙管齊下之餘，再加上有氧運動，想必一定能縮短目標達成的時間。但是，成功的前提是沒有心理負擔。如果抱著「今天太忙，沒時間走路」「雖然累得

要死，但下班後還得去游泳」之類的想法就ＮＧ。因為讓肌肉過度疲勞、被時間壓力逼得喘不過氣而感到內心受挫，都很容易讓人在目標達成後，因為終於從壓力中解脫，導致快速復胖的悲劇發生。不過，有氧運動畢竟是有益健康的活動，只要身體和時間上允許，而且是不會造成心理負擔的程度，還是值得鼓勵。

····哪一種做起來比較容易，效果又好呢？····

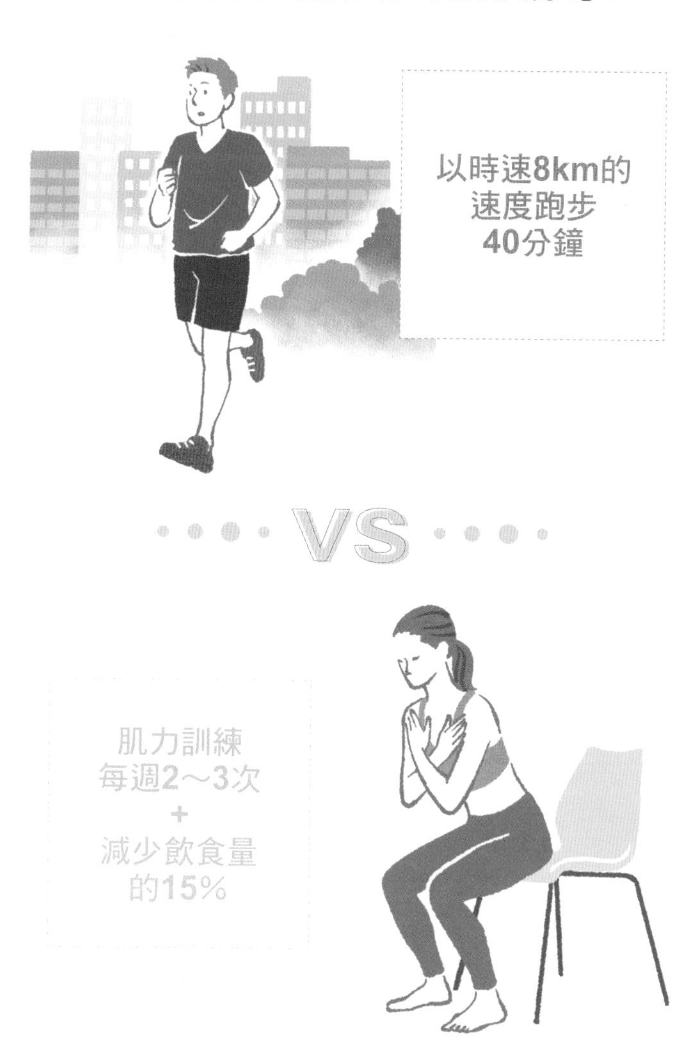
以時速8km的
速度跑步
40分鐘
VS
肌力訓練
每週2～3次
+
減少飲食量
的15%

檢視全身的肌肉

以下為各位介紹在30天減重中登場的
運動和日常生活中主要使用的肌肉。

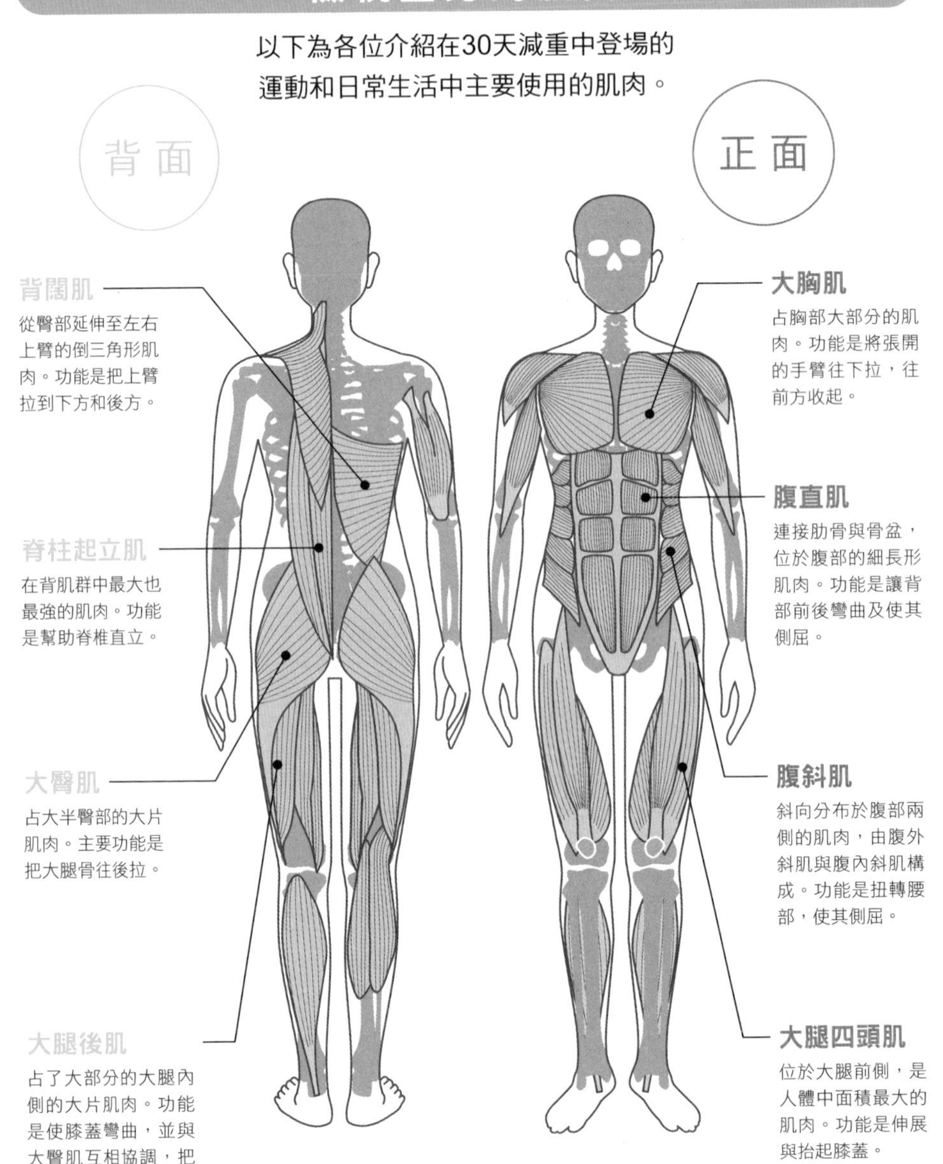

背面
正面
背闊肌
從臀部延伸至左右上臂的倒三角形肌肉。功能是把上臂拉到下方和後方。
脊柱起立肌
在背肌群中最大也最強的肌肉。功能是幫助脊椎直立。
大臀肌
占大半臀部的大片肌肉。主要功能是把大腿骨往後拉。
大腿後肌
占了大部分的大腿內側的大片肌肉。功能是使膝蓋彎曲，並與大臀肌互相協調，把大腿骨往後拉。
大胸肌
占胸部大部分的肌肉。功能是將張開的手臂往下拉，往前方收起。
腹直肌
連接肋骨與骨盆，位於腹部的細長形肌肉。功能是讓背部前後彎曲及使其側屈。
腹斜肌
斜向分布於腹部兩側的肌肉，由腹外斜肌與腹內斜肌構成。功能是扭轉腰部，使其側屈。
大腿四頭肌
位於大腿前側，是人體中面積最大的肌肉。功能是伸展與抬起膝蓋。

自我檢核量表

※填寫方式請參照P31。

月　日(日)　體重：　kg　體脂肪率：　%

	開始時間	所需時間	主食	主菜	副菜	湯品
早餐	：	分				
午餐	：	分				
晚餐	：	分				
點心	：	分				

月　日(一)　體重：　kg　體脂肪率：　%

	開始時間	所需時間	主食	主菜	副菜	湯品
早餐	：	分				
午餐	：	分				
晚餐	：	分				
點心	：	分				

月　日(二)　體重：　kg　體脂肪率：　%

	開始時間	所需時間	主食	主菜	副菜	湯品
早餐	：	分				
午餐	：	分				
晚餐	：	分				
點心	：	分				

月　日(三)　體重：　kg　體脂肪率：　%

	開始時間	所需時間	主食	主菜	副菜	湯品
早餐	：	分				
午餐	：	分				
晚餐	：	分				
點心	：	分				

月　日(四)　體重：　kg　體脂肪率：　%

	開始時間	所需時間	主食	主菜	副菜	湯品
早餐	：	分				
午餐	：	分				
晚餐	：	分				
點心	：	分				

月　日(五)　體重：　kg　體脂肪率：　%

	開始時間	所需時間	主食	主菜	副菜	湯品
早餐	：	分				
午餐	：	分				
晚餐	：	分				
點心	：	分				

月　日(六)　體重：　kg　體脂肪率：　%

	開始時間	所需時間	主食	主菜	副菜	湯品
早餐	：	分				
午餐	：	分				
晚餐	：	分				
點心	：	分				

1週的回顧

每天都要針對當天的每個項目進行檢核，
已完成的就打勾！

DAY 6 □

做伸展運動

Daily Checks

□每餐與兩餐之間喝水
□記錄飲食內容

DAY 7 □

知道瘦得健康的重要性

Daily Checks

□每餐與兩餐之間喝水
□記錄飲食內容
□伸展運動（腹部）

DAY 8 □

將減重「可視化」

Daily Checks

□每餐與兩餐之間喝水
□記錄飲食內容
□伸展運動（腹部）

DAY 9 □

臀部伸展運動

Daily Checks

□每餐與兩餐之間喝水
□記錄飲食內容
□伸展運動（腹部）
□將減重「可視化」

DAY 10 □

每餐都有肉類或魚肉當作主食

Daily Checks

□每餐與兩餐之間喝水
□記錄飲食內容
□伸展運動（腹部、臀部）
□將減重「可視化」

DAY 16 □

把酒精當作主食看待

Daily Checks

□每餐與兩餐之間喝水
□記錄飲食內容
□伸展運動（腹部、臀部、拱背）
□將減重「可視化」
□每餐都有肉類或魚肉當作主食

DAY 17 □

慢慢地坐在椅子上

Daily Checks

□每餐與兩餐之間喝水
□記錄飲食內容
□伸展運動（腹部、臀部、拱背）
□將減重「可視化」
□每餐都有肉類或魚肉當作主食

DAY 18 □

不是替結果，而是為過程打分數

Daily Checks

□每餐與兩餐之間喝水
□記錄飲食內容
□伸展運動（腹部、臀部、拱背）
□將減重「可視化」
□每餐都有肉類或魚肉當作主食

DAY 19 □

停止傷身的情緒性進食

Daily Checks

□每餐與兩餐之間喝水
□記錄飲食內容
□伸展運動（腹部、臀部、拱背）
□將減重「可視化」
□每餐都有肉類或魚肉當作主食

DAY 20 □

對自已心懷期待

Daily Checks

□每餐與兩餐之間喝水
□記錄飲食內容
□伸展運動（腹部、臀部、拱背）
□將減重「可視化」
□每餐都有肉類或魚肉當作主食

DAY 26 □

鍛鍊背肌以提升代謝

Daily Checks

□每餐與兩餐之間喝水
□記錄飲食內容
□伸展運動（腹部、臀部、拱背）
□將減重「可視化」
□每餐都有肉類或魚肉當作主食

DAY 27 □

增加NEAT

Daily Checks

□每餐與兩餐之間喝水
□記錄飲食內容
□伸展運動（腹部、臀部、拱背）
□將減重「可視化」
□每餐都有肉類或魚肉當作主食

DAY 28 □

點心聰明選，安心吃

Daily Checks

□每餐與兩餐之間喝水
□記錄飲食內容
□伸展運動（腹部、臀部、拱背）
□將減重「可視化」
□每餐都有肉類或魚肉當作主食
□增加NEAT

DAY 29 □

加入腹肌運動

Daily Checks

□每餐與兩餐之間喝水
□記錄飲食內容
□伸展運動（腹部、臀部、拱背）
□將減重「可視化」
□每餐都有肉類或魚肉當作主食
□增加NEAT

DAY 30 □

為了避免三分鐘熱度的心理建設

Daily Checks

□每餐與兩餐之間喝水
□記錄飲食內容
□伸展運動（腹部、臀部、拱背）
□將減重「可視化」
□每餐都有肉類或魚肉當作主食
□增加NEAT

※請影印本表格再使用

自　我　檢　核　量　表

DAY 1 □	DAY 2 □	DAY 3 □	DAY 4 □	DAY 5 □
重建有關減重的知識	每餐與兩餐之間一定要喝水	記錄飲食的內容（自我檢核）	紓緩壓力	1天吃4餐
Daily Checks	Daily Checks	Daily Checks	Daily Checks	Daily Checks
		□每餐與兩餐之間喝水	□每餐與兩餐之間喝水	□每餐與兩餐之間喝水
			□記錄飲食內容	□記錄飲食內容

DAY 11 □	DAY 12 □	DAY 13 □	DAY 14 □	DAY 15 □
對外發表減重宣言	擁有品質良好的睡眠	減少糖類的攝取	利用拱背伸展運動美姿	將泡澡的效果發揮到極致
Daily Checks	Daily Checks	Daily Checks	Daily Checks	Daily Checks
□每餐與兩餐之間喝水	□每餐與兩餐之間喝水	□每餐與兩餐之間喝水	□每餐與兩餐之間喝水	□每餐與兩餐之間喝水
□記錄飲食內容	□記錄飲食內容	□記錄飲食內容	□記錄飲食內容	□記錄飲食內容
□伸展運動（腹部、臀部）	□伸展運動（腹部、臀部）	□伸展運動（腹部、臀部）	□伸展運動（腹部、臀部）	□伸展運動（腹部、臀部、拱背）
□將減重「可視化」	□將減重「可視化」	□將減重「可視化」	□將減重「可視化」	□將減重「可視化」
□每餐都有肉類或魚肉當作主食	□每餐都有肉類或魚肉當作主食	□每餐都有肉類或魚肉當作主食	□每餐都有肉類或魚肉當作主食	□每餐都有肉類或魚肉當作主食

DAY 21 □	DAY 22 □	DAY 23 □	DAY 24 □	DAY 25 □
把樓梯化為訓練裝備	即使外食，也要實踐三菜一湯	養成更添魅力的站姿、走路方式	攝取3K食材	挑戰爬樓梯
Daily Checks	Daily Checks	Daily Checks	Daily Checks	Daily Checks
□每餐與兩餐之間喝水	□每餐與兩餐之間喝水	□每餐與兩餐之間喝水	□每餐與兩餐之間喝水	□每餐與兩餐之間喝水
□記錄飲食內容	□記錄飲食內容	□記錄飲食內容	□記錄飲食內容	□記錄飲食內容
□伸展運動（腹部、臀部、拱背）	□伸展運動（腹部、臀部、拱背）	□伸展運動（腹部、臀部、拱背）	□伸展運動（腹部、臀部、拱背）	□伸展運動（腹部、臀部、拱背）
□將減重「可視化」	□將減重「可視化」	□將減重「可視化」	□將減重「可視化」	□將減重「可視化」
□每餐都有肉類或魚肉當作主食	□每餐都有肉類或魚肉當作主食	□每餐都有肉類或魚肉當作主食	□每餐都有肉類或魚肉當作主食	□每餐都有肉類或魚肉當作主食

國家圖書館出版品預行編目資料

最強瘦身教科書：30天就會瘦！1天1頁跟著做，養成易瘦體質不復胖！ / 坂詰真二監修；藍嘉楹譯. -- 初版. -- 臺中市：晨星出版有限公司, 2024.03

面；公分. —（知的！；226）

譯自：1日1ページで痩せるダイエット最強の教科書

ISBN 978-626-320-765-3（平裝）

1.CST: 減重

411.94　　113000029

知的！226

最強瘦身教科書：

30天就會瘦！1天1頁跟著做，養成易瘦體質不復胖！

1日1ページで痩せるダイエット最強の教科書

監修者　坂詰真二
內文圖版　宮島 薰、益子航平（I'll Products）
插畫　Kei、nicospyder、福島康子
譯者　藍嘉楹
編輯　吳雨書
封面設計　ivy_design
美術設計　曾麗香

創辦人　陳銘民
發行所　晨星出版有限公司
407台中市西屯區工業30路1號1樓
TEL：（04）23595820　FAX：（04）23550581
http://star.morningstar.com.tw
行政院新聞局局版台業字第2500號
法律顧問　陳思成律師
初版　西元2024年03月15日　初版1刷

讀者服務專線　TEL：（02）23672044 /（04）23595819#212
讀者傳真專線　FAX：（02）23635741 /（04）23595493
讀者專用信箱　service @morningstar.com.tw
網路書店　http://www.morningstar.com.tw
郵政劃撥　15060393（知己圖書股份有限公司）

印刷　上好印刷股份有限公司

掃描QR code填回函，
成為晨星網路書店會員，
即送「晨星網路書店Ecoupon優惠券」
一張，同時享有購書優惠。

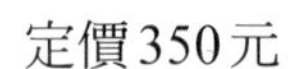

定價350元

ISBN 978-626-320-765-3

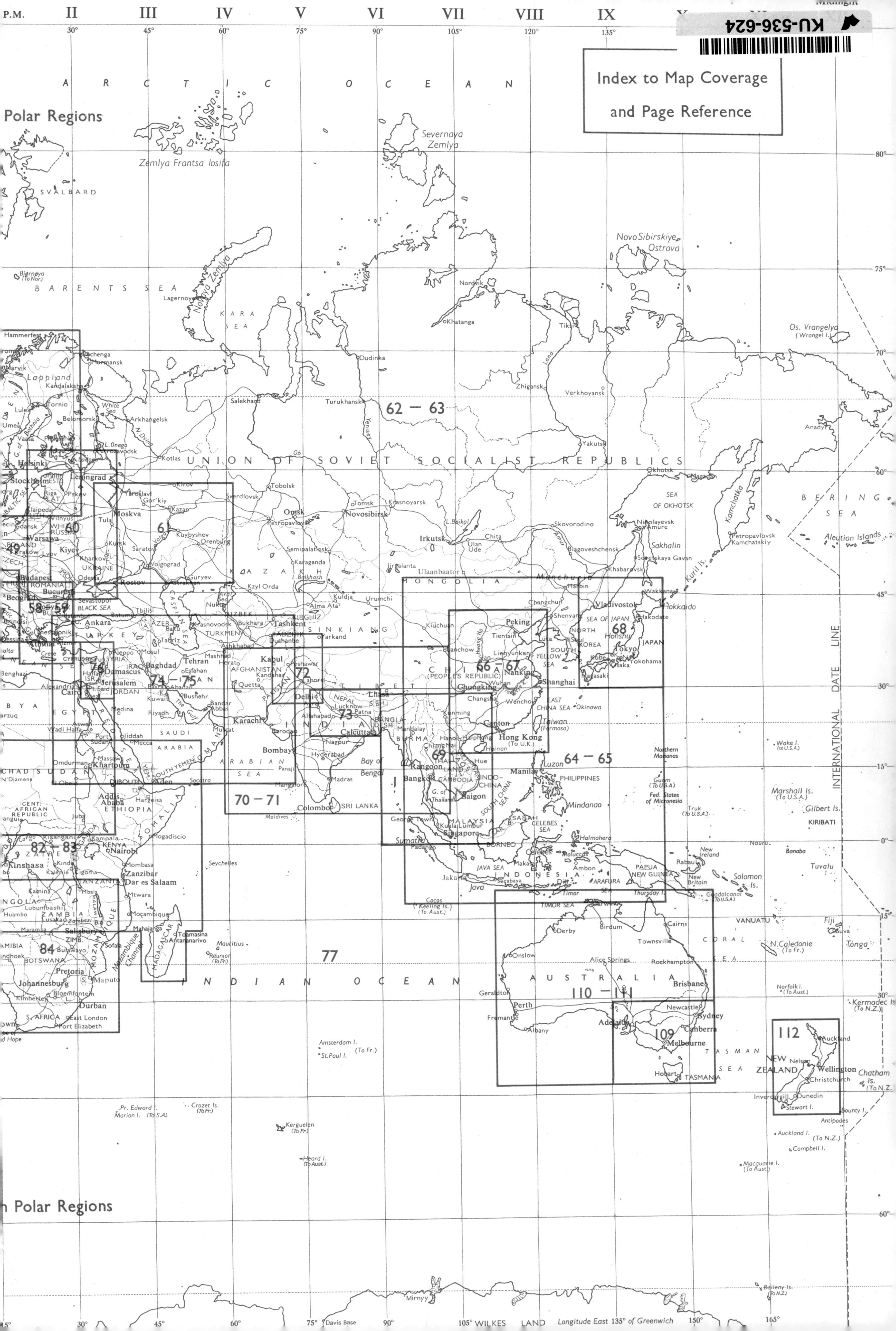
Index to Map Coverage
and Page Reference
Polar Regions
ARCTIC OCEAN
Zemlya Frantsa Iosifa
Severnaya Zemlya
SVALBARD
BARENTS SEA
KARA SEA
Novo Sibirskiye Ostrova
UNION OF SOVIET SOCIALIST REPUBLICS
62 — 63
61
60
49
58
59
76
74 — 75
72
73
70 — 71
66
67
68
69
64 — 65
82 — 83
84
77
110 — 111
109
112
SEA OF OKHOTSK
BERING SEA
Aleutian Islands
SEA OF JAPAN
JAPAN
KOREA
YELLOW SEA
EAST CHINA SEA
CHINA (PEOPLE'S REPUBLIC)
MONGOLIA
SINKIANG
TIBET
INDIA
ARABIAN SEA
Bay of Bengal
SRI LANKA
BURMA
THAILAND
CAMBODIA
INDO-CHINA
SOUTH CHINA SEA
PHILIPPINES
MALAYSIA
INDONESIA
JAVA SEA
BORNEO
CELEBES SEA
PAPUA NEW GUINEA
ARAFURA SEA
TIMOR SEA
AUSTRALIA
CORAL SEA
TASMAN SEA
NEW ZEALAND
INDIAN OCEAN
SAUDI ARABIA
TURKEY
AFGHANISTAN
PAKISTAN
IRAN
IRAQ
SYRIA
JORDAN
EGYPT
SUDAN
ETHIOPIA
SOMALIA
KENYA
TANZANIA
ZAIRE
ZAMBIA
MOZAMBIQUE
MADAGASCAR
BOTSWANA
S. AFRICA
INTERNATIONAL DATE LINE
Longitude East 135° of Greenwich
WILKES LAND
Polar Regions

— R.E. HAWORTH 1983. —

WORLD ATLAS

JOHN C. BARTHOLOMEW, M.A., F.R.S.E.
DIRECTOR, THE GEOGRAPHICAL INSTITUTE, EDINBURGH

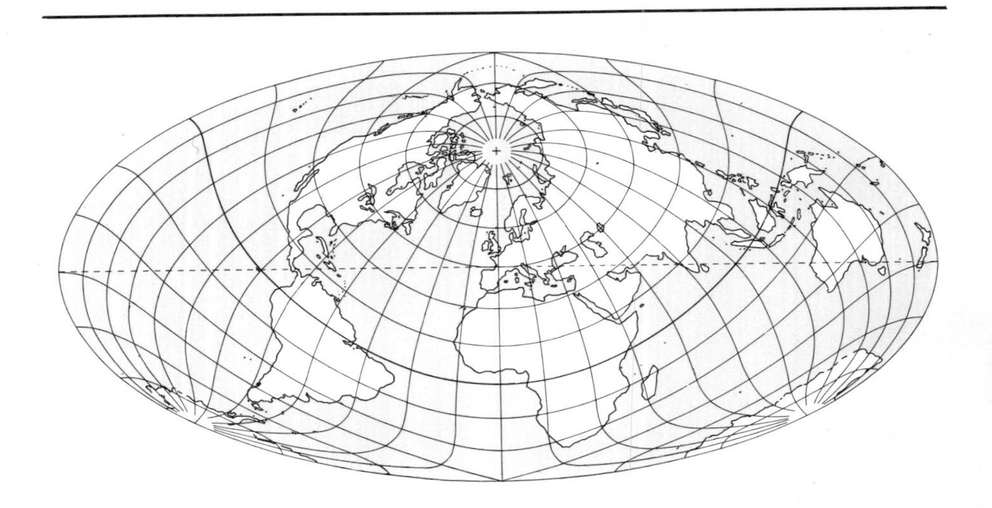

JOHN BARTHOLOMEW & SON LTD
EDINBURGH

As Edinburgh World Atlas
First Edition – 1954
Eighth Edition – 1973
As The World Atlas
Ninth Edition – 1974
Tenth Edition – 1975
Eleventh Edition - 1977
Reprinted - 1979
Twelfth Edition - 1982

PRINTED IN GREAT BRITAIN
AT THE GEOGRAPHICAL INSTITUTE, EDINBURGH
ISBN 0 7028 0404 5
8947

FOREWORD

THIS Atlas, planned originally for academic purposes, has become so popular among general readers throughout the world, on account of its fresh scientific approach to many world problems, that it is now issued as a library and general reference atlas under the present modified title.

A humanistic viewpoint is given to all continental areas by showing density of population along with its vegetational, climatic and physical backgrounds. Special introductory maps show racial distinctions along with mineral and agricultural resources of the world.

Students of cartography will find matter of interest in the new projections employed. These to the number of four are designed to show more realistic relations of the inhabited land masses, as in the *Nordic* Projection on pages 22-23, which reveals the proximity of the Soviet Union to the United States; another, the *Regional* on pages 14-15, claims to show conformal properties (truth to shape) in the best manner possible; while another, the *Atlantis* on page 11, is ideal for displaying world air communications centred on the Atlantic Ocean.

Place-names are spelt on the most rational system possible, *viz.*, to conform with the local usage of the country in question; traditional or English forms are given in brackets where these are of sufficient importance.

A new form of co-ordinate system for the ready location of positions has been introduced and is explained on page 1; being related to time, it is known as the "Hour System".

THE GEOGRAPHICAL INSTITUTE,
EDINBURGH, July 1954.

JOHN BARTHOLOMEW.

PREFACE TO SEVENTH EDITION

Recent strides in the advancement of our knowledge of the earth and its resources are reflected in a series of new world maps illustrating structure, seismology, relief, continental drift, minerals, energy, food and soils. The British Isles likewise have a comparable series of new maps.

In conformity with the metrication of units of measurement, all temperature maps have been redrawn in degrees Celsius (°C) and spot heights have been altered from feet to metres.

JOHN C. BARTHOLOMEW

EDINBURGH, September 1970.

CONTENTS

The contraction "M" is used to denote scale of map in millionths.

PAGE		
1	GEOGRAPHICAL CO-ORDINATES	
2–3	GEOGRAPHICAL TERMS	
4	CLIMATIC TABLES	
5	STATES AND POPULATION	
6	WORLD EXPLORATION (Old World)	
7	WORLD EXPLORATION (New World)	
8–9	MAP PROJECTIONS	
10	MAP PROJECTIONS (modern)	
11	WORLD AIRWAYS	
12	ASTRONOMICAL CHARTS	
	THE WORLD	
13	(*a*) STRUCTURE	1:130 M.
	(*b*) SEISMOLOGY	1:130 M.
14–15	PHYSIOGRAPHY Drainage Regions, Continental Drift	1:90 M.
16–17	TEMPERATURE AND AIR MOVEMENTS Air Pressure and Winds, January, July Temperature, January, July Air Masses and Fronts Storm Tracks Temperature Extremes Amount of Cloud	
18–19	RAINFALL AND OCEANOGRAPHY Climatic Regions Length of Growing Seasons	
20–21	ECONOMIC RESOURCES Minerals Food Energy Soils	
22–23	ETHNOLOGY Cephalic Index, Religions	1:140 M.
24–25	STATES OF THE WORLD Changes of Sovereignty Time Zones	
26	NORTH POLAR REGIONS Temperature, January, July	1:30 M.
27	SOUTH POLAR REGIONS Temperature, January, July	1:30 M.
	EURASIA	
28	VEGETATION Rainfall, January, July	1:45 M.
29	POPULATION Temperature, January, July	1:45 M.
30–31	EURASIA Races	1:30 M.
	EUROPE	
32–33	EUROPE	1:15 M.
34	NORTH-WEST EUROPE	1:10 M.
35	BRITISH ISLES Geology Structure and Land Use	1:6 M.
36	Climate Population Energy Industry	1:8 M.
37	NORTH ENGLAND Isle of Man	1:1¼ M.
38–39	SOUTH ENGLAND AND WALES Channel Islands	1:1¼ M.
40–41	SCOTLAND Shetland, Fair Isle, St Kilda	1:1¼ M.
42–43	IRELAND Population	1:1¼ M.
44	THE LOW COUNTRIES	1:1¼ M.
45	SWITZERLAND	1:1¼ M.
46–47	SCANDINAVIA AND THE BALTIC Iceland, The Faeroes	1:4½ M.
48–49	GERMANY, POLAND & CZECHOSLOVAKIA	1·3 M.
50–51	CENTRAL EUROPE & MEDITERRANEAN	1:10 M.
52–53	IBERIAN PENINSULA	1:3 M.
54–55	FRANCE AND NORTH ALGERIA Corsica	1:3 M.
	EUROPE—*continued*	
56-57	ITALY AND THE ADRIATIC	1:3 M.
58-59	THE BALKANS AND LOWER DANUBE	1:3 M.
60	EUROPEAN RUSSIA	1:6 M.
61	VOLGA BASIN	1:6 M.
	ASIA	
62-63	SOVIET UNION	1:17½ M.
64-65	THE FAR EAST	1:15 M.
66-67	EAST CHINA	1:6 M.
68	JAPAN	1:6 M.
69	INDO-CHINA Singapore	1:10 M.
70-71	INDIA, PAKISTAN AND SRI LANKA Races, Population, Religions	1:10 M.
72	PUNJAB AND KASHMIR	1:4 M·
73	PLAIN OF THE GANGES	1:4 M.
74-75	THE MIDDLE EAST	1:10 M.
76	THE LEVANT COAST	1:2½ M.
77	INDIAN OCEAN Islands	1:40 M.
	AFRICA	
78	VEGETATION Rainfall, January, July	1:35 M.
79	POPULATION Temperature, January, July	1:35 M.
80-81	NORTH-WEST AFRICA Azores, Cape Verde	1:12½ M.
82-83	CENTRAL AND EAST AFRICA Ascension, St Helena, Madagascar	1:12½ M.
84	SOUTH AFRICA The Cape, Witwatersrand	1:12½ M.
	NORTH AMERICA	
85	ATLANTIC OCEAN	1:48 M.
86	VEGETATION Rainfall, January, July	1:34 M.
87	POPULATION Temperature, January, July	1:34 M.
88-89	CANADA	1:12½ M.
90	GULF OF ST LAWRENCE	1:5 M.
91	GREAT LAKES	1:5 M.
92	PACIFIC COAST	1:5 M.
93	NORTH CENTRAL STATES	1:5 M.
94-95	MIDDLE WEST STATES	1:5 M.
96	MIDDLE ATLANTIC STATES	1:2½ M.
97	SOUTHERN STATES	1:5 M.
98-99	UNITED STATES OF AMERICA Hawaiian Is., San Francisco, Alaska, New York	1:12½ M.
100	MEXICO	1:10 M.
101	THE CARIBBEAN The Panama Canal	1:10 M.
	SOUTH AMERICA	
102	VEGETATION Rainfall, January, July	1:32 M.
103	ARGENTINA AND CHILE South America Population	1:12½ M.
104-105	BRAZIL & NORTH ANDEAN STATES South America Temperature, Jan., July	1:12½ M.
	AUSTRALASIA	
106-107	PACIFIC OCEAN Islands	1:45 M.
108	VEGETATION Temperature, January, July Rainfall, January, July	1:28 M.
109	SOUTH-EAST AUSTRALIA Tasmania	1:5 M.
110-111	AUSTRALIA Population	1:12½ M.
112	NEW ZEALAND Population	1:5 M.

INDEX OF GEOGRAPHICAL NAMES

GEOGRAPHICAL CO-ORDINATES

THE most ancient function of geography has probably been to describe the location of places on the earth's surface. Thus it came about that early Greek philosophers, absorbed in conjectures as to the size and shape of the world they lived in, hit on the method of measuring its estimated circumference by 360 degrees to the circle. Any locality could then be determined by reference to a prime meridian and the number of degrees from the Equator. This method was adopted by Claudius Ptolemy of Alexandria in his tables and maps; and with modifications is much the same as the system of latitude and longitude in use to-day. That it should have survived so long is testimony of its efficiency, especially for navigational purposes. For more ordinary use, however, it is surprising that a simpler and more easily quoted system has not been adopted. True, there have been attempts in that direction. The circle has been divided into 100, which would help if all maps were so printed. More noteworthy are the systems of Military and National Grids, which served an essential purpose during both World Wars. For civilian and international use, however, these grids stand at great disadvantage. Being imposed in right-angled pattern on a particular projection of limited area, they are not suitable for extending to other areas. For instance, a grid planned for Great Britain on Transverse Mercator's Projection would not at the same time be suitable for Germany. Moreover, unless the grid were printed on all maps in common use it would be of little service to the man-in-the-street.

To avoid these disadvantages, therefore, the system used in this atlas has been devised. It has the merit of being international. It is related to the World Grid, based on Greenwich, and can thus be used on any map, if necessary without being specially so printed. It avoids the confusing factor of reading east and west of a prime meridian. Its formula is compact and simple to understand. Finally, it is capable of infinite precision by the use of decimal subdivision.

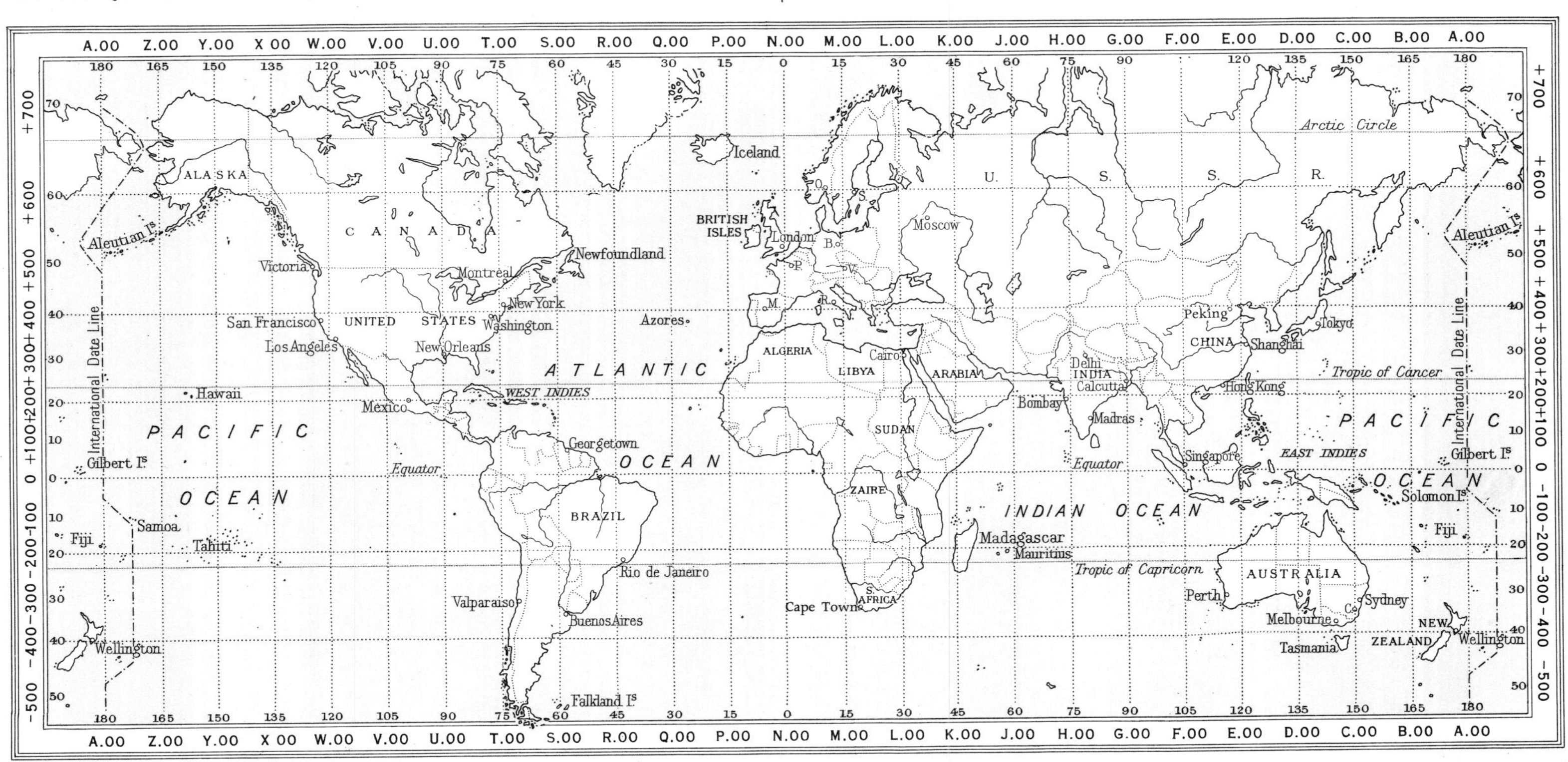

RULES FOR USE OF "HOUR" CO-ORDINATES

1. The World is divided into twenty-four *hour* zones, each of 15° longitude and denoted by a letter of the alphabet, omitting **I** and **O** which may be confused with numerals. Starting point of the **A** zone is the meridian 180° E. of Greenwich, associated with the International Date Line. All readings are made East to West, *i.e.*, with transit of the Sun, Greenwich being **N**.

2. Every *hour* zone of 15° is subdivided longitudinally, *i.e.*, by *Westings* into 90 units, reading likewise East to West. For greater precision these may be divided into further decimal parts. The units are marked in the top and bottom borders of each map.

   It will be found that 60 units *Westing* = 10° of longitude

06	,,	= 1°	,,
01	,,	= 10′	,,
001	,,	= 1′	,,
0001	,,	= 6″	,,

3. In the co-ordinate of latitude the quadrant from Equator to Pole is divided into 90 parts, each of which is then subdivided into 10 units.

   Thus 100 units *Northing* = 10° of latitude

010	,,	= 1°	,,
001	,,	= 6′	,,
0001	,,	= 36″	,,

   The coupling sign + or − marks this co-ordinate, meaning North or South respectively from the Equator. These *Northing* or *Southing* units are marked on the East and West sides of the Atlas maps. Further decimal subdivisions may also be used.

4. The complete co-ordinate is given by the *hour* figure or *Westing*, followed by the latitude figure or *Northing*,

   thus **M 89 + 522** = Cambridge, England
   and **T 12 + 389** = Washington, D.C.

   As the *hour* letter and the + or − are both treated as if they were decimal points, it is important to include the initial 0's so that all readings less than 10 should be written 05, 001, or as the case may be.

5. Readings apply to the space between the last digit given and the next digit; but, where greater precision on a larger scale is required, as in the case of the annexed One-Inch section of the English Lake District readings may be made to several places of decimals. Here the Church at Grasmere becomes **N 1813 + 54456**.

6. The above system, as used in this Atlas, is intended to assist travellers, writers, or scientific and commercial interests in their work. Free permission is accordingly given by the author for its use anywhere without restriction. It may be described as Bartholomew's Hour System of Geographical Co-ordinates.

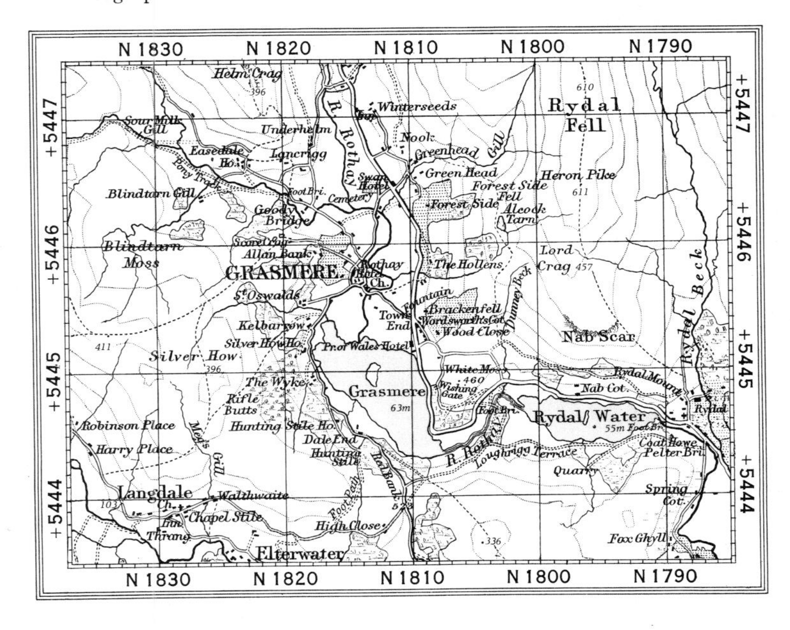

GEOGRAPHICAL TERMS

Abad *(Persian)*, town.
Aborigines, the earliest inhabitants of a country.
Ada *(Turkish)*, island.
Aiguille *(French)*, needle; applied to certain pinnacle-shaped mountain peaks.
Ain, Bir *(Arabic)*, a well or spring.
Ainu, a race inhabiting N. Hokkaido and S. Sakhalin.
Air Mass, an extensive body of air, moving or stationary, having throughout similar characteristics of temperature and humidity.
Akaba *(Arabic)*, pass.
Alf, älv, elf, elv *(Swedish* and *Norse)*, river.
Alluvium, fine sand or silt deposited, largely during flood periods, by streams and rivers.
Anticline, an arch of strata on both sides of which the rocks dip downwards.
Anticyclone, a high pressure system occurring in the zone of the "Westerlies", usually accompanied by fine weather. Wind tends to move outwards in clockwise direction in the Northern Hemisphere, anticlockwise in the Southern.
Antipodes, that part of the earth diametrically opposite to our feet, on the same meridian, but with latitude and seasons reversed, *e.g.* New Zealand is the antipodes of Great Britain.
Arctic Circle, constituted by the parallel 66°32′ N., separating North Temperate and North Frigid Zones. North of this at mid-summer the sun does not set during the 24 hours, while at mid-winter it does not rise. In the Southern Hemisphere the same conditions apply S. of the **Antarctic Circle**, 66°32′ S.
Artesian Well, a water supply obtained by tapping porous rock strata from which the water rises by natural pressure. Derived from Artois in France.
Atolls, circular coral reefs enclosing a central lagoon connected with the outside sea by an opening. Found mostly in the Pacific Ocean.
Avalanches, masses of loosened snow and ice mixed with earth and stone, precipitated with destructive force down mountain sides.
Axis, the imaginary line running from pole to pole through the centre of and on which the earth revolves.
Aztecs, the highly civilised dominant race in Mexico at the time of the Spanish invasion in 1519.
Bahia *(Portuguese* and *Spanish)*, bay.
Bahr *(Arabic)*, sea, lake, river.
Bal, Bally, Baile *(Celtic)*, town, village.
Ban *(Siamese)*, village.
Bandar, Nagar, Pura *(Indian)*, town.
Bantu, *i.e.*, "people"; correlated races of Africa between lat. 5° N. and 25° S. They include Xhosas and Zulus.
Bar, gravel, sand or mud deposited across the mouth of a river by currents or wave action; often impedes navigation.
Bas *(French)*, low, low-lying.
Basin, area of land drained by a river, and its tributaries.
Basin of Inland Drainage, an area of land which has no surface drainage outlet to the sea.
Basques, an ancient race with a distinct language inhabiting N.E. Spain and S.W. France, on the shores of the Bay of Biscay.
Basutos, a branch of the Bantu race occupying Lesotho.
Batang *(Malay)*, river.
Beaches, Raised, small platforms of land, formerly sea shore, now left dry through a rise of the land level.
Beaufort Scale, a scale of 13 symbols used in weather maps to portray the force of the wind from calm to more than 120 kilometres per hour.
Bedouins, nomadic tribes of Arabia and North Africa.
Beled *(Arabic)*, country, village.
Ben, Beinn *(Celtic)*, mountain.
Bender *(Persian)*, harbour, landing-place.
Black Earth, fertile soil in S. Russia and parts of Romania and Hungary on which heavy grain crops are grown.
Boers, descendants of the early Dutch colonists in South Africa.
Bora, a cold, dry, northerly wind, blowing in winter and spring along the Dalmatian coast of the Adriatic Sea.
Bore or **Eagre**, a tidal wave arising in the estuaries of certain rivers.
Boulder Clay, a glacial deposit, consisting of boulders of various sizes embedded in finer material, laid down under a glacier or ice cap and often found to great depths in glaciated valleys.
Brdo *(Czech.)*, a hill.
Brunn *(German)*, a spring, well.
Bugt, Bukt *(Danish* and *Swedish)*, a bay.
Buran, snow blizzards of winter occuring in Russia and Siberia.
Burun *(Turkish)*, a headland, promontory.
Bush, The, interior uncultivated scrubland.
Bushmen, or in Afrikaans **Boesmanne** an aboriginal Negrito nomadic race of south central Africa, now mostly in the Kalahari desert.
Butte *(French* and *Amer.)*, an isolated hill or peak.
Cabo *(Portuguese* and *Spanish)*, a cape.
Campo *(Italian* and *Spanish)*, a plain.
Campos, grasslands of S.E. Brazil.
Cañan or Canyon *(Spanish)*, a deep gorge or ravine with lofty sides. Formed by rapid erosion of the softer strata in a dry region, *e.g.*, Colorado Canon.
Catingas, open forest lands on the plateaux of Eastern Brazil, north of 15° S. Drier and warmer than the adjoining **Cerrados**; they contain cactus, mimosa and other types of dry vegetation.
Cephalic Index, the shape of the head expressed by a number which is obtained by giving the breadth of the head as a percentage of its length.
Cerrados, semi-dry plateaux of S.E. Brazil covered with grass and trees of stunted growth.
Chart, map of the sea for use of navigators.
Chinook, a warm, dry west wind blowing down the east slopes of the Rocky Mountains.
Chotts, *see* Shotts.
Chow *(Chinese)*, town of the second rank.
Chrebet *(Russian)*, a chain; mountain range.
Cidade *(Portuguese)*, town.
Cima, Pizzo *(Italian)*, mountain peak.
Cirrus Clouds, very lofty (eight to ten kilometres high) fibrous looking clouds, associated with fine weather.
Città *(Italian)*, town, city.
Ciudad *(Spanish)*, city, town.
Climate, the generalisation of day to day weather conditions.
Col *(French)*, **Colle** *(Italian)*, a pass or neck.
Cold Front, the sloping boundary between an advancing mass of cold air and warmer air under which the cold air forms a wedge.
Continental Shelf, a sea-covered platform extending from the coast-line of all continents. It varies in width and the edge is usually marked by the isobath for 200 metres.
Contour, a line on a map joining all points which are situated at the same height above sea-level.
Cordillera *(Spanish)*, mountain range.
Crater, the cup-shaped cavity forming the mouth of a volcano.
Creek *(Amer.)*, a stream or small river.
Crevasse, rent or fissure in a glacier or ice sheet.
Cumulus Clouds, massive rounded clouds (approx. 1500 metres high), associated with hot weather and rising air-currents.
Cycle of Erosion, the development of the landscape by the various processes of denudation from the youthful stage, after a period of instability and mountain building, through maturity till the surface is reduced to a peneplane.
Cyclone, a low pressure system, or **depression**, generally associated with stormy or wet weather. Winds tend to blow inwards in anti-clockwise direction in N. Hemisphere; clockwise in South.
Daban *(Mongolian)*, a pass.
Dagh *(Turkish)*, mountain.
Dake, Take *(Japanese)*, mountain.
Dal *(Norwegian, Swedish)*, valley.
Darya *(Persian)*, sea, stream, river.
Date Line, this follows approximately the 180° meridian from Greenwich, and marks the point where according to international convention the day begins. A ship crossing this line eastwards goes back a day, while westward it goes forward a day.
Declination, the deviation of the compass needle from True North.
Delta, a triangular or finger-shaped tract of mud and detritus deposited by a river at its mouth when it no longer has sufficient speed to keep them in suspension.
Denudation, the slow process of laying bare and levelling down the physical features of the earth's surface by natural forces.
Depression, a localised and mobile low pressure system occuring in the zone of the "Westerlies" associated with rain and stormy weather.
Derbend *(Persian, Turkish)*, pass.
Desert, a barren area of land, practically devoid of rainfall or vegetation.
Dip, the angle between the downward slope of a stratum of rock and the horizontal.
Dogger Bank, important fishing ground in North Sea, depth varies from 11 to 36 metres.
Doldrums, nautical term for a region of calms and baffling winds near the equator between the N.E. and S.E. Trade Winds.
Dolina *(Slav.)*, a large hollow or basin caused by the dissolving of limestone. Cultivated if not occupied by a pond.
Donga *(Afrikaans)*, ravine, gulley.
Dorp *(Dutch)*, **Dorf** *(German)*, village.
Dunes, mounds formed by wind-blown sand; capable of considerable advances over level ground unless arrested by the planting of suitable vegetation.
Earthquake, disturbance of the earth's surface generally occuring along faults or lines of weakness in the earth's crust. Sometimes cause great destruction, especially on alluvial ground.
Eiland *(Dutch)*' island.
Ennis *(Irish)*, island.
Equator, imaginary line circumscribing the globe midway between the poles and at its greatest circumference (40 074.72 km). It constitutes the zero from which latitudes N. and S. are calculated.
Equinox, one of the two periods of the year when day and night are of equal duration owing to the sun's crossing the Equator. 20th March and 22nd September.
Erosion, the wearing away of surface features of the earth by the action of wind, water or ice.
Escarpment, the steep face of a hill or range which on the other side slopes gently downwards *e.g.*, Cotswold and Chiltern escarpments.
Eskimos or **Esquimaux**, an aboriginal race inhabiting the Arctic coasts of America, especially of Greenland and Alaska. They live chiefly by fishing.
Estuary, the lower reaches of a river affected by the tides.
Falu *(Hungarian)*, village.
Fault, a break or crack in the earth's surface.
Fell *(Norwegian*, **Fjeld**; *Swedish*, **Fjäll**), mountain.
Fen *(Anglo-Saxon)*, swampy or boggy land.
Fiume *(Italian)*, river.
Fjord, old glacial valley filled by the sea. Sides often steepened by faulting.
Flood Plain, the generally flat area in the bottom of a valley which is covered by water when the river draining it is in flood.
Föhn, a dry warm wind in the valleys of the Alps, blowing in winter from the south.
Fork, the junction of two streams or rivers of approximately the same size.
Fu *(Chinese)*, town of importance.
Ganga *(Indian)*, river.
Gap, *see* **Pass.**
Gawa, Kawa *(Japanese)*, river.
Gebel, Jebel *(Arabic)*, rock, mountain.
Geysers, intermittent spouting hot springs associated with volcanic activity as in Iceland.
Glaciers, rivers of ice originating in snowfields, and moving slowly down valleys until they melt, or on reaching the sea break off as icebergs.
Gol, Song *(Mongolian)*, river.
Gora *(Slav.)*, mountain.
Gorod, Grad *(Slav.)*, town.
Gran Chaco, "the great hunting place", is an extensive area between Argentina, Bolivia and Paraguay consisting for the most part of swampy plains with varied vegetation; rich in animal and bird life.
Grand Banks, submarine banks situated south-east of Newfoundland. One of the best cod fishing grounds in the world.
Great Circle, a circle on the earth's surface whose plane passes through the centre of the earth.
Great Circle Route, shortest distance between two points on the earth, hence used for preference by shipping and air services.
Growing Season, that part of the year during which plant growth is possible. The main factors limiting the length of the period are the occurrence of killing frosts and drought.
Guba *(Russian)*, bay.
Gulch *(Amer.)*, a narrow, deep ravine.
Gulf Stream, great warm water current originating in the Gulf of Mexico and flowing across the Atlantic to North-West Europe.
Gunung *(Malay)*, mountain.
Hachures, closely drawn lines sometimes used on maps to denote ground relief. They should follow the direction of slope and vary in intensity with the gradient.
Haf *(Swedish)*, sea.
Hai, Hu *(Chinese)*, sea or lake.
Hamn *(Swedish)*, harbour.
Harmattan, a hot dry wind laden with clouds of reddish dust from the desert blowing over the Guinea Lands in December, January and February. It is an extension of the N.E. Trade wind.
Havn *(Danish)*, harbour.
Havre *(French)*, harbour, port.
Hegy *(Hungarian)*, mountain.
Height of Land *(Amer.)*, a watershed or divide.
Hinterland, region inland from a coast. Often deciding factor in location or growth of a port.
Ho *(Chinese)*, river.
Hoek *(Dutch)*, cape.
Höhe *(German)*, height, hill.
Horse Latitudes, regions of calms and variable winds between 25° and 40° N. and S. on the polar margins of the Trade Winds.
Horst, a block of rock left upstanding by the down faulting of rocks on either side. Exact opposite of rift valley.
Hottentots, an indigenous race in western South Africa.
Hsi *(Chinese)*, west.
Hsien *(Chinese)*, town of the third class.
Humidity, the amount of water vapour in the air. Relative Humidity is percentage of moisture contained as compared with that contained in air completely saturated at the given temperature.
Hurricane or **Typhoon**, a violent and destructive tropical cyclone which occasionally blows in the Gulf of Mexico and the China Seas (where it is known as Typhoon) in August, September or October.
Icebergs, detached masses of ice floating in the Polar Seas, carried along by ocean currents. Originate from glaciers, terminating in the sea. Danger to navigation in Atlantic.
Inch, Innis *(Celtic)*, island.

GEOGRAPHICAL TERMS—*continued*

Irmak *(Turkish)*, river.
Isla *(Spanish)*, **Isola** *(Italian)*, island.
Isobars, lines connecting points having the same barometric pressure at a given time.
Isobaths, lines connecting points of the ocean of equal depths.
Isohyets, lines connecting points with equal rainfall over given period.
Isotherms, lines connecting points of equal temperature at a given time.
Jaur, Javr, Järvi *(Finnish)*, lake.
Jesero *(Serbian)*, lake.
Joch *(German)*, mountain ridge; pass.
Joki *(Finnish)*, river.
Jug *(Serbian)*, **Yug** *(Russian)*, south.
Kahli *(Arabic)*, desert.
Kampong *(Malay)*, village.
Karroos, terraced plains between the mountains in South Africa. Desert in dry season, but develop vegetation in wet season and are used as sheep pasture.
Karst, the porous limestone region of the Dinaric Alps north-east of Adriatic Sea. Also applied to similar types of country in other lands where the river system disappears underground.
Kato *(Greek)*, under.
Khamsin *(Arabic)*, "Fifty"), name given to Sirocco in Lower Egypt where it blows for fifty days between April and June.
Kiang *(Chinese)*, river.
Koppie *(S. African)*, a small hill.
Kraal, a native dwelling in South Africa.
Kuh *(Persian)*, mountain.
Kul *(Turkish)*, lake.
Kum or **Qum** *(Turkish)*, sand.
La *(Tibetan)*, pass.
Lac *(French)*, **Lacul** *(Romanian)*, lake.
Lago *(Italian, Portuguese, Spanish)*, lake.
Lande *(French)*, heath or waste land.
Latitude, the angular distance of a place N. or S. of the equator measured on its meridian. Each degree represents sixty geographical or nautical miles equal to 69.172 statute miles (111.319 km).
Levante *(Italian)*, east.
Levees, embankments, natural or artificial, erected along the banks of rivers and built, as on the Mississippi, to prevent flooding.
Llanos, grasslands of the N.W. Orinoco Basin.
Loch, Lough *(Celtic)*, lake.
Loess, a post glacial wind-blown soil of great fertility; found in N. European Plain and in the Hwang Ho Valley of China.
Long Forties, a portion of the North Sea, so known to fishermen because the depth of water approximates 40 fathoms (73 metres).
Longitude, the angular distance of any place on the globe eastward or westward from a standard meridian, as in Great Britain that of Greenwich. Each degree of longitude represents 4 minutes of time, so that 15° of longitude represent an hour.
Magyars, native name of Hungarians.
Mallee, type of Australian scrub growing in the Murray-Darling and other areas. It is characterised by low-growing eucalyptus and other gum trees.
Maoris, the aboriginal inhabitants of New Zealand.
Marais *(French)*, marsh.
Mean Annual Rainfall, the average amount of rain which falls in a year. The average is deduced from observations taken over a considerable period.
Meander, the winding about of a river in its flood plain when it has reached its base line of erosion but still has energy for further erosion.
Medine *(Arabic)*, town.
Mer *(French)*, **Meer** *(German)*, sea.
Meridian, an imaginary line represented by a portion of a circle passing through the earth's two poles and on which all places have noon at the same time.
Miasto *(Polish)*, village.
Mile (geographical) = 1 minute of latitude, or 6080 feet (1.15 statute miles)(1.9 kilometres).
Millibar, a standard unit of barometric pressure. Average pressure is approximately 1013 millibars or 76 cms of mercury.
Mistral, a violent, dry, cold wind blowing in winter down the Rhône Valley which acts as a funnel when a depression lies over the Mediterranean.
Monsoon, seasonal winds blowing over the S.E. half of Asia. General direction October to March from N.E., April to September from S.W.
Mont *(French)*, **Monte** *(Italian)*, mount.
Monte, a type of deciduous hardwood forest situated in the higher portions of the **Gran Chaco,** moister than **Cerrados.**
Montagna *(Italian)*, mountain range.
Moraine, the waste material deposited by a glacier.
More *(Russian)*, sea.
Muang *(Siamese)*, town.
Myo *(Burmese)*, town.
Nagar *(Indian)*, town.
Nahr *(Arabic)*, river.
Nam *(Siamese)*, river.
Nan *(Chinese)*, south.
Näs *(Scandinavian)*, cape.
Natural Scale, *see* Representative Fraction.
Neap-Tides, period of lowest tide-range, when sun and moon are at right angles, as seen from the earth.
Negeri *(Malay)*, town.
Nejd *(Arabic)*, high plain.
Nimbus, dark water-laden rain cloud.
Nor *(Mongol.)*, lake.
Nos *(Russian)*, cape.
Oasis, fertile spot in a desert owing its existence to a spring or well.
Occluded Front, a line along which warm air of the atmosphere has been raised from the earth's surface by the junction of cold and warm fronts.
Ola *(Mongolian)*, mountain range.
Oxbow Lake, remains of a pronounced meander which has been short circuited by the river cutting through its neck. They occur on a river like the Mississippi.
Ozero *(Russian)*, lake.
Pack Ice, sea ice which has drifted from its original position. It takes the form of floes of various sizes and can be either loosely or tightly packed together.
Pampa *(Argentina)*, dreary expanse of treeless grass plain, and salt steppe, lat. 30° to 40° S., between the Andes and the Atlantic Ocean.
Pampero, a cold south-westerly wind that sweeps over the pampas in Central South America.
Pass, a depression or **Gap** in a mountain range which serves as way for communication between the lands on either side.
Peneplane, the almost level surface which, if the normal course of denudation is undisturbed, results from the erosion of a landscape by running water. The gradient of a river draining a peneplane is just great enough for the flow of water to be maintained.
Pizzo *(Italian)*, peak.
Plain, an area of flat or undulating ground usually at low level.
Planina *(Bulg., Serb.)*, mountain range.
Plateau, an area of relatively flat ground at considerable attitude, sometimes called a Tableland.
Polder, land recovered from the sea in Holland, and protected by dykes from being again flooded.
Ponente *(Italian)*, evening, west.
Pont, Ponte *(French, Span., Italian)*, bridge.
Potomos *(Greek)*, river.
Prairie, a series of grassy plains stretching eastwards from the Rocky Mountains in Canada and U.S.A.
Primeval Forest, a forest which has not been interfered with by man and is allowed to remain in its natural state.
Pristan *(Russian)*, port, harbour.
Projection, is the process of transferring the outline of the features on the earth's spherical surface on to a flat surface, thus constituting a map.
Pueblo *(Spanish)*, village.
Pulau *(Malay)*, island.
Puna, a high plateau between the E. and W. Andes in Bolivia and Peru.
Pur, Pura *(Indian)*, town.
Ras *(Arabic)*, cape.
Reef, a ridge of rock or coral generally covered by sea, but exposed at low tide.
Representative Fraction, a fraction representing a distance of unit lengths on a map over its corresponding length on the earth's surface.
Ria, river valley drowned by the sea owing to a fall in the land level.
Rieka *(Slav.)*, river.
Rift Valley, valley with steep walls caused by the sinking of land between two parallel geological faults.
Rio *(Portuguese, Spanish)*, river.
River Capture, process by which one river having more rapid powers of erosion than another cuts into the head waters of the latter and steals certain of its tributaries.
Riviera, narrow strip of sea coast between Toulon and Spezia, noted for mild climate in winter.
Roaring Forties, nautical name of steady north-westerly winds between lat. 40° and 60° S. Equivalent to Westerlies of N. Hemisphere.
Ross *(Celtic)*, promontory.
Saki *(Japanese)*, cape.
Sargasso Sea, an area of calms and floating seaweed in the N. Atlantic, east of the Bahamas and the Antilles Current.
Savannas, grasslands of the sub-tropics.
Sea Level, the mean level of the sea between high and low tide.
Selo *(Russian)*, village.
Selva *(Portuguese)*, forest. The name of Selvas is given to the vast rain forests of the Amazon basin.
Shan *(Chinese)*, mountain range.
Shotts *(Arabic)*, salt marshy lakes of N. Algeria and Tunisia.
Sierra *(Spanish)*, **Serra** *(Portuguese)*, mountain range.
Silt, material, finer than sand, which is often carried in suspension by rivers and deposited by them, on flood plains and deltas, when the river has lost the force required to hold the load.
Sirocco, a hot southerly wind blowing off Africa in Southern Mediterranean Countries.
Sjö *(Swedish)*, lake.
Slieve *(Irish)*, mountain.
Snow Line, the lower limit in altitude of the region which is never free from snow.
Spring Tides, period of highest tides at new or at full moon time, *i.e.* when sun and moon are pulling in line with the earth.
Stad, Stadt *(Dutch, Swedish, German)*, town.
Steppe, large expanses of grassland as in European Russia and S.W. Siberia.
Strath *(Celtic)*, broad valley of a river.
Stratus, cloud in the form of a level or horizontal sheet.
Sudd, large floating islands of vegetable matter which impede navigation on the Upper White Nile.
Syd *(Danish-Norwegian)*, south.
Sziget *(Hungarian)*, island.
Taiga, coniferous forest belt south of the Tundra, chiefly used for hunting.
Tanjong *(Malay)*, cape.
Tind *(Norwegian)*, peak.
Trade Winds, regular steady winds in the tropics, between latitudes 30° N. and 30° S. blowing to the equator, from N.E. in N. Hemisphere and S.E. in Southern.
Tributary, a river or stream which flows into and thus becomes part of a larger river.
Tropics, the parallels 23½° N., **Tropic of Cancer,** and 23½° S., **Tropic of Capricorn,** are "turning points" in the apparent seasonal movements of the sun. On June 22nd at noon it is vertically over all points on the Northern Tropic, on December 22nd at noon it is vertically over all points on the Southern Tropic.
Tundra, treeless plains along Arctic and Antarctic coasts; hard frozen in winter, and only partly thawed in summer; scanty vegetation of lichens and mosses.
Tung *(Chinese)*, east.
Ula *(Mongol.)*, mountain.
Vatn *(Norwegian)*, lake.
Veld, grassy plain in South Africa.
Volcano, a vent in the earth's crust through which molten rock, ashes and steam are ejected from the hot interior.
Wadi, Oued *(Arabic)*, a water-course.
Wallace's Line, an imaginary line dividing the characteristic flora and fauna of Asia from that of Australasia. It passes between the islands of Bali and Lombok, thence through the Strait of Macassar between Borneo and Celebes and south of the Philippine Islands. Named after Alfred Russel Wallace the noted scientist.
Warm Front, the sloping boundary in the atmosphere between an advancing mass of warm air and colder air over which the warm air rises.
Watershed, the land-form separating head streams of two river systems. Also known as **waterparting** or **divide.**
Westerlies, predominantly westerly winds in the northern and southern hemispheres N. of 30° N. and S. of 30° S.
Zee *(Dutch)*, sea.

CLIMATIC TABLES

A selection of characteristic stations in different parts of the world, giving Mean Temperature in degrees Celsius (°C), and Mean Rainfall in millimetres for each month of the year.

Climatic Type	Station	Lat.	Alt in m.		Jan.	Feb.	Mar.	April	May	June	July	Aug.	Sept.	Oct.	Nov.	Dec.	Year
SUB-POLAR -	Nome, Alaska	64.30N	7	°C	−17.1	−14.6	−13.2	−8.2	1.3	7.1	10.1	9.7	5.1	−1.7	−9.8	−14.3	−3.8
				mm	**25**	**28**	**23**	**15**	**23**	**30**	**74**	**76**	**58**	**38**	**25**	**28**	**445**
	North Cape, Norway	71.6 N	6	°C	−3.6	−4.2	−3.4	−0.3	2.8	6.8	9.9	10.0	6.6	2.1	−1.1	−2.9	1.9
				mm	**58**	**61**	**58**	**46**	**48**	**46**	**66**	**58**	**84**	**76**	**74**	**66**	**747**
	Stanley Harbour, Falkland Is.	51.41S	2	°C	9.7	9.8	8.6	6.7	4.7	3.1	2.6	3.0	4.1	5.3	6.8	8.3	6.1
				mm	**71**	**58**	**56**	**61**	**76**	**61**	**56**	**53**	**33**	**38**	**53**	**71**	**686**
WEST MARITIME	Ben Nevis, Scotland	56.48N	1344	°C	−4.4	−4.6	−4.5	−2.3	0.7	4.2	4.7	4.4	3.3	−0.8	−2.0	−3.9	−0.5
				mm	**480**	**340**	**391**	**221**	**196**	**193**	**279**	**348**	**394**	**386**	**399**	**478**	**4105**
	Christchurch, N.Z.	43.31S	6	°C	16.3	15.9	14.5	11.9	8.8	6.4	5.9	6.8	9.4	11.7	13.6	15.7	11.4
				mm	**56**	**46**	**53**	**51**	**66**	**71**	**46**	**46**	**41**	**41**	**46**	**51**	**640**
	Edinburgh, Scotland	55.55N	80	°C	3.9	4.2	5.2	7.4	10.1	13.2	14.8	14.6	12.6	9.2	6.3	4.4	8.8
				mm	**43**	**41**	**48**	**36**	**51**	**48**	**69**	**79**	**51**	**66**	**53**	**53**	**635**
	Paris, France	48.50N	50	°C	2.5	3.9	6.2	10.3	13.4	16.9	18.6	18.0	15.0	10.3	6.0	2.9	10.3
				mm	**36**	**28**	**36**	**38**	**48**	**53**	**51**	**48**	**48**	**53**	**48**	**41**	**528**
	Valdivia, Chile	39.46S	43	°C	15.3	14.9	13.7	11.9	10.8	9.2	7.8	7.9	9.6	10.6	11.8	13.7	11.4
				mm	**74**	**81**	**163**	**236**	**389**	**445**	**391**	**343**	**185**	**127**	**112**	**122**	**2667**
	Valentia, Ireland	51.56N	9	°C	6.9	6.8	7.2	8.9	11.1	13.7	14.9	14.9	13.7	10.8	8.6	7.5	10.4
				mm	**140**	**132**	**114**	**94**	**79**	**81**	**97**	**122**	**104**	**142**	**140**	**165**	**1415**
	Victoria, B.C.	48.24N	26	°C	3.8	4.6	6.3	8.8	11.6	13.9	15.7	15.4	13.3	10.2	6.9	5.1	9.6
				mm	**117**	**81**	**64**	**41**	**30**	**23**	**10**	**15**	**46**	**64**	**147**	**147**	**787**
SEMI-CONTINENTAL	Chicago, Illinois	41.53N	251	°C	−3.6	−2.8	2.6	8.6	14.7	20.0	23.3	22.7	19.1	12.7	5.3	−0.9	10.1
				mm	**53**	**53**	**66**	**74**	**91**	**84**	**86**	**76**	**79**	**66**	**61**	**53**	**841**
	Nashville, Tennessee	36.10N	175	°C	3.8	4.9	9.7	14.9	20.2	24.4	26.1	25.3	22.2	15.8	9.4	5.1	15.2
				mm	**119**	**107**	**130**	**112**	**97**	**107**	**104**	**89**	**89**	**61**	**89**	**99**	**1204**
	Warsaw, Poland	52.13N	119	°C	−3.1	−1.9	1.8	7.9	14.1	17.2	18.8	17.5	13.5	7.9	2.2	−1.2	7.9
				mm	**33**	**25**	**33**	**41**	**51**	**61**	**86**	**66**	**46**	**41**	**36**	**36**	**478**
COLD CONTINENTAL	Moscow, U.S.S.R.	55.50N	146	°C	−10.8	−9.0	−4.3	3.4	11.8	15.6	18.0	15.8	9.7	3.7	−2.8	−7.9	3.6
				mm	**33**	**30**	**36**	**36**	**46**	**66**	**81**	**79**	**53**	**53**	**46**	**41**	**599**
	Verkhoyansk, U.S.S.R.	67.33N	101	°C	−50.5	−44.0	−31.0	−13.3	1.6	13.1	15.6	10.0	1.9	−15.0	−36.5	−46.4	−16.2
				mm	**5**	**3**	**0**	**3**	**5**	**13**	**30**	**23**	**5**	**5**	**5**	**5**	**99**
	Winnipeg, Manitoba	49.53N	232	°C	−15.6	−17.7	−9.4	3.2	11.1	16.8	19.1	17.7	12.1	4.8	−5.9	−14.5	1.4
				mm	**23**	**18**	**30**	**36**	**51**	**79**	**79**	**56**	**56**	**36**	**28**	**23**	**513**
EAST MARITIME -	Miyako, Japan	39.38N	30	°C	−0.6	−0.3	2.6	8.2	12.3	16.0	19.9	22.1	18.5	12.6	7.2	2.2	10.0
				mm	**69**	**66**	**89**	**99**	**119**	**127**	**135**	**178**	**216**	**170**	**81**	**64**	**1412**
	St John's, Newfoundland	47.34N	38	°C	−4.7	−5.3	−2.4	1.6	6.1	10.6	15.2	15.4	12.1	7.4	2.8	−1.7	4.8
				mm	**137**	**127**	**117**	**109**	**91**	**91**	**97**	**94**	**97**	**137**	**152**	**137**	**1382**
PRAIRIE STEPPE	Bahia Blanca, Argentina	38.43S	15	°C	23.2	22.2	19.4	15.3	11.5	8.4	8.1	9.4	12.2	14.9	18.6	21.7	15.4
				mm	**51**	**56**	**66**	**56**	**30**	**23**	**25**	**25**	**41**	**58**	**51**	**53**	**533**
	Calgary, Alberta	51.2 N	1033	°C	−10.9	−9.2	−3.7	4.6	9.5	13.5	16.2	15.2	10.4	5.4	−2.4	−7.0	3.4
				mm	**13**	**15**	**18**	**20**	**58**	**74**	**66**	**64**	**33**	**18**	**18**	**13**	**401**
	Semipalatinsk, U.S.S.R.	50.26N	180	°C	−17.5	−16.8	−9.8	3.5	14.0	20.0	22.2	19.6	12.7	3.4	−6.6	−14.4	2.5
				mm	**13**	**5**	**10**	**10**	**20**	**23**	**28**	**10**	**15**	**15**	**15**	**20**	**185**
MANCHURIAN -	Peking, China	39.55N	40	°C	−4.7	−1.5	5.0	13.7	19.9	24.5	26.0	24.7	19.8	12.5	3.6	−2.6	11.7
				mm	**3**	**5**	**5**	**15**	**36**	**76**	**239**	**160**	**66**	**15**	**8**	**3**	**632**
HUMID TEMPERATE -	Brisbane, Australia	27.28S	42	°C	25.1	24.7	23.5	21.3	18.1	15.7	14.7	15.8	18.5	21.0	23.1	24.7	20.5
				mm	**160**	**157**	**142**	**91**	**71**	**66**	**58**	**53**	**53**	**66**	**94**	**122**	**1135**
	Charleston, S. Carolina	32.47N	15	°C	9.9	10.7	14.2	17.7	22.3	25.6	27.0	26.7	24.6	19.4	14.3	10.6	18.6
				mm	**79**	**84**	**86**	**74**	**86**	**122**	**180**	**168**	**127**	**91**	**61**	**74**	**1229**
	Wuhan, China	30.35N	36	°C	3.8	4.5	9.6	16.2	21.7	25.7	28.6	28.5	24.4	18.2	12.1	6.3	16.6
				mm	**53**	**28**	**71**	**122**	**127**	**178**	**218**	**117**	**56**	**99**	**28**	**15**	**1113**
MEDITERRANEAN	Adelaide, Australia	34.55S	43	°C	23.4	23.3	21.1	17.8	14.3	11.9	10.8	12.1	13.9	16.6	19.4	21.7	17.2
				mm	**20**	**15**	**28**	**46**	**71**	**76**	**66**	**61**	**46**	**46**	**25**	**20**	**521**
	Athens, Greece	37.58N	107	°C	9.1	9.7	11.3	14.8	19.1	23.5	26.7	26.4	22.9	18.9	14.1	11.2	17.4
				mm	**53**	**43**	**30**	**23**	**20**	**18**	**8**	**13**	**18**	**41**	**66**	**66**	**394**
	Gibraltar	36.6 N	15	°C	12.8	13.3	14.1	15.9	18.2	20.8	23.0	23.8	22.2	18.7	15.8	13.4	17.6
				mm	**130**	**107**	**122**	**69**	**43**	**13**	**0**	**3**	**36**	**84**	**163**	**140**	**897**
	Marseilles, France	43.18N	75	°C	6.9	7.9	10.0	12.8	16.3	19.7	22.2	21.3	19.4	14.8	10.6	7.6	14.1
				mm	**41**	**38**	**48**	**56**	**43**	**28**	**18**	**20**	**61**	**97**	**71**	**53**	**574**
	Sacramento, California	38.35N	22	°C	8.1	10.2	12.6	14.7	18.0	21.6	22.9	22.3	20.6	16.0	11.6	8.4	15.6
				mm	**97**	**71**	**71**	**38**	**18**	**3**	**0**	**0**	**8**	**20**	**48**	**97**	**472**
SEMI-ARID -	Alice Springs, Australia	23.38S	587	°C	28.5	27.8	24.8	20.1	15.4	12.4	11.4	14.7	18.6	22.9	26.1	27.9	20.9
				mm	**46**	**43**	**30**	**20**	**18**	**15**	**10**	**10**	**10**	**18**	**25**	**41**	**284**
	Denver, Colorado	39.45N	1613	°C	−1.2	−0.2	3.8	8.6	13.7	19.6	22.3	21.6	16.9	10.3	4.0	−0.2	9.9
				mm	**10**	**13**	**25**	**53**	**61**	**36**	**46**	**36**	**25**	**25**	**15**	**18**	**363**
	Kabul, Afghanistan	34.35N	1905	°C	−0.7	2.1	8.2	14.9	20.0	22.9	24.8	24.2	20.4	14.6	10.4	4.7	13.9
				mm	**25**	**20**	**119**	**56**	**15**	**5**	**5**	**5**	**0**	**3**	**25**	**5**	**284**
	Karachi, Pakistan	24.51N	4	°C	18.5	20.2	23.9	27.0	29.3	30.4	29.1	28.0	27.8	26.7	23.3	19.7	25.3
				mm	**15**	**10**	**8**	**3**	**3**	**18**	**71**	**43**	**15**	**0**	**3**	**3**	**188**
	Madrid, Spain	40.24N	655	°C	4.6	6.5	8.7	12.2	16.1	20.8	25.1	24.8	19.6	13.4	8.4	5.0	13.7
				mm	**33**	**33**	**41**	**41**	**43**	**33**	**10**	**13**	**38**	**46**	**51**	**41**	**422**
	Tombouctou, Mali	16.37N	250	°C	21.7	23.1	28.4	33.1	34.7	34.3	31.8	30.3	31.8	31.6	27.1	21.7	29.1
				mm	**0**	**0**	**3**	**0**	**8**	**23**	**89**	**71**	**28**	**10**	**0**	**0**	**229**
DESERT -	Esfahān, Iran	32.40N	1773	°C	1.2	5.3	9.4	15.6	20.7	25.2	27.8	25.6	22.4	16.1	9.1	4.4	15.2
				mm	**18**	**13**	**23**	**15**	**5**	**0**	**0**	**0**	**0**	**3**	**15**	**23**	**114**
	Swakopmund, Namibia	22.40S	6	°C	17.0	17.3	17.4	15.5	15.9	14.7	13.6	12.7	13.4	14.5	14.8	16.4	15.2
				mm	**0**	**3**	**5**	**0**	**0**	**0**	**0**	**0**	**0**	**3**	**0**	**5**	**18**
	Yuma, Arizona	32.45N	43	°C	12.6	15.1	18.1	21.2	24.9	29.3	32.7	32.3	28.8	22.4	16.1	13.2	22.3
				mm	**13**	**10**	**8**	**3**	**0**	**0**	**5**	**15**	**8**	**5**	**8**	**10**	**84**
DRY TROPICAL -	Bombay, India	18.55N	11	°C	24.2	24.3	26.4	28.4	29.9	28.9	27.4	27.1	27.2	28.0	27.0	25.2	27.0
				mm	**3**	**0**	**3**	**0**	**18**	**523**	**693**	**406**	**300**	**61**	**10**	**0**	**2017**
	Cuyaba, Brazil	15.36S	165	°C	27.2	27.1	27.1	26.8	25.3	24.1	24.4	25.7	27.8	27.6	27.8	28.4	26.4
				mm	**251**	**211**	**211**	**102**	**53**	**5**	**5**	**30**	**51**	**114**	**152**	**206**	**1389**
	Darwin, N. Australia	12.28S	30	°C	28.8	28.6	28.9	28.9	27.7	26.1	25.2	26.3	28.1	29.6	29.9	29.5	28.1
				mm	**404**	**330**	**257**	**104**	**18**	**3**	**3**	**3**	**13**	**56**	**122**	**262**	**1570**
	Manila, Philippines	14.35N	14	°C	24.8	25.3	26.6	28.1	28.6	27.8	27.1	27.1	26.8	26.6	25.8	25.1	26.5
				mm	**20**	**10**	**20**	**33**	**114**	**234**	**439**	**406**	**363**	**170**	**132**	**76**	**2032**
	Veracruz, Mexico	19.10N	15	°C	21.9	22.9	23.8	26.1	27.2	27.5	27.6	27.7	26.9	24.7	23.8	21.6	25.2
				mm	**10**	**15**	**15**	**3**	**109**	**318**	**376**	**226**	**295**	**229**	**81**	**51**	**1727**
WET TROPICAL -	Georgetown, Guyana	6.50N	23	°C	25.8	25.8	26.1	26.4	26.3	26.0	26.1	26.5	27.2	27.3	26.9	26.1	26.4
				mm	**201**	**117**	**183**	**152**	**282**	**297**	**251**	**165**	**79**	**79**	**170**	**282**	**2253**
	Lagos, Nigeria	6.27N	8	°C	27.2	27.9	28.5	28.1	27.7	26.3	25.6	25.4	25.8	26.4	27.4	27.5	26.9
				mm	**28**	**53**	**94**	**147**	**267**	**472**	**272**	**71**	**135**	**196**	**66**	**20**	**1819**
	Singapore	1.24N	3	°C	25.7	26.1	26.8	27.1	27.5	27.3	27.2	27.0	26.9	26.7	26.3	25.9	26.7
				mm	**216**	**155**	**165**	**175**	**183**	**170**	**173**	**216**	**180**	**208**	**254**	**264**	**2360**
MOUNTAIN -	Bogota, Colombia	4.36N	2661	°C	14.2	14.4	14.8	14.8	14.7	14.5	14.0	13.9	13.9	14.4	14.6	14.5	14.4
				mm	**58**	**61**	**104**	**145**	**114**	**61**	**51**	**56**	**61**	**163**	**117**	**66**	**1057**
	Darjeeling, India	27.3 N	2248	°C	4.5	5.3	9.8	13.4	14.6	15.5	16.4	16.1	15.2	12.9	8.8	5.4	11.5
				mm	**20**	**28**	**51**	**104**	**198**	**615**	**805**	**660**	**465**	**135**	**5**	**5**	**3094**
	Johannesburg, S. Africa	26.11S	1806	°C	19.2	18.6	17.4	15.4	12.4	10.4	10.3	12.4	15.2	17.0	17.5	18.4	15.3
				mm	**157**	**132**	**112**	**43**	**20**	**3**	**13**	**13**	**25**	**66**	**127**	**137**	**843**
	Mexico City, Mexico	19.26N	2278	°C	12.2	13.8	15.8	17.9	18.3	17.7	16.9	16.7	16.2	14.8	13.6	11.9	15.5
				mm	**5**	**5**	**15**	**15**	**48**	**99**	**104**	**119**	**104**	**46**	**13**	**5**	**587**

STATES AND POPULATIONS

	area (sq. km)	POPULATION
AFGHANISTAN	657 500	17 600 000
ALBANIA	28 748	2 170 000
ALGERIA	2 381 730	14 600 000
ANDORRA	453	20 000
ANGOLA	1 246 700	5 673 000
ARGENTINA	2 778 412	24 000 000
AUSTRALIA	7 686 900	12 959 000
Australian Capital Terr.	2 432	158 000
New South Wales	801 432	4 663 000
Northern Territory	1 347 515	93 000
Queensland	1 727 520	1 869 000
South Australia	984 381	1 186 000
Tasmania	68 332	392 200
Victoria	227 620	3 546 000
Western Australia	2 527 623	1 053 000
AUSTRIA	83 849	7 456 000
BAHAMAS, THE	11 400	171 000
BAHRAIN	598	216 000
BANGLADESH	142 776	75 000 000
BARBADOS	430	238 141
BELGIUM	30 513	9 676 000
BELIZE	22 963	126 000
BENIN	112 600	2 800 000
BERMUDA	53	55 000
BHUTAN	46 600	1 000 000
BOLIVIA	1 098 580	5 100 000
BOTSWANA	600 000	700 000
BRAZIL	8 511 965	98 000 000
BRUNEI	5 765	142 000
BULGARIA	110 912	8 490 000
BURMA	678 034	28 870 000
BURUNDI	27 834	3 800 000
CAMBODIA	181 305	7 200 000
CAMEROON	475 500	6 200 000
CANADA	9 976 169	21 568 000
Alberta	661 188	1 627 900
British Columbia	948 600	2 184 600
Manitoba	650 090	988 200
New Brunswick	73 437	634 600
Newfoundland	404 519	522 100
Northwest Territories	3 379 689	34 800
Nova Scotia	55 490	789 000
Ontario	1 068 587	7 703 000
Prince Edward Island	5 657	111 600
Quebec	1 549 677	6 027 800
Saskatchewan	651 903	926 200
Yukon	536 327	18 400
CAPE VERDE	4 033	272 000
CENT. AFRICAN REP.	623 018	1 520 000
CHAD	1 284 000	3 710 000
CHILE	756 945	10 000 000
CHINA	9 560 975	750 000 000
Inner Mongolia	450 000	9 000 000
Sinkiang	1 646 790	8 000 000
Tibet	1 221 600	1 250 000
COLOMBIA	1 138 914	22 500 000
CONGO	342 000	1 000 000
COSTA RICA	50 900	1 800 000
CUBA	114 524	8 553 395
CYPRUS	9 255	600 000
CZECHOSLOVAKIA	127 870	14 362 000
DENMARK	43 069	4 976 000
DJIBOUTI	23 000	81 000
DOMINICAN REP.	48 442	4 200 000
ECUADOR	281 341	6 500 000
EGYPT	1 000 253	34 700 000
EL SALVADOR	21 393	3 700 000
EQUATORIAL GUINEA	28 051	290 000
ETHIOPIA	1 221 900	26 400 000
FAEROES	1 373	38 000
FALKLAND ISLANDS	11 961	2 105
FIJI	18 272	533 000
FINLAND	337 032	4 706 000
FRANCE	549 430	51 600 000
FRENCH GUIANA	91 000	51 000
GABON	267 000	500 000
GAMBIA, THE	11 295	364 000
EAST GERMANY	108 173	17 042 000
WEST GERMANY	248 533	61 682 000
GHANA	238 539	9 600 000
GIBRALTAR	6	26 833
GREECE	131 944	9 000 000
GREENLAND	2 175 600	47 000
GUATEMALA	108 889	5 500 000
GUINEA	245 857	3 920 000
GUINEA-BISSAU	36 125	560 000
GUYANA	214 970	700 000
HAITI	27 750	5 000 000
HONDURAS	112 088	2 700 000
HONG KONG	1 032	4 078 000
HUNGARY	93 030	10 415 000

	area (sq. km)	POPULATION
ICELAND	103 000	200 000
INDIA	3 287 593	638 388 000
INDONESIA	1 904 334	129 000 000
IRAN	1 648 180	30 550 000
IRAQ	438 446	9 800 000
IRELAND, Rep. of	68 893	3 000 000
ISRAEL	20 700	3 080 000
ITALY	301 224	55 000 000
IVORY COAST	322 463	4 500 000
JAMAICA	11 525	2 040 000
JAPAN	372 077	106 958 000
JORDAN	97 740	2 467 000
KENYA	582 600	11 800 000
KIRIBATI	655	70 000
KOREA, NORTH	127 158	14 500 000
KOREA, SOUTH	98 431	33 400 000
KUWAIT	16 000	800 000
LAOS	236 800	2 962 000
LEBANON	10 400	2 855 000
LESOTHO	30 340	1 200 000
LIBERIA	111 000	1 300 000
LIBYA	1 759 540	2 100 000
LIECHTENSTEIN	160	21 350
LUXEMBOURG	2 586	345 000
MADAGASCAR	594 180	7 655 000
MALAWI	126 338	4 530 000
MALAYSIA	333 507	10 800 000
MALI	1 240 000	5 300 000
MALTA	316	326 000
MAURITANIA	1 030 700	1 400 000
MAURITIUS	1 865	836 000
MEXICO	1 967 183	52 500 000
MONACO	15	23 000
MONGOLIA	1 565 000	1 290 000
MOROCCO	458 730	15 700 000
MOZAMBIQUE	784 961	8 234 000
NAMIBIA (S.W. Africa)	824 293	852 000
NEPAL	141 400	11 500 000
NETHERLANDS	40 893	13 270 000
NETHERLANDS ANTILLES	1 019	225 000
NEW HEBRIDES	14 760	84 000
NEW ZEALAND	268 680	2 900 000
NICARAGUA	148 000	2 210 000
NIGER	1 267 000	4 200 000
NIGERIA	923 773	58 000 000
NORWAY	324 219	3 918 000
OMAN	212 000	660 000
PAKISTAN	803 994	58 000 000
PANAMA	75 650	1 826 000
PAPUA-NEW GUINEA	461 700	2 467 000
PARAGUAY	406 752	2 500 000
PERU	1 285 215	14 400 000
PHILIPPINES	299 400	40 600 000
POLAND	312 700	32 900 000
PORTUGAL	92 082	9 700 000
PUERTO RICO	8 891	2 770 000
QATAR	22 000	80 000
ROMANIA	237 500	20 600 000
RWANDA	26 330	3 800 000
SAN MARINO	61	19 000
SAUDI ARABIA	2 263 600	7 200 000
SENEGAL	197 161	3 925 000
SIERRA LEONE	73 326	2 550 000
SOLOMON IS.	29 785	163 000
SOMALIA	637 660	2 790 000
SOUTH AFRICA	1 221 042	22 700 000
Cape of Good Hope	721 004	5 363 000
Natal	86 967	2 980 000
Orange Free State	129 153	1 387 000
Transvaal	283 918	6 273 000
SPAIN	504 748	34 600 000
SRI LANKA	65 610	13 033 000
SUDAN	2 505 813	16 700 000
SURINAM	17 400	385 000
SWAZILAND	173 400	408 000
SWEDEN	449 793	8 127 000
SWITZERLAND	41 288	6 270 000
SYRIA	185 680	6 600 000
TAIWAN	35 961	14 990 000
TANZANIA	939 700	14 000 000
THAILAND	514 000	38 000 000
TOGO	56 000	2 004 711
TRINIDAD & TOBAGO	5 128	1 070 000
TUNISIA	164 150	5 300 000
TURKEY	780 576	37 010 000
TUVALU	24.6	10 000
UGANDA	236 037	9 764 000
UNION OF SOVIET SOCIALIST REPS.	22 400 000	246 300 000
Armenian S.S.R.	29 759	2 600 000

	area (sq. km)	POPULATION
Azerbaijan S.S.R.	86 853	5 300 000
Byelorussian S.S.R.	207 588	9 100 000
Estonian S.S.R.	45 092	1 357 000
Georgian S.S.R.	69 670	4 800 000
Kazakh S.S.R.	2 717 000	13 500 000
Kirghiz S.S.R.	198 652	3 100 000
Latvian S.S.R.	64 000	2 365 000
Lithuanian S.S.R.	65 190	3 129 000
Moldavian S.S.R.	33 800	3 700 000
Russian S.F.S.R.	17 077 962	130 090 000
Tadzhik S.S.R.	143 072	3 100 000
Turkmen S.S.R.	487 956	2 300 000
Ukrainian S.S.R.	604 000	47 900 000
Uzbek S.S.R.	447 000	12 500 000
UNITED ARAB EMIRATES	83 660	180 000
UNITED KINGDOM OF GT. BRITAIN & N. IRELAND	230 608	55 356 000
England and Wales	130 362	48 604 000
Scotland	78749	5 224 000
Northern Ireland	14147	1 528 000
Channel Islands	195	125 240
Isle of Man	588	49 743
UNITED STATES OF AMERICA	9 363 353	209 000 000
Alabama	133 167	3 444 165
Alaska	1 518 800	302 173
Arizona	295 022	1 772 482
Arkansas	137 539	1 923 295
California	411 012	19 953 134
Colorado	269 998	2 207 259
Connecticut	12 973	3 032 217
Delaware	5 328	548 104
District of Columbia	174	756 510
Florida	151 670	6 789 443
Georgia	152 488	4 589 575
Hawaii	16 705	769 913
Idaho	216 412	713 008
Illinois	146 075	11 113 976
Indiana	93 993	5 193 669
Iowa	145 791	2 825 041
Kansas	213 063	2 249 071
Kentucky	104 623	3 219 311
Louisiana	125 674	3 643 180
Maine	86 027	993 663
Maryland	27 394	3 922 399
Massachusetts	21 386	5 689 170
Michigan	150 779	8 875 083
Minnesota	217 735	3 805 069
Mississippi	123 584	2 216 912
Missouri	180 486	4 677 399
Montana	381 084	694 409
Nebraska	200 017	1 483 791
Nevada	286 296	488 738
New Hampshire	24 097	737 681
New Jersey	20 295	7 168 164
New Mexico	315 113	1 016 000
New York	128 401	18 241 266
North Carolina	136 197	5 082 059
North Dakota	183 022	617 716
Ohio	106 765	10 652 017
Oklahoma	181 090	2 559 253
Oregon	251 180	2 091 385
Pennsylvania	117 412	11 793 909
Rhode Island	3 144	949 723
South Carolina	80 432	2 590 516
South Dakota	199 551	666 257
Tennessee	109 412	3 924 164
Texas	692 403	11 196 730
Utah	219 932	1 059 273
Vermont	24 887	444 732
Virginia	105 816	4 648 494
Washington	176 617	3 409 169
West Virginia	62 629	1 744 237
Wisconsin	145 438	4 417 933
Wyoming	253 597	332 416
UPPER VOLTA	274 122	5 600 000
URUGUAY	186 926	3 000 000
VATICAN CITY	0.44	1 000
VENEZUELA	912 050	11 000 000
VIETNAM	329 650	41 000 000
YEMEN	195 000	5 750 000
YEMEN, SOUTH	160 300	1 280 000
YUGOSLAVIA	255 804	20 800 000
ZAIRE	2 345 409	22 800 000
ZAMBIA	752 262	4 500 000
ZIMBABWE	389 361	6 930 000

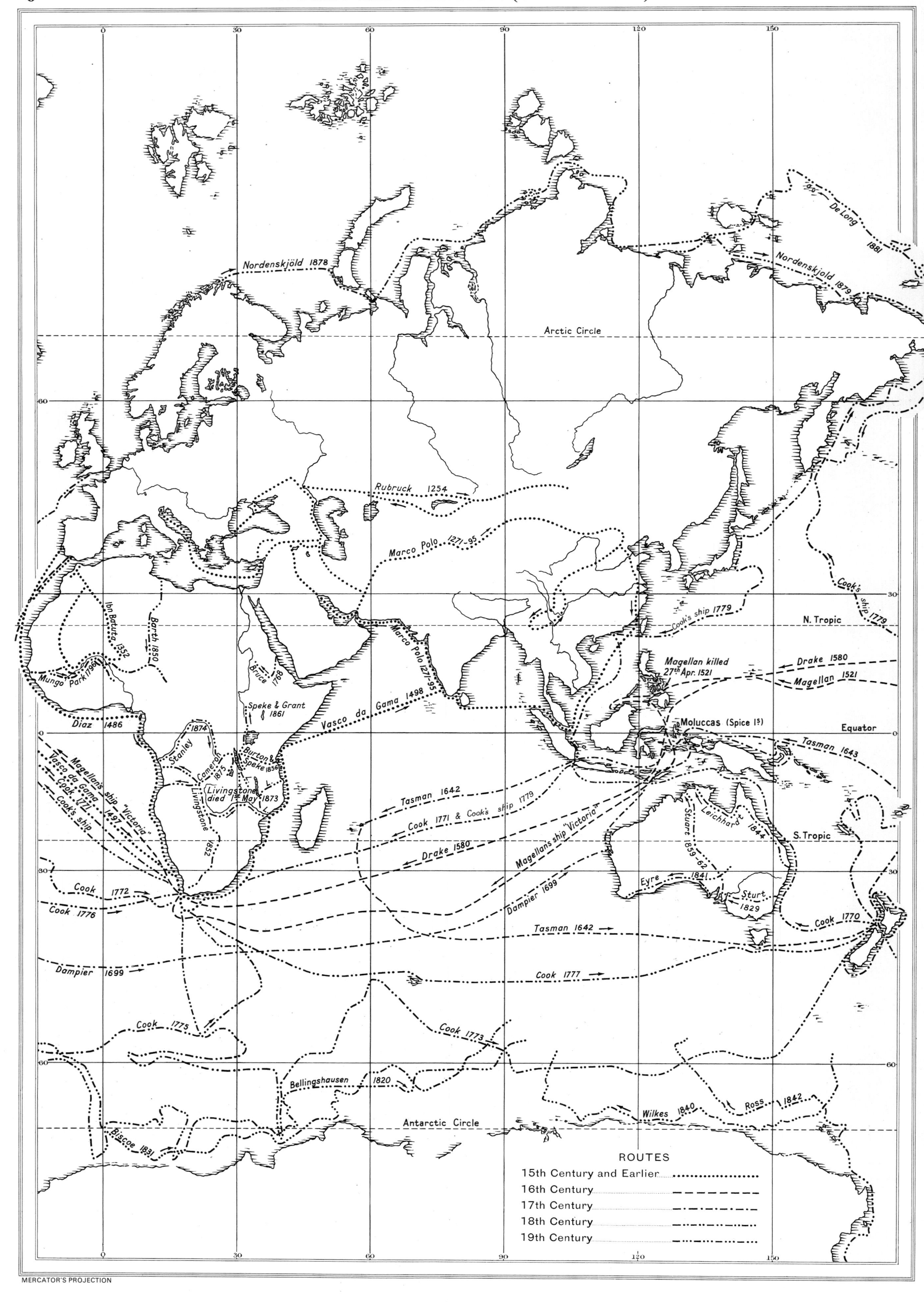
Nordenskjöld 1878
De Long 1881
Nordenskjöld 1879
Arctic Circle
Rubruck 1254
Marco Polo 1271-95
Cook's ship 1779
N. Tropic
Ibn Batuta 1352
Barth 1850
Mungo Park 1796
Bruce 1768
Magellan killed 27th Apr. 1521
Drake 1580
Magellan 1521
Speke & Grant 1861
Vasco da Gama 1498
Diaz 1486
Moluccas (Spice Is)
Equator
Tasman 1643
Stanley
1874
Cameron 1875
Burton & Speke 1856
Livingstone died 1st May 1873
Livingstone 1852
Magellan's ship "Victoria"
Vasco da Gama 1497
Cook 1772
Cook's ship
Tasman 1642
Cook 1771 & Cook's ship 1779
Drake 1580
Magellans ship "Victoria"
Stuart 1859-62
Leichhardt 1844
S. Tropic
Eyre 1841
Sturt 1829
Dampier 1699
Cook 1772
Cook 1776
Cook 1770
Tasman 1642
Dampier 1699
Cook 1777
Cook 1775
Cook 1773
Bellingshausen 1820
Wilkes 1840
Ross 1842
Antarctic Circle
Biscoe 1831
ROUTES
15th Century and Earlier
16th Century
17th Century
18th Century
19th Century
MERCATOR'S PROJECTION

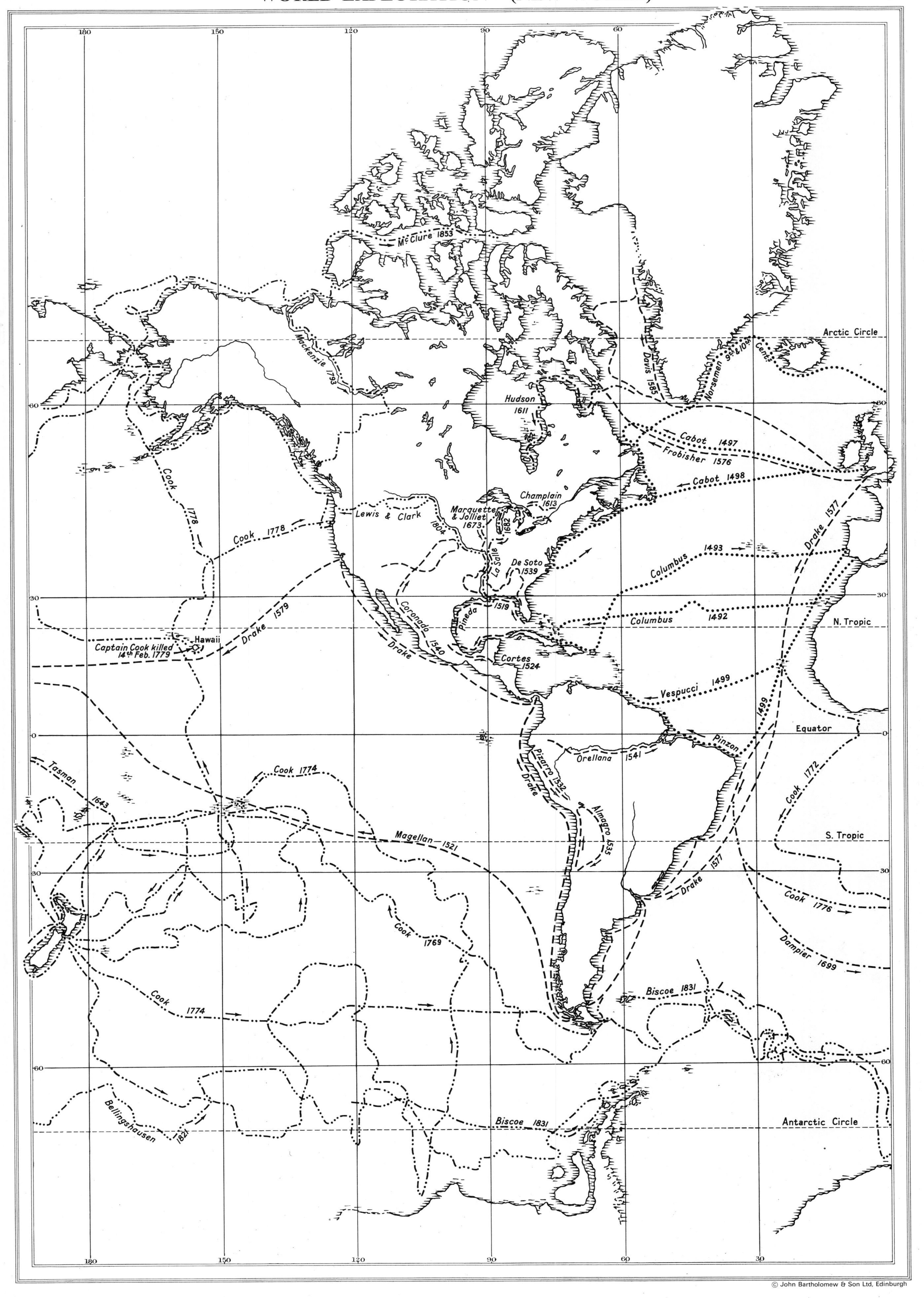
180
150
120
90
60
30
0
Arctic Circle
N. Tropic
Equator
S. Tropic
Antarctic Circle
Mc Clure 1853
Mackenzie 1793
Davis 1585
Norsemen 9th & 10th Cents.
Hudson 1611
Cabot 1497
Frobisher 1576
Cabot 1498
Cook
1778
Cook 1778
Lewis & Clark 1804
Marquette & Jolliet 1673
Champlain 1613
1682
La Salle
De Soto 1539
Columbus 1493
Drake 1577
Columbus 1492
Pineda 1519
Coronado 1540
Drake 1579
Hawaii
Captain Cook killed 14th Feb. 1779
Drake
Cortes 1524
Vespucci 1499
1499
Pinzon
Orellana 1541
Pizarro 1532
Drake
Almagro 1535
Tasman 1643
Cook 1774
Magellan 1521
Cook 1772
Drake 1577
Cook 1776
Dampier 1699
Cook 1769
Cook 1774
Biscoe 1831
Biscoe 1831
Bellingshausen 1821

STEREOGRAPHIC PROJECTION

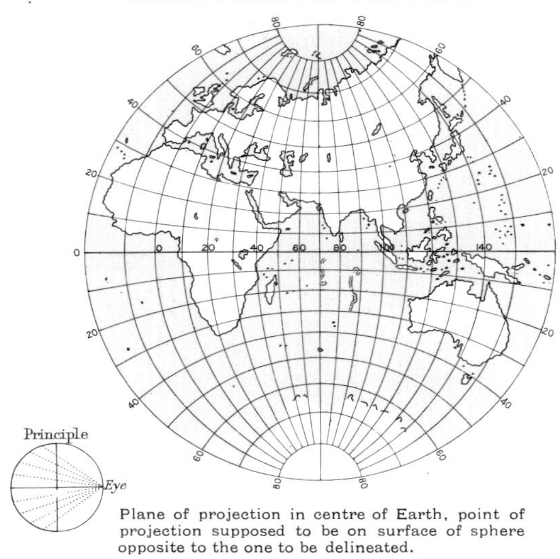

Plane of projection in centre of Earth, point of projection supposed to be on surface of sphere opposite to the one to be delineated.

ORTHOGRAPHIC PROJECTION

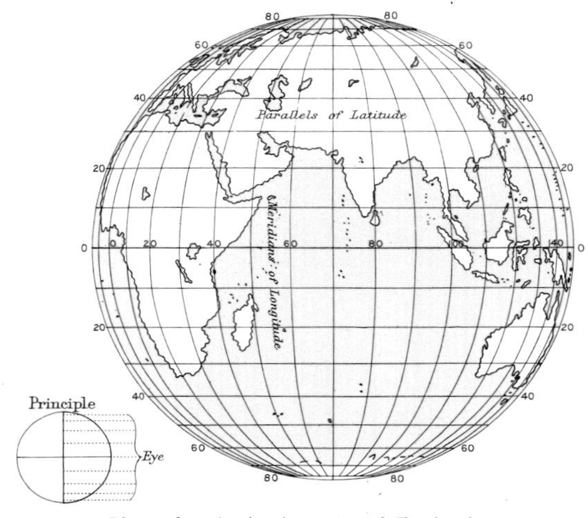

Plane of projection in centre of Earth, the eye or point of projection supposed to be at infinite distance so that lines of projection are all parallel.

EQUIDISTANT OR GLOBULAR PROJECTION

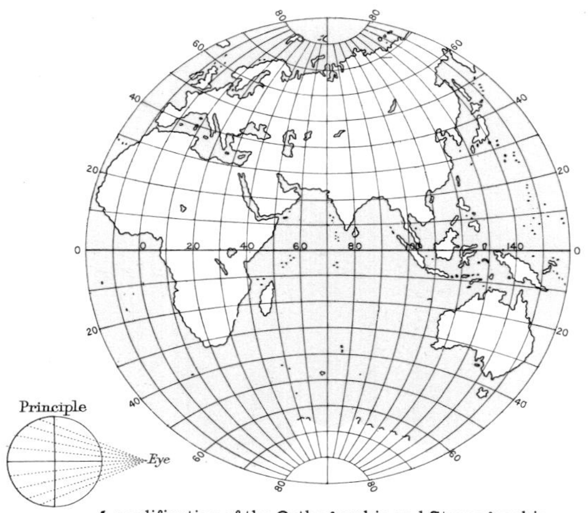

A modification of the Orthographic and Stereographic in which the point of projection is supposed to be removed to a point outside of the opposite surface of the sphere.

POLAR PROJECTIONS

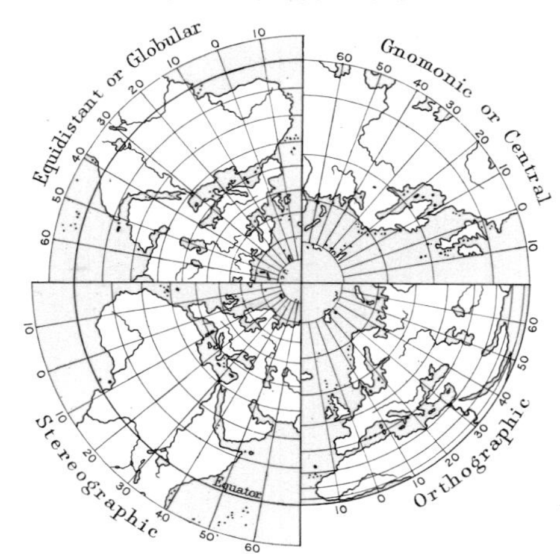

The Gnomonic Projection cannot be made to include the whole hemisphere. The Stereographic and Globular Projections can be extended to include more than the hemisphere.

MERCATOR'S PROJECTION

The plane of projection is the surface of an imaginary cylinder surrounding the globe and touching its surface at the Equator. At the Equator its scale agrees with the globe, but as each parallel of latitude becomes a great circle equal to the Equator, the scale increases as we go North and South. The latitude is, however, increased in same proportion as the longitude. Mercator's projection is the only one which gives the true direction of one point in relation to another, and is therefore most used for the purposes of navigation.

GALL'S STEREOGRAPHIC PROJECTION

This is another Cylindrical Projection, but the cylinder, instead of touching the sphere only at the Equator as in Mercator's, is supposed to be sunk into its surface so that it cuts its surface half way between the Equator and the poles, and thus coincides with the two parallels of 45° N. and S. Lat. The parallels are projected stereographically.

SANSON'S (SINUSOIDAL) PROJECTION

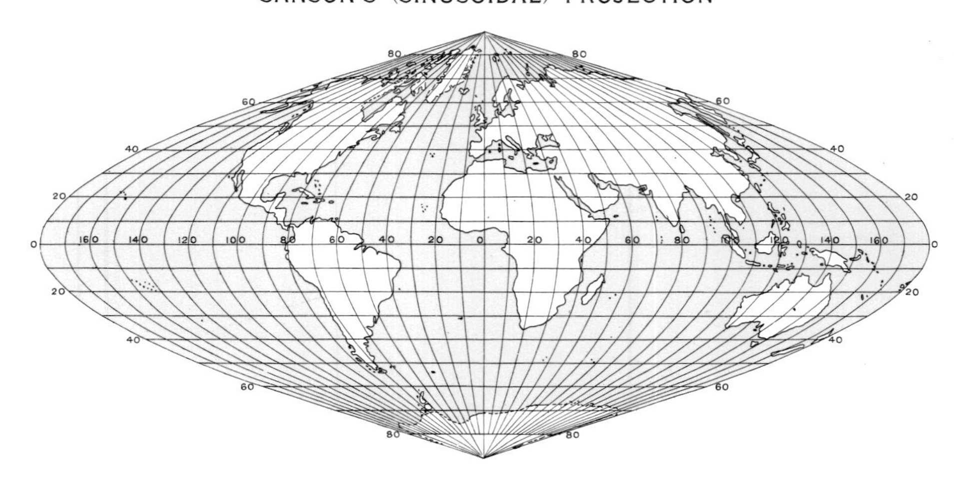

The parallels are drawn at their true distances from the Equator and along each of these. correct distances are measured through which the meridians are drawn. The projection is obviously equal-area.

MOLLWEIDE'S HOMOLOGRAPHIC PROJECTION

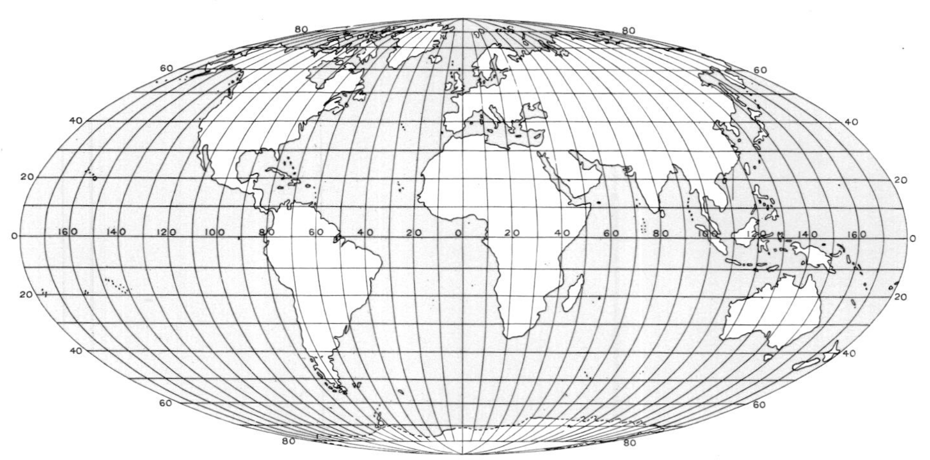

This is an equal area projection. The complete circle on the map is made to equal the world hemisphere. Parallels are so drawn that the zone enclosed by them bears the same relation to the area of the circle as the similar zone on the Earth bears to the hemisphere. The meridians are ellipses cutting the parallels at equal distances.

CONIC PROJECTION WITH ONE STANDARD PARALLEL

Diagram showing the principle of the projection. Cone A.B.C. imposed upon sphere and touching it at P.P.

Portion of surface of cone spread out representing map. P′P′ the parallel where cone coincides with the sphere.

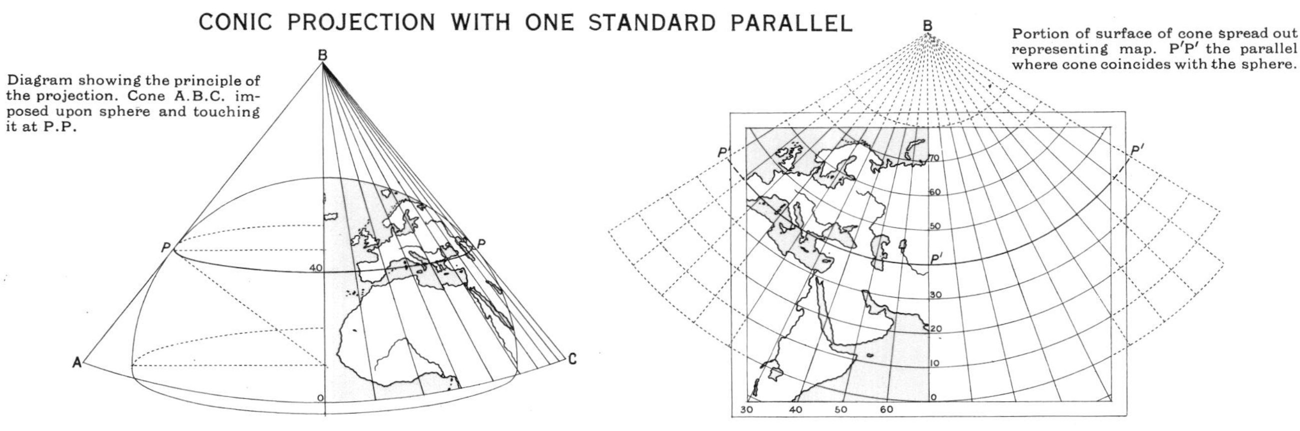

The plane of projection is the surface of an imaginary cone imposed on the sphere and touching its surface along the parallel of 40° P.P. Distances measured along that parallel on the map are absolutely correct as they exactly coincide with the globe. But the scale is distorted to the North and South of tangential parallel according to distance away from it.

LENGTH OF DEGREES OF LONGITUDE AT VARIOUS DEGREES OF LATITUDE

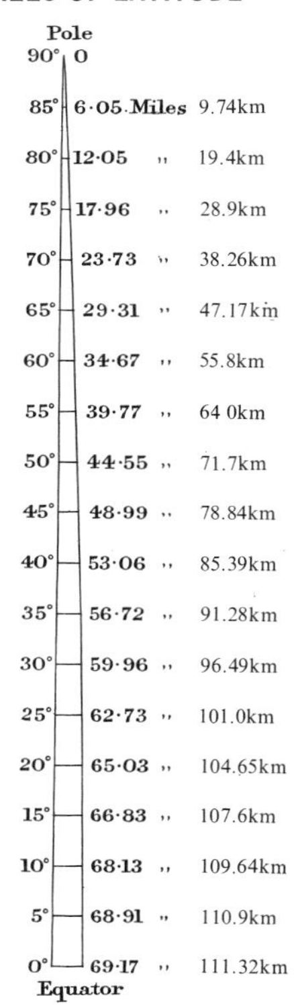

Latitude	Miles	km
90° (Pole)	0	
85°	6·05 Miles	9.74km
80°	12·05	19.4km
75°	17·96	28.9km
70°	23·73	38.26km
65°	29·31	47.17km
60°	34·67	55.8km
55°	39·77	64.0km
50°	44·55	71.7km
45°	48·99	78.84km
40°	53·06	85.39km
35°	56·72	91.28km
30°	59·96	96.49km
25°	62·73	101.0km
20°	65·03	104.65km
15°	66·83	107.6km
10°	68·13	109.64km
5°	68·91	110.9km
0° (Equator)	69·17	111.32km

CONIC PROJECTION WITH TWO STANDARD PARALLELS

Diagram showing the principle of the projection. Cone A.B.C. imposed upon sphere and touching it at P.P. P′P′.

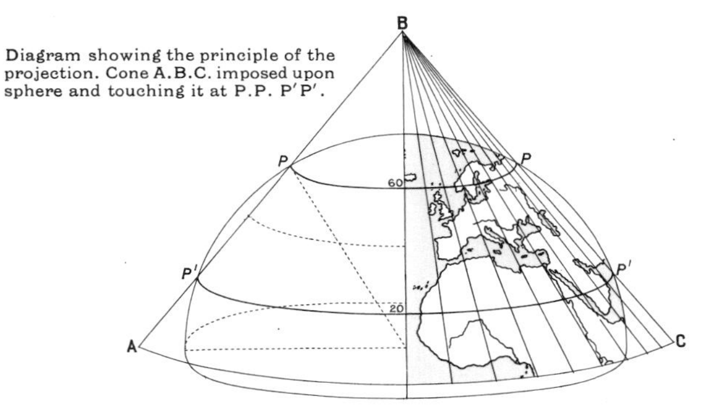

Portion of surface of cone spread out representing map. P.P. P′P′ the parallels where the cone coincides with the sphere.

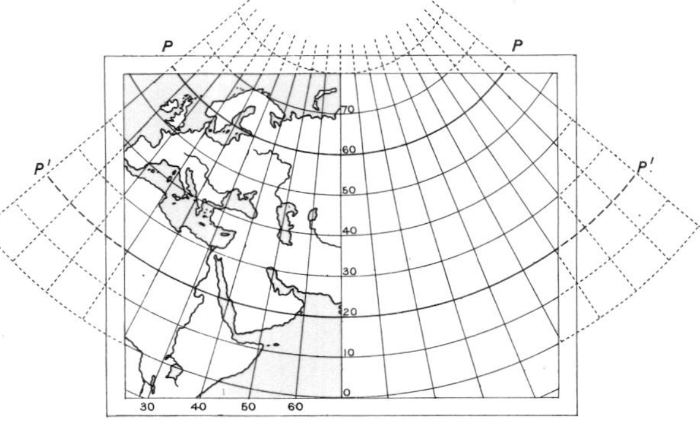

In this case the cone is supposed to cut the sphere along two parallels PP. and P′P′, which, however, are plotted their true distance apart (*i.e.* the distance along the arc PP′, not the chord). The map has therefore the advantage of coinciding with the globe along two parallels instead of one as in the Simple Conic.

BONNE'S PROJECTION

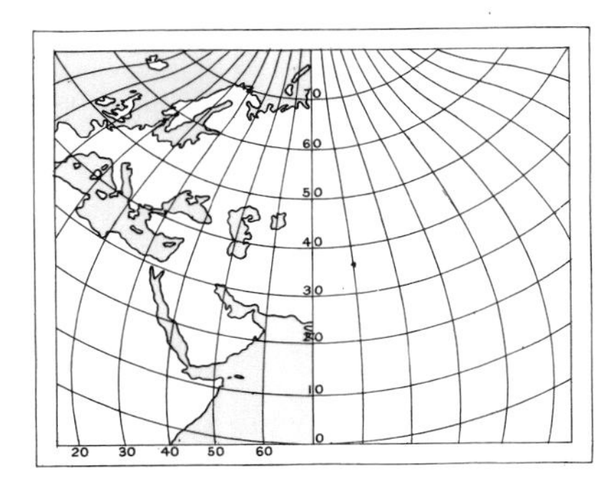

This is a development of the Conic Projection and differs from the pure Conic in that instead of distances being correctly measured along one parallel, true distances are measured along each parallel.

VAN DER GRINTEN'S PROJECTION

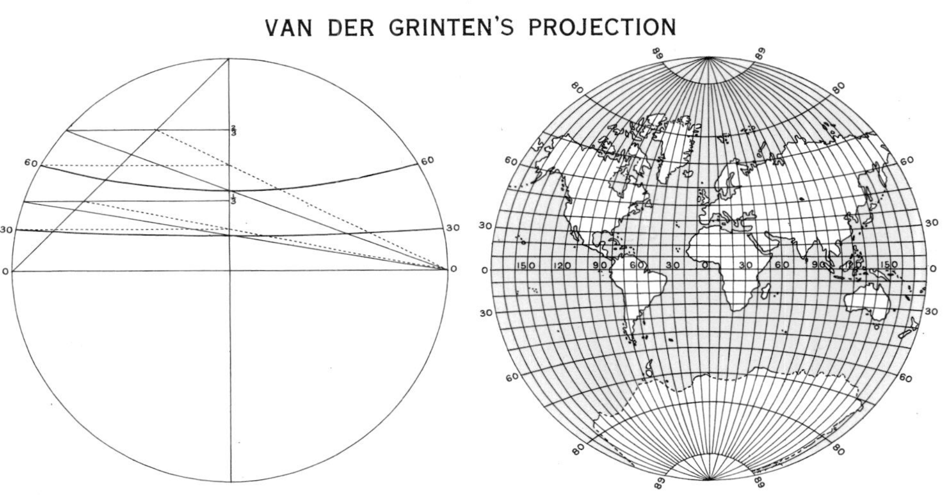

This projection strikes a mean between Mercator's and Mollweide's. It has neither the great exaggeration of land areas towards the Pole, of the former, nor the excessive angular distortion of the latter.

COVERING OF A 2½ INCH WORLD GLOBE IN GORES

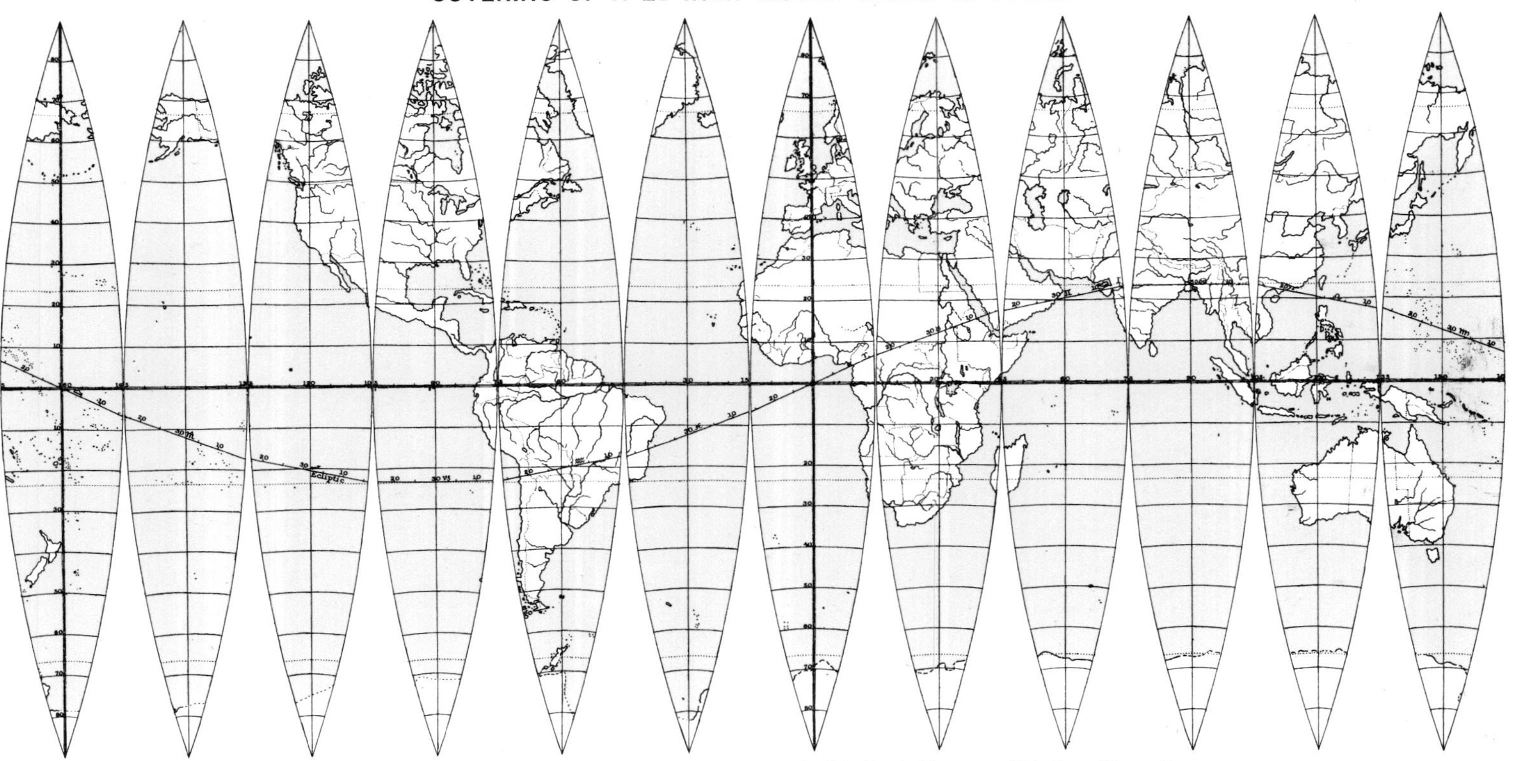

Note—These Gores are designed to be cut out and mounted on a Globe 2½ inches in diameter, which they will exactly cover.

MAP PROJECTIONS

LAMBERT'S AZIMUTHAL PROJECTION

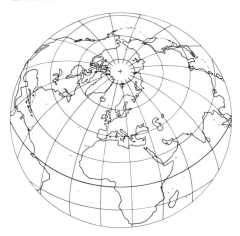

This projection is calculated from a selected central point as in a Polar, the crossing of degree lines being calculated to retain equal-area properties. It gives excellent treatment of large continental masses, but necessarily leads to some distension in circumferential areas.

AITOFF'S PROJECTION

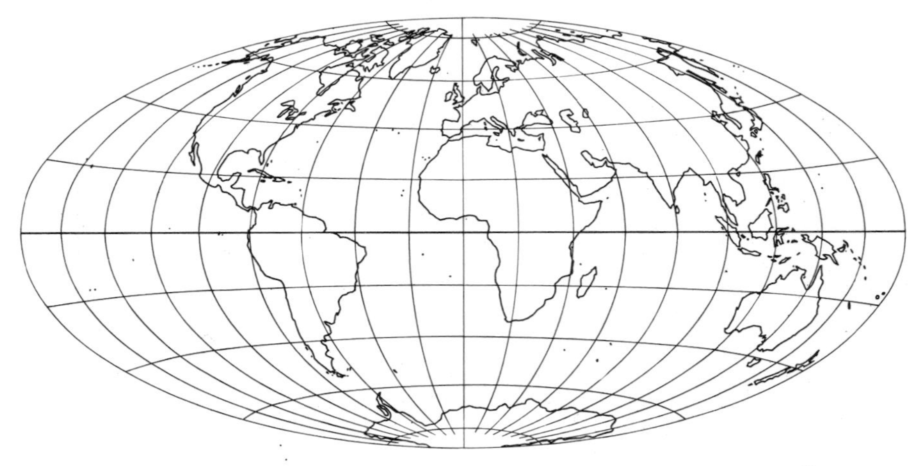

This is developed from Lambert's equal-area treatment of the hemisphere. Co-ordinates on the "X" axis are doubled while those on the "Y" remain as they were. The result is an ellipse containing an equal-area grid which may be subdivided for the whole world.

BARTHOLOMEW'S ATLANTIS PROJECTION

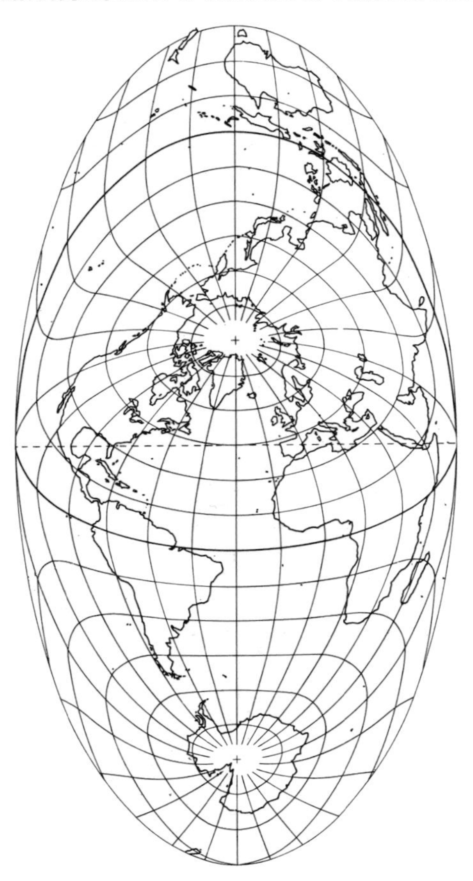

A novel application of Mollweide's Homolographic, the main axis being taken as a transverse great circle running through the poles. The minor axis lies on an oblique great circle touching 45°N. It is equal-area and shows the land masses in unbroken formation with regard to the N. Atlantic Ocean.

BARTHOLOMEW'S NORDIC PROJECTION

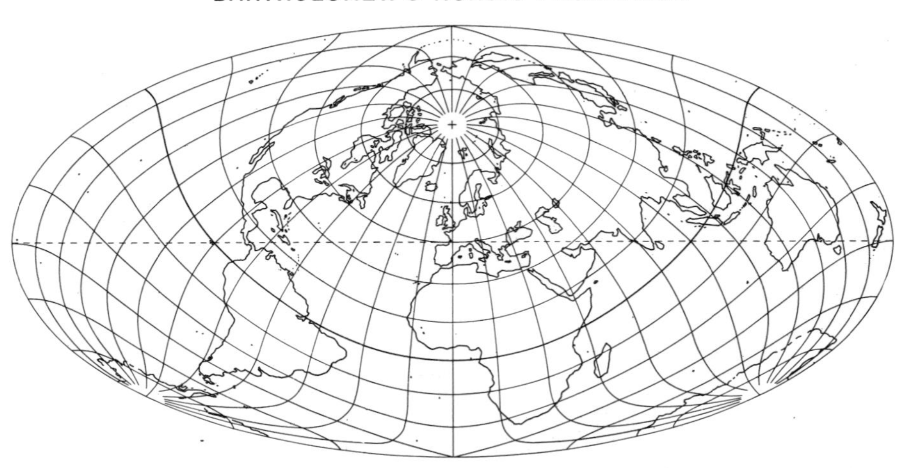

Like Aitoff's, this is a development of Lambert's Azimuthal. The main axis, however, instead of following the Equator becomes an oblique great circle, in this case touching 45° N. and 45° S. It is equal-area and gives a good basis for distributional maps, particularly in the north temperate and circum-polar areas.

BARTHOLOMEW'S RE-CENTRED SINUSOIDAL PROJECTION

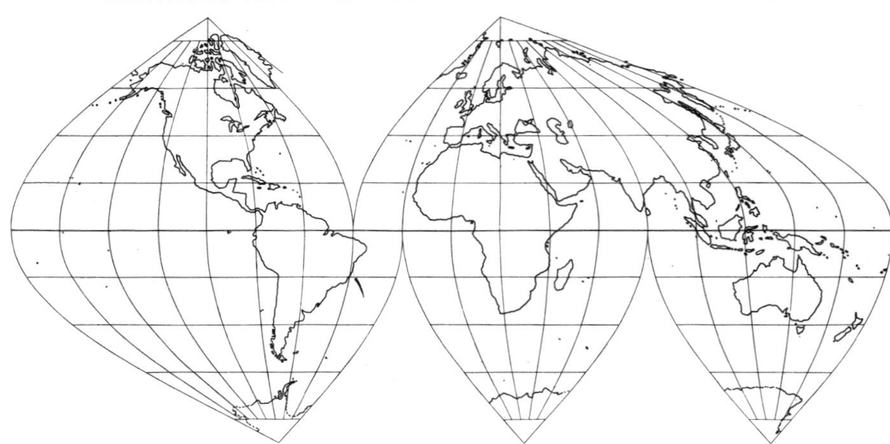

The equal-area properties and simple construction of the Sinusoidal are here applied to each continental mass separately so as to preserve optimum conformity. It was developed from Prof. Paul Goode's idea of the "Interrupted Homolographic" over which it claims certain advantages for purposes of land distribution.

TETRAHEDRAL PROJECTION

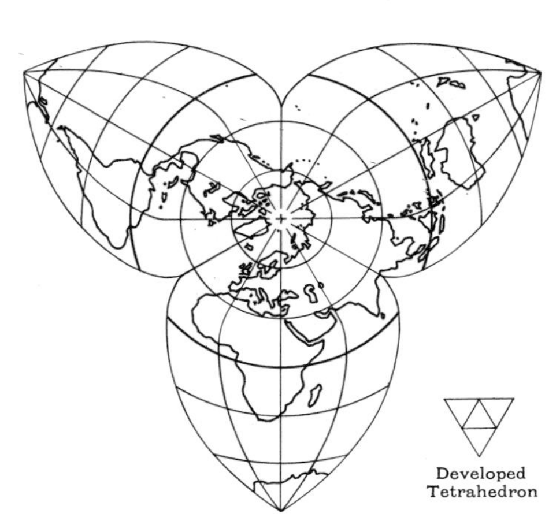

Developed Tetrahedron

One of the simplest yet most natural developments of the Globe. Prof. J. W. Gregory was first to point out the Earth's affinity to a tetrahedron, whose edges represented the main lines of mountain folding.

BARTHOLOMEW'S REGIONAL PROJECTION

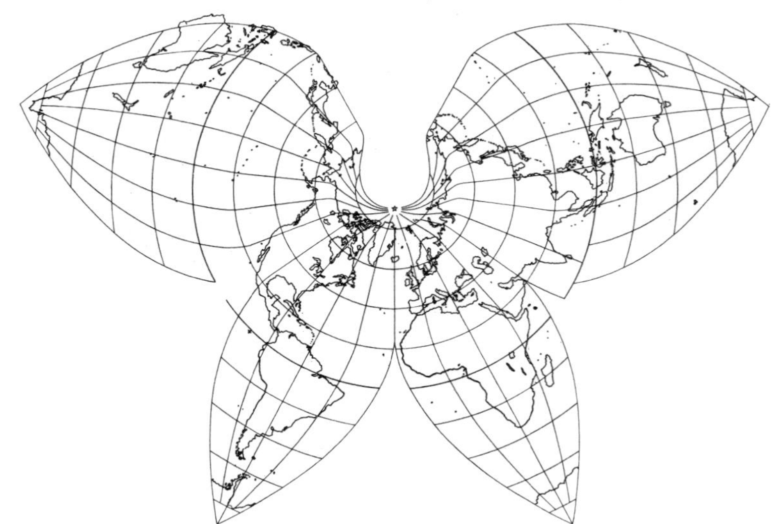

This arrangement claims to combine the best conformal properties with those as near equal-area as possible. It recognises that the chief field of man's development is in the North Temperate Zone and from a cone cutting the globe along two selected parallels it is continued on interrupted lines to complete the Earth.

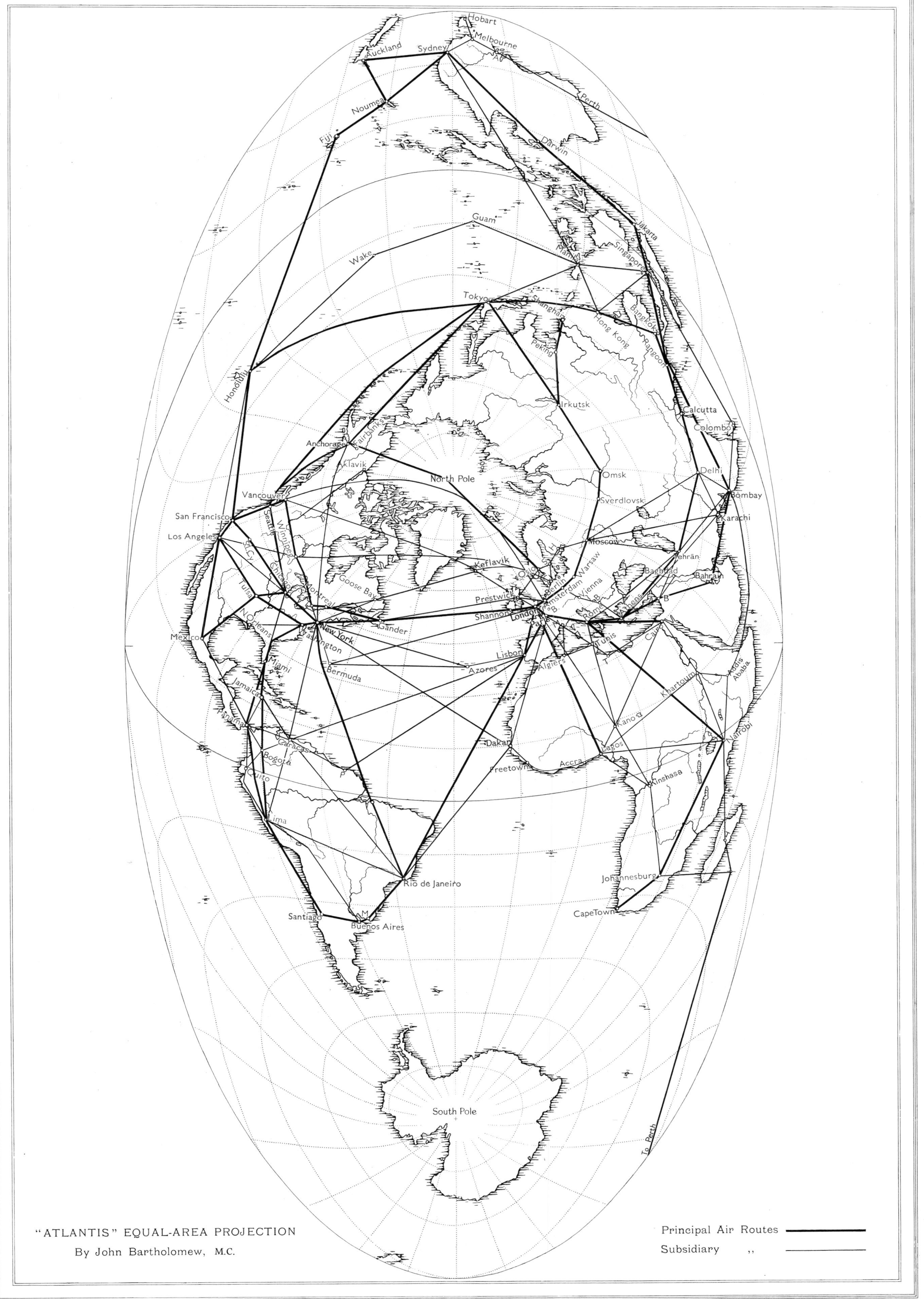
Hobart
Melbourne
Sydney
Auckland
Perth
Noumea
Fiji
Darwin
Guam
Wake
Jakarta
Singapore
Manila
Tokyo
Shanghai
Hong Kong
Bangkok
Rangoon
Peking
Honolulu
Irkutsk
Calcutta
Colombo
Anchorage
Fairbanks
Aklavik
North Pole
Omsk
Delhi
Bombay
Sverdlovsk
Karachi
Vancouver
San Francisco
Seattle
Winnipeg
Los Angeles
Moscow
Tehran
Keflavik
Baghdad
Bahrain
Goose Bay
Montreal
Chicago
Tulsa
Prestwick
Shannon
London
Amsterdam
Berlin
Warsaw
Vienna
Rome
Athens
N. Orleans
New York
Washington
Gander
Mexico
Lisbon
Tunis
Cairo
Miami
Bermuda
Azores
Algiers
Jamaica
Khartoum
Addis Ababa
Panama
Kano
Nairobi
Caracas
Dakar
Bogota
Lagos
Quito
Freetown
Accra
Kinshasa
Lima
Rio de Janeiro
Johannesburg
Santiago
Buenos Aires
CapeTown
South Pole
To Perth
"ATLANTIS" EQUAL-AREA PROJECTION
By John Bartholomew, M.C.
Principal Air Routes
Subsidiary ,,
© John Bartholomew & Son Ltd, Edinburgh

1:120M

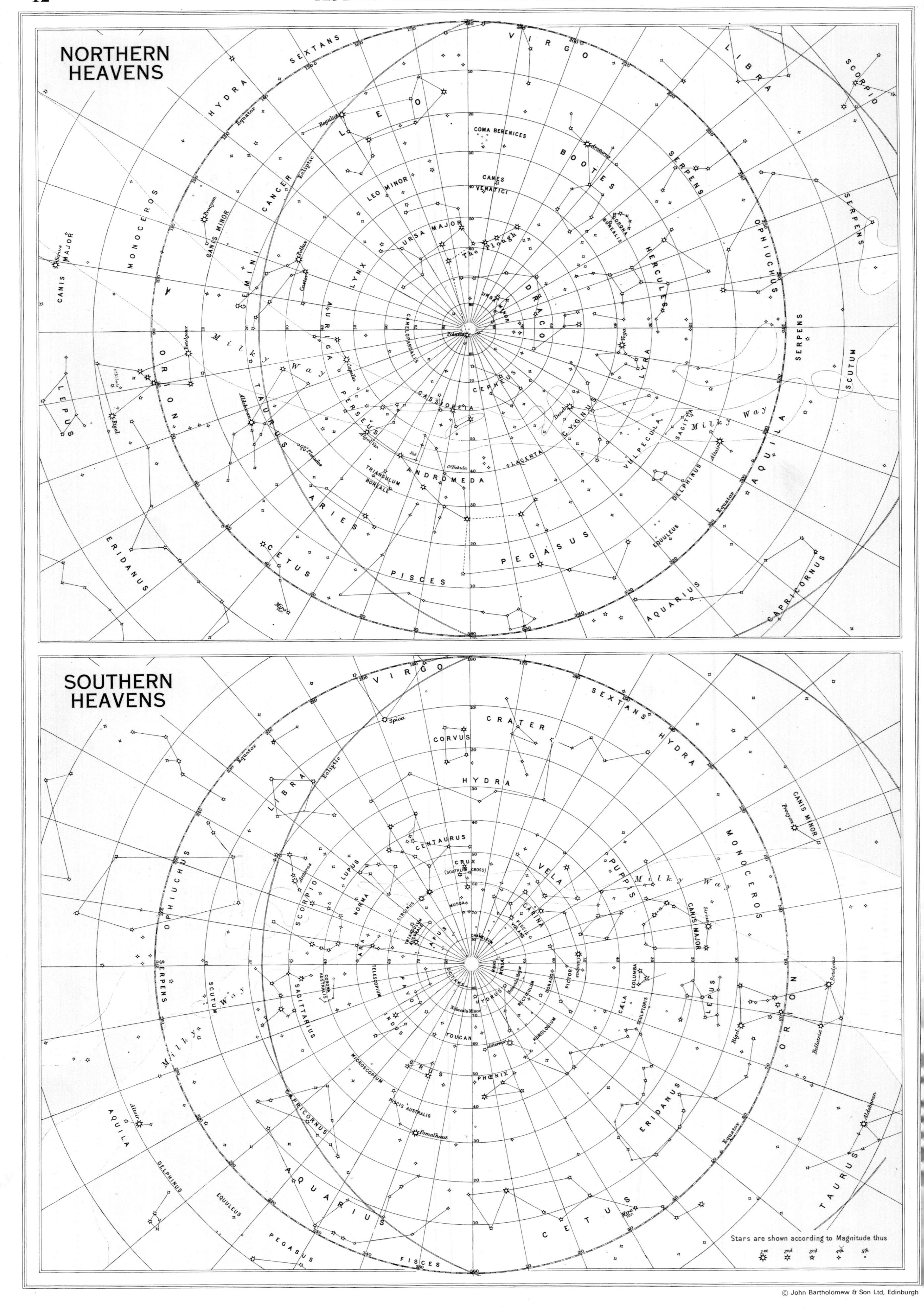
NORTHERN HEAVENS
SOUTHERN HEAVENS
Stars are shown according to Magnitude thus
1st 2nd 3rd 4th 5th

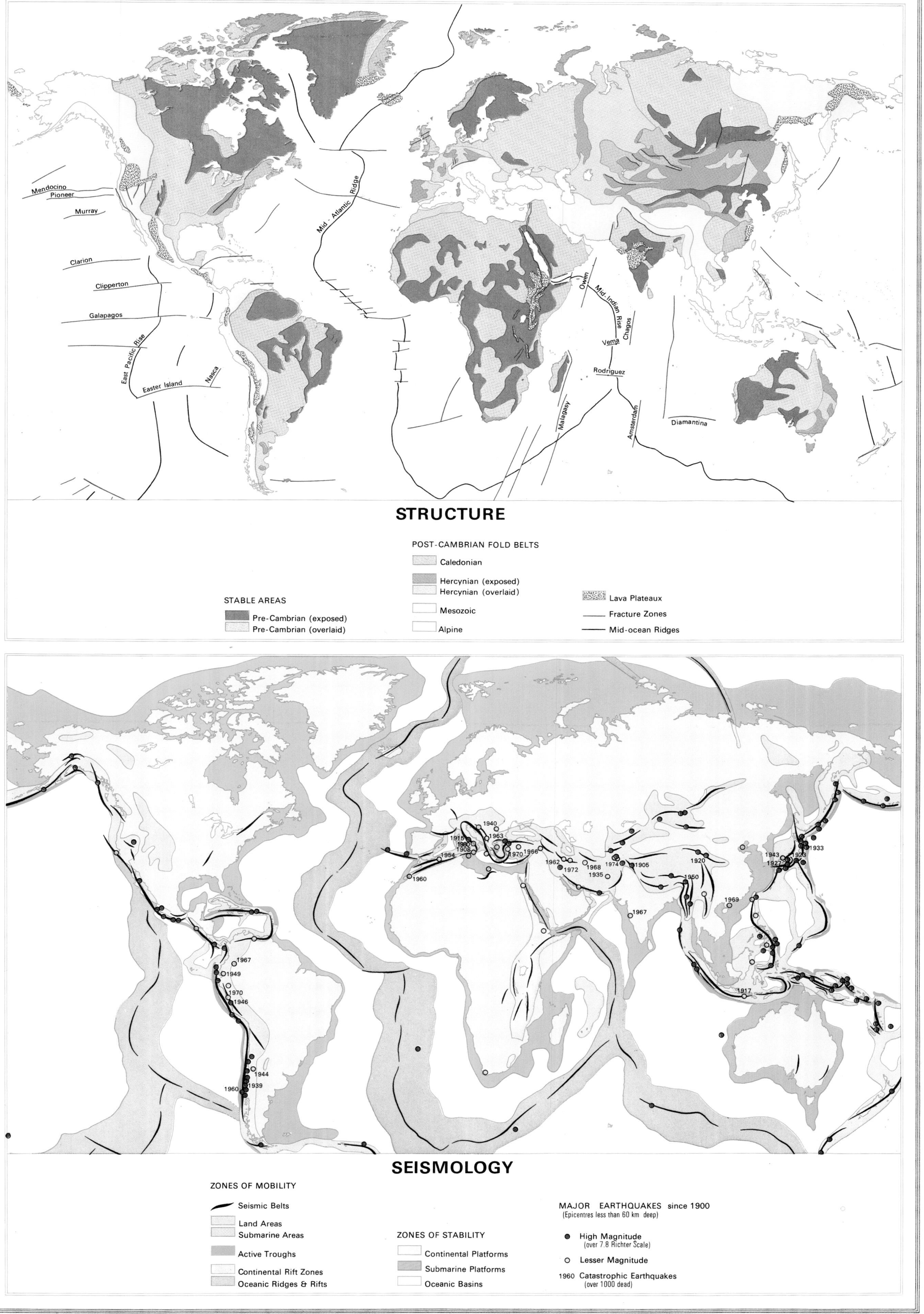
Mendocino
Pioneer
Murray
Clarion
Clipperton
Galapagos
East Pacific Rise
Easter Island
Nasca
Mid - Atlantic Ridge
Owen
Mid-Indian Rise
Chagos
Vema
Rodriguez
Malagasy
Amsterdam
Diamantina
STRUCTURE
POST-CAMBRIAN FOLD BELTS
Caledonian
Hercynian (exposed)
Hercynian (overlaid)
Mesozoic
Alpine
STABLE AREAS
Pre-Cambrian (exposed)
Pre-Cambrian (overlaid)
Lava Plateaux
Fracture Zones
Mid-ocean Ridges
SEISMOLOGY
ZONES OF MOBILITY
Seismic Belts
Land Areas
Submarine Areas
Active Troughs
Continental Rift Zones
Oceanic Ridges & Rifts
ZONES OF STABILITY
Continental Platforms
Submarine Platforms
Oceanic Basins
MAJOR EARTHQUAKES since 1900
(Epicentres less than 60 km deep)
High Magnitude
(over 7.8 Richter Scale)
Lesser Magnitude
1960 Catastrophic Earthquakes
(over 1000 dead)

1:140M

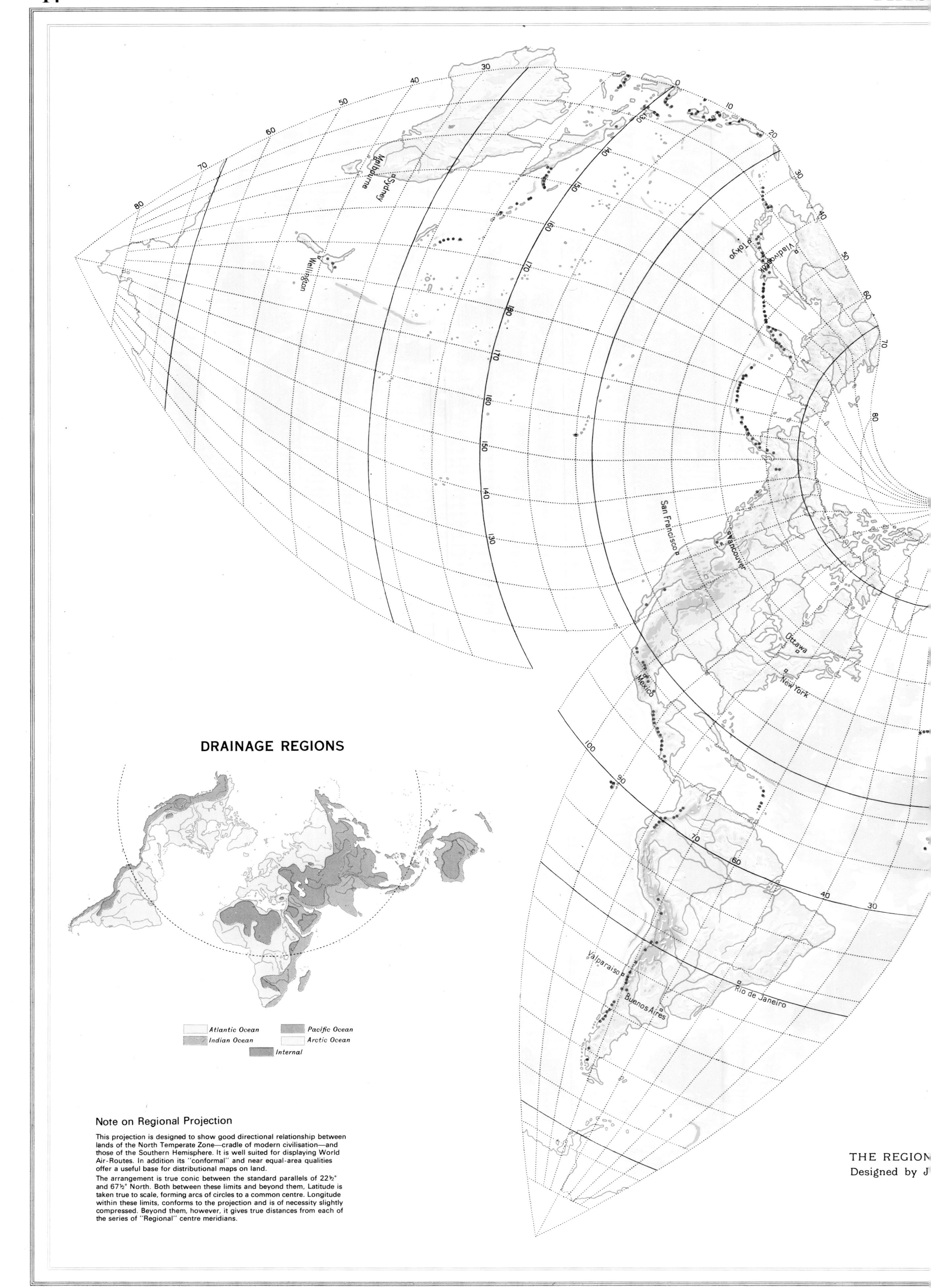

Note on Regional Projection

This projection is designed to show good directional relationship between lands of the North Temperate Zone—cradle of modern civilisation—and those of the Southern Hemisphere. It is well suited for displaying World Air-Routes. In addition its "conformal" and near equal-area qualities offer a useful base for distributional maps on land.

The arrangement is true conic between the standard parallels of 22½° and 67½° North. Both between these limits and beyond them, Latitude is taken true to scale, forming arcs of circles to a common centre. Longitude within these limits, conforms to the projection and is of necessity slightly compressed. Beyond them, however, it gives true distances from each of the series of "Regional" centre meridians.

Metres	7000	5000	4000	3000	1000	0
Feet	22960	16400	13120	9840	3280	0

Land Depression

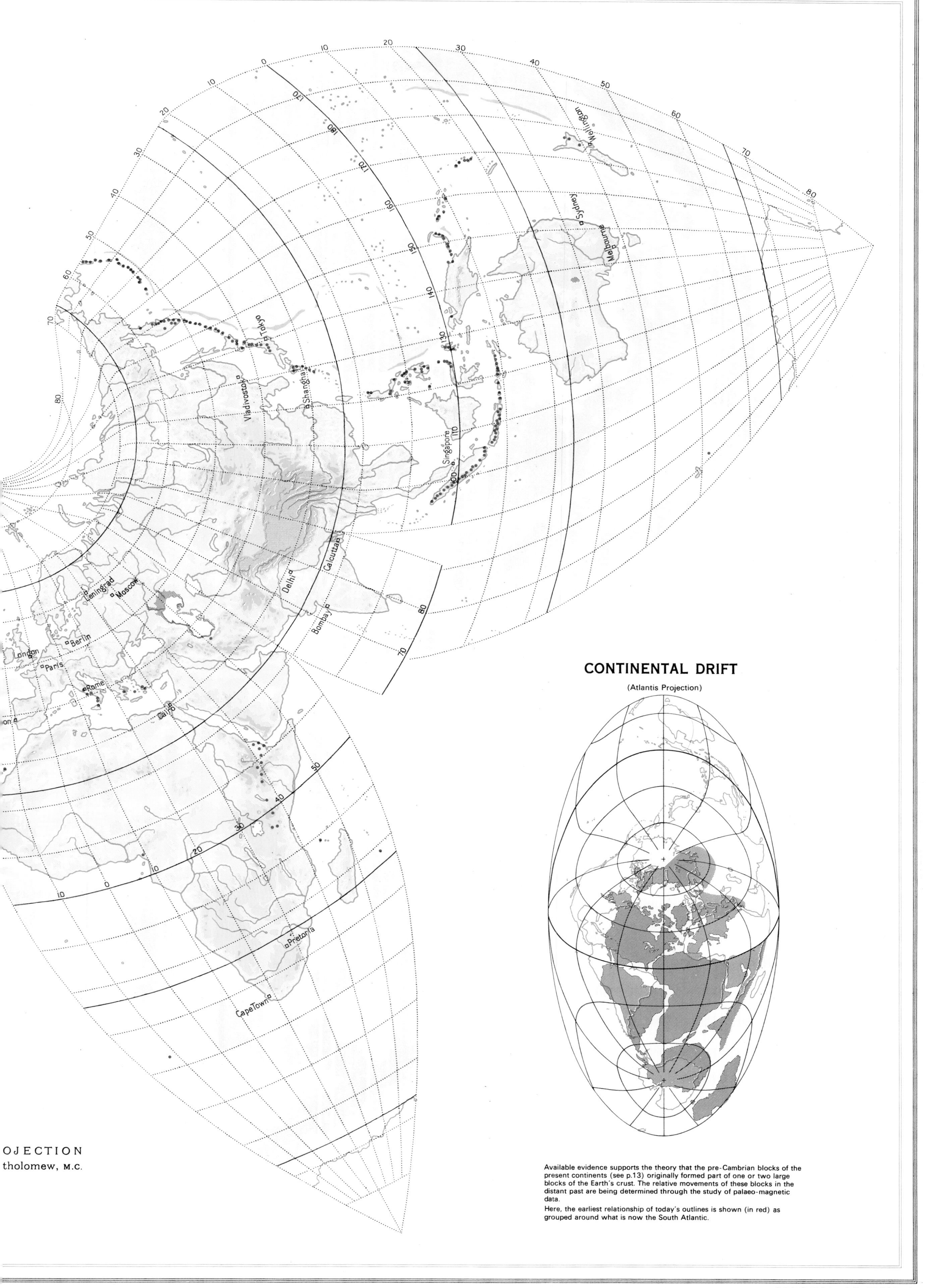

CONTINENTAL DRIFT

(Atlantis Projection)

Available evidence supports the theory that the pre-Cambrian blocks of the present continents (see p.13) originally formed part of one or two large blocks of the Earth's crust. The relative movements of these blocks in the distant past are being determined through the study of palaeo-magnetic data.

Here, the earliest relationship of today's outlines is shown (in red) as grouped around what is now the South Atlantic.

0	200	500	1000	2000	4000	Metres
0	660	1640	3280	6560	13120	Feet

• Active Volcanoes

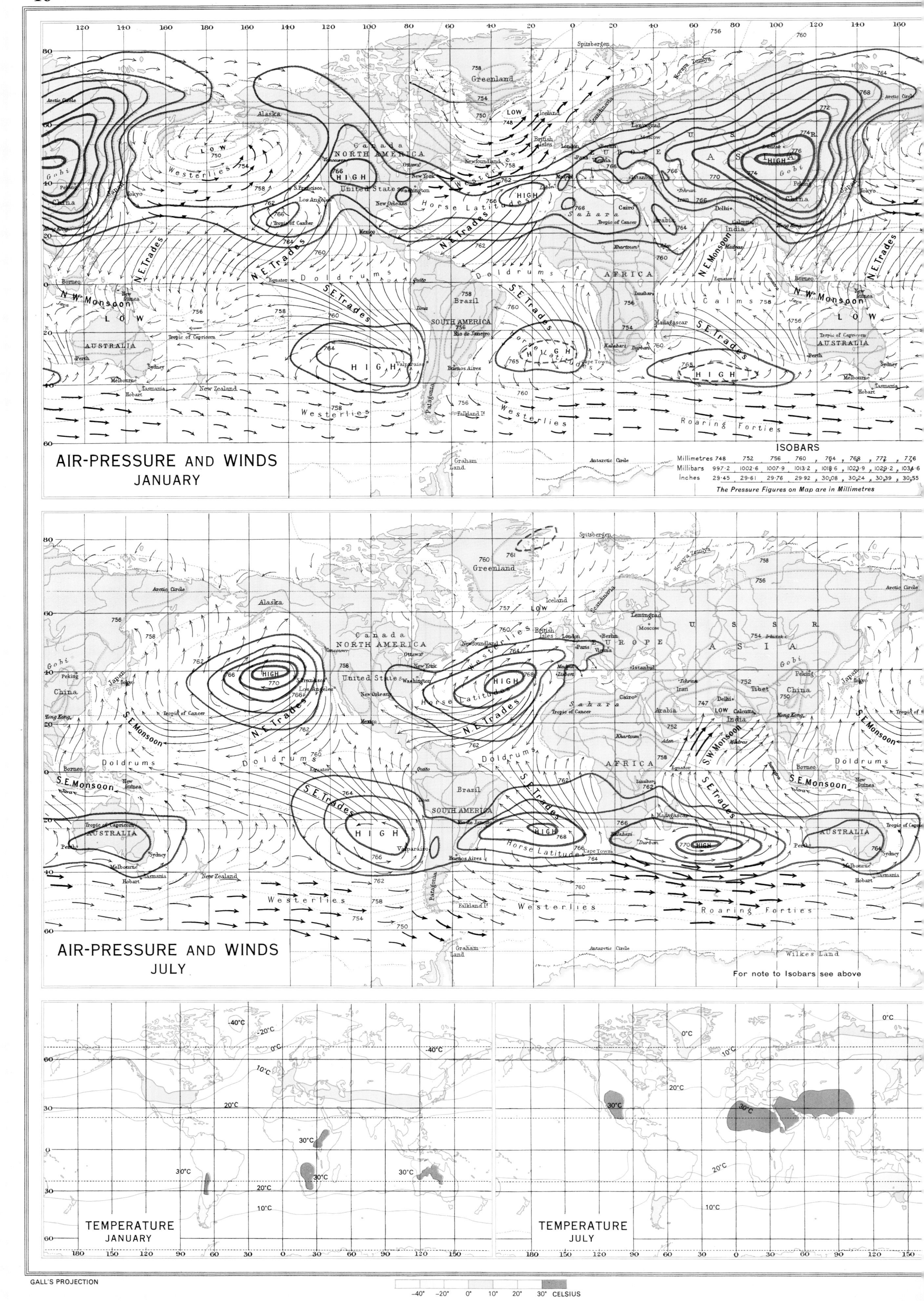
AIR-PRESSURE AND WINDS
JANUARY
ISOBARS
Millimetres 748 752 756 760 764 768 772 776
Millibars 997·2 1002·6 1007·9 1013·2 1018·6 1023·9 1029·2 1034·6
Inches 29·45 29·61 29·76 29·92 30·08 30·24 30·39 30·55
The Pressure Figures on Map are in Millimetres
Westerlies
Horse Latitudes
N.E. Trades
S.E. Trades
Doldrums
N.W. Monsoon
N.E. Monsoon
Calms
Roaring Forties
HIGH
LOW
AIR-PRESSURE AND WINDS
JULY
For note to Isobars see above
S.E. Monsoon
S.W. Monsoon
TEMPERATURE
JANUARY
TEMPERATURE
JULY
GALL'S PROJECTION
-40° -20° 0° 10° 20° 30° CELSIUS

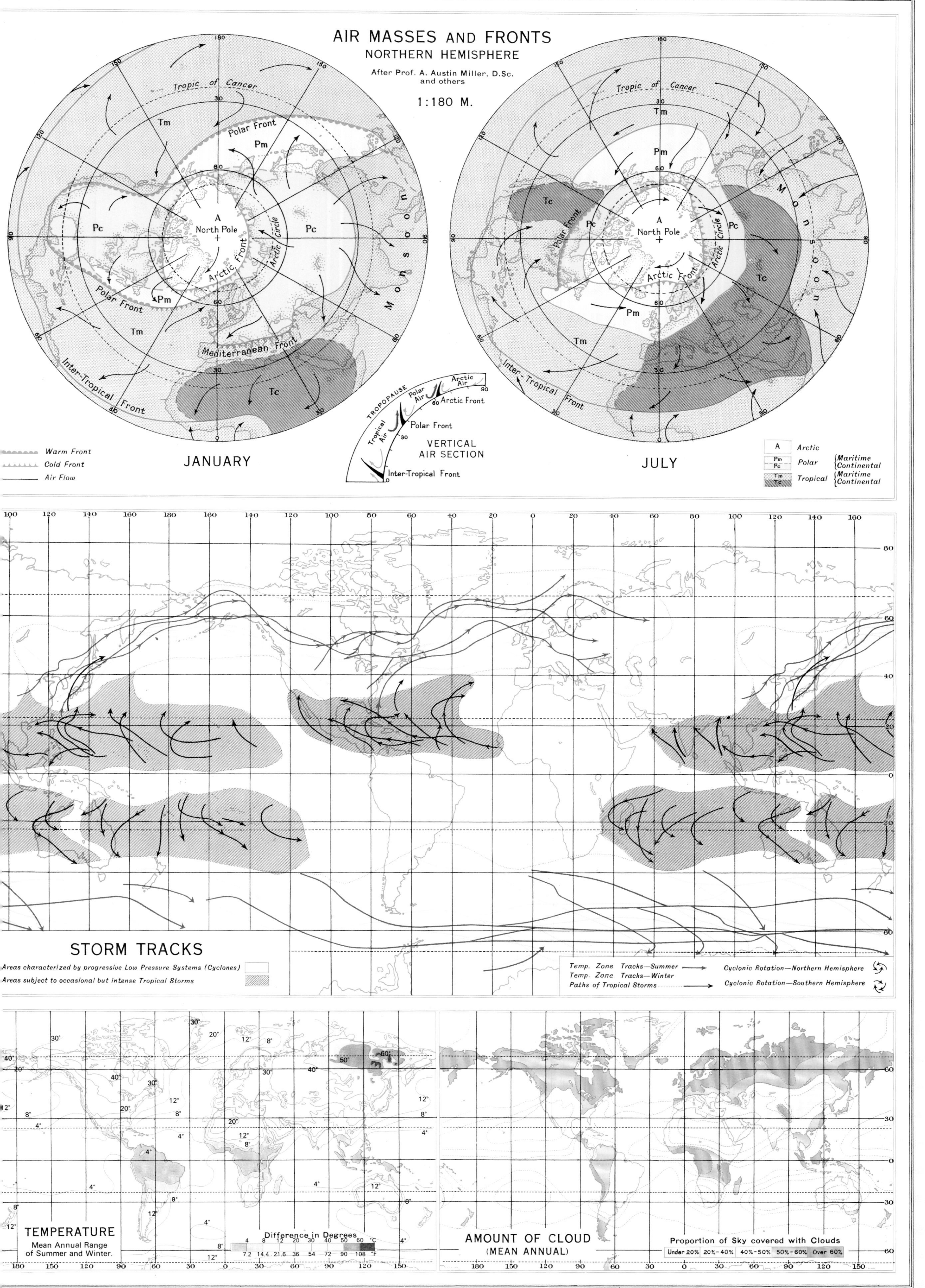
AIR MASSES AND FRONTS
NORTHERN HEMISPHERE
After Prof. A. Austin Miller, D.Sc. and others
1:180 M.
JANUARY
JULY
Tropic of Cancer
Polar Front
Arctic Front
Arctic Circle
Mediterranean Front
Inter-Tropical Front
Monsoon
North Pole
VERTICAL AIR SECTION
Tropopause
Arctic Air
Polar Air
Tropical Air
Arctic Front
Polar Front
Inter-Tropical Front
Warm Front
Cold Front
Air Flow
A Arctic
Pm Pc Polar Maritime Continental
Tm Tc Tropical Maritime Continental
STORM TRACKS
Areas characterized by progressive Low Pressure Systems (Cyclones)
Areas subject to occasional but intense Tropical Storms
Temp. Zone Tracks—Summer
Temp. Zone Tracks—Winter
Paths of Tropical Storms
Cyclonic Rotation—Northern Hemisphere
Cyclonic Rotation—Southern Hemisphere
TEMPERATURE
Mean Annual Range of Summer and Winter.
Difference in Degrees
4 8 12 20 30 40 50 60 °C
7.2 14.4 21.6 36 54 72 90 108 °F
AMOUNT OF CLOUD
(MEAN ANNUAL)
Proportion of Sky covered with Clouds
Under 20% 20%-40% 40%-50% 50%-60% Over 60%

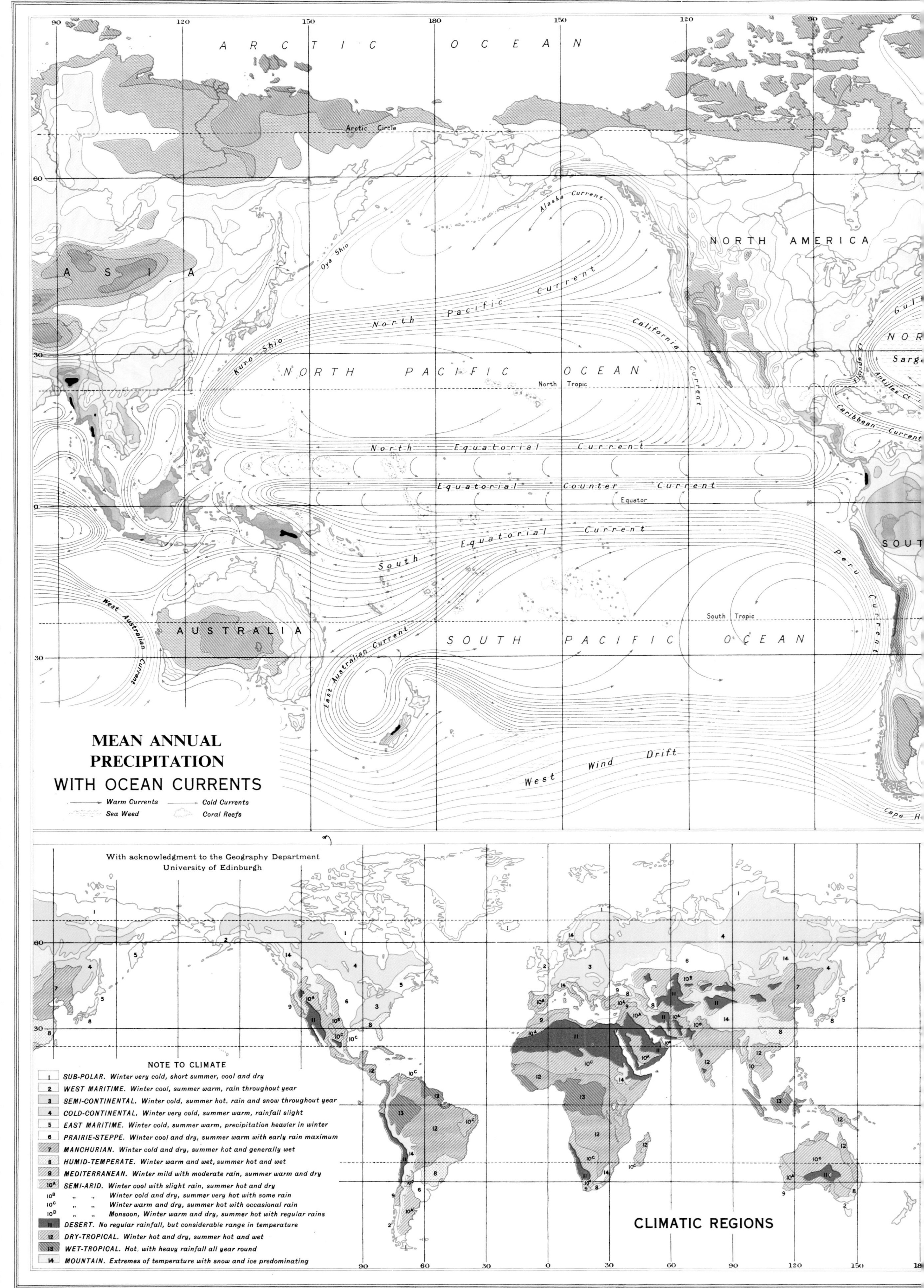
MEAN ANNUAL
PRECIPITATION
WITH OCEAN CURRENTS
Warm Currents
Cold Currents
Sea Weed
Coral Reefs
ARCTIC OCEAN
Arctic Circle
ASIA
NORTH AMERICA
AUSTRALIA
NORTH PACIFIC OCEAN
SOUTH PACIFIC OCEAN
North Tropic
South Tropic
Equator
Oya Shio
Kuro Shio
North Pacific Current
Alaska Current
California Current
North Equatorial Current
Equatorial Counter Current
South Equatorial Current
Peru Current
East Australian Current
West Australian Current
West Wind Drift
Florida Ct.
Antilles Ct.
Caribbean Current
With acknowledgment to the Geography Department
University of Edinburgh
NOTE TO CLIMATE
1 SUB-POLAR. Winter very cold, short summer, cool and dry
2 WEST MARITIME. Winter cool, summer warm, rain throughout year
3 SEMI-CONTINENTAL. Winter cold, summer hot, rain and snow throughout year
4 COLD-CONTINENTAL. Winter very cold, summer warm, rainfall slight
5 EAST MARITIME. Winter cold, summer warm, precipitation heavier in winter
6 PRAIRIE-STEPPE. Winter cool and dry, summer warm with early rain maximum
7 MANCHURIAN. Winter cold and dry, summer hot and generally wet
8 HUMID-TEMPERATE. Winter warm and wet, summer hot and wet
9 MEDITERRANEAN. Winter mild with moderate rain, summer warm and dry
10A SEMI-ARID. Winter cool with slight rain, summer hot and dry
10B " " Winter cold and dry, summer very hot with some rain
10C " " Winter warm and dry, summer hot with occasional rain
10D " " Monsoon. Winter warm and dry, summer hot with regular rains
11 DESERT. No regular rainfall, but considerable range in temperature
12 DRY-TROPICAL. Winter hot and dry, summer hot and wet
13 WET-TROPICAL. Hot, with heavy rainfall all year round
14 MOUNTAIN. Extremes of temperature with snow and ice predominating
CLIMATIC REGIONS

GALL'S PROJECTION

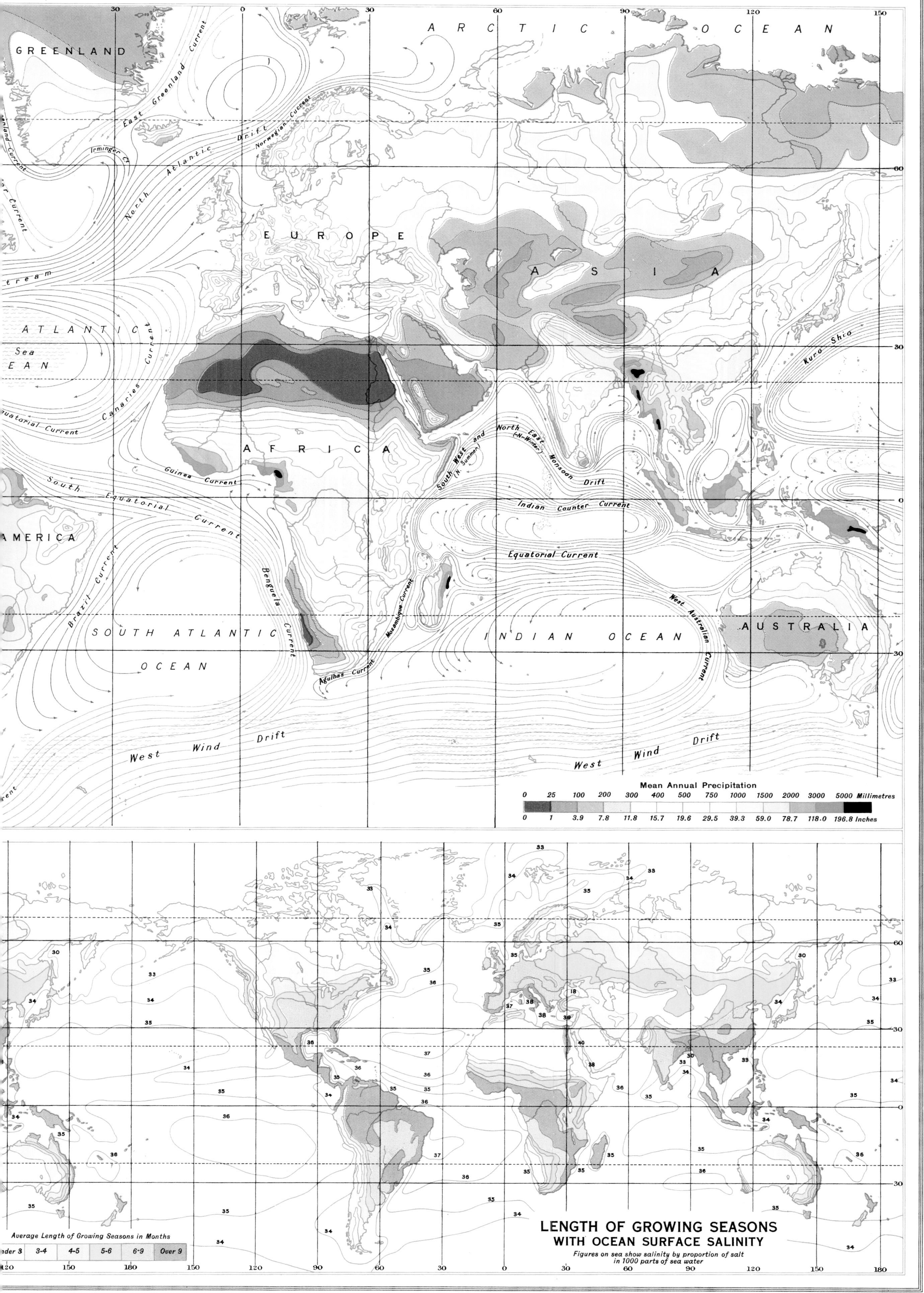
ARCTIC OCEAN
GREENLAND
East Greenland Current
Irminger Ct
Norwegian Current
North Atlantic Drift
EUROPE
ASIA
ATLANTIC
Sea
OCEAN
Canaries Current
Equatorial Current
AFRICA
Guinea Current
South Equatorial Current
AMERICA
Brazil Current
Benguela Current
SOUTH ATLANTIC OCEAN
Mozambique Current
Agulhas Current
South West (N. Summer) and North East (N. Winter) Monsoon Drift
Indian Counter Current
Equatorial Current
Kuro Shio
West Australian Current
INDIAN OCEAN
AUSTRALIA
West Wind Drift
West Wind Drift
Mean Annual Precipitation
0 25 100 200 300 400 500 750 1000 1500 2000 3000 5000 Millimetres
0 1 3.9 7.8 11.8 15.7 19.6 29.5 39.3 59.0 78.7 118.0 196.8 Inches
Average Length of Growing Seasons in Months
Under 3 3-4 4-5 5-6 6-9 Over 9
LENGTH OF GROWING SEASONS
WITH OCEAN SURFACE SALINITY
Figures on sea show salinity by proportion of salt in 1000 parts of sea water

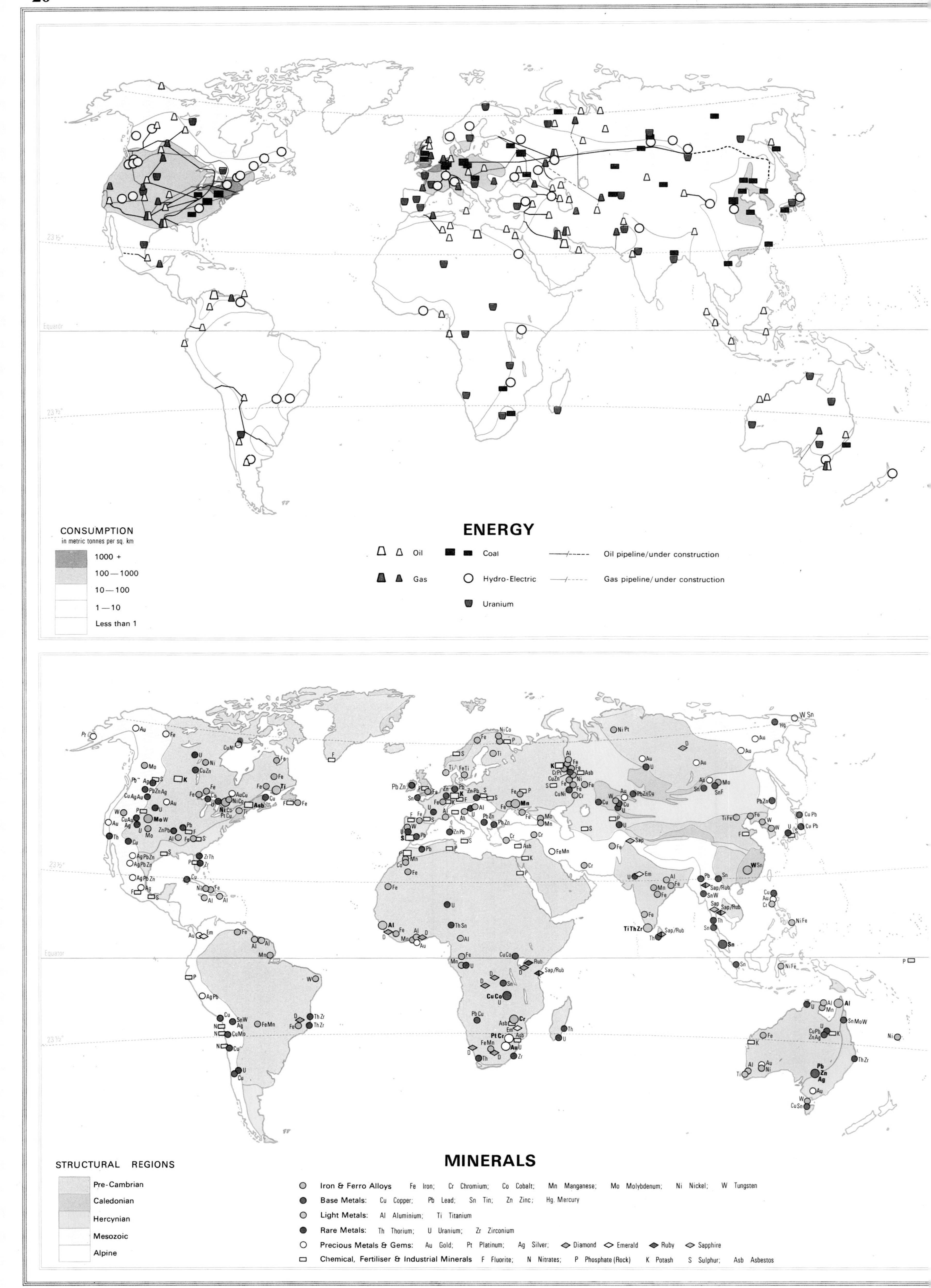
ENERGY
CONSUMPTION
in metric tonnes per sq. km
1000 +
100—1000
10—100
1—10
Less than 1
Oil
Gas
Coal
Hydro-Electric
Uranium
Oil pipeline/under construction
Gas pipeline/under construction
Equator
MINERALS
STRUCTURAL REGIONS
Pre-Cambrian
Caledonian
Hercynian
Mesozoic
Alpine
Iron & Ferro Alloys Fe Iron; Cr Chromium; Co Cobalt; Mn Manganese; Mo Molybdenum; Ni Nickel; W Tungsten
Base Metals: Cu Copper; Pb Lead; Sn Tin; Zn Zinc; Hg. Mercury
Light Metals: Al Aluminium; Ti Titanium
Rare Metals: Th Thorium; U Uranium; Zr Zirconium
Precious Metals & Gems: Au Gold; Pt Platinum; Ag Silver; Diamond Emerald Ruby Sapphire
Chemical, Fertiliser & Industrial Minerals F Fluorite; N Nitrates; P Phosphate (Rock) K Potash S Sulphur; Asb Asbestos

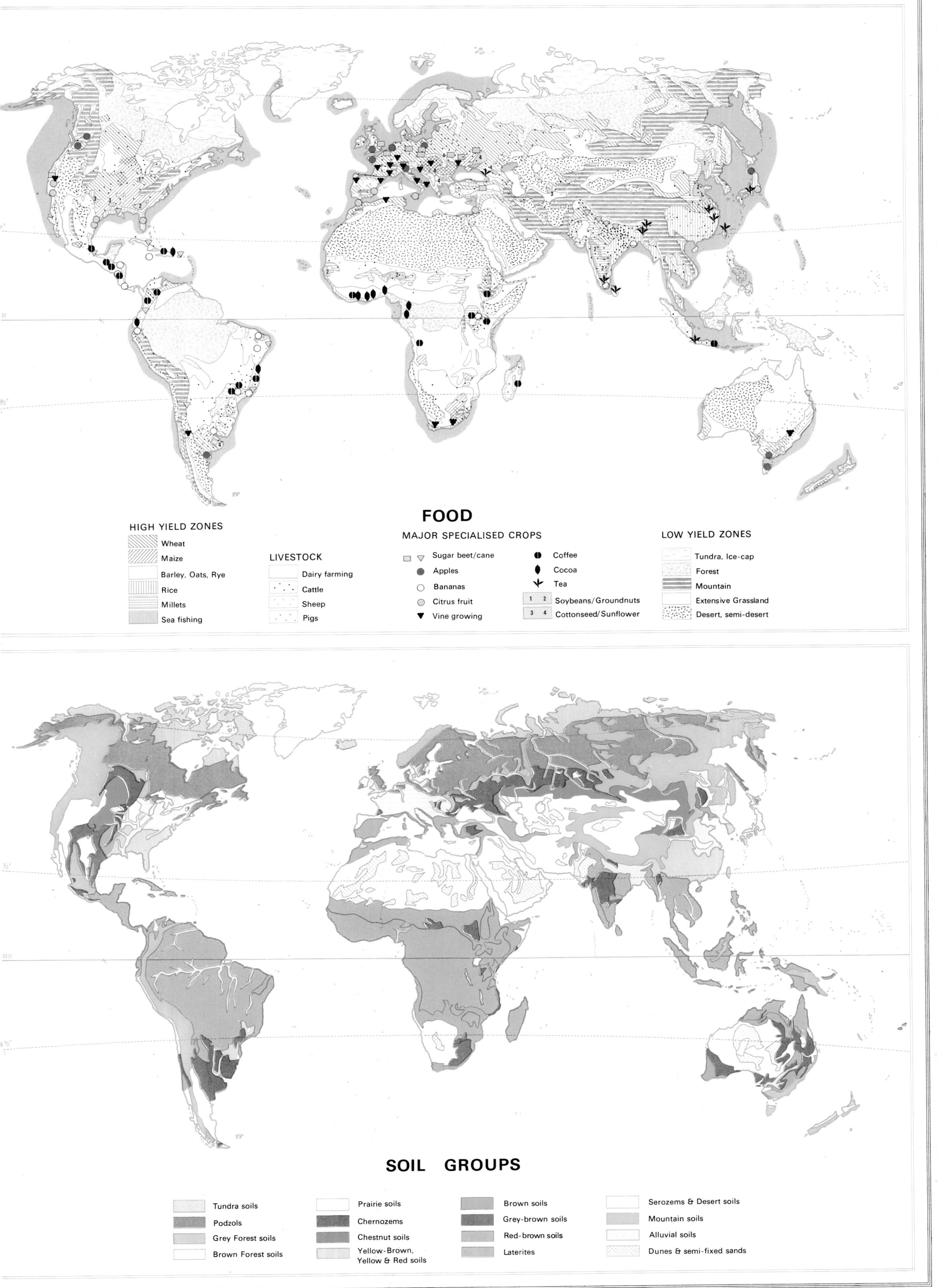
FOOD
HIGH YIELD ZONES
Wheat
Maize
Barley, Oats, Rye
Rice
Millets
Sea fishing
LIVESTOCK
Dairy farming
Cattle
Sheep
Pigs
MAJOR SPECIALISED CROPS
Sugar beet/cane
Apples
Bananas
Citrus fruit
Vine growing
Coffee
Cocoa
Tea
1 2 Soybeans/Groundnuts
3 4 Cottonseed/Sunflower
LOW YIELD ZONES
Tundra, Ice-cap
Forest
Mountain
Extensive Grassland
Desert, semi-desert
SOIL GROUPS
Tundra soils
Podzols
Grey Forest soils
Brown Forest soils
Prairie soils
Chernozems
Chestnut soils
Yellow-Brown, Yellow & Red soils
Brown soils
Grey-brown soils
Red-brown soils
Laterites
Serozems & Desert soils
Mountain soils
Alluvial soils
Dunes & semi-fixed sands

1:135M

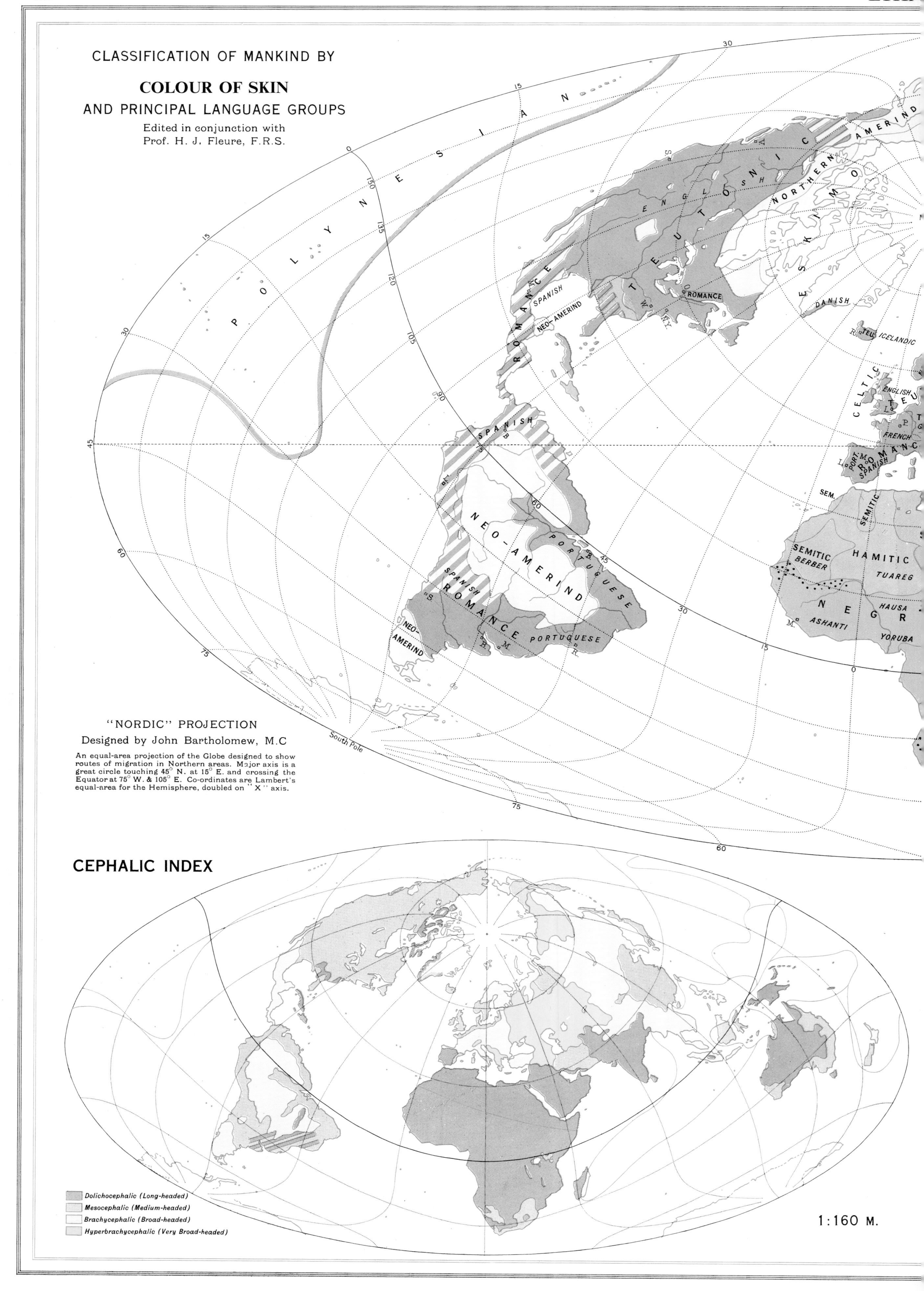
CLASSIFICATION OF MANKIND BY
COLOUR OF SKIN
AND PRINCIPAL LANGUAGE GROUPS
Edited in conjunction with
Prof. H. J. Fleure, F.R.S.
POLYNESIAN
TEUTONIC
ENGLISH
ROMANCE
SPANISH
NEO-AMERIND
NORTHERN AMERIND
ESKIMO
DANISH
ICELANDIC
CELTIC
FRENCH
SEMITIC
BERBER
HAMITIC
TUAREG
HAUSA
ASHANTI
YORUBA
NEGR
PORTUGUESE
"NORDIC" PROJECTION
Designed by John Bartholomew, M.C
An equal-area projection of the Globe designed to show routes of migration in Northern areas. Major axis is a great circle touching 45° N. at 15° E. and crossing the Equator at 75° W. & 105° E. Co-ordinates are Lambert's equal-area for the Hemisphere, doubled on "X" axis.
South Pole
CEPHALIC INDEX
Dolichocephalic (Long-headed)
Mesocephalic (Medium-headed)
Brachycephalic (Broad-headed)
Hyperbrachycephalic (Very Broad-headed)
1:160 M.

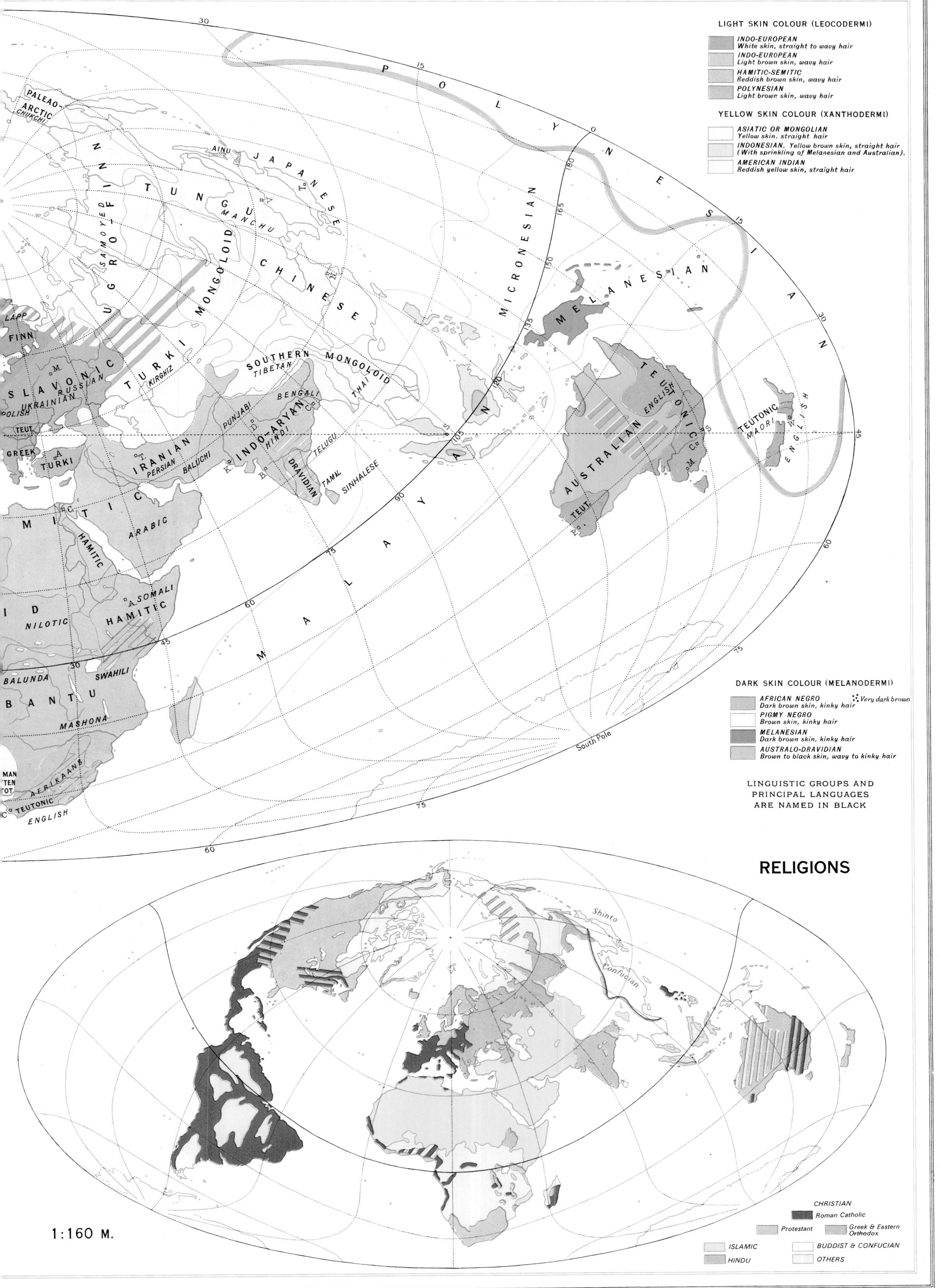
LIGHT SKIN COLOUR (LEOCODERMI)
INDO-EUROPEAN
White skin, straight to wavy hair
INDO-EUROPEAN
Light brown skin, wavy hair
HAMITIC-SEMITIC
Reddish brown skin, wavy hair
POLYNESIAN
Light brown skin, wavy hair
YELLOW SKIN COLOUR (XANTHODERMI)
ASIATIC OR MONGOLIAN
Yellow skin, straight hair
INDONESIAN. Yellow brown skin, straight hair
(With sprinkling of Melanesian and Australian).
AMERICAN INDIAN
Reddish yellow skin, straight hair
DARK SKIN COLOUR (MELANODERMI)
AFRICAN NEGRO
Dark brown skin, kinky hair
Very dark brown
PIGMY NEGRO
Brown skin, kinky hair
MELANESIAN
Dark brown skin, kinky hair
AUSTRALO-DRAVIDIAN
Brown to black skin, wavy to kinky hair
LINGUISTIC GROUPS AND
PRINCIPAL LANGUAGES
ARE NAMED IN BLACK
POLYNESIAN
MICRONESIAN
MELANESIAN
MALAYAN
PALEAO-ARCTIC
CHUKCHI
AINU
JAPANESE
TUNGU
MANCHU
UGRO-FINN
SAMOYED
MONGOLOID
CHINESE
TURKI
KIRGHIZ
SOUTHERN MONGOLOID
TIBETAN
THAI
BENGALI
PUNJABI
INDO-ARYAN
HINDI
TELUGU
DRAVIDIAN
TAMIL
SINHALESE
IRANIAN
PERSIAN
BALUCHI
LAPP
FINN
SLAVONIC
RUSSIAN
UKRAINIAN
POLISH
TEUT
GREEK
TURKI
SEMITIC
ARABIC
HAMITIC
SOMALI
NILOTIC
SWAHILI
BALUNDA
BANTU
MASHONA
AFRIKAANS
TEUTONIC
ENGLISH
AUSTRALIAN
TEUTONIC
ENGLISH
TEUT
MAORI
South Pole
RELIGIONS
Shinto
Confucian
CHRISTIAN
Roman Catholic
Protestant
Greek & Eastern Orthodox
ISLAMIC
HINDU
BUDDHIST & CONFUCIAN
OTHERS
1:160 M.

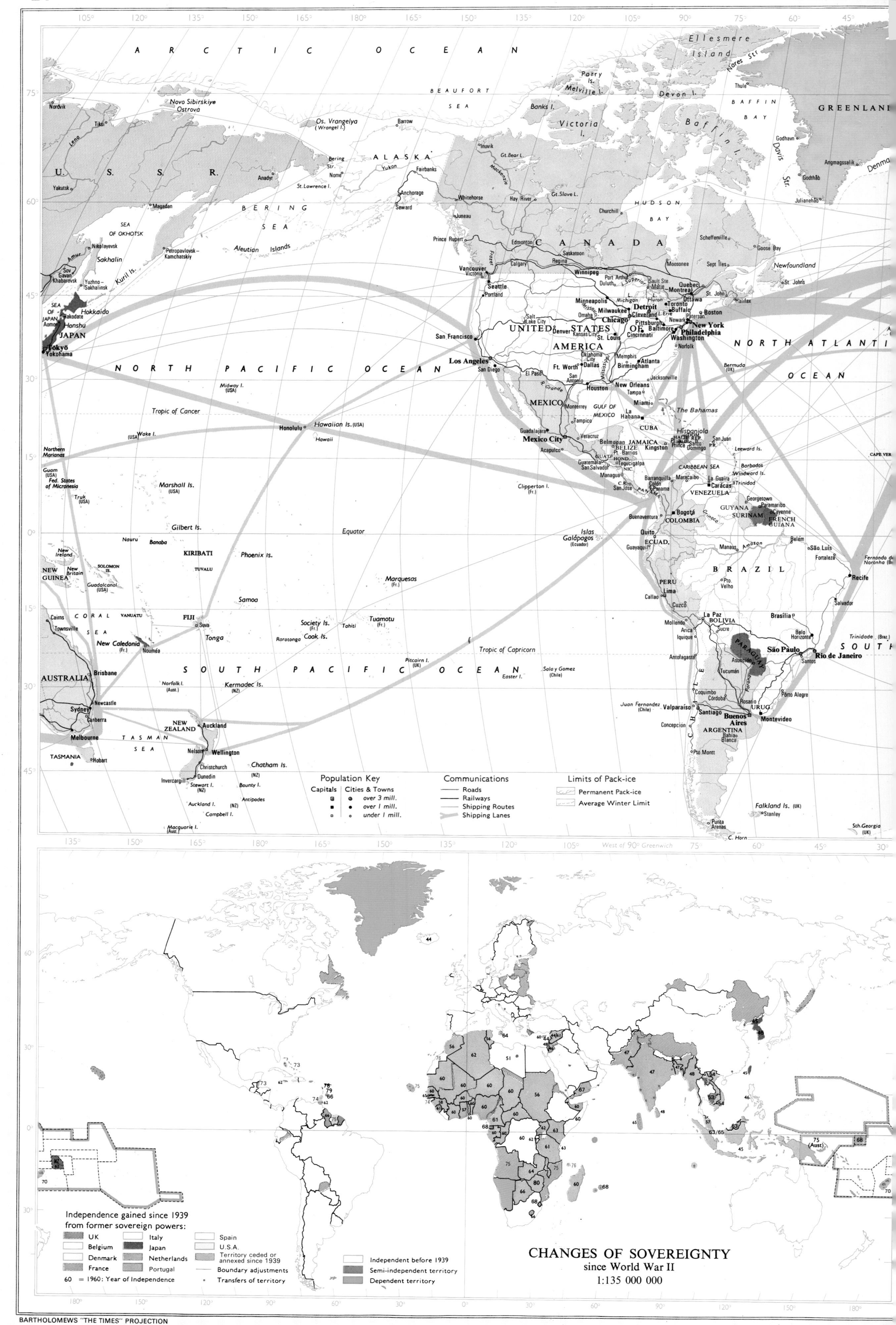
ARCTIC OCEAN
BEAUFORT SEA
BERING SEA
SEA OF OKHOTSK
HUDSON BAY
BAFFIN BAY
GREENLAND
ALASKA
CANADA
UNITED STATES OF AMERICA
MEXICO
U. S. S. R.
JAPAN
NORTH PACIFIC OCEAN
SOUTH PACIFIC OCEAN
NORTH ATLANTIC OCEAN
CARIBBEAN SEA
GULF OF MEXICO
CORAL SEA
TASMAN SEA
AUSTRALIA
NEW ZEALAND
BRAZIL
ARGENTINA
COLOMBIA
VENEZUELA
PERU
BOLIVIA
Tropic of Cancer
Equator
Tropic of Capricorn
Population Key
Capitals
Cities & Towns
over 3 mill.
over 1 mill.
under 1 mill.
Communications
Roads
Railways
Shipping Routes
Shipping Lanes
Limits of Pack-ice
Permanent Pack-ice
Average Winter Limit
West of 90° Greenwich
Independence gained since 1939
from former sovereign powers:
UK
Belgium
Denmark
France
Italy
Japan
Netherlands
Portugal
Spain
U.S.A.
Territory ceded or annexed since 1939
Boundary adjustments
Transfers of territory
60 = 1960: Year of Independence
Independent before 1939
Semi-independent territory
Dependent territory
CHANGES OF SOVEREIGNTY
since World War II
1:135 000 000

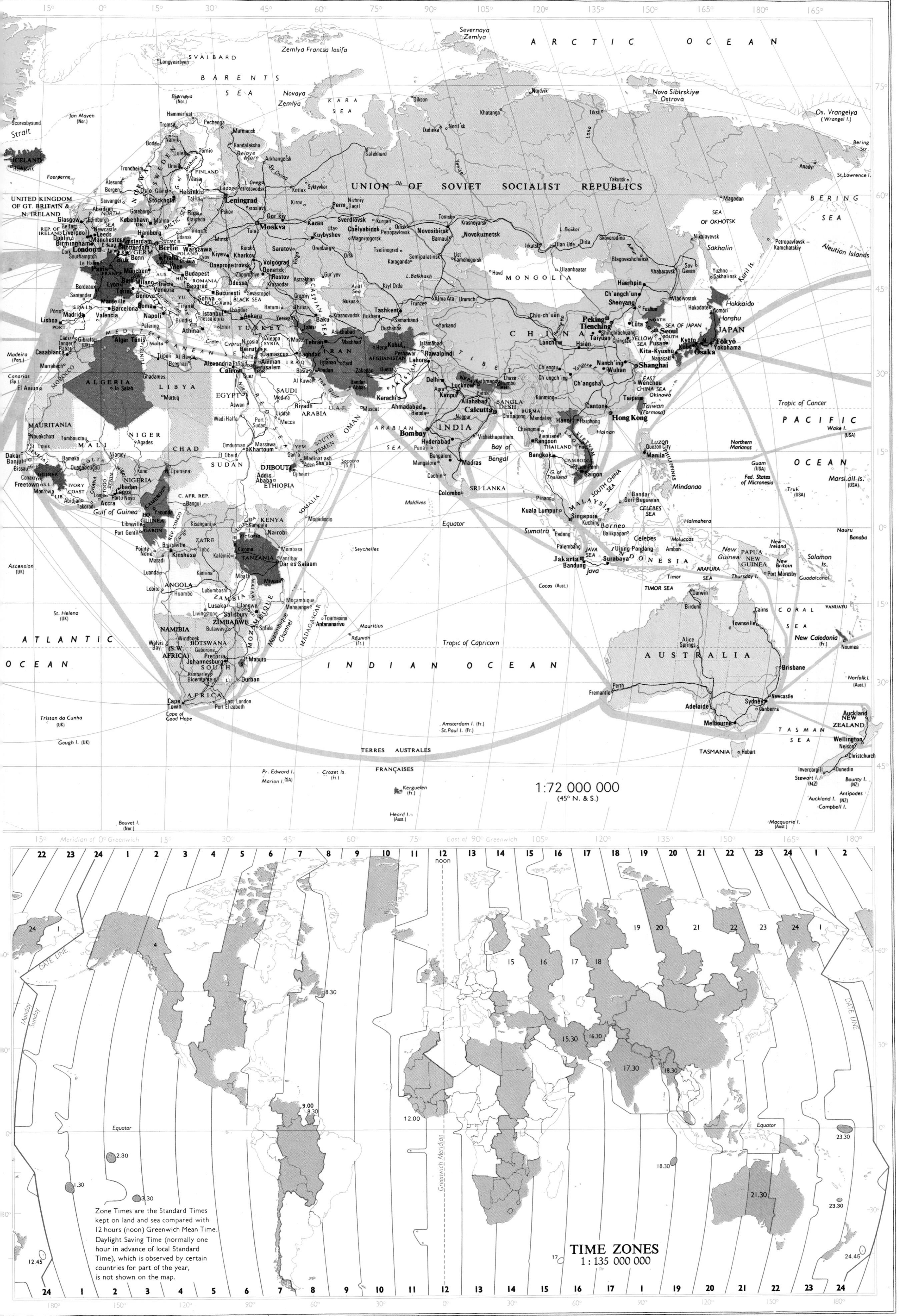
ARCTIC OCEAN
Severnaya Zemlya
Zemlya Frantsa Iosifa
SVALBARD
BARENTS SEA
Novaya Zemlya
KARA SEA
Novo Sibirskiye Ostrova
Os. Vrangelya (Wrangel I.)
Bering Str.
UNION OF SOVIET SOCIALIST REPUBLICS
BERING SEA
SEA OF OKHOTSK
Aleutian Islands
Sakhalin
Kuril Is.
UNITED KINGDOM OF GT. BRITAIN & N. IRELAND
ICELAND
Leningrad
Moskva
Novosibirsk
MONGOLIA
CHINA
Peking
Shanghai
Hokkaido
Honshu
JAPAN
Tōkyō
Osaka
Seoul
SEA OF JAPAN
Taiwan (Formosa)
Hong Kong
TURKEY
IRAN
AFGHANISTAN
PAKISTAN
TIBET
INDIA
Bombay
Calcutta
Madras
Bay of Bengal
ARABIAN SEA
SRI LANKA
SAUDI ARABIA
MEDITERRANEAN SEA
ALGERIA
LIBYA
EGYPT
Cairo
MAURITANIA
MALI
NIGER
CHAD
SUDAN
ETHIOPIA
NIGERIA
CAMEROON
Gulf of Guinea
ZAIRE
KENYA
TANZANIA
ANGOLA
ZAMBIA
ZIMBABWE
NAMIBIA (S.W. AFRICA)
BOTSWANA
SOUTH AFRICA
MOZAMBIQUE
MADAGASCAR
Cape Town
Cape of Good Hope
ATLANTIC OCEAN
INDIAN OCEAN
Tropic of Capricorn
Equator
Tropic of Cancer
PACIFIC OCEAN
Luzon
Manila
PHILIPPINES
Mindanao
MALAYSIA
Singapore
Borneo
Sumatra
Jakarta
Java
INDONESIA
PAPUA NEW GUINEA
TIMOR SEA
ARAFURA SEA
CORAL SEA
AUSTRALIA
Perth
Adelaide
Melbourne
Sydney
Brisbane
TASMANIA
TASMAN SEA
NEW ZEALAND
Wellington
New Caledonia (Fr.)
TERRES AUSTRALES FRANÇAISES
Kerguelen (Fr.)
1:72 000 000
(45° N. & S.)
TIME ZONES
1 : 135 000 000
Greenwich Meridian
DATE LINE
Monday
Sunday
noon
Zone Times are the Standard Times kept on land and sea compared with 12 hours (noon) Greenwich Mean Time. Daylight Saving Time (normally one hour in advance of local Standard Time), which is observed by certain countries for part of the year, is not shown on the map.

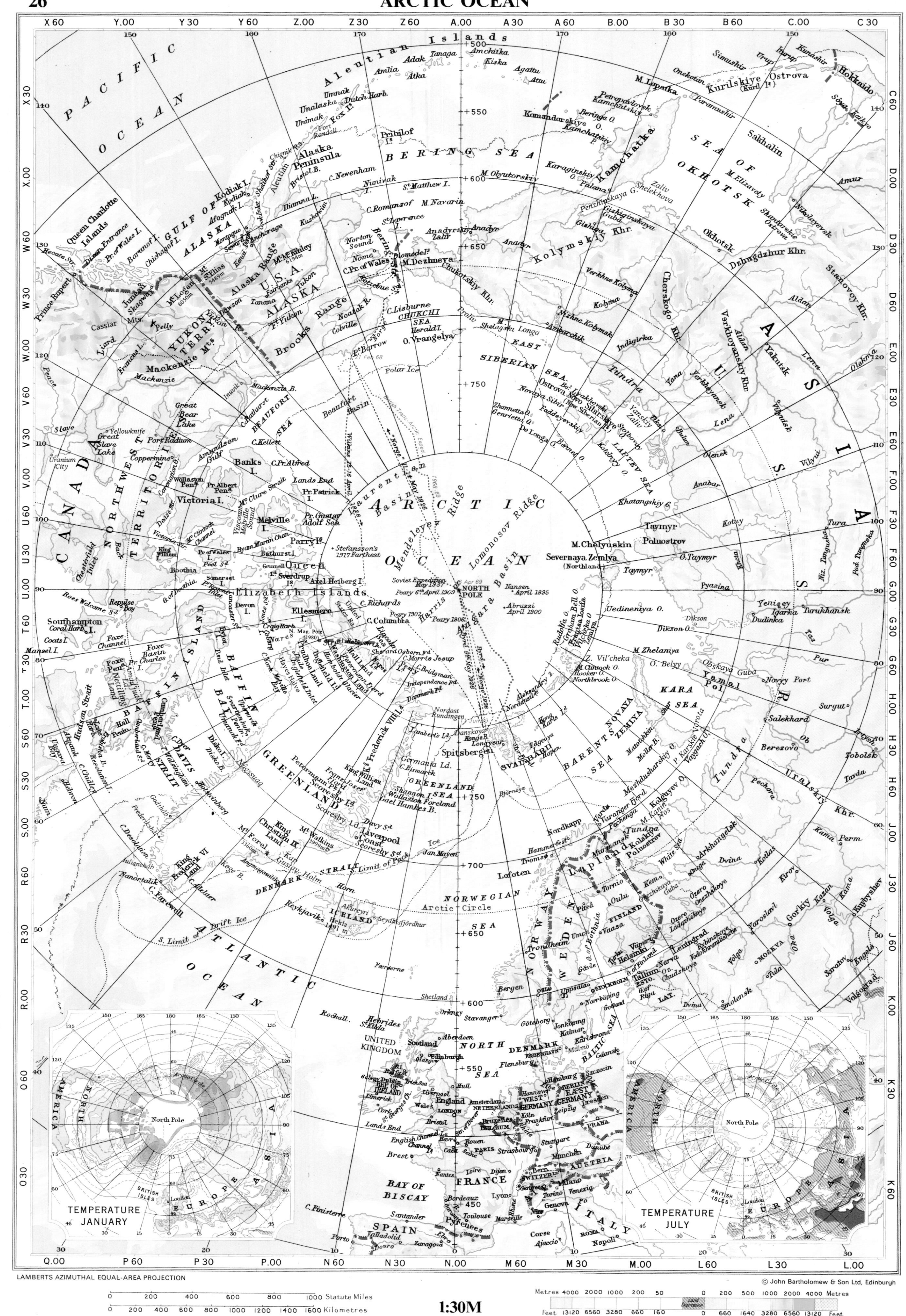
ARCTIC OCEAN
PACIFIC OCEAN
ATLANTIC OCEAN
Aleutian Islands
BERING SEA
SEA OF OKHOTSK
CHUKCHI SEA
EAST SIBERIAN SEA
LAPTEV SEA
KARA SEA
BARENTS SEA
NORWEGIAN SEA
NORTH SEA
BALTIC SEA
BAY OF BISCAY
BEAUFORT SEA
BAFFIN BAY
DAVIS STRAIT
DENMARK STRAIT
GREENLAND SEA
GREENLAND
ICELAND
Spitsbergen
SVALBARD
NOVAYA ZEMLYA
Severnaya Zemlya
NORTH POLE
Lomonosov Ridge
Mendeleyev Ridge
ASIA
U.S.S.R.
CANADA
ALASKA
U.S.A.
NORTHWEST TERRITORIES
YUKON TERR.
BAFFIN ISLAND
Queen Elizabeth Islands
Ellesmere I.
Victoria I.
Banks I.
Kamchatka
Sakhalin
Kurilskiye Ostrova
Hokkaido
O. Vrangelya
Brooks Range
Alaska Range
Mackenzie Mts
Arctic Circle
NORWAY
SWEDEN
FINLAND
UNITED KINGDOM
FRANCE
SPAIN
ITALY
DENMARK
AUSTRIA
EAST GERMANY
WEST GERMANY
TEMPERATURE JANUARY
TEMPERATURE JULY
North Pole
LAMBERTS AZIMUTHAL EQUAL-AREA PROJECTION
© John Bartholomew & Son Ltd, Edinburgh
1:30M
Statute Miles
Kilometres
Metres 4000 2000 1000 200 50 0 200 500 1000 2000 4000 Metres
Land Depression
Feet 13120 6560 3280 660 160 0 660 1640 3280 6560 13120 Feet
C° F°
30 86
20 68
10 50
0 32
10 14
20 -4
30 -22
40 -40

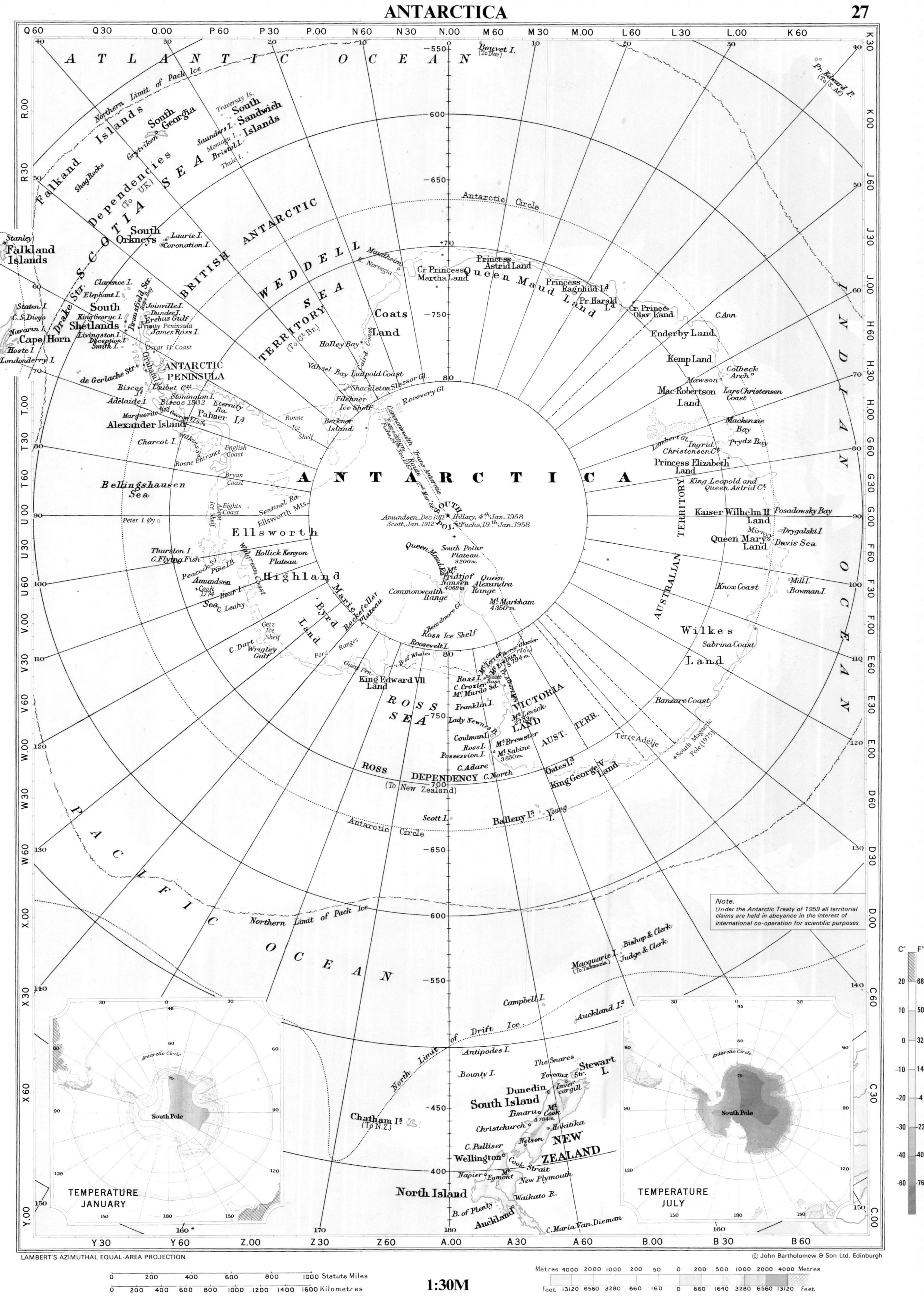

LAMBERT'S AZIMUTHAL EQUAL-AREA PROJECTION

0 200 400 600 800 1000 Statute Miles

0 200 400 600 800 1000 1200 1400 1600 Kilometres

1:30M

Metres 4000 2000 1000 200 50 0 200 500 1000 2000 4000 Metres

Feet 13120 6560 3280 660 160 0 660 1640 3280 6560 13120 Feet

Antarctic Bases (1970-71) are shown by a red dot.

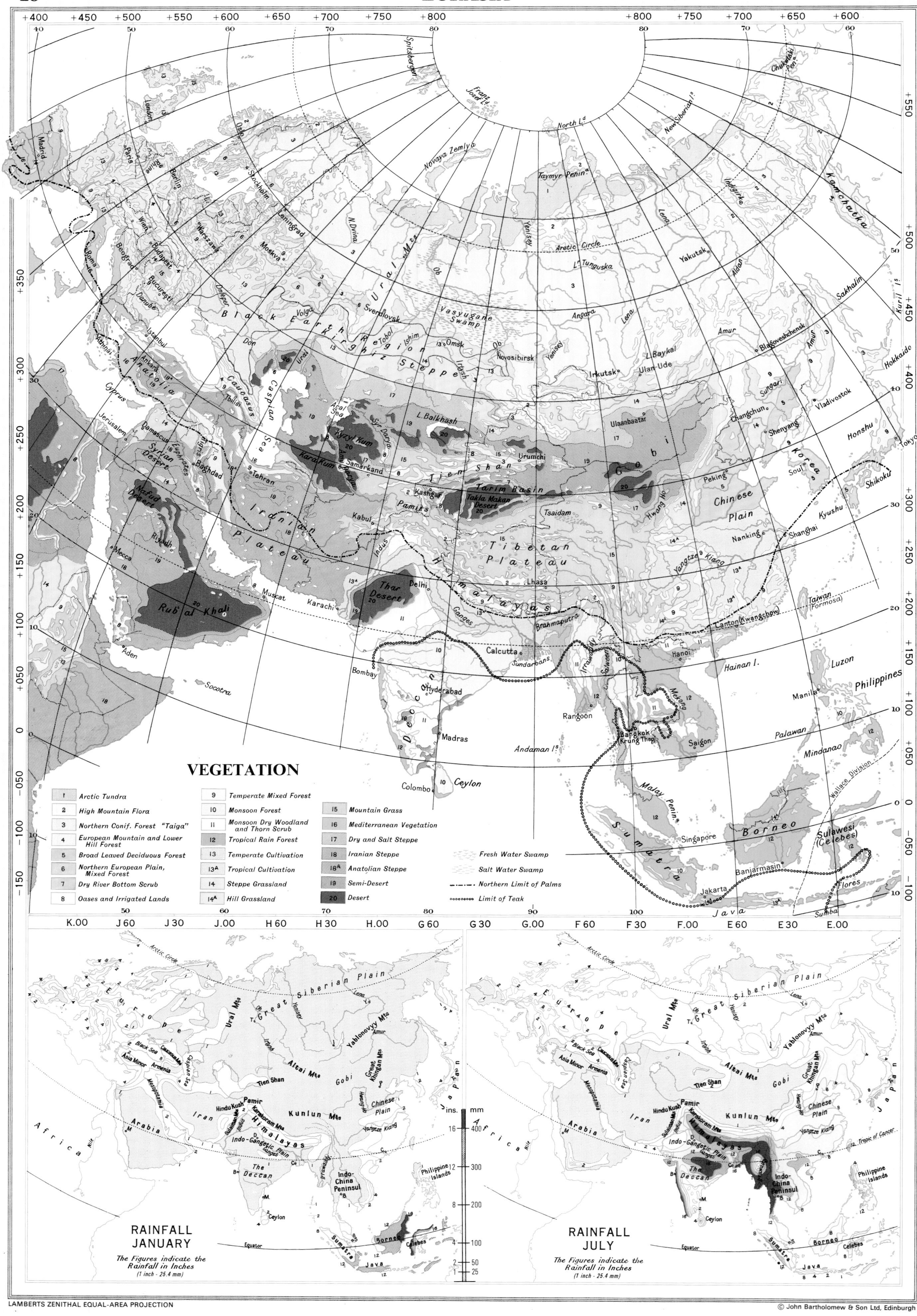
VEGETATION
1 Arctic Tundra
2 High Mountain Flora
3 Northern Conif. Forest "Taiga"
4 European Mountain and Lower Hill Forest
5 Broad Leaved Deciduous Forest
6 Northern European Plain, Mixed Forest
7 Dry River Bottom Scrub
8 Oases and Irrigated Lands
9 Temperate Mixed Forest
10 Monsoon Forest
11 Monsoon Dry Woodland and Thorn Scrub
12 Tropical Rain Forest
13 Temperate Cultivation
13A Tropical Cultivation
14 Steppe Grassland
14A Hill Grassland
15 Mountain Grass
16 Mediterranean Vegetation
17 Dry and Salt Steppe
18 Iranian Steppe
18A Anatolian Steppe
19 Semi-Desert
20 Desert
Fresh Water Swamp
Salt Water Swamp
Northern Limit of Palms
Limit of Teak
RAINFALL JANUARY
The Figures indicate the Rainfall in Inches
(1 inch - 25.4 mm)
RAINFALL JULY
The Figures indicate the Rainfall in Inches
(1 inch - 25.4 mm)
ins. mm
16 400
12 300
8 200
4 100
2 50
1 25
LAMBERTS ZENITHAL EQUAL-AREA PROJECTION
0 200 400 600 800 1000 Statute Miles
1:45M
0 200 400 600 800 1000 1200 1400 1600 Kilometres

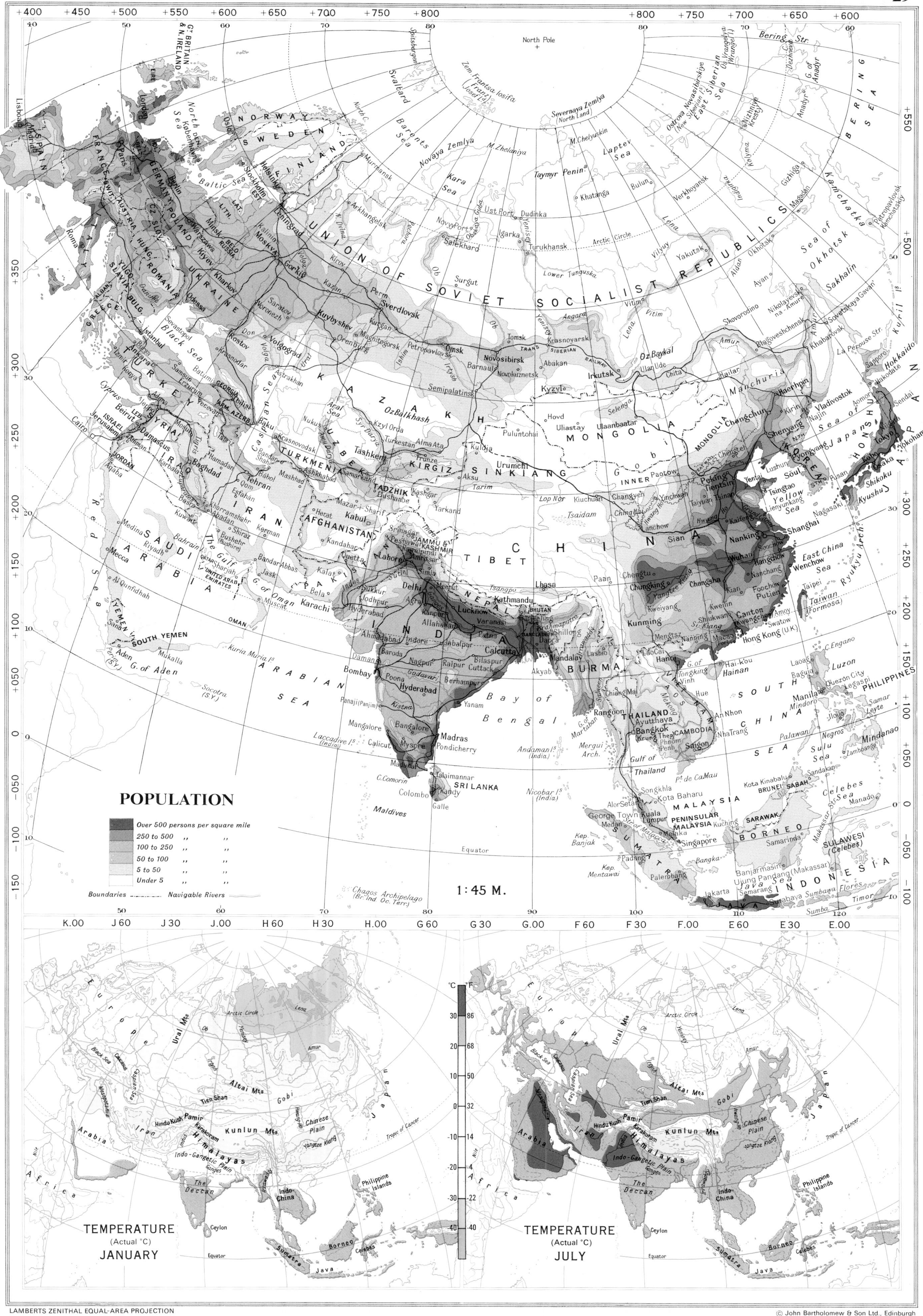

0 200 400 600 800 1000 Statute Miles **1:45M** 0 200 400 600 800 1000 1200 1400 1600 Kilometres

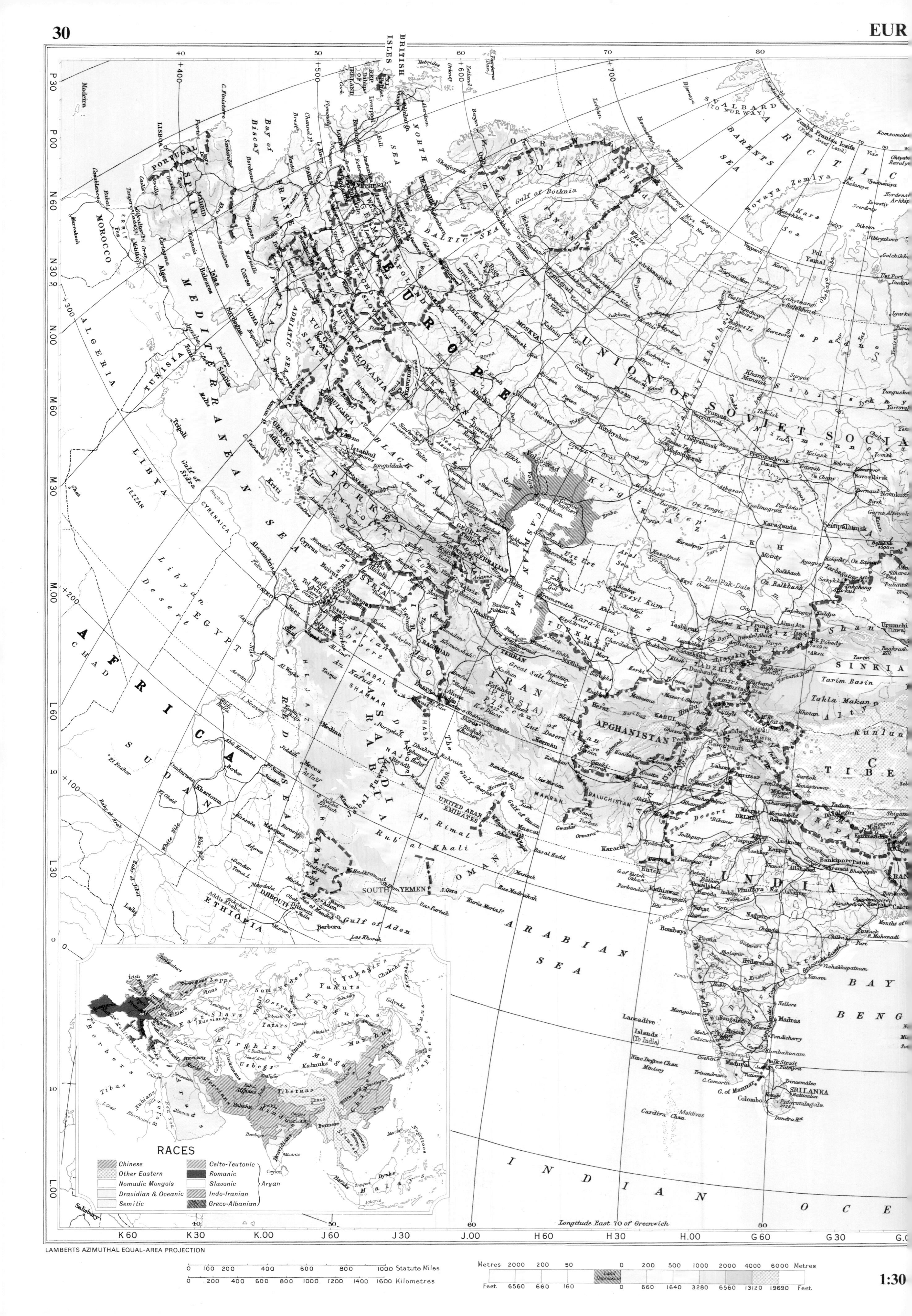
EUROPE
UNION OF SOVIET SOCIA
AFRICA
ARCTIC
BARENTS SEA
NORTH SEA
BALTIC SEA
BLACK SEA
CASPIAN SEA
MEDITERRANEAN SEA
RED SEA
ARABIAN SEA
INDIAN OCEAN
BAY OF BENG
Gulf of Aden
Gulf of Bothnia
Bay of Biscay
SVALBARD (TO NORWAY)
Novaya Zemlya
Kara Sea
White Sea
Aral Sea
BRITISH ISLES
IRELAND
NETHERLANDS
DENMARK
NORWAY
SWEDEN
FINLAND
PORTUGAL
SPAIN
FRANCE
ITALY
POLAND
ROMANIA
BULGARIA
GREECE
HUNGARY
YUGOSLAVIA
TURKEY
SYRIA
IRAN (PERSIA)
AFGHANISTAN
BALUCHISTAN
INDIA
NEPAL
SRI LANKA
TIBET
SINKIA
SAUDI ARABIA
OMAN
SOUTH YEMEN
UNITED ARAB EMIRATES
QATAR
DJIBOUTI
ETHIOPIA
SUDAN
EGYPT
LIBYA
TUNISIA
ALGERIA
MOROCCO
CHAD
Libyan Desert
Syrian Desert
Great Salt Desert
Lut Desert
Thar Desert
Rub' al Khali
Tarim Basin
Takla Makan
Kara-kum
Kyzyl Kum
Laccadive Islands (To India)
Maldives
MOSKVA
LONDON
PARIS
MADRID
LISBOA
Istanbul
Baghdad
Tehran
Kabul
Delhi
Bombay
Madras
Colombo
Karachi
Mecca
Medina
Khartoum
Cairo
Alexandria
Tripoli
Longitude East 70 of Greenwich
RACES
Chinese
Other Eastern
Nomadic Mongols
Dravidian & Oceanic
Semitic
Celto-Teutonic
Romanic
Slavonic
Indo-Iranian
Greco-Albanian
Aryan
LAMBERTS AZIMUTHAL EQUAL-AREA PROJECTION
0 100 200 400 600 800 1000 Statute Miles
0 200 400 600 800 1000 1200 1400 1600 Kilometres
Metres 2000 200 50 0 200 500 1000 2000 4000 6000 Metres
Land Depression
Feet 6560 660 160 0 660 1640 3280 6560 13120 19690 Feet
1:30

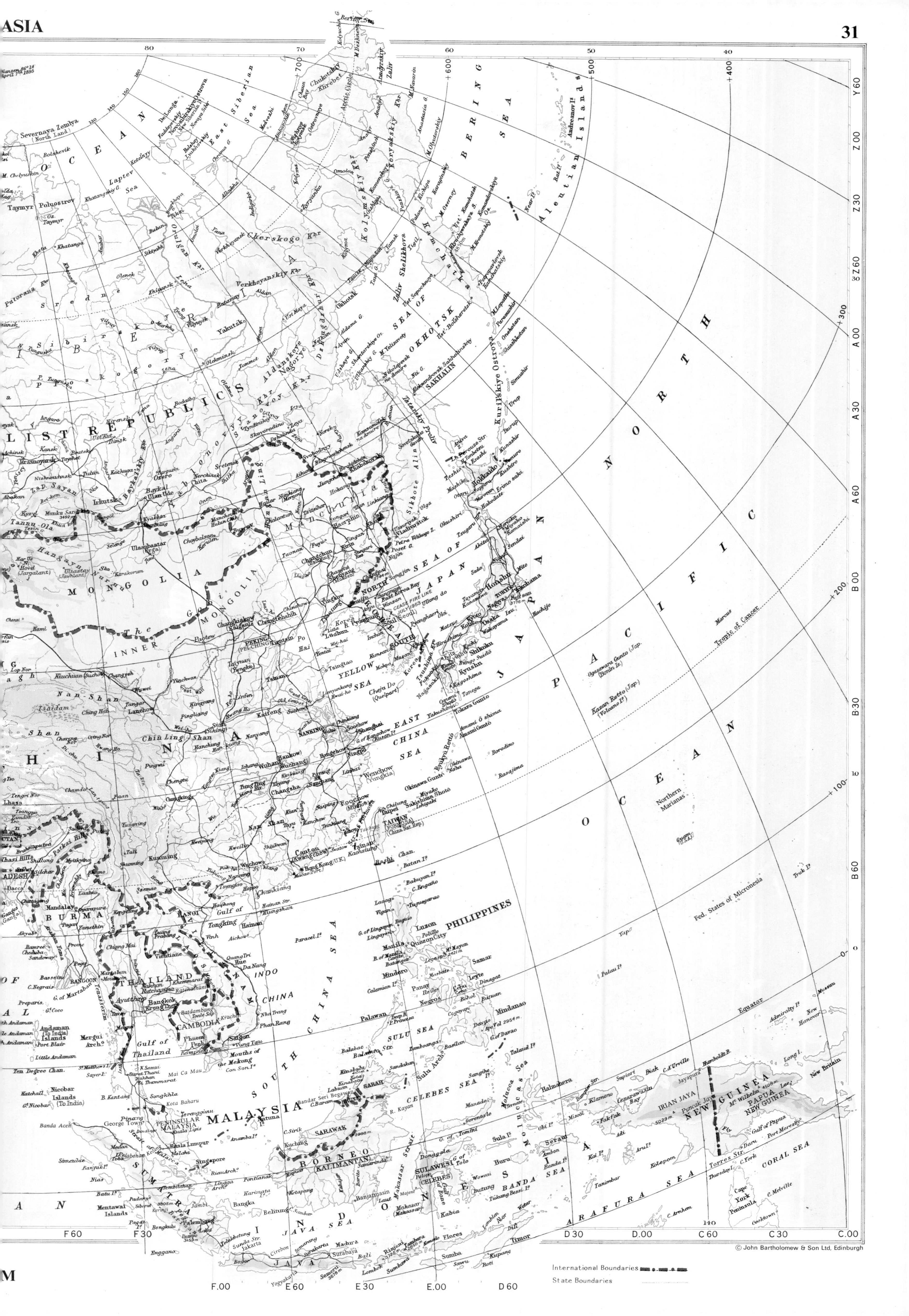
BERING SEA
Aleutian Islands
SEA OF OKHOTSK
NORTH PACIFIC OCEAN
SEA OF JAPAN
YELLOW SEA
EAST CHINA SEA
SOUTH CHINA SEA
SULU SEA
CELEBES SEA
BANDA SEA
JAVA SEA
ARAFURA SEA
CORAL SEA
East Siberian Sea
Laptev Sea
Kamchatka
SAKHALIN
Kuril'skiye Ostrova
Hokkaido
Honshu
Kyushu
Shikoku
TOKYO
MONGOLIA
INNER MONGOLIA
Manchuria
CHINA
NORTH KOREA
SOUTH KOREA
PEKING (PEI-CHING)
Shanghai
NANKING
Hong Kong (UK)
TAIWAN (FORMOSA) (China Nat. Rep.)
PHILIPPINES
Luzon
Mindanao
BURMA
THAILAND
Bangkok (Krung Thep)
LAOS
Vientiane
HANOI
Saigon
CAMBODIA
MALAYSIA
PENINSULAR MALAYSIA
Singapore
SARAWAK
SABAH
BORNEO (KALIMANTAN)
SULAWESI (CELEBES)
SUMATRA
JAVA
Jakarta
Halmahera
IRIAN JAYA
NEW GUINEA
PAPUA NEW GUINEA
Gulf of Thailand
Gulf of Tongking
Tropic of Cancer
Equator
Fed. States of Micronesia
Northern Marianas
Guam (U.S.A.)
Marcus
Palau Is.
Andaman Islands (To India)
Nicobar Islands (To India)
International Boundaries
State Boundaries

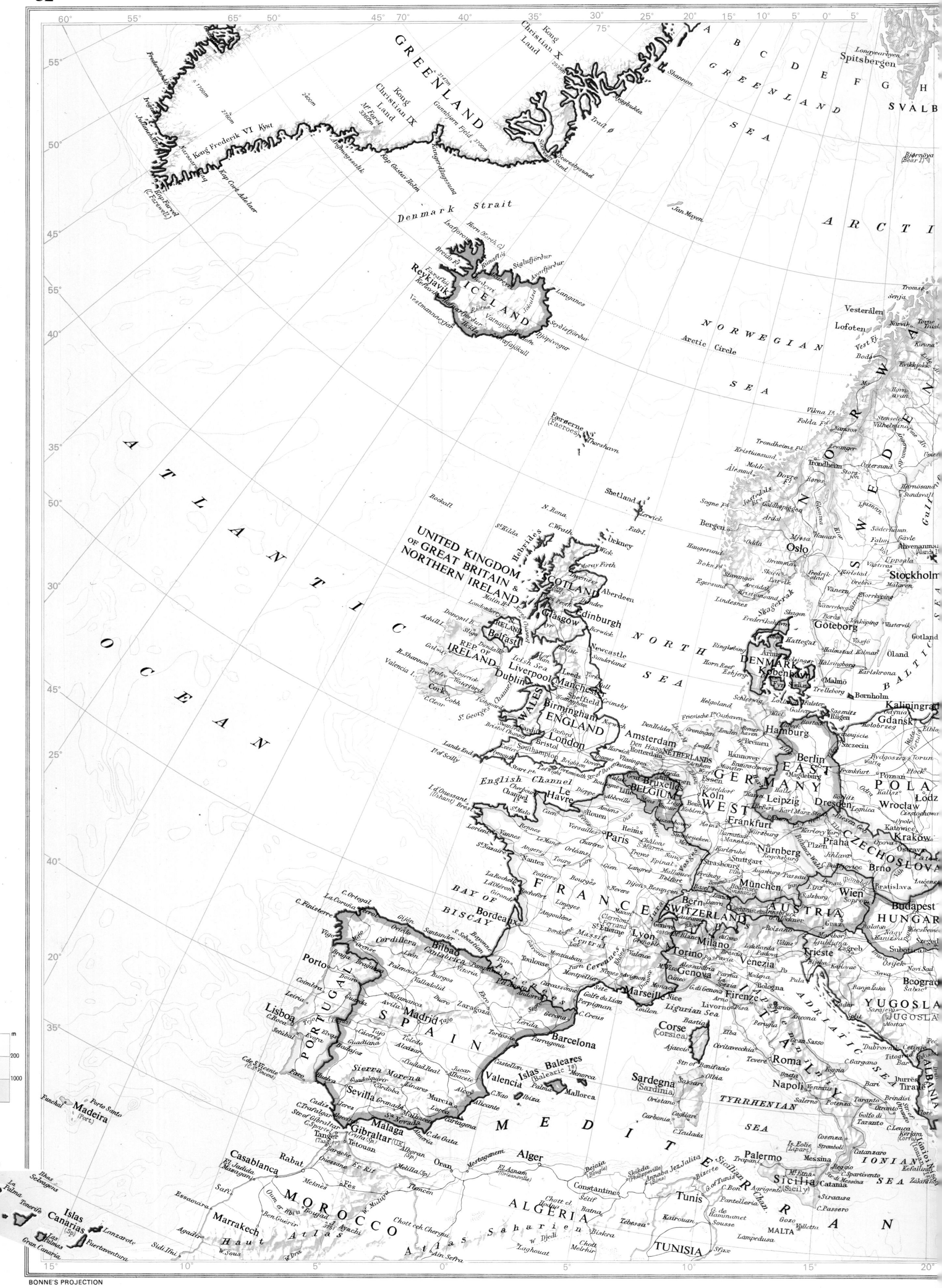

BONNE'S PROJECTION

1:15

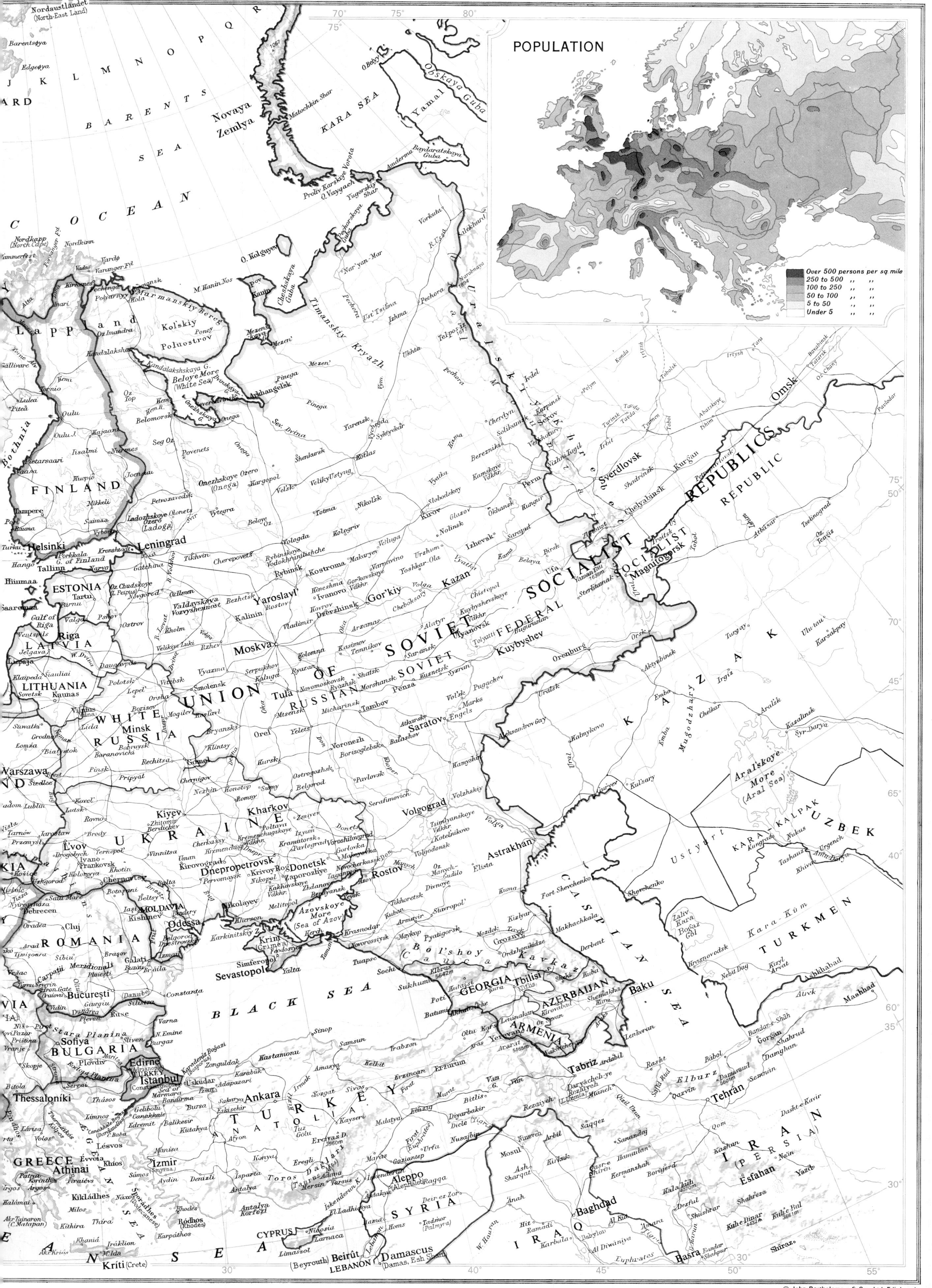

POPULATION
Over 500 persons per sq mile
250 to 500
100 to 250
50 to 100
5 to 50
Under 5
BARENTS SEA
OCEAN
KARA SEA
Novaya Zemlya
Yamal
Obskaya Guba
Kol'skiy Poluostrov
Beloye More (White Sea)
Arkhangel'sk
Timanskiy Kryazh
FINLAND
Helsinki
Leningrad
ESTONIA
Tallinn
Tartu
LATVIA
Riga
LITHUANIA
Kaunas
Vilnius
WHITE RUSSIA
Minsk
Warszawa
Moskva
Yaroslavl'
Gor'kiy
Kazan
Kuybyshev
Sverdlovsk
Chelyabinsk
Magnitogorsk
Omsk
Perm
Ufa
Orenburg
Tula
Tambov
Saratov
Volgograd
Astrakhan
UNION OF SOVIET SOCIALIST REPUBLICS
RUSSIAN SOVIET FEDERAL SOCIALIST REPUBLIC
KAZAKH
UKRAINE
Kiyev
Kharkov
L'vov
Dnepropetrovsk
Donetsk
Rostov
Odessa
MOLDAVIA
Kishinev
Sevastopol
Krim (Crimea)
Azovskoye More (Sea of Azov)
BLACK SEA
CASPIAN SEA
Aral'skoye More (Aral Sea)
KARA-KALPAK
UZBEK
TURKMEN
GEORGIA
Tbilisi
AZERBAIJAN
Baku
ARMENIA
Yerevan
Bol'shoy Kavkaz
ROMANIA
Bucureşti
BULGARIA
Sofiya
GREECE
Athinai
Thessaloniki
Istanbul
Ankara
İzmir
TURKEY
ANATOLIA
CYPRUS
Nicosia
SYRIA
Aleppo
Damascus
LEBANON
Beirut
IRAQ
Baghdad
Basra
IRAN (PERSIA)
Tehrān
Tabriz
Esfahan
Elburz
Mashhad
Kriti (Crete)
0 100 200 300 400 500 Statute Miles
© John Bartholomew & Son Ltd. Edinburgh

M

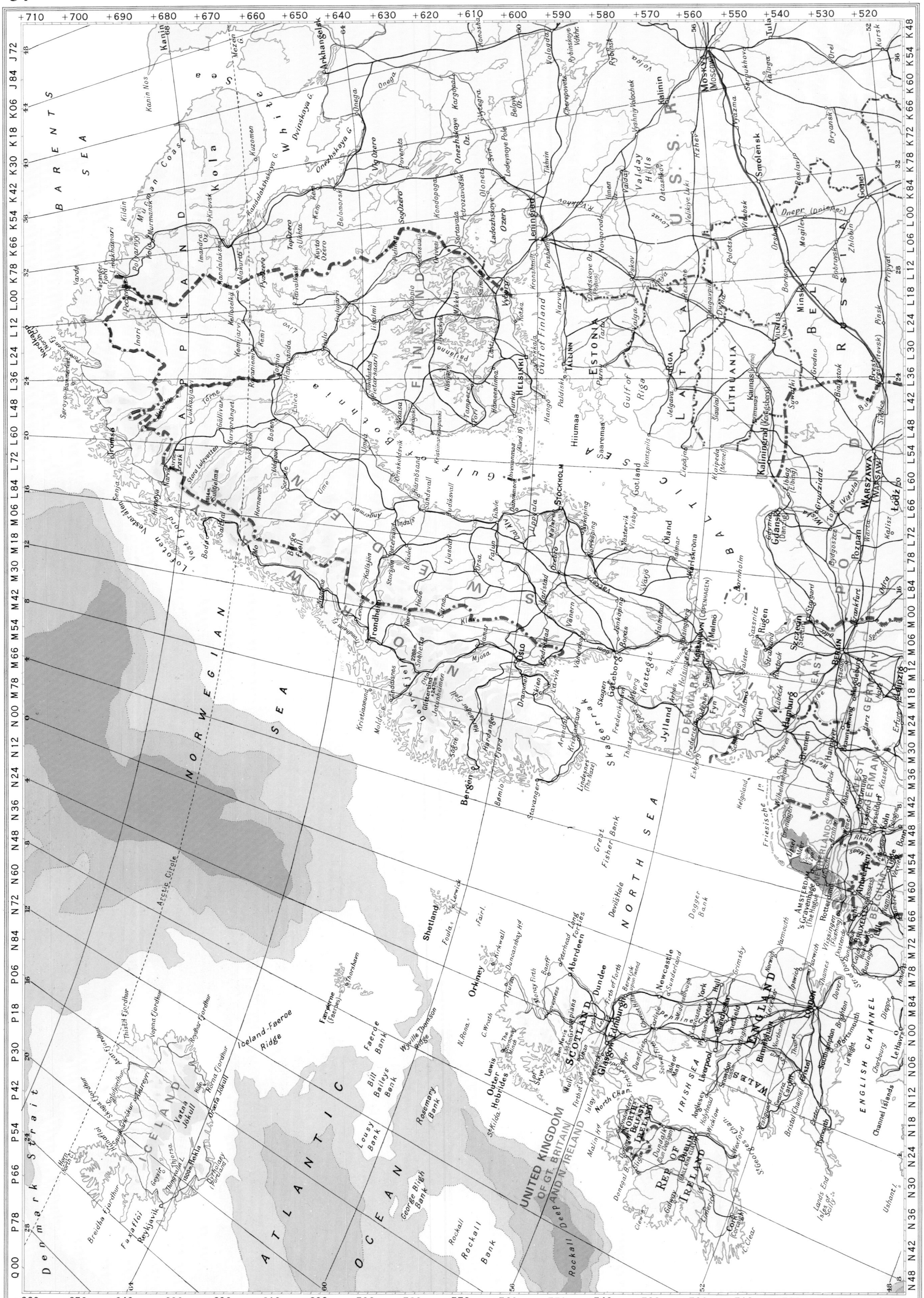

NORTH-WEST EUROPE

BONNE'S PROJECTION

0 100 200 300 400 Statute Miles

0 100 200 300 400 500 600 Kilometres

1:10M

Metres 3000 2000 1000 500 200 100 50 | Land Depression | 0 200 500 1000 2000 Metres

Feet 9840 6560 3280 1640 660 330 160 | | 0 660 1640 3280 6560 Feet

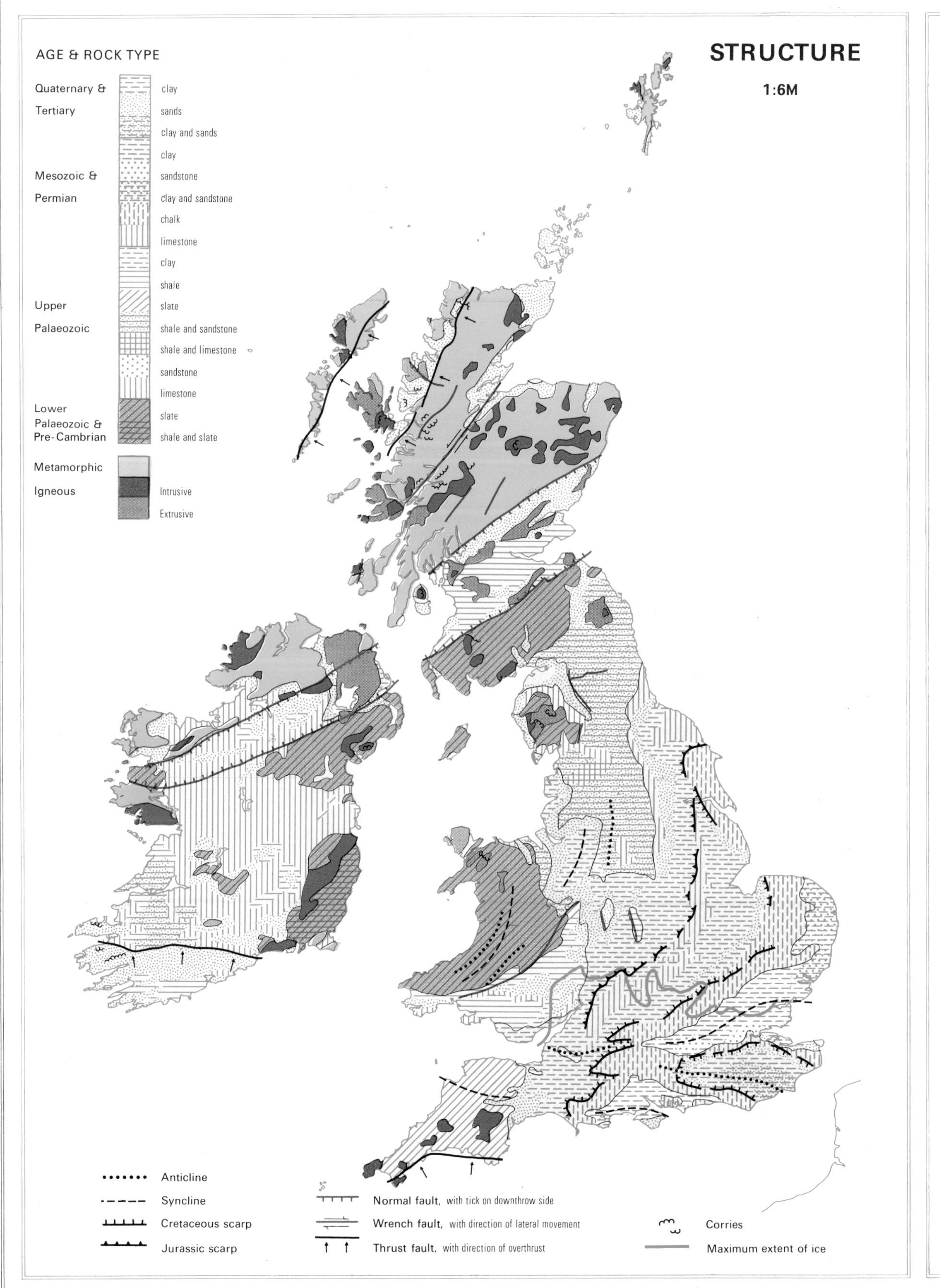
STRUCTURE
1:6M
AGE & ROCK TYPE
Quaternary & Tertiary
clay
sands
clay and sands
Mesozoic & Permian
clay
sandstone
clay and sandstone
chalk
limestone
Upper Palaeozoic
clay
shale
slate
shale and sandstone
shale and limestone
sandstone
limestone
Lower Palaeozoic & Pre-Cambrian
slate
shale and slate
Metamorphic
Igneous
Intrusive
Extrusive
Anticline
Syncline
Cretaceous scarp
Jurassic scarp
Normal fault, with tick on downthrow side
Wrench fault, with direction of lateral movement
Thrust fault, with direction of overthrust
Corries
Maximum extent of ice

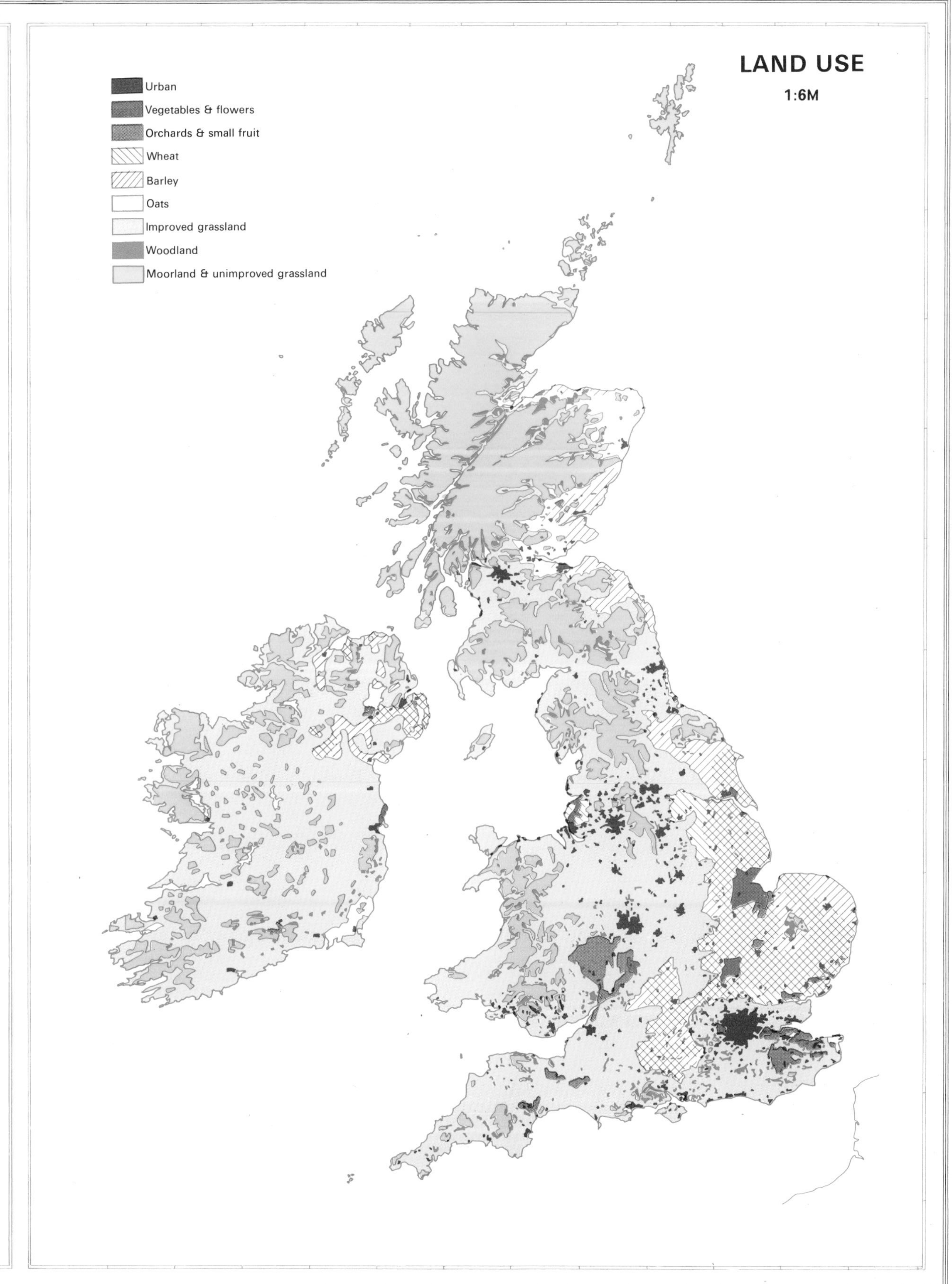
LAND USE
1:6M
Urban
Vegetables & flowers
Orchards & small fruit
Wheat
Barley
Oats
Improved grassland
Woodland
Moorland & unimproved grassland

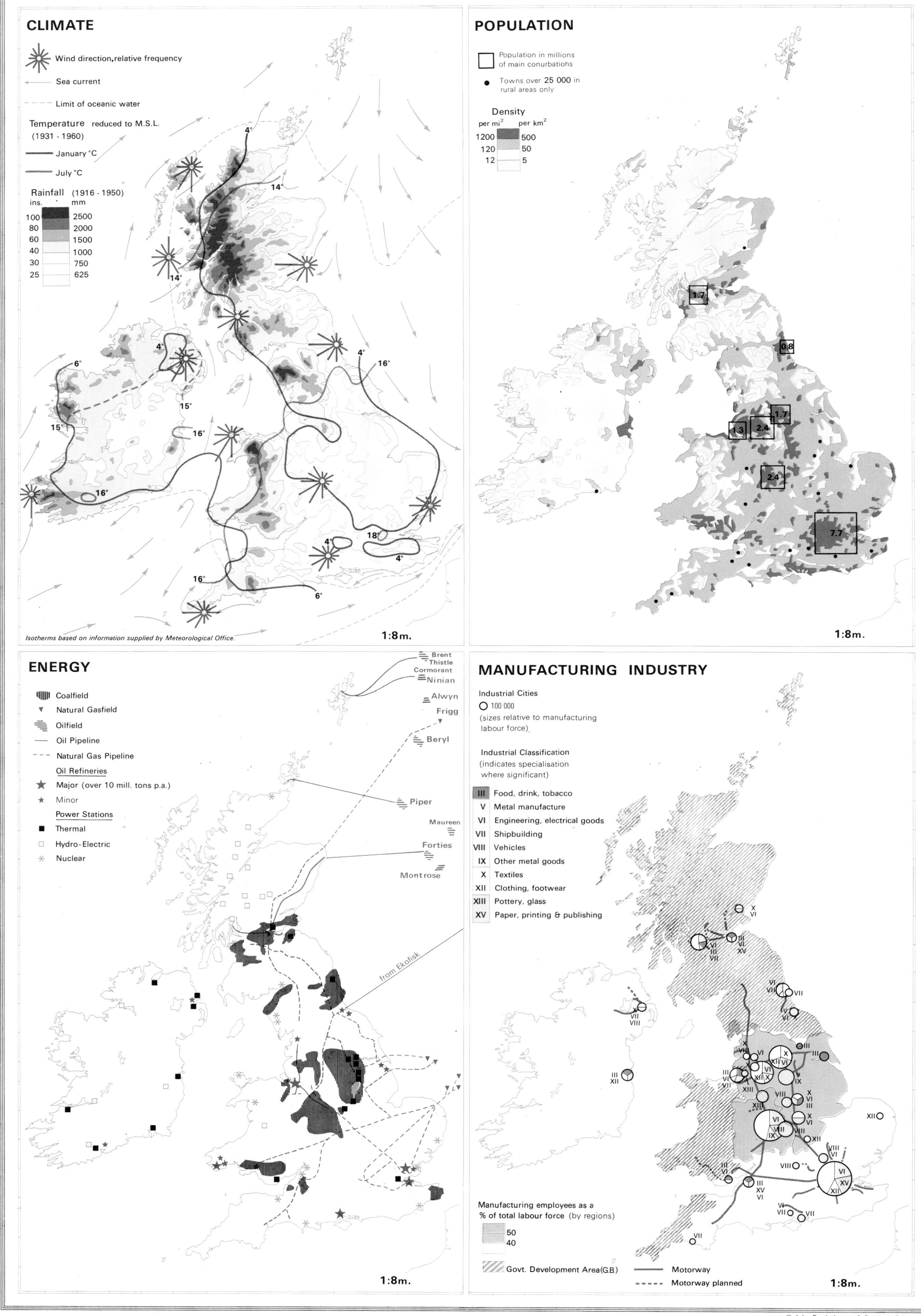
CLIMATE
Wind direction, relative frequency
Sea current
Limit of oceanic water
Temperature reduced to M.S.L. (1931 - 1960)
January °C
July °C
Rainfall (1916 - 1950)
ins. mm
100 2500
80 2000
60 1500
40 1000
30 750
25 625
Isotherms based on information supplied by Meteorological Office.
1:8m.
POPULATION
Population in millions of main conurbations
Towns over 25 000 in rural areas only
Density
per mi² per km²
1200 500
120 50
12 5
1.7
0.8
1.7
1.3
2.4
2.4
7.7
1:8m.
ENERGY
Coalfield
Natural Gasfield
Oilfield
Oil Pipeline
Natural Gas Pipeline
Oil Refineries
Major (over 10 mill. tons p.a.)
Minor
Power Stations
Thermal
Hydro-Electric
Nuclear
Brent
Thistle
Cormorant
Ninian
Alwyn
Frigg
Beryl
Piper
Maureen
Forties
Montrose
from Ekofisk
1:8m.
MANUFACTURING INDUSTRY
Industrial Cities
100 000
(sizes relative to manufacturing labour force)
Industrial Classification
(indicates specialisation where significant)
III Food, drink, tobacco
V Metal manufacture
VI Engineering, electrical goods
VII Shipbuilding
VIII Vehicles
IX Other metal goods
X Textiles
XII Clothing, footwear
XIII Pottery, glass
XV Paper, printing & publishing
Manufacturing employees as a % of total labour force (by regions)
50
40
Govt. Development Area (G.B.)
Motorway
Motorway planned
1:8m.

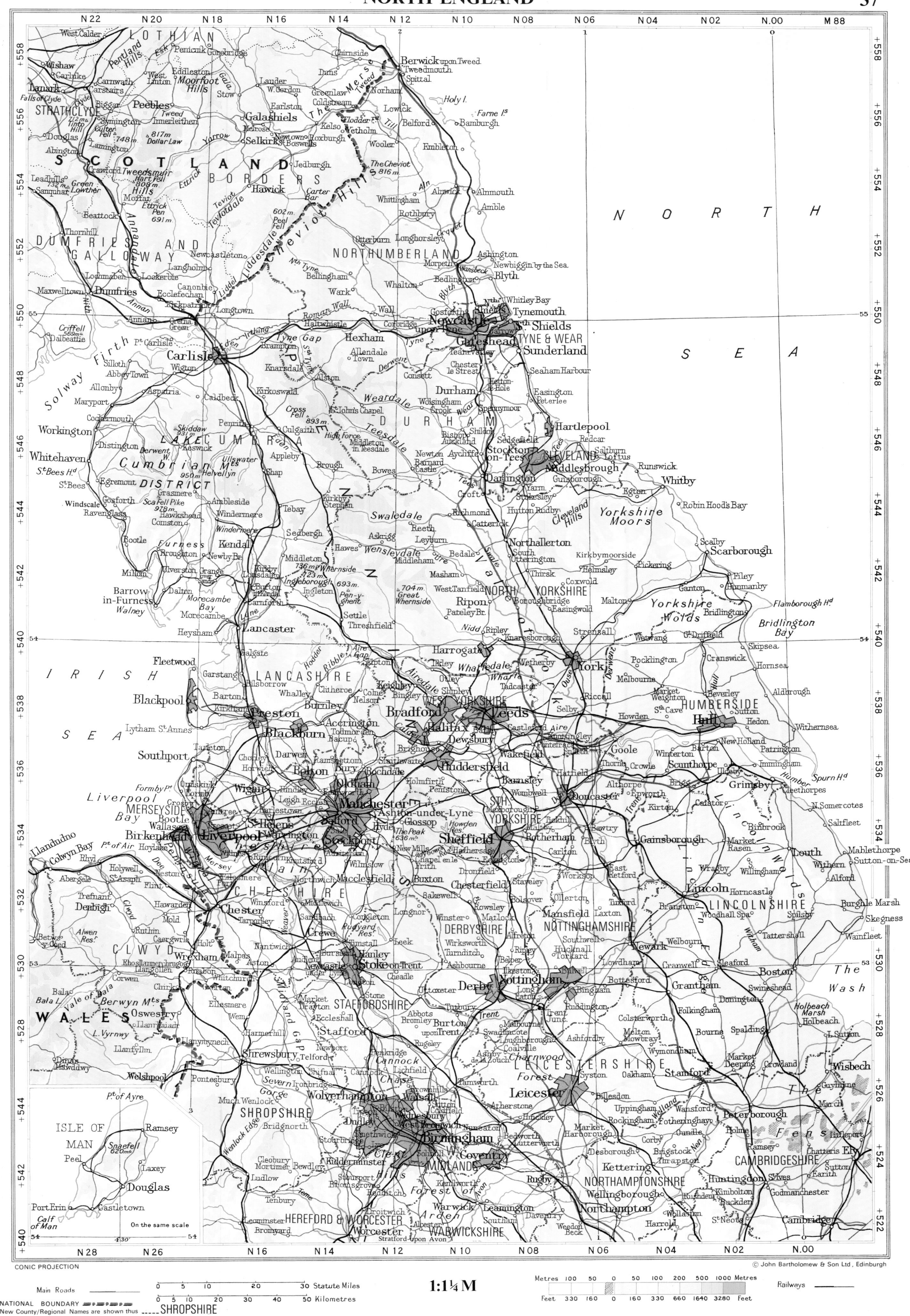
LOTHIAN
SCOTLAND
BORDERS
STRATHCLYDE
DUMFRIES AND GALLOWAY
NORTHUMBERLAND
TYNE & WEAR
DURHAM
CUMBRIA
LAKE DISTRICT
Cumbrian Mts
CLEVELAND
NORTH YORKSHIRE
Yorkshire Moors
Yorkshire Wolds
LANCASHIRE
WEST YORKSHIRE
STH. YORKSHIRE
HUMBERSIDE
MERSEYSIDE
CHESHIRE
DERBYSHIRE
NOTTINGHAMSHIRE
LINCOLNSHIRE
CLWYD
WALES
STAFFORDSHIRE
SHROPSHIRE
LEICESTERSHIRE
NORTHAMPTONSHIRE
CAMBRIDGESHIRE
HEREFORD & WORCESTER
WARWICKSHIRE
W. MIDLANDS
ISLE OF MAN
NORTH SEA
IRISH SEA
Solway Firth
Liverpool Bay
The Wash
The Fens
Cheviot Hills
The Cheviot 816 m
Berwick upon Tweed
Newcastle upon Tyne
Gateshead
Sunderland
Tynemouth
Sth. Shields
Carlisle
Durham
Hartlepool
Middlesbrough
Stockton on-Tees
Darlington
Whitby
Scarborough
Workington
Whitehaven
Kendal
Lancaster
Barrow in-Furness
Morecambe
Blackpool
Preston
Blackburn
Bradford
Leeds
Harrogate
York
Hull
Halifax
Huddersfield
Wakefield
Doncaster
Sheffield
Manchester
Liverpool
Birkenhead
Stockport
Bolton
Wigan
St. Helens
Chester
Wrexham
Stoke on Trent
Derby
Nottingham
Lincoln
Grimsby
Scunthorpe
Leicester
Birmingham
Wolverhampton
Coventry
Shrewsbury
Northampton
Peterborough
Cambridge
Douglas
Ramsey
Castletown
Peel
Snaefell 620 m
Calf of Man
On the same scale
CONIC PROJECTION
© John Bartholomew & Son Ltd, Edinburgh
1:1¼ M
Main Roads
Railways
NATIONAL BOUNDARY
New County/Regional Names are shown thus SHROPSHIRE
Statute Miles
Kilometres
Metres
Feet

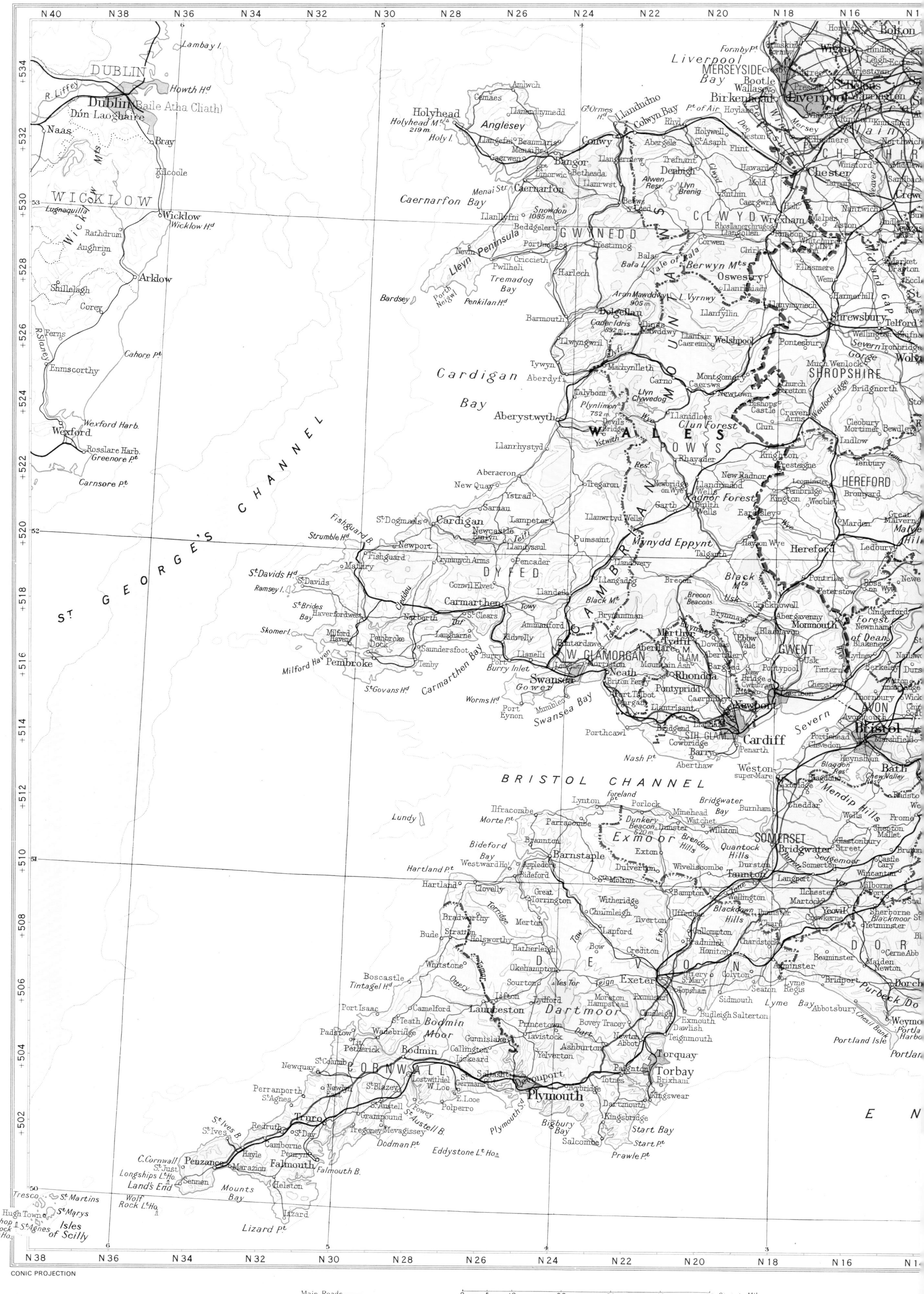
DUBLIN
Dublin
(Baile Atha Cliath)
Dún Laoghaire
Howth Hd
Lambay I.
R. Liffey
Naas
Bray
Kilcoole
WICKLOW
Wicklow
Wicklow Hd
Lugnaquilla
Rathdrum
Aughrim
Arklow
Shillelagh
Corey
Ferns
R. Slaney
Enniscorthy
Cahore Pt
Wexford
Wexford Harb.
Rosslare Harb.
Greenore Pt
Carnsore Pt
ST GEORGE'S CHANNEL
Holyhead
Holyhead Mt
219 m.
Holy I.
Anglesey
Amlwch
Cemaes
Llangefni
Beaumaris
Menai Br.
Bangor
Menai Str.
Caernarfon
Caernarfon Bay
Snowdon
1085 m.
Beddgelert
Lleyn Peninsula
Nevin
Pwllheli
Criccieth
Porthmadog
Tremadog Bay
Bardsey
Penkilan Hd
Harlech
Llandudno
Gt Ormes Hd
Colwyn Bay
Conwy
Llanrwst
Betws y Coed
Bethesda
Abergele
Rhyl
Prestatyn
St Asaph
Holywell
Flint
Denbigh
Ruthin
Mold
Hawarden
Chester
Wrexham
CLWYD
GWYNEDD
Ffestiniog
Bala
Bala L.
Corwen
Llangollen
Berwyn Mts
Oswestry
Chirk
Ellesmere
Aran Mawddwy
905 m.
L. Vyrnwy
Dolgellau
Cader Idris
892 m.
Barmouth
Llwyngwril
Dyfi
Tywyn
Aberdyfi
Machynlleth
Welshpool
Shrewsbury
Telford
Llanfair Caereinion
Montgomery
Newtown
Caersws
Carno
Llyn Clywedog
Llanidloes
Plynlimon
752 m.
Cardigan Bay
Aberystwyth
Devil's Bridge
Ystwyth
WALES
POWYS
Rhayader
Clun Forest
Clun
Bishops Castle
Church Stretton
Craven Arms
SHROPSHIRE
Wenlock Edge
Much Wenlock
Bridgnorth
Ludlow
Knighton
Presteigne
New Radnor
Radnor Forest
Llandrindod Wells
Builth Wells
Kington
Leominster
HEREFORD
Hereford
Ledbury
Llanrhystyd
Aberaeron
New Quay
Tregaron
Lampeter
Cardigan
Newcastle Emlyn
Fishguard
Newport
Strumble Hd
St Davids Hd
St Davids
Ramsey I.
St Brides Bay
Skomer I.
Haverfordwest
Milford Haven
Pembroke
Pembroke Dock
Tenby
Saundersfoot
St Govans Hd
DYFED
Carmarthen
Carmarthen Bay
Llanelli
Ammanford
Kidwelly
Burry Port
Swansea
Gower
Worms Hd
Port Eynon
Mumbles
Swansea Bay
W. GLAMORGAN
Neath
Port Talbot
Bridgend
Porthcawl
Pontypridd
Rhondda
Merthyr Tydfil
Caerphilly
Cardiff
Newport
Barry
Penarth
Cowbridge
STH GLAM.
Brecon
Brecon Beacons
Black Mts
Black Mt
Mynydd Eppynt
Abergavenny
Monmouth
GWENT
Pontypool
Chepstow
Forest of Dean
Severn
AVON
Bristol
Clevedon
Bath
Weston super-Mare
Nash Pt
BRISTOL CHANNEL
Lundy
Ilfracombe
Morte Pt
Lynton
Porlock
Minehead
Dunkery Beacon
520 m.
Exmoor
Brendon Hills
Quantock Hills
Bridgwater
Bridgwater Bay
Burnham
Cheddar
Mendip Hills
Wells
Glastonbury
Taunton
SOMERSET
Yeovil
Bideford
Bideford Bay
Barnstaple
Hartland Pt
Hartland
Clovelly
Great Torrington
Bude
Holsworthy
Okehampton
Tiverton
Crediton
Exeter
DEVON
Dartmoor
Tavistock
Ashburton
Newton Abbot
Torquay
Torbay
Paignton
Brixham
Dartmouth
Kingsbridge
Salcombe
Start Bay
Start Pt
Prawle Pt
Plymouth
Plymouth Sd
Bigbury Bay
Eddystone Lt Ho.
Exmouth
Sidmouth
Lyme Regis
Lyme Bay
Bridport
Dorchester
Weymouth
Portland Isle
Boscastle
Tintagel Hd
Launceston
Bodmin
Bodmin Moor
Liskeard
Looe
Polperro
Fowey
St Austell
St Austell B.
Mevagissey
Dodman Pt
CORNWALL
Padstow
Newquay
Perranporth
St Agnes
Truro
Redruth
Camborne
Falmouth
Falmouth B.
Helston
Lizard
Lizard Pt
St Ives
St Ives B.
Hayle
Penzance
Marazion
Mounts Bay
Sennen
Land's End
Longships Lt Ho.
C. Cornwall
St Just
Wolf Rock Lt Ho.
Isles of Scilly
St Marys
St Martins
Tresco
Hugh Town
Bishop Rock Lt Ho.
St Agnes
CONIC PROJECTION
Main Roads
Railways
0 5 10 20 30 40 50 Statute Miles
0 5 10 20 30 40 50 60 70 80 Kilometres
1:1¼

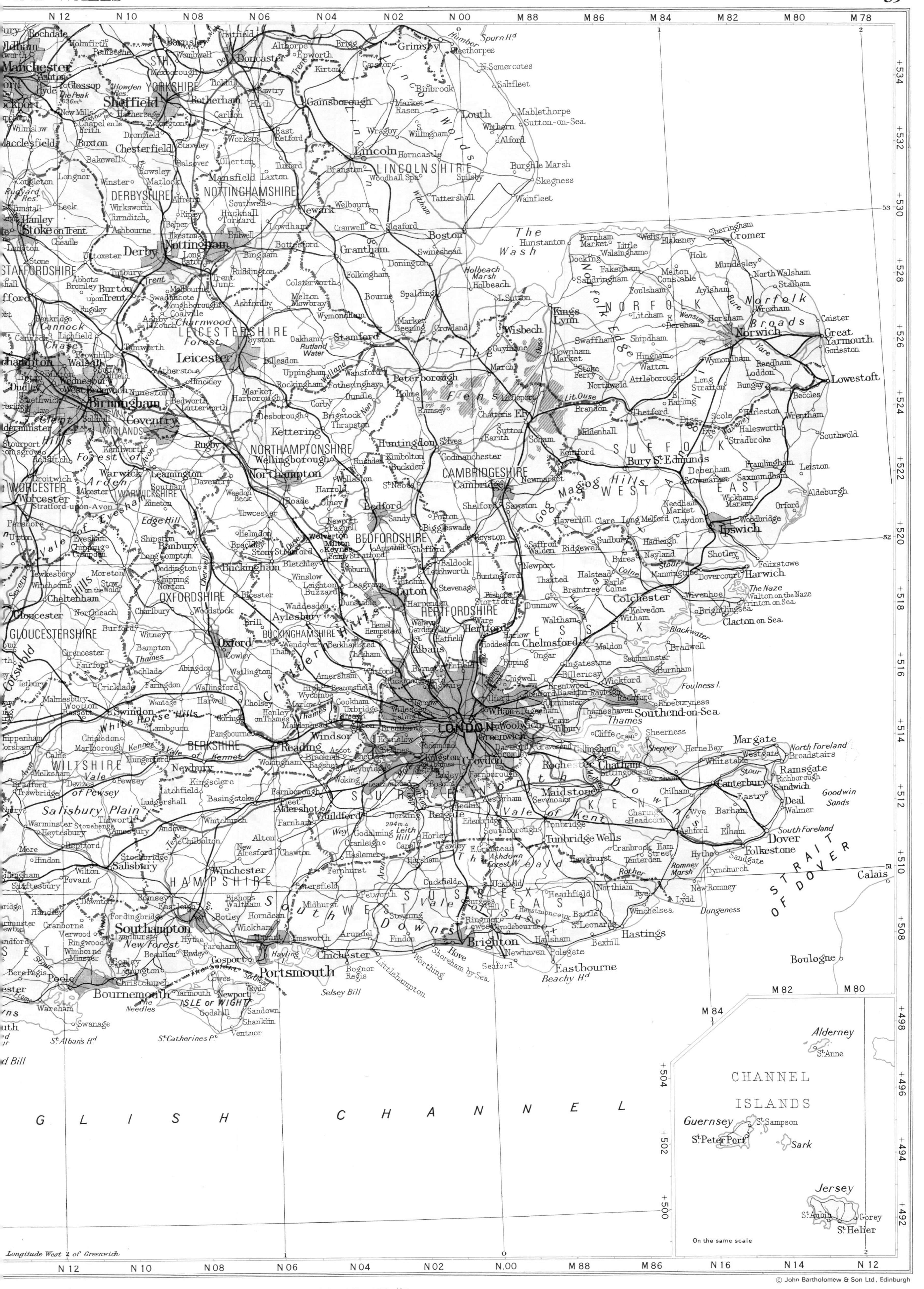

© John Bartholomew & Son Ltd, Edinburgh

M

Metres 200 100 50 0 50 100 200 500 1000 Metres
Feet 660 330 160 0 160 330 660 1640 3280 Feet

NATIONAL BOUNDARY
COUNTY/REGION BOUNDARY CUMBRIA

SHETLAND
Muckle Flugga
Herma Ness
Norwick
Haroldswick
Unst
Balta
Baltasound
Uyeasound
Uyea
Fetlar
Funzie
Cullivoe
Mid Yell
Yell
Otterswick
Burravoe
Hogsa Ness
Out Skerries
Whalsay
Dalsetter
Yell Sound
Mossbank
Lunna
Neap
Ulsta
Isbister
Voe
Laxo
Bressay
I. of Noss
Lerwick
Cunningsburgh
Mousa
Sandwick
Grutness
Sumburgh Hd.
Mainland
The Faither
Hillswick
St. Magnus Bay
Muckle Roe
Tresta
Walls
Reawick
Scalloway
West Burra
Rerwick
Fitful Hd.
Stenness
Papa Stour
Sandness
Vaila

ORKNEY
North Ronaldsay
North Ronaldsay Firth
Start Pt.
Sanday
Sanday Sound
Stronsay
Auskerry
Lower Whitehall
Papa Westray
The North Sound
Eday
Egilsay
Stronsay Firth
Shapinsay
Copinsay
Mull Hd.
Pierowall
Westray
Westray Firth
Rousay
Kirkwall
Mainland
St. Marys
Burray
St. Margaret's Hope
South Ronaldsay
Brough Ness
Pentland Skerries
John o' Groats
Duncansby Hd.
Pomona
Scapa Flow
Flotta
Swona
Stroma
Pentland Firth
Brough Hd.
Birsay
Marwick Hd.
Loch of Harray
Loch of Stenness
Stromness
Hoy Sd.
Hoy
Hurliness
Rora Hd.
Dunnet Hd.
Dunnet B.

Sinclairs B.
Wick
Castletown
Lybster
Thurso
Scrabster
Halkirk
Watten
Latheron
Berriedale
Helmsdale
Morven 705m.
Kinbrace
Strath Halladale
Dounreay
Melvich
Strathy Pt.
Brora
Golspie
Dornoch
Dornoch Firth
Tarbat Ness
Hill of Fearn
Tain
Lairg
Invershin
Bonar Bridge
Ardgay
Tongue
Kyle of Tongue
Ben Loyal 763 m.
Ben Hope 927 m.
Ben Klibreck
L. Naver
Durness
L. Eriboll
Foinaven 908 m.
Altnaharra
L. More
Loch Shin
Ben More Assynt 998m.
Inchnadamph
Oykel
C. Wrath
Loch Inchard
Loch Laxford
Scourie
Eddrachillis Bay
Pt. of Stoer
Lochinver
Canisp 847m.
Suilven 731m.
Enard Bay
Coigach
Rubha Coigeach
Ullapool
Loch Broom
Ben Dearg 1081m.
Summer Is.
An Teallach 1062m.
Gruinard Bay
Greenstone Pt.
Aultbea
Fionn Loch
Loch Ewe
Poolewe
Gairloch
Loch Maree
Kinlochewe
Slioch
Rubha Reidh
North Minch
Minch

Fraserburgh
Kinnairds Hd.
Rattray Hd.
Peterhead
Buchan Ness
Cruden B.
Boddam
Strichen
Buchan
Port Erroll
Ellon
Newburgh
Aberdeen
Girdle Ness
Stonehaven
Rosehearty
New Pitsligo
Turriff
New Deer
Oldmeldrum
Inverurie
Dyce
Kintore
Peterculter
Dee
Banff
Macduff
Deveron
Portsoy
Cullen
Aberchirder
Huntly
GRAMPIAN
Insch
Alford
Echt
Torphins
Banchory
Michalls
Lumsden
Don
Tarland
Aboyne
Rhynie
Keith
Portgordon
Buckie
Fochabers
Lossiemouth & Branderburgh
Elgin
Lossie
Dufftown
Rothes
Craigellachie
Spey
Tomintoul
Cock Br.
Ballater
Balmoral Castle
Gairn
Braemar
Lochnagar
Burghead
Findhorn
Forres
Moray Firth
Dava
Nethybridge
Boat of Garten
Grantown on Spey
Cairngorm
Ben Macdui
Cairn Toul
Braeriach
Linn of Dee
Nairn
Cawdor
Findhorn
Strath Dearn
Cromarty
Rosemarkie
Fortrose
Invergordon
Cromarty Firth
Inverness
Black Isle
Dingwall
Alness
Strathpeffer
Beauly
Carrbridge
Aviemore
Kincraig
Kingussie
Newtonmore
Tomatin
Strath Nairn
Monadhliath Mts
Caledonian Canal
Loch Ness
Foyers
Falls of Foyers
Drumnadrochit
Glen Urquhart
Fort Augustus
Caledonian Canal
Laggan
Dalwhinnie
Ben Wyvis 1045 m.
Garve
Strath Conon
Orrin
Glen Strathfarrar
Glen Cannich
Glen Affric
Glen Moriston
L. Oich
Creag Meagaidh 1128 m.
Glen Garry
L. Lochy
Gairlochy
Sgurr Mor 1109 m.
Meall a' Chrasgaidh
L. Fannich
Achnasheen
Glen Carron
L. Monar
Falls of Glomach
Mam Soul 1177m.
Ben Attow 1031 m.
L. Cluanie
L. Loyne
L. Quoich
L. Arkaig
HIGHLAND
NORTH WEST HIGHLANDS
Lochcarron
Strome Ferry
Dornie
Glenelg
The Saddle 1011 m.
L. Hourn
L. Nevis
L. Morar
Kyle of Lochalsh
Plockton
Applecross
Shieldaig
L. Torridon
Inner Sound
Rona
Raasay
Scalpay
Sound of Raasay
Sound of Sleat
Mallaig
Ardvasar
Sleat
Broadford
Sligachan
Cuillin Hills
Portree
SKYE
The Storr 719 m.
Uig
Kilmaluag
Quiraing
Rubha Hunish
Bracadale
Dunvegan
Loch Snizort
L. Dunvegan
L. Bracadale
L. Coruisk
Soay
Cuillin Sound
Rum
Canna
Little Minch

Butt of Lewis
Port of Ness
Tolsta Hd.
Broad B.
Eye Peninsula
Barvas
Stornoway
L. Erisort
Carloway
LEWIS
Gt. Bernera
L. Langavat
Harris
Clisham 800 m.
Tarbert
E. L. Tarbert
W. L. Tarbert
Leverburgh
Rodel
Taransay
Scarp
Sound of Harris
Lochmaddy
North Uist
Pabbay
Berneray
Sound of Monach
Monach Is.
Benbecula
South Uist
Lochboisdale
Eriskay
Sd. of Barra
Barra
Castlebay
Shiant Is.
Sound of Shiant
Flannan Is. or Seven Hunters
WESTERN ISLES
OUTER HEBRIDES
North Rona
Sula Sgeir
Sule Skerry
Stack Skerry
ATLANTIC OCEAN

St. Kilda
Boreray
Soay
Fair Isle

CONIC PROJECTION

Main Roads
Railways

0 5 10 20 30 40 50 Statute Miles
0 5 10 20 30 40 50 60 70 80 Kilometres

1:1¼

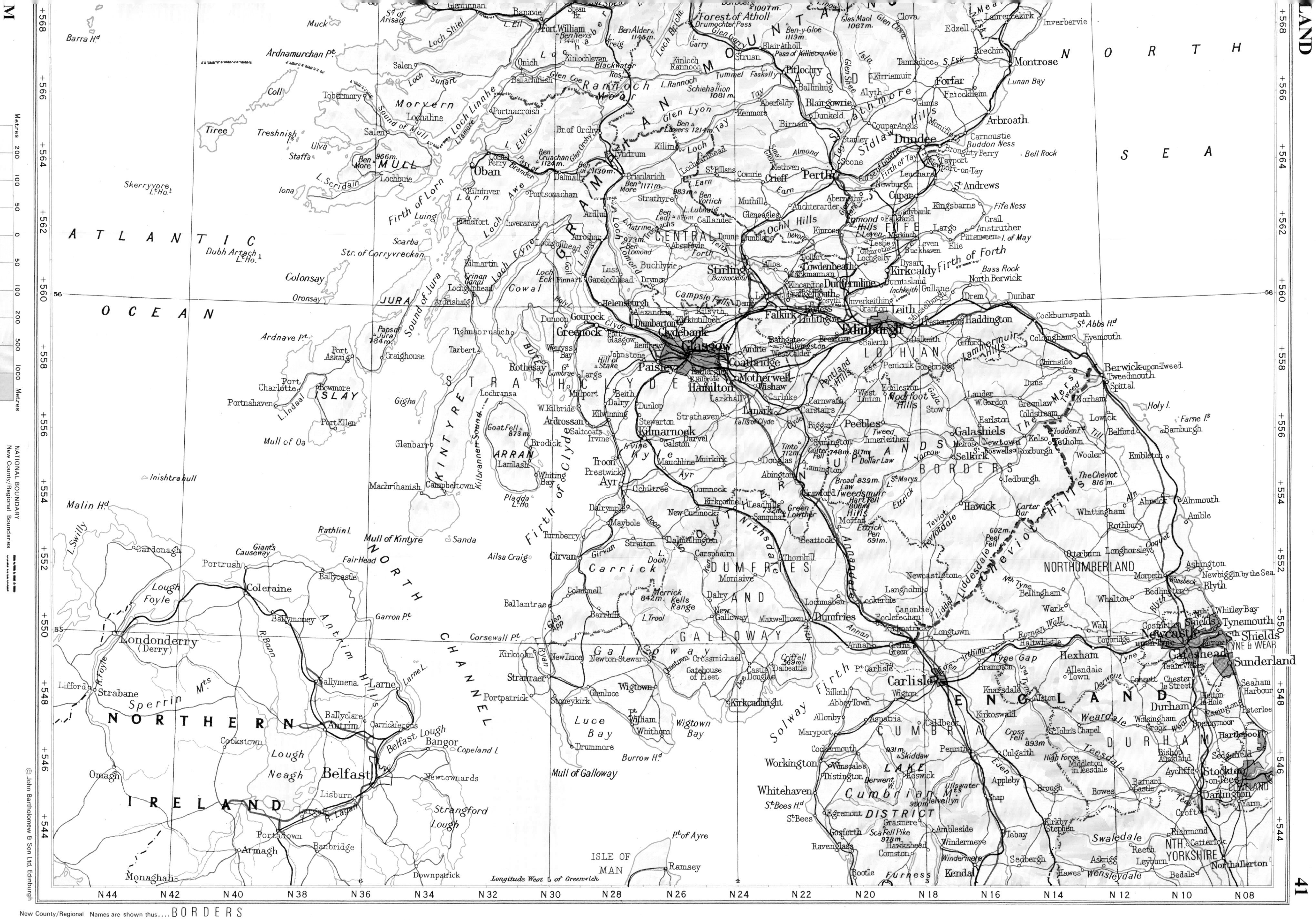
NORTH SEA
ATLANTIC OCEAN
NORTH CHANNEL
NORTHERN IRELAND
ENGLAND
GRAMPIAN MOUNTAINS
TAYSIDE
CENTRAL
FIFE
LOTHIAN
STRATHCLYDE
SOUTHERN UPLANDS
BORDERS
DUMFRIES AND GALLOWAY
NORTHUMBERLAND
CUMBRIA
DURHAM
LAKE DISTRICT
Cumbrian Mts
Cheviot Hills
Firth of Forth
Firth of Clyde
Firth of Lorn
Solway Firth
Sound of Jura
Sound of Mull
Loch Linnhe
Lough Neagh
Lough Foyle
Luce Bay
Wigtown Bay
MULL
JURA
ISLAY
ARRAN
BUTE
KINTYRE
ISLE OF MAN
Colonsay
Coll
Tiree
Glasgow
Edinburgh
Leith
Dundee
Perth
Stirling
Dunfermline
Kirkcaldy
Paisley
Greenock
Motherwell
Coatbridge
Hamilton
Kilmarnock
Ayr
Oban
Fort William
Dumfries
Carlisle
Newcastle upon Tyne
Gateshead
Sunderland
Tynemouth
Durham
Darlington
Stockton-on-Tees
Hartlepool
Berwick-upon-Tweed
Londonderry (Derry)
Coleraine
Belfast
Armagh
Omagh
Larne
Bangor
Longitude West 5 of Greenwich
Metres 200 100 50 0 50 100 200 500 1000 Metres
Feet 660 330 160 0 160 330 660 1640 3280 Feet
NATIONAL BOUNDARY
New County/Regional Boundaries
© John Bartholomew & Son Ltd. Edinburgh
New County/Regional Names are shown thus....BORDERS

M

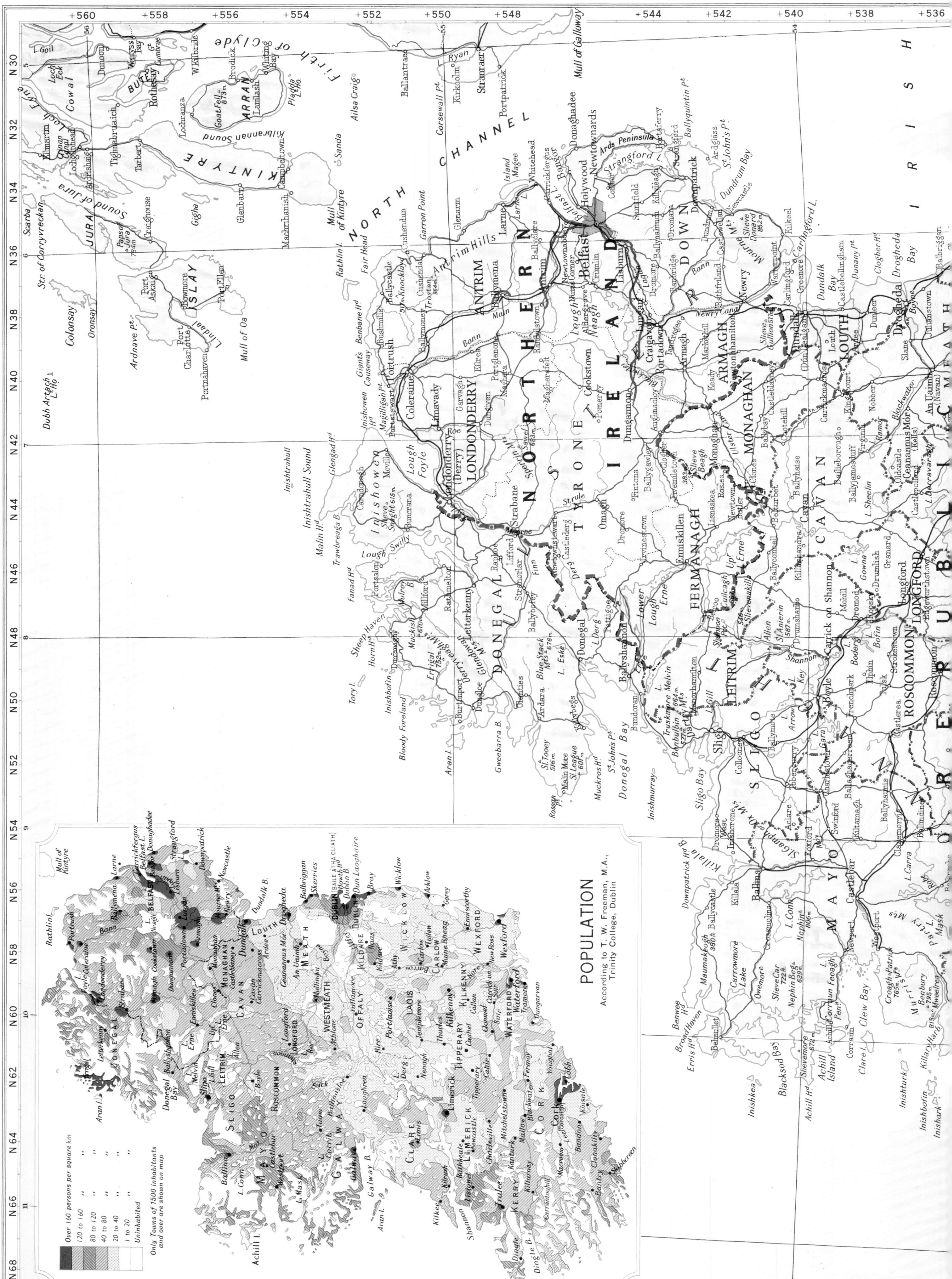

POPULATION

According to T. W. Freeman, M.A., Trinity College, Dublin

Over 160 persons per square km
120 to 160
80 to 120
40 to 80
20 to 40
1 to 20
Uninhabited

Only Towns of 1500 inhabitants and over are shown on map

CONIC PROJECTION

Main Roads

Railways

0 5 10 20 30 40 50 Statute Miles

0 5 10 20 30 40 50 60 70 80 Kilometres

1:1½

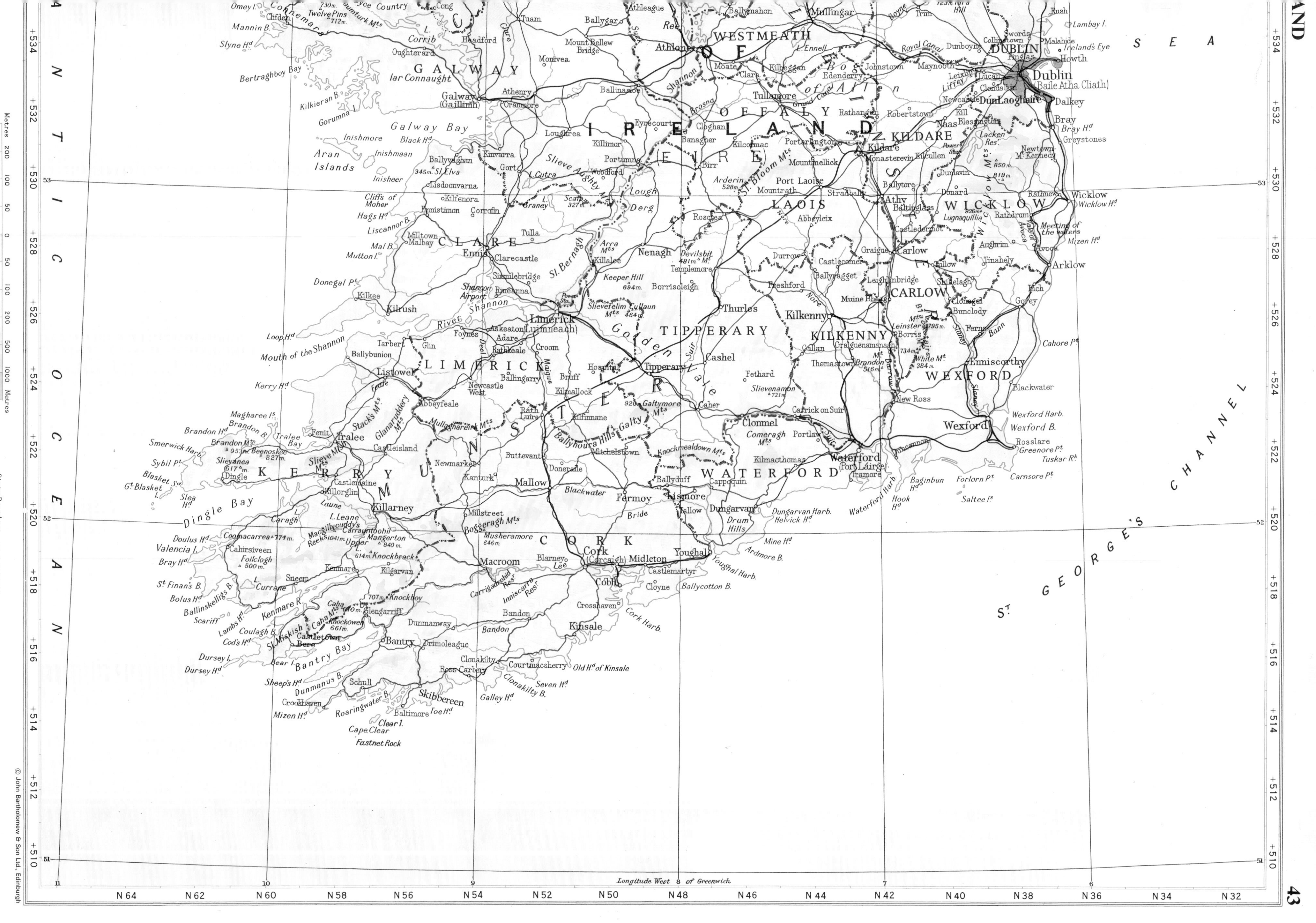
IRELAND
EIRE
SEA
ST GEORGE'S CHANNEL
ATLANTIC OCEAN
LEINSTER
MUNSTER
WESTMEATH
OFFALY
KILDARE
WICKLOW
LAOIS
CARLOW
KILKENNY
WEXFORD
WATERFORD
TIPPERARY
LIMERICK
CLARE
GALWAY
KERRY
CORK
Dublin
(Baile Átha Cliath)
DUBLIN
Dún Laoghaire
Dalkey
Bray
Greystones
Howth
Malahide
Ireland's Eye
Lambay I.
Rush
Trim
Maynooth
Dunboyne
Mullingar
Athlone
Athleague
Tuam
Galway
(Gaillimh)
Galway Bay
Aran Islands
Inishmore
Inishmaan
Inisheer
Iar Connaught
Oughterard
L. Corrib
Headford
Monivea
Athenry
Oranmore
Loughrea
Kinvarra
Gort
Ennis
Clarecastle
Lisdoonvarna
Kilfenora
Ennistimon
Corrofin
Tulla
Sixmilebridge
Shannon Airport
Kilrush
Kilkee
Cliffs of Moher
Hags Hd
Loop Hd
Mouth of the Shannon
Kerry Hd
Limerick
(Luimneach)
Askeaton
Foynes
Adare
Rathkeale
Croom
Newcastle West
Abbeyfeale
Listowel
Tarbert
Glin
Ballybunion
Tralee
Tralee Bay
Fenit
Castleisland
Brandon Mt
953m.
Brandon Hd
Slievanea
617m.
Dingle
Dingle Bay
Blasket Sd.
Gt Blasket I.
Slea Hd
Castlemaine
Killorglin
Killarney
Macgillycuddy's Reeks
1041m.
Carrauntoohil
Mangerton
840 m.
Kenmare
Kenmare R.
Sneem
Cahirsiveen
Valencia I.
Doulus Hd
Bray Hd
Bolus Hd
Ballinskelligs B.
Scariff
Caha Mts
Castletown Bere
Bantry
Bantry Bay
Bear I.
Dursey I.
Dursey Hd
Sheep's Hd
Dunmanus B.
Mizen Hd
Crookhaven
Schull
Roaringwater B.
Baltimore
Toe Hd
Clear I.
Cape Clear
Fastnet Rock
Skibbereen
Ross Carbery
Clonakilty
Clonakilty B.
Galley Hd
Courtmacsherry
Old Hd of Kinsale
Seven Hd
Kinsale
Bandon
Dunmanway
Drimoleague
Glengarriff
Kilgarvan
Macroom
Millstreet
Boggeragh Mts
Musheramore
646m.
Cork
(Corcaigh)
Cobh
Crosshaven
Cork Harb.
Blarney
Lee
Midleton
Castlemartyr
Cloyne
Ballycotton B.
Youghal
Youghal Harb.
Ardmore B.
Mine Hd
Mallow
Kanturk
Newmarket
Buttevant
Doneraile
Blackwater
Fermoy
Bride
Lismore
Tallow
Ballyduff
Cappoquin
Dungarvan
Dungarvan Harb.
Helvick Hd
Drum Hills
Waterford
(Port Láirge)
Tramore
Waterford Harb.
Hook Hd
Baginbun Hd
Saltee Is
Forlorn Pt
Carnsore Pt
Rosslare
Greenore Pt
Tuskar Rk
Wexford
Wexford Harb.
Wexford B.
New Ross
Enniscorthy
Blackwater
Cahore Pt
Gorey
Bunclody
Ferns
Clonmel
Comeragh Mts
Carrick on Suir
Portlaw
Kilmacthomas
Knockmealdown Mts
Mitchelstown
Galty Mts
Galtymore
Ballyhoura Hills
Kilfinnane
Kilmallock
Bruff
Hospital
Tipperary
Golden Vale
Cashel
Caher
Fethard
Slievenamon
721m
Thurles
Templemore
Devilsbit
Borrisoleigh
Nenagh
Keeper Hill
694m.
Killaloe
Arra Mts
L. Derg
Portumna
Woodford
Birr
Roscrea
Banagher
Cloghan
Kilcormac
Tullamore
Clara
Moate
Kilbeggan
Edenderry
Bog of Allen
Ballinasloe
Eyrecourt
Killimor
Slieve Aughty Mts
Port Laoise
Mountmellick
Portarlington
Mountrath
Abbeyleix
Slieve Bloom Mts
Arderin
528m.
Stradbally
Athy
Ballitore
Kildare
Monasterevin
Kilcullen
Naas
Newbridge
Robertstown
Rathangan
Kilkenny
Freshford
Castlecomer
Ballyragget
Durrow
Callan
Thomastown
Graiguenamanagh
Brandon
516m.
Carlow
Leighlinbridge
Muine Bheag
Tullow
Shillelagh
Borris
Blackstairs Mts
Mt Leinster
795m.
White Mt
Baltinglass
Castledermot
Donard
Dunlavin
Blessington
Wicklow Mts
Lugnaquillia
926m.
Rathdrum
Avoca
Meeting of the Waters
Aughrim
Tinahely
Arklow
Wicklow
Wicklow Hd
Mizen Hd
Newtown Mt Kennedy
Shannon
Suir
Nore
Barrow
Slaney
Liffey
Royal Canal
Grand Canal
Longitude West 8 of Greenwich
Metres 200 100 50 0 50 100 200 500 1000 Metres
Feet 660 330 160 0 160 330 660 1640 3280 Feet
State Boundary
County Boundaries
M

BENELUX COUNTRIES

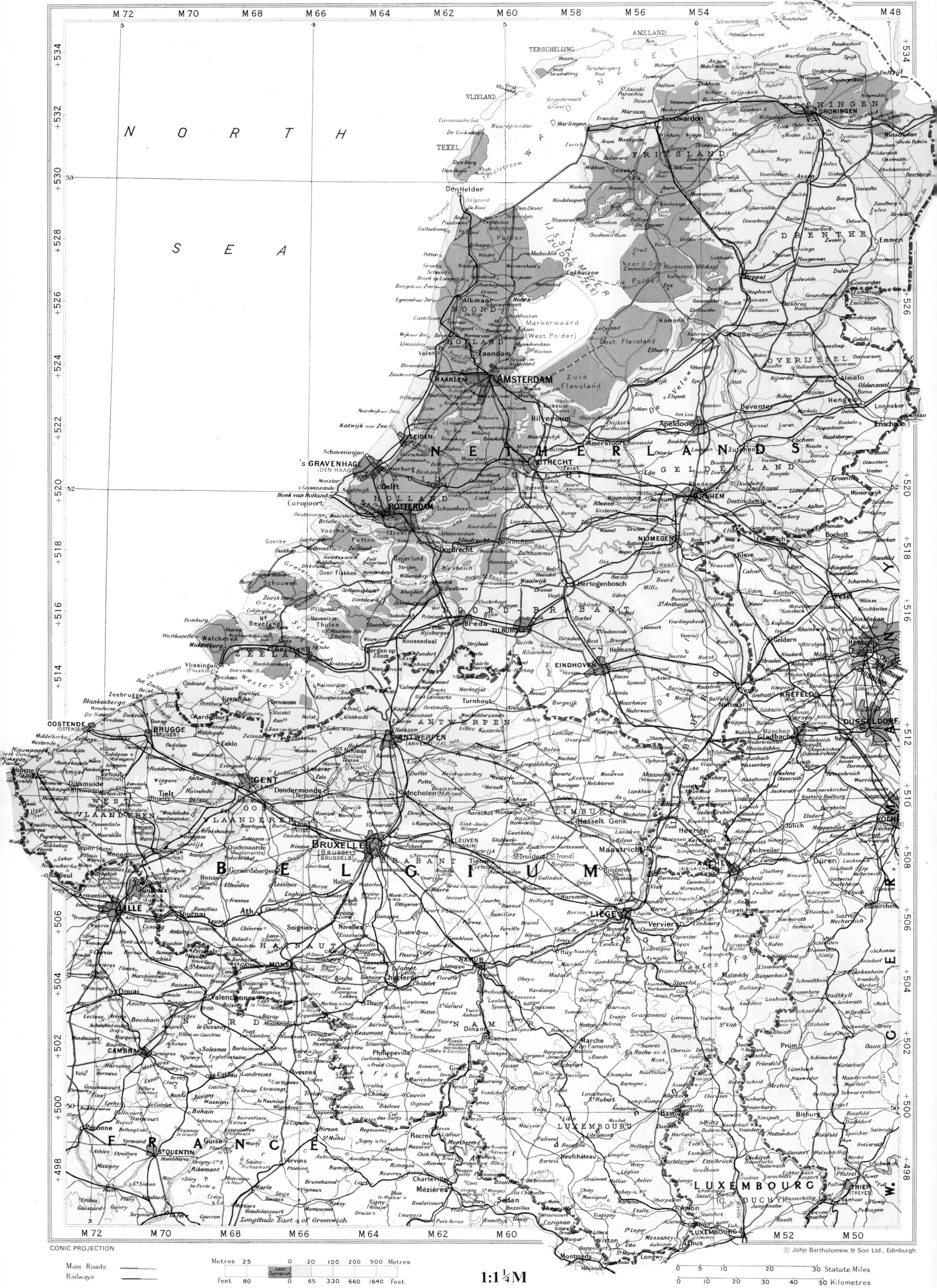

CONIC PROJECTION

Main Roads

Railways

Metres 25 0 20 100 200 500 Metres

Land Depression

Feet 80 0 65 330 660 1640 Feet

1:1¼M

0 5 10 20 30 Statute Miles

0 10 20 30 40 50 Kilometres

Longitude East of Greenwich

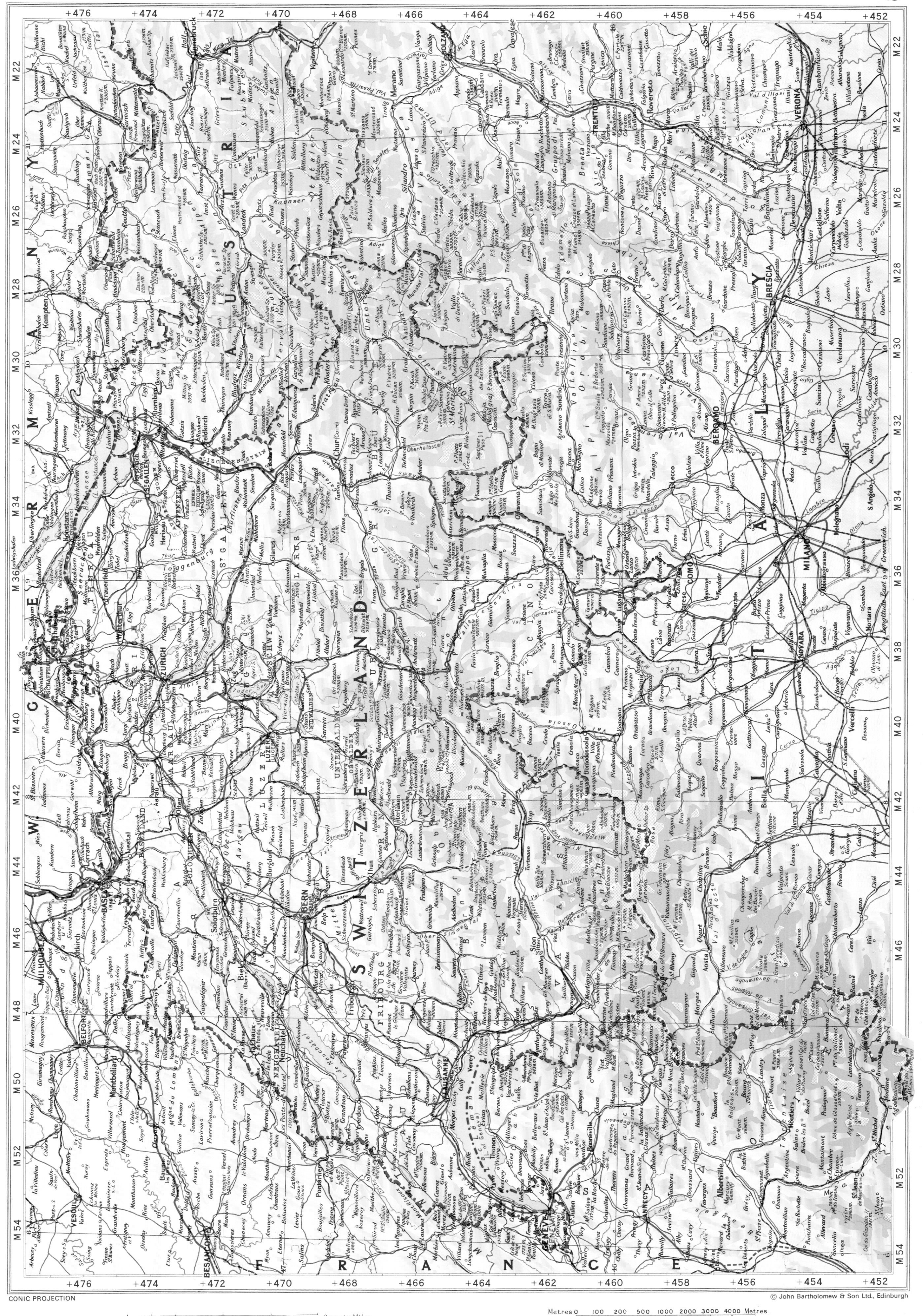

SWITZERLAND
GERMANY
AUSTRIA
ITALY
FRANCE
ZÜRICH
BERN
BASEL
LUZERN
GENÈVE
LAUSANNE
MILANO
NOVARA
BERGAMO
BRESCIA
VERONA
TRENTO
BOLZANO
COMO
CONIC PROJECTION
© John Bartholomew & Son Ltd., Edinburgh
Statute Miles
Kilometres
1:1¼M
Metres 0 100 200 500 1000 2000 3000 4000 Metres
Feet 0 330 660 1640 3280 6560 9840 13120 Feet

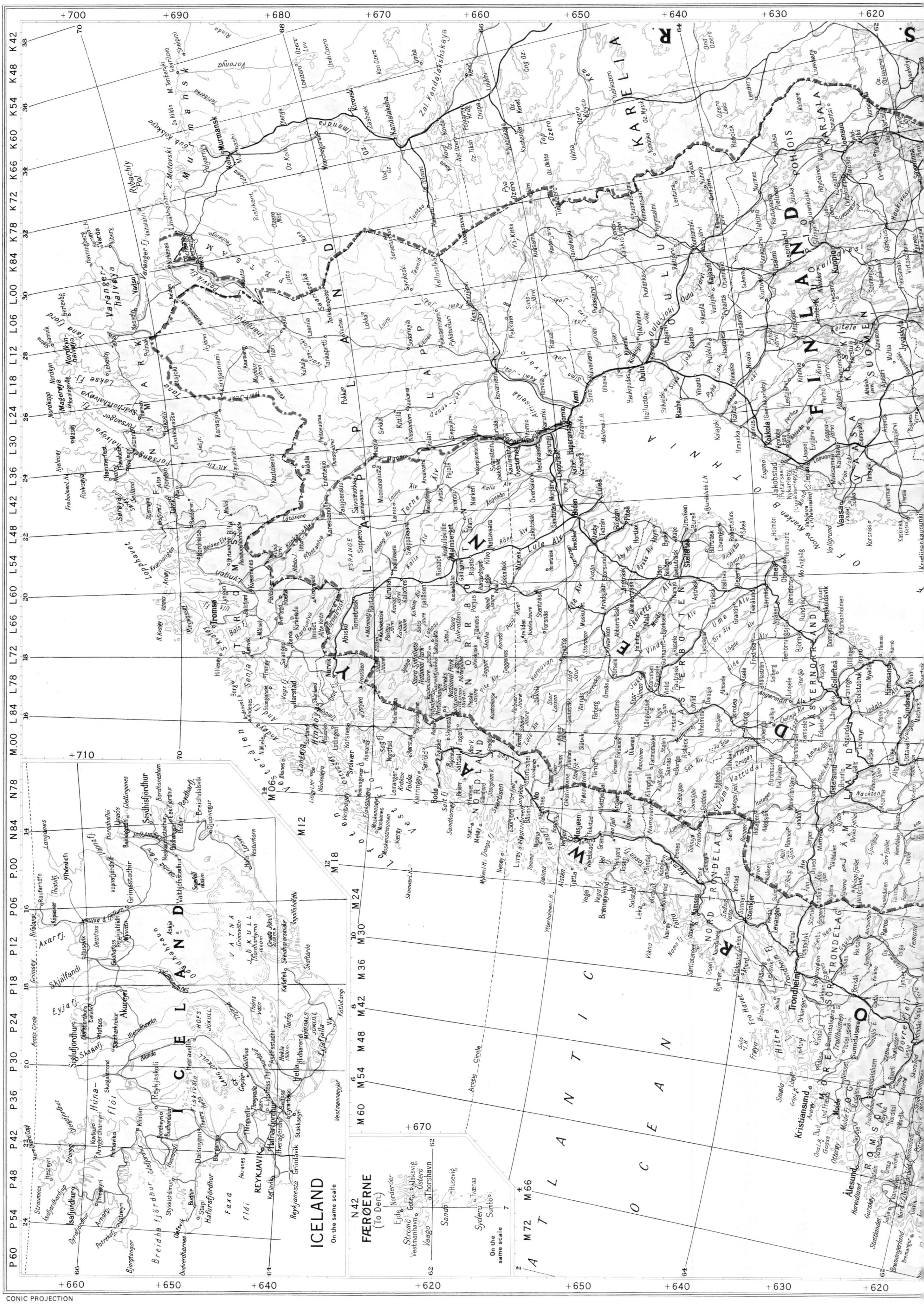

ICELAND
On the same scale

N42
FÆRØERNE
(To Den.)
On the same scale

CONIC PROJECTION

Main Roads
Railways

0 20 40 60 80 100 120 140 160 180 Statute Miles
0 20 40 80 120 160 200 240 280 Kilometres

1:4½

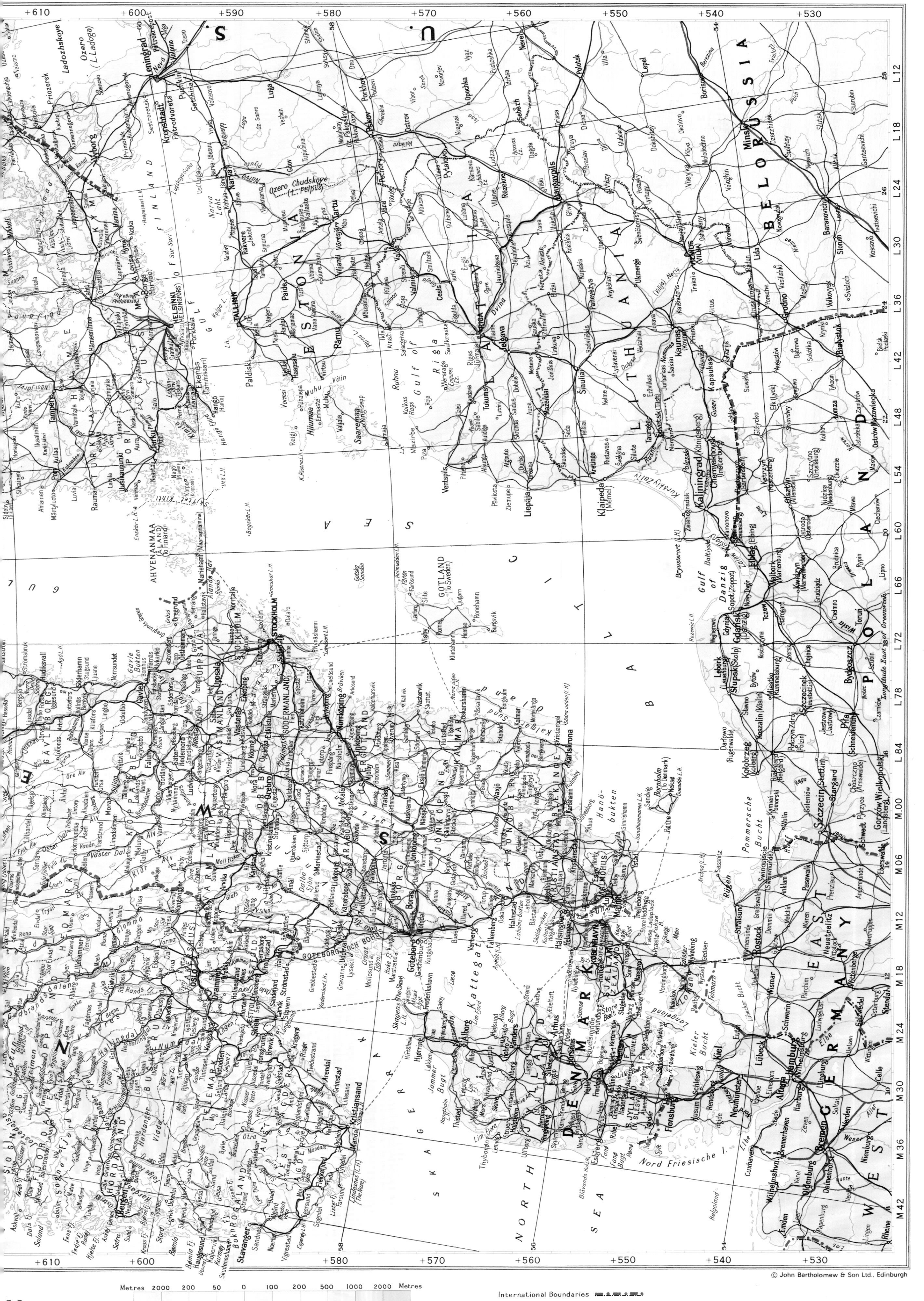
Metres 2000 200 50 0 100 200 500 1000 2000 Metres
Feet 6560 660 160 0 330 660 1640 3280 6560 Feet
International Boundaries
State Boundaries

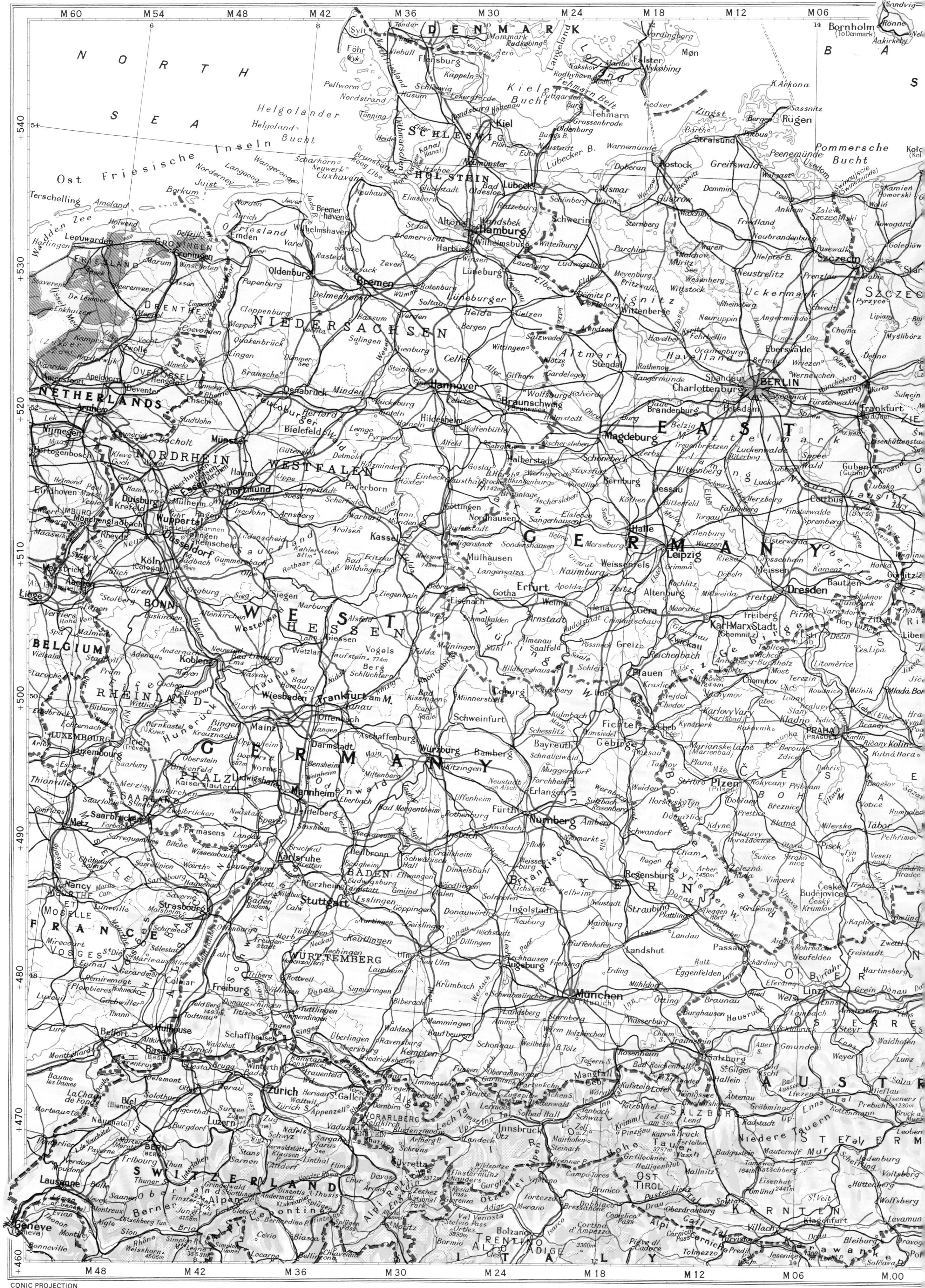

Main Roads

Railways

0 10 20 30 40 50 60 70 80 90 100 110 120 Statute Miles

0 10 20 40 60 80 100 120 140 160 180 Kilometres

1:3

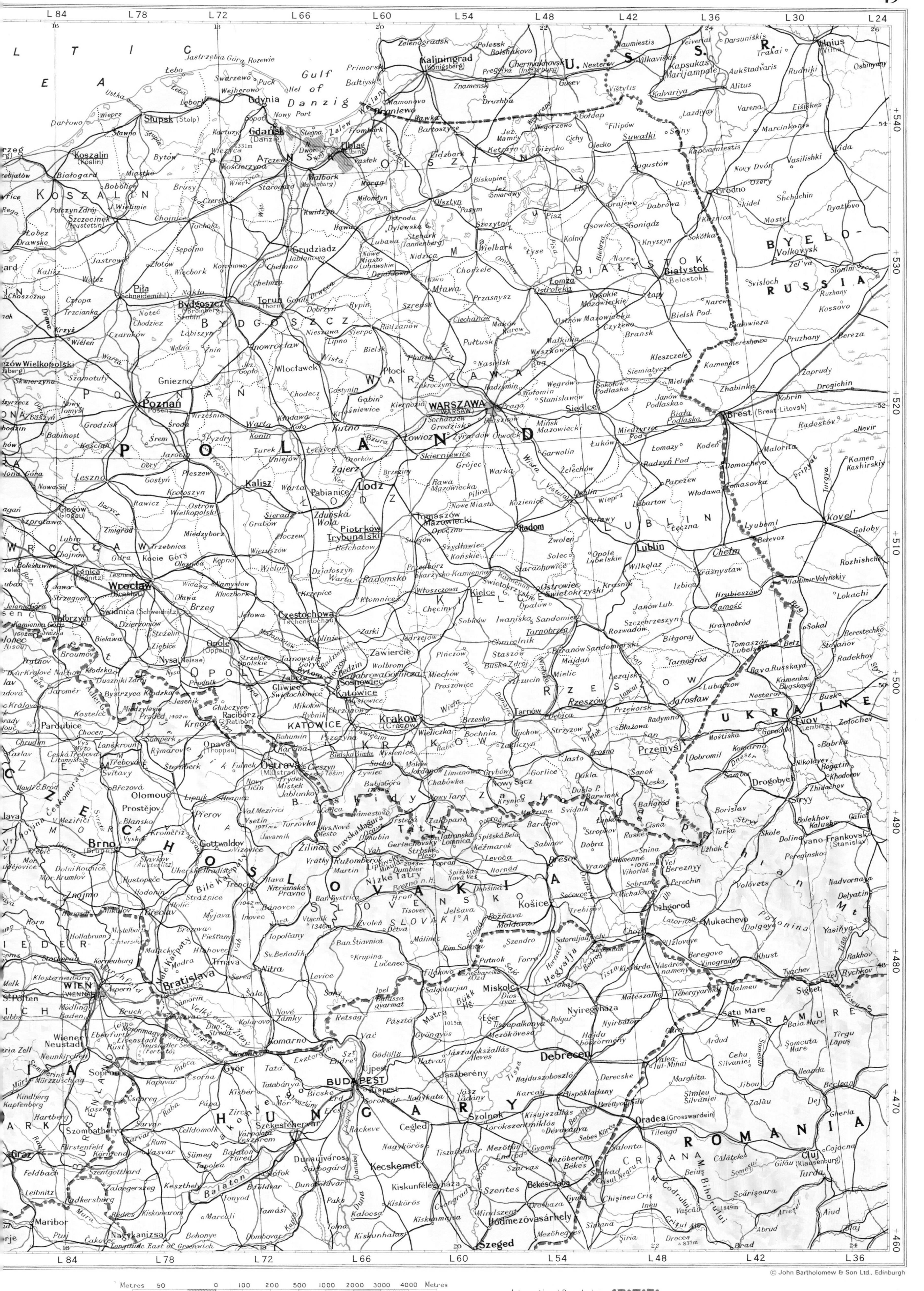

Metres 50 0 100 200 500 1000 2000 3000 4000 Metres
Land Depression
Feet 100 0 330 660 1640 3280 6560 9840 13120 Feet

International Boundaries
State Boundaries

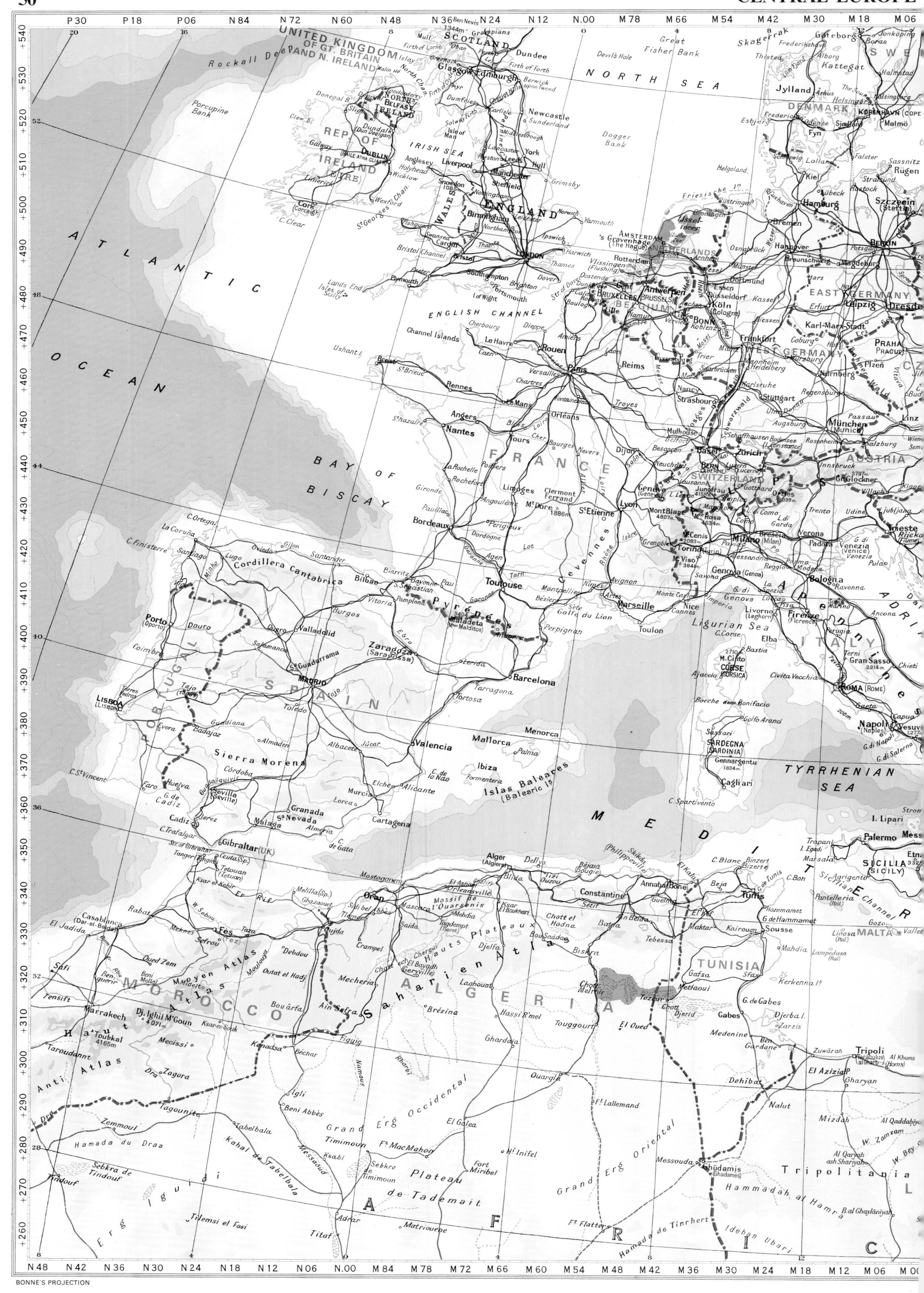

BONNE'S PROJECTION

International Boundaries
State Boundaries
Main Roads
Railways

0 100 200 300 400 Statute Miles

0 100 200 300 400 500 600 Kilometres

1:10

Metres	5000	4000	3000	2000	1000	500	200	100	50	Land Depression	0	200	500	1000	2000	3000	4000	Metres
Feet	16400	13120	9840	6560	3280	1640	660	330	160		0	660	1640	3280	6560	9840	13120	Feet

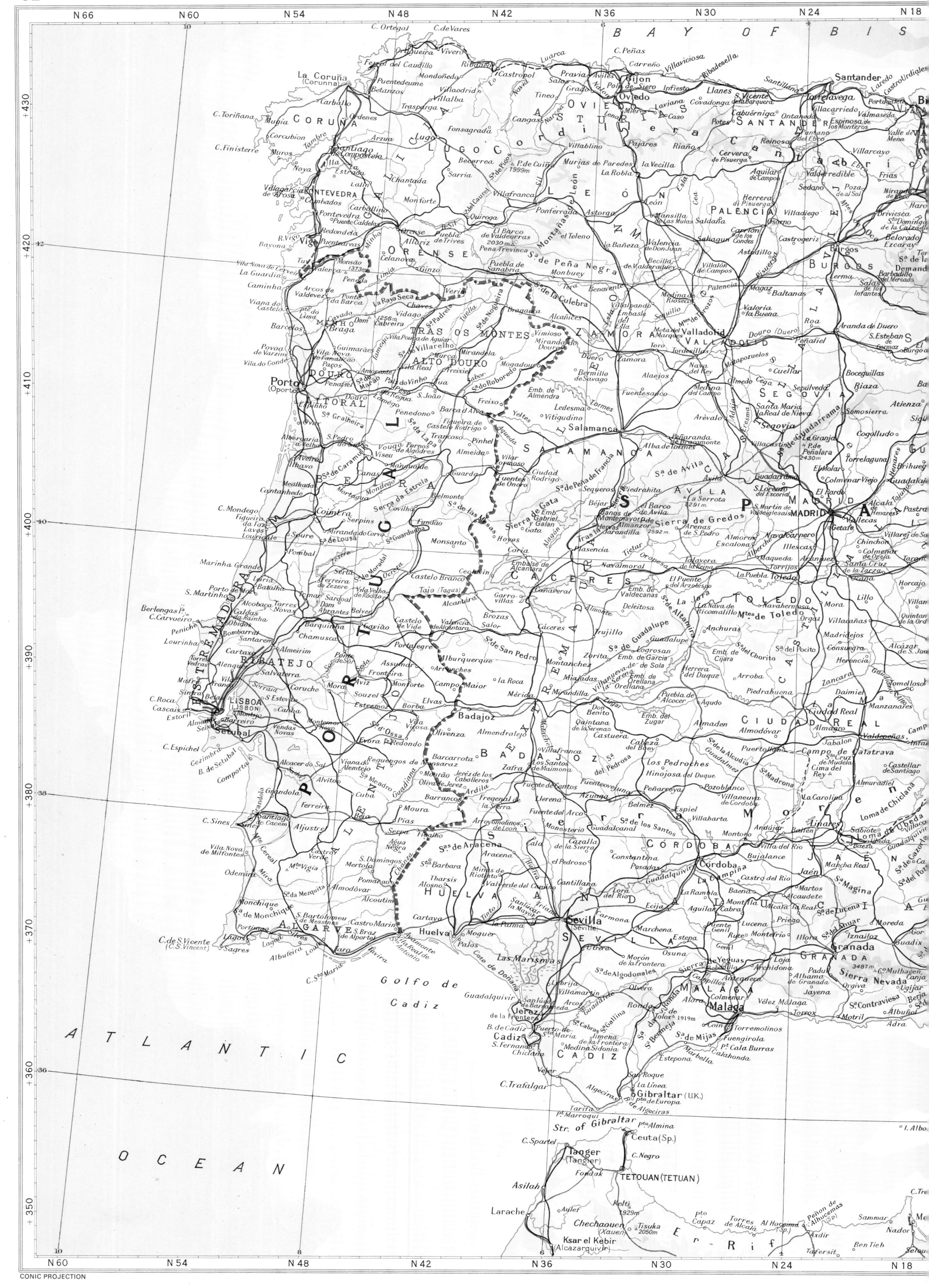

Main Roads

Railways

0 10 20 30 40 50 60 70 80 90 100 110 120 Statute Miles

0 10 20 40 60 80 100 120 140 160 180 Kilometres

1:3

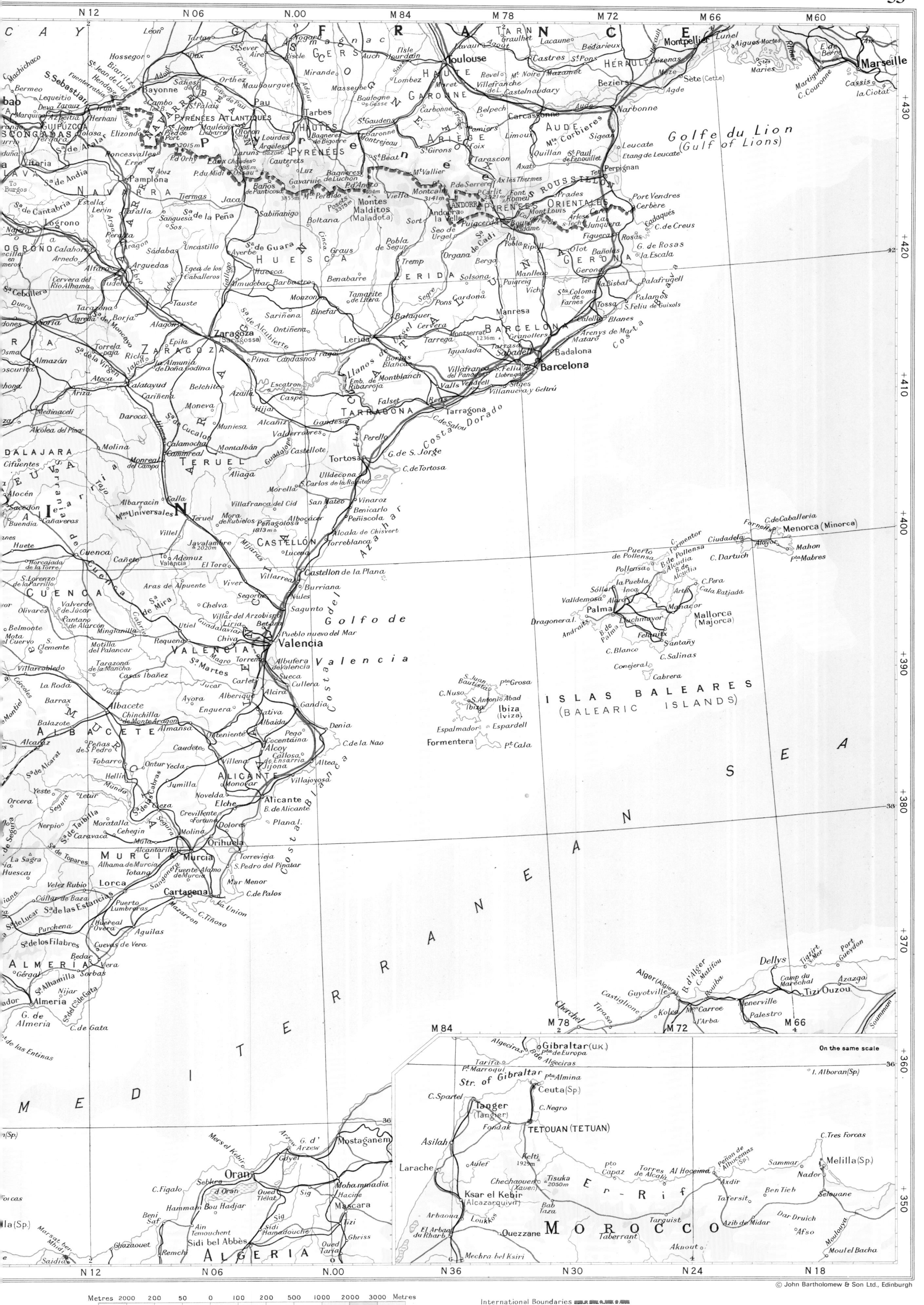

Metres	2000	200	50	0	100	200	500	1000	2000	3000	Metres
Feet	6560	660	160	0	330	660	1640	3280	6560	9840	Feet

International Boundaries

State Boundaries

M

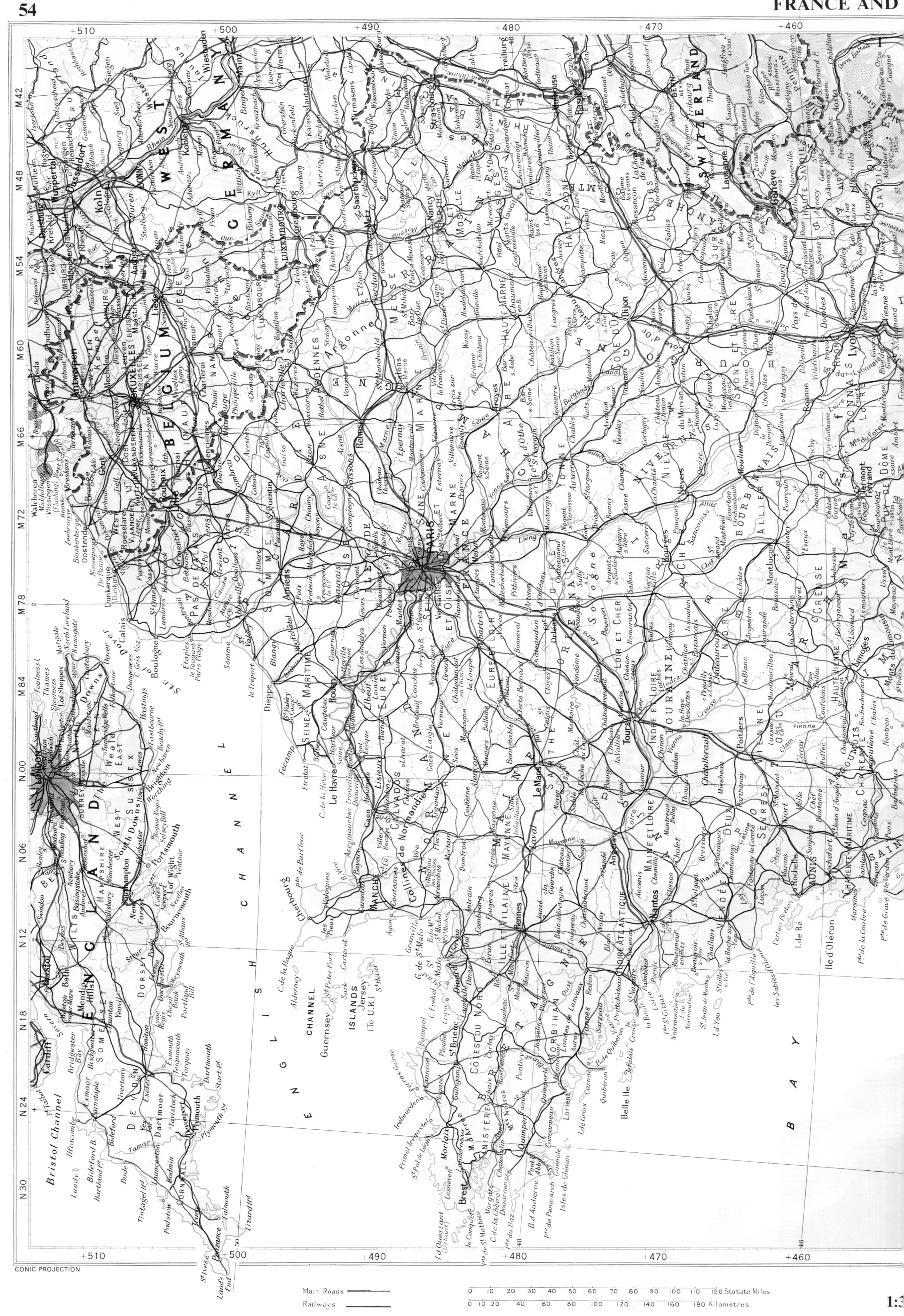
CONIC PROJECTION
Main Roads
Railways
0 10 20 30 40 50 60 70 80 90 100 110 120 Statute Miles
0 10 20 40 60 80 100 120 140 160 180 Kilometres
1:3
+510
+500
+490
+480
+470
+460
M42
M48
M54
M60
M66
M72
M78
M84
N00
N06
N12
N18
N24
N30
ENGLISH CHANNEL
CHANNEL ISLANDS
(To U.K.)
BAY
WEST GERMANY
BELGIUM
SWITZERLAND
LUXEMBOURG
ENGLAND
PARIS
LONDON
Bristol Channel
Guernsey
Jersey
Alderney
Sark
Le Havre
Rouen
Caen
Cherbourg
Brest
Nantes
Tours
Orléans
Dijon
Lyon
Genève
Lausanne
Bruxelles
Antwerpen
Köln
Düsseldorf
Wiesbaden
Mainz
Strasbourg
Nancy
Metz
Reims
Amiens
Lille
Calais
Boulogne
Dunkerque
Oostende
Dover
Plymouth
Portsmouth
Southampton
Cardiff
Bristol
Exeter
Rennes
Le Mans
Poitiers
Limoges
Angers
Lorient
Quimper
Saint-Nazaire
La Rochelle
Bourges
Nevers
Clermont Ferrand
Besançon
Mulhouse
Basel
Troyes
Chartres
Evreux
Dieppe
Fécamp
Granville
St Malo
Morlaix
Belle Ile
I. de Ré
Ile d'Oléron
Lundy
Isles of Scilly
Land's End
Lizard Hd
Start Pt
Ushant

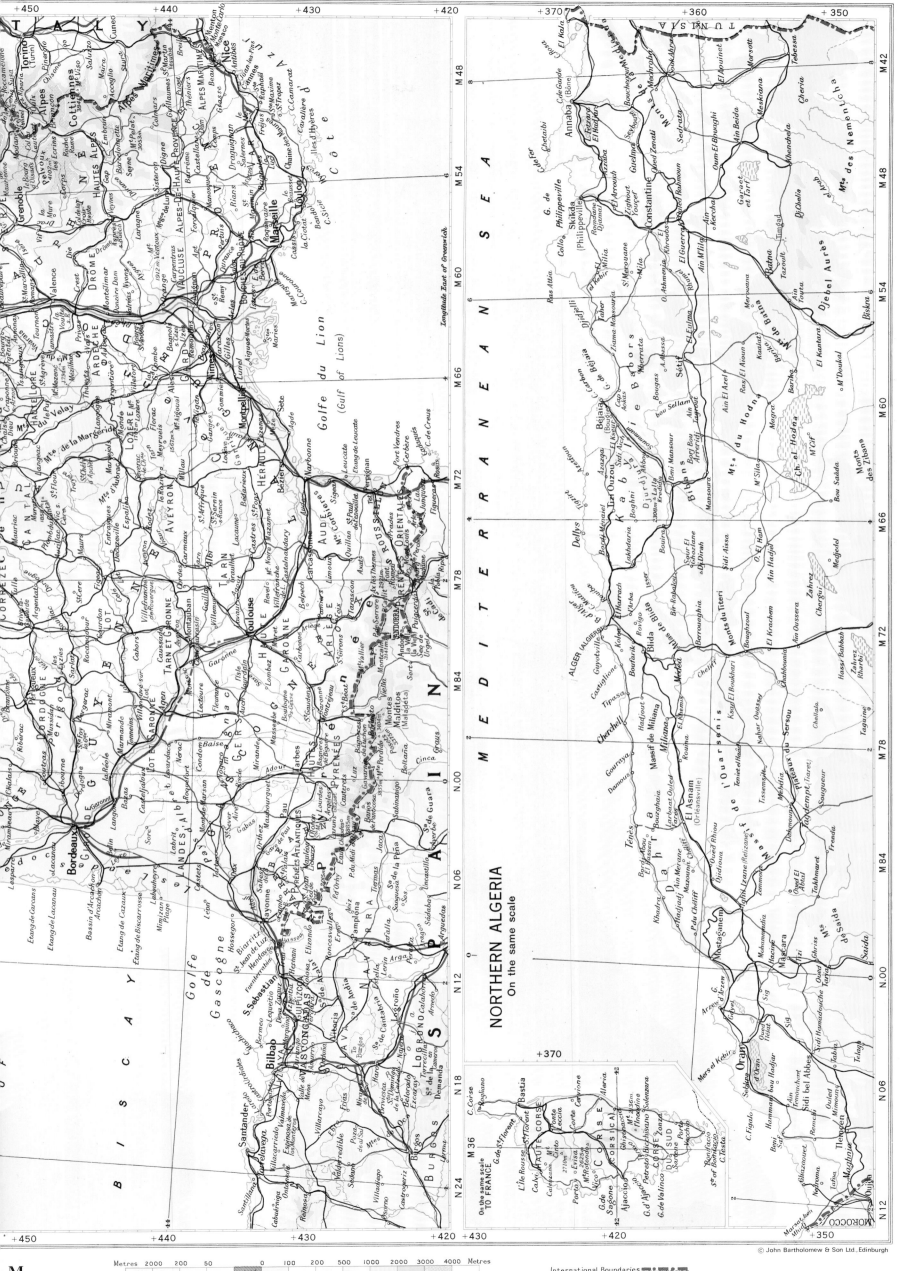
NORTHERN ALGERIA
On the same scale
M E D I T E R R A N E A N S E A
Golfe du Lion
(Gulf of Lions)
Golfe de Gascogne
B I S C A Y
S P A I N
Longitude East of Greenwich
On the same scale TO FRANCE
CORSE (CORSICA)
Ajaccio
Bastia
ALGER (ALGIERS)
Oran
Constantine
Annaba (Bône)
Skikda (Philippeville)
Sétif
Batna
Biskra
Tlemcen
Mostaganem
Blida
Médéa
Dellys
Béjaïa
Djidjelli
El Asnam (Orléansville)
Sidi bel Abbes
Mascara
Saïda
Massif de l'Ouarsenis
Ch. el Hodna
Djebel Aurès
Mts des Nementcha
Monts du Titeri
TUNISIA
MOROCCO
Bordeaux
Toulouse
Marseille
Montpellier
Nîmes
Narbonne
Perpignan
Nice
Toulon
Grenoble
Torino (Turin)
Bilbao
Santander
S. Sebastian
Pamplona
Vitoria
Logroño
Burgos
ANDORRA
PYRENEES ORIENTALES
International Boundaries
State Boundaries
Metres 2000 200 50 0 100 200 500 1000 2000 3000 4000 Metres
Land Depression
Feet 6560 660 160 0 330 660 1640 3280 6560 9840 13120 Feet
© John Bartholomew & Son Ltd. Edinburgh

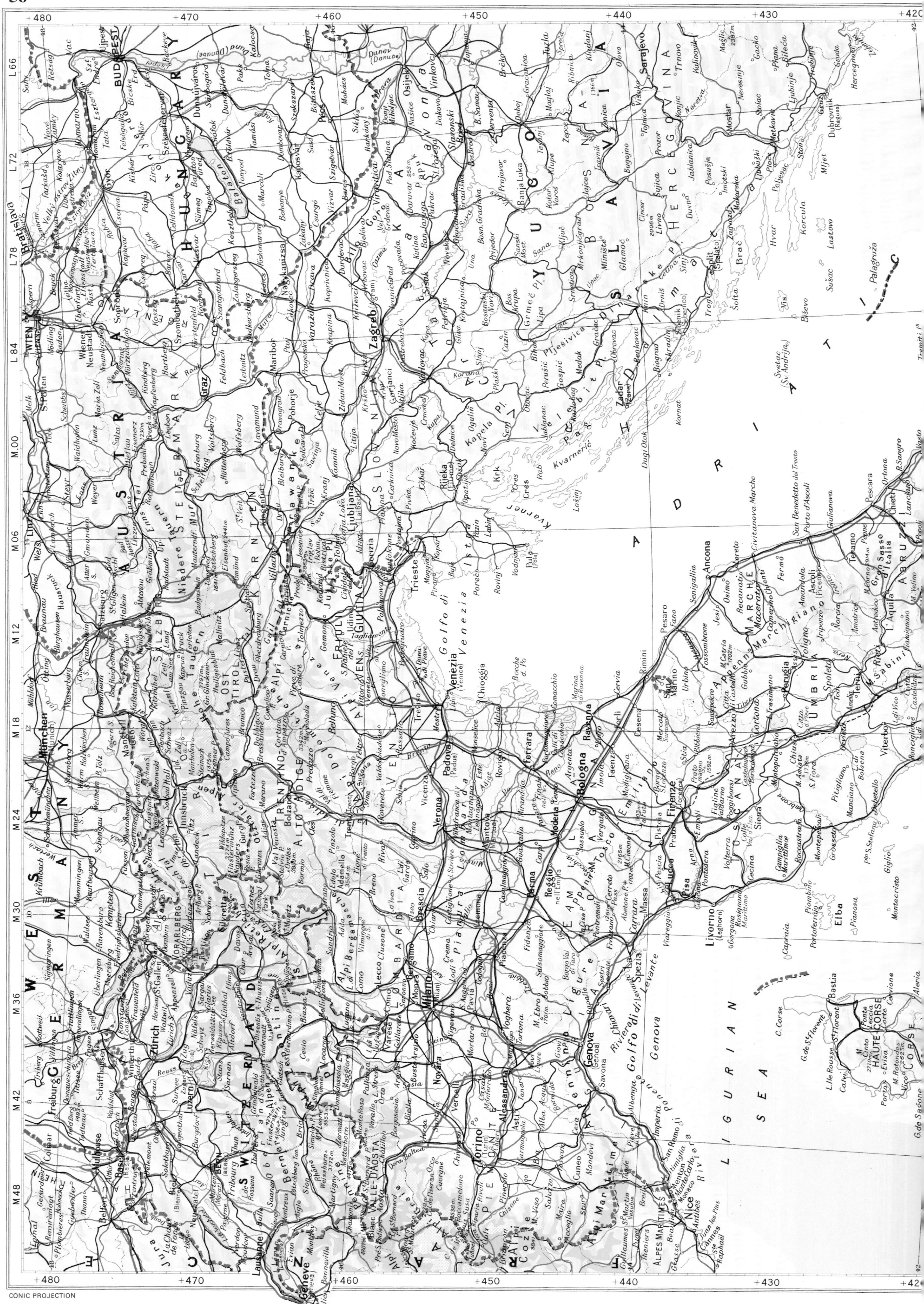

CONIC PROJECTION

Main Roads

Railways

0 10 20 30 40 50 60 70 80 90 100 110 120 Statute Miles

0 10 20 40 60 80 100 120 140 160 180 Kilometres

1:3

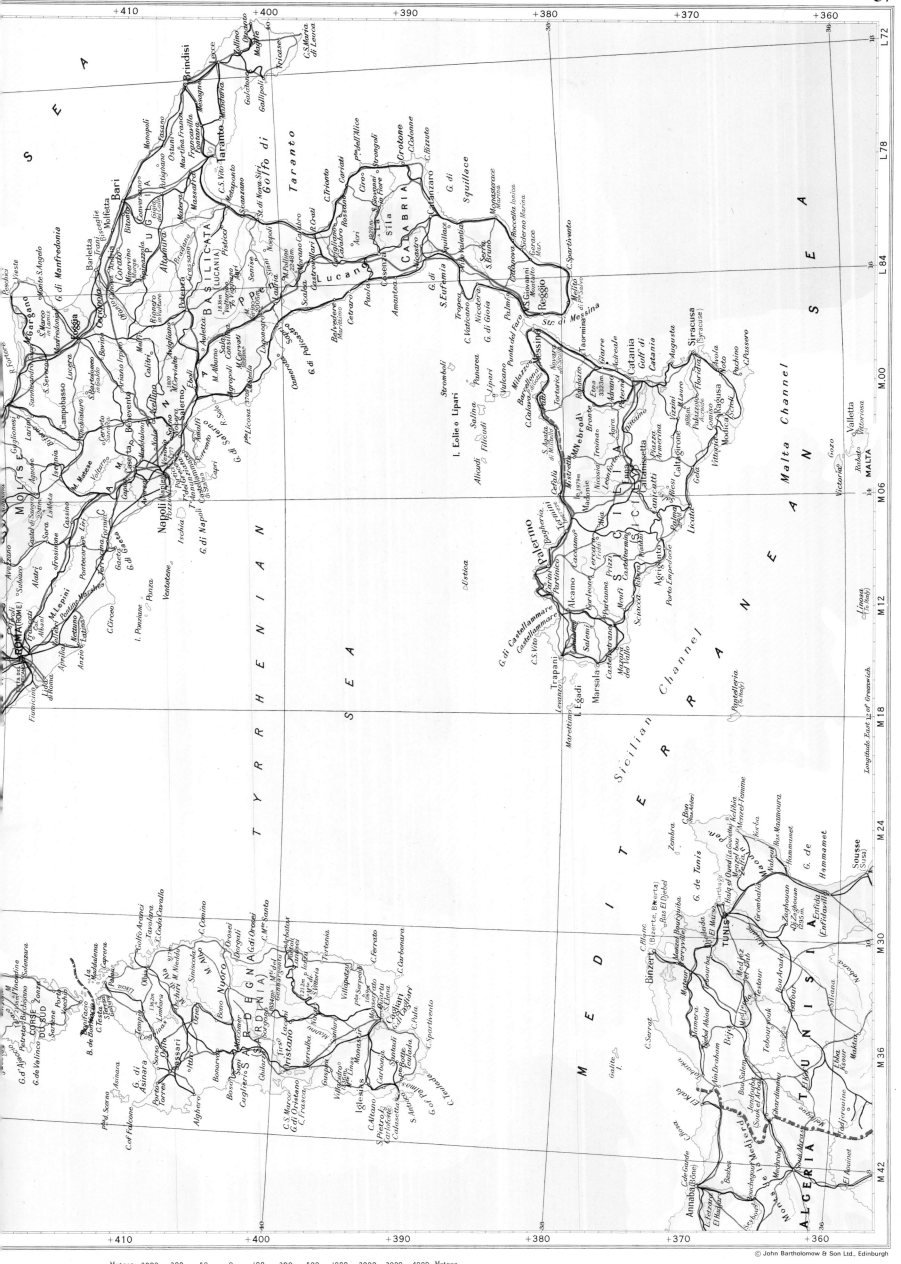

© John Bartholomew & Son Ltd., Edinburgh

Metres 2000 200 50 0 100 200 500 1000 2000 3000 4000 Metres

Feet 6560 660 160 0 330 660 1640 3280 6560 9840 13120 Feet

International Boundaries

State Boundaries

M

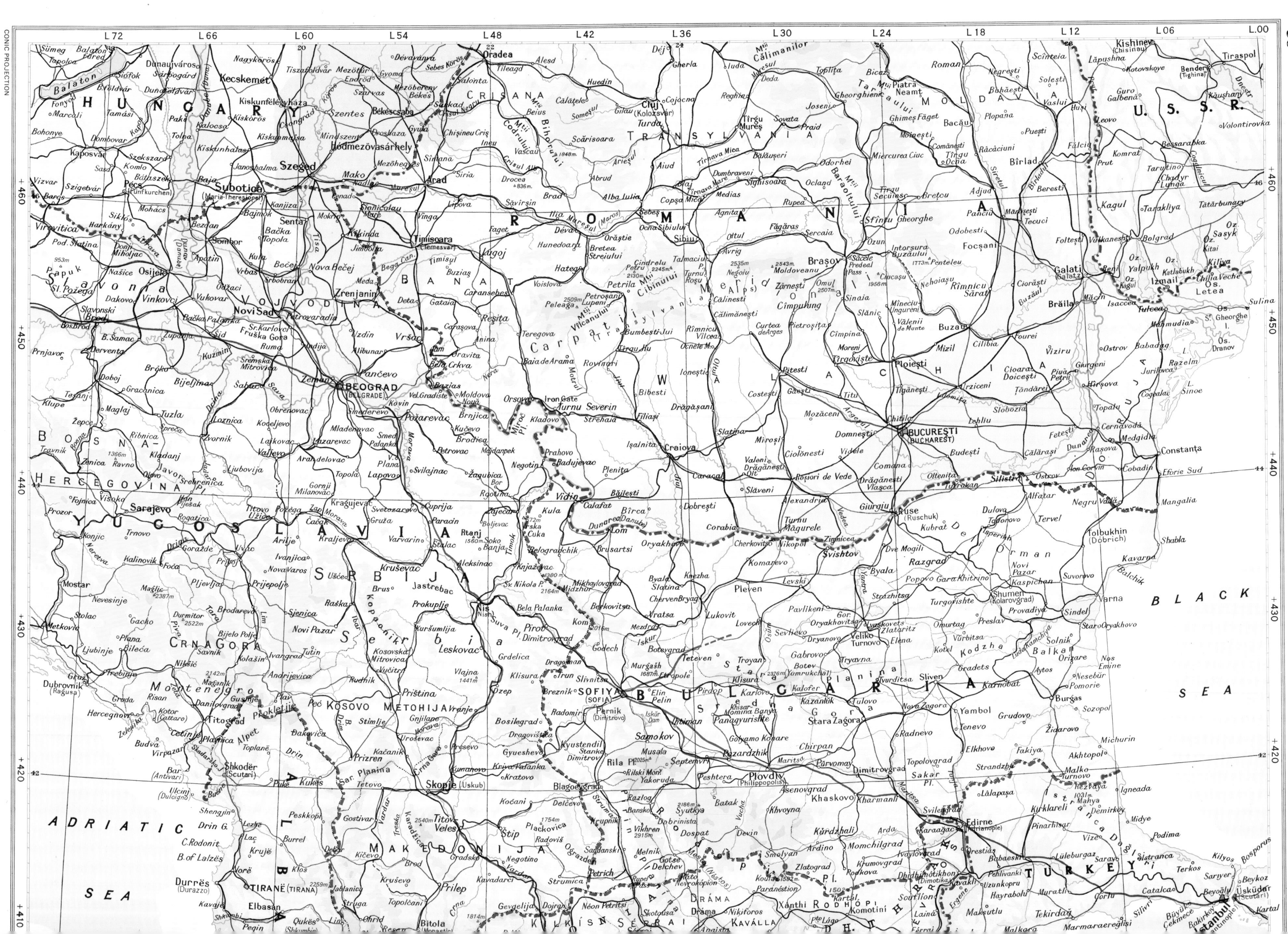

CONIC PROJECTION

Main Roads

Railways

0 10 20 30 40 50 60 70 80 90 100 110 120 Statute Miles

0 10 20 40 60 80 100 120 140 160 180 Kilometres

1:3

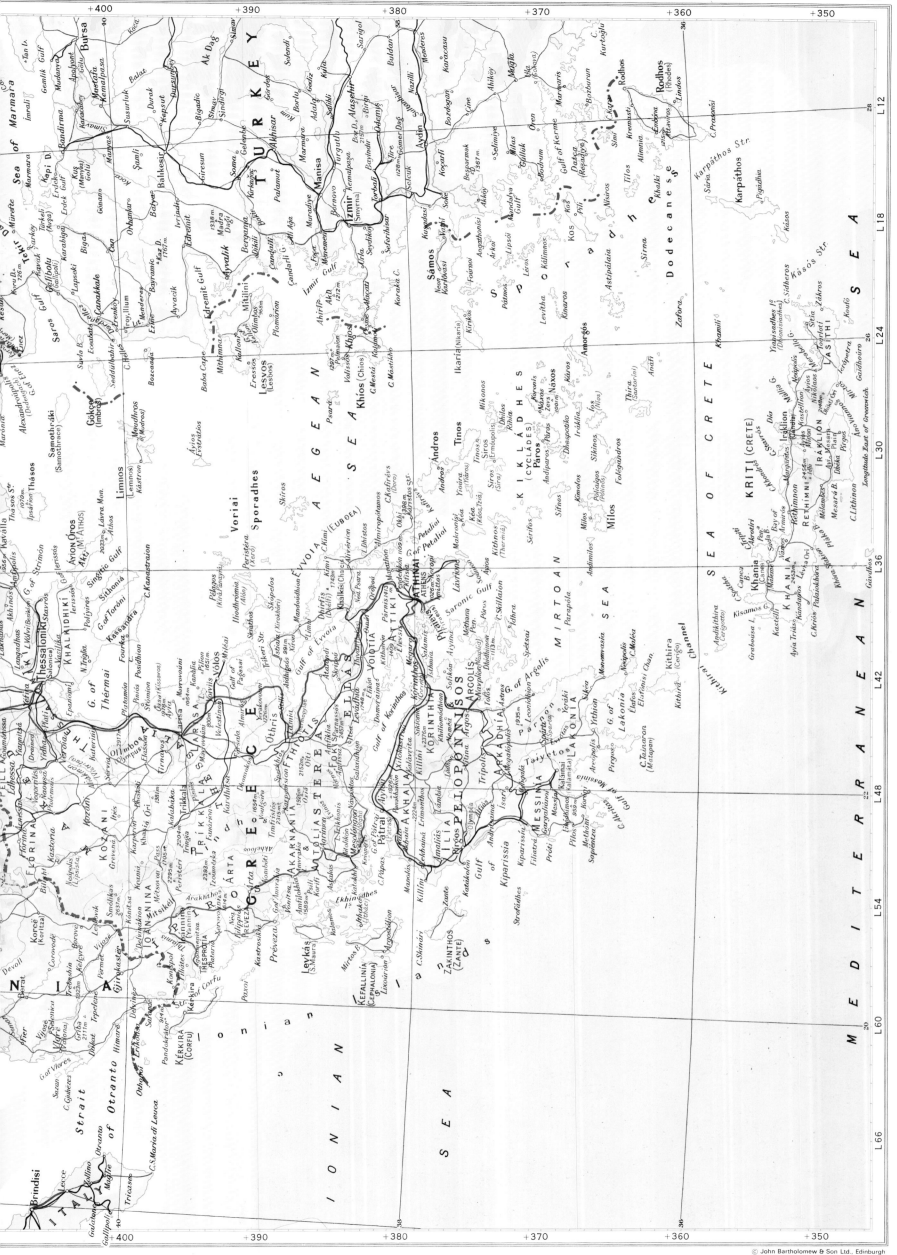

M

Metres	2000	200	50	0	100	200	500	1000	2000	Metres
Feet	6560	660	160	0	330	660	1640	3280	6560	Feet

International Boundaries

State Boundaries

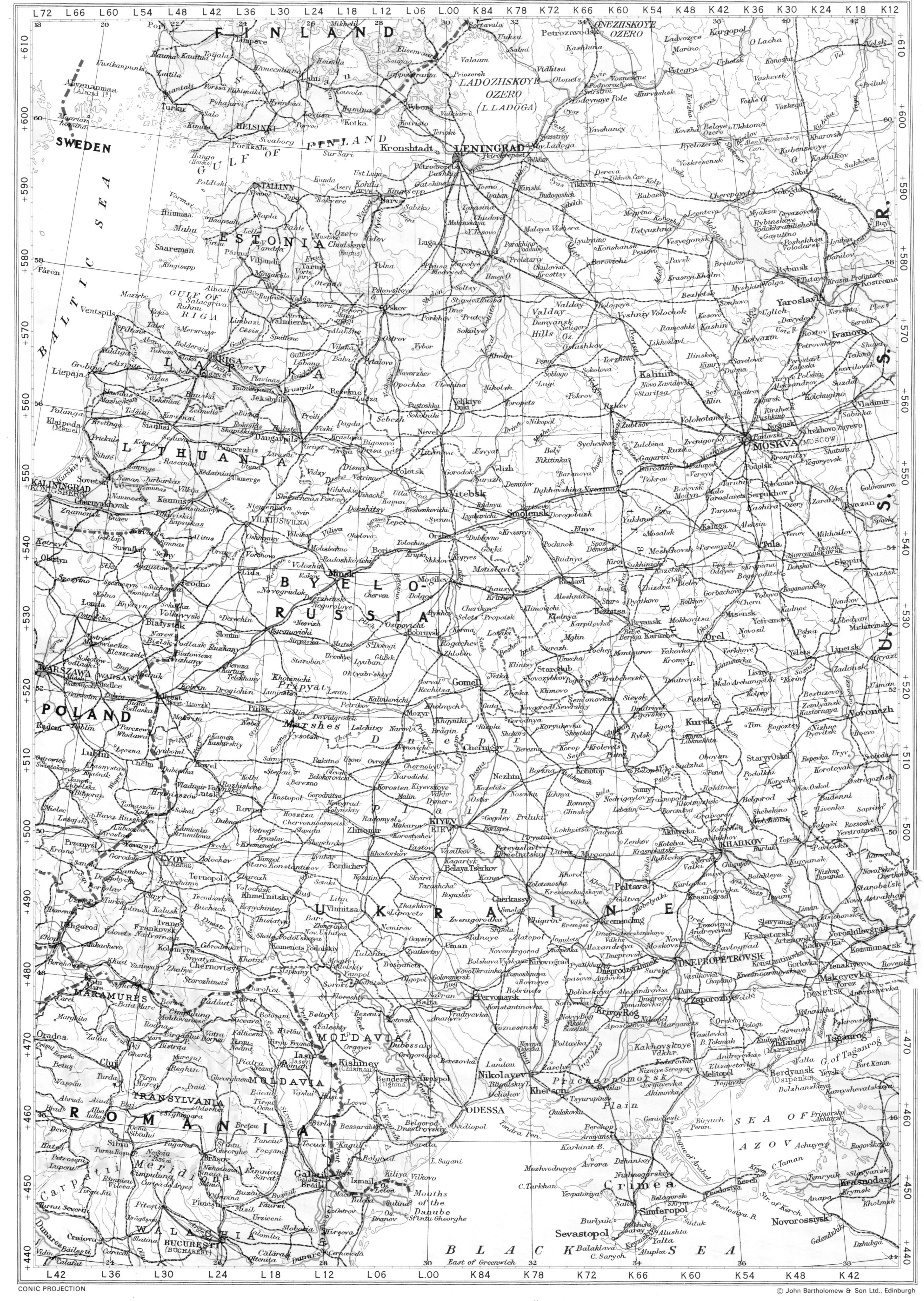
FINLAND
SWEDEN
GULF OF FINLAND
BALTIC SEA
ESTONIA
LATVIA
LITHUANIA
BYELO-RUSSIA
POLAND
UKRAINE
MOLDAVIA
ROMANIA
TRANSYLVANIA
WALACHIA
MARAMURES
Crimea
SEA OF AZOV
BLACK SEA
GULF OF RIGA
LADOZHSKOYE OZERO (L.LADOGA)
ONEZHSKOYE OZERO
U. S. S. R.
Central Russian Upland
Valday Hills
Pripyat Marshes
Dnepr
Carpathians
Mouths of the Danube
HELSINKI
LENINGRAD
TALLINN
RIGA
KALININGRAD (KÖNIGSBERG)
VILNIUS (VILNA)
Minsk
WARSZAWA (WARSAW)
MOSKVA (MOSCOW)
KIYEV (KIEV)
KHARKOV
DNEPROPETROVSK
ODESSA
Kishinev (Chişinău)
LVOV (LEMBERG)
BUCUREŞTI (BUCHAREST)
Sevastopol
Simferopol
Novorossiysk
Krasnodar
Voronezh
Kursk
Orel
Tula
Ryazan
Kalinin
Smolensk
Vitebsk
Gomel
Mogilev
Brest
Poltava
Nikolayev
Kherson
Zaporozhye
Taganrog
DONETSK
Yaroslavl
Vologda
Rybinsk
Kostroma
Ivanovo
Vladimir
Novgorod
Pskov
East of Greenwich
CONIC PROJECTION
© John Bartholomew & Son Ltd., Edinburgh
0 20 40 60 80 100 120 140 160 180 Statute Miles
0 20 40 80 120 160 200 240 280 Kilometres
1:6M
Metres 200 50 0 100 200 500 1000 2000 Metres
Feet 660 160 0 330 660 1640 3280 6560 Feet

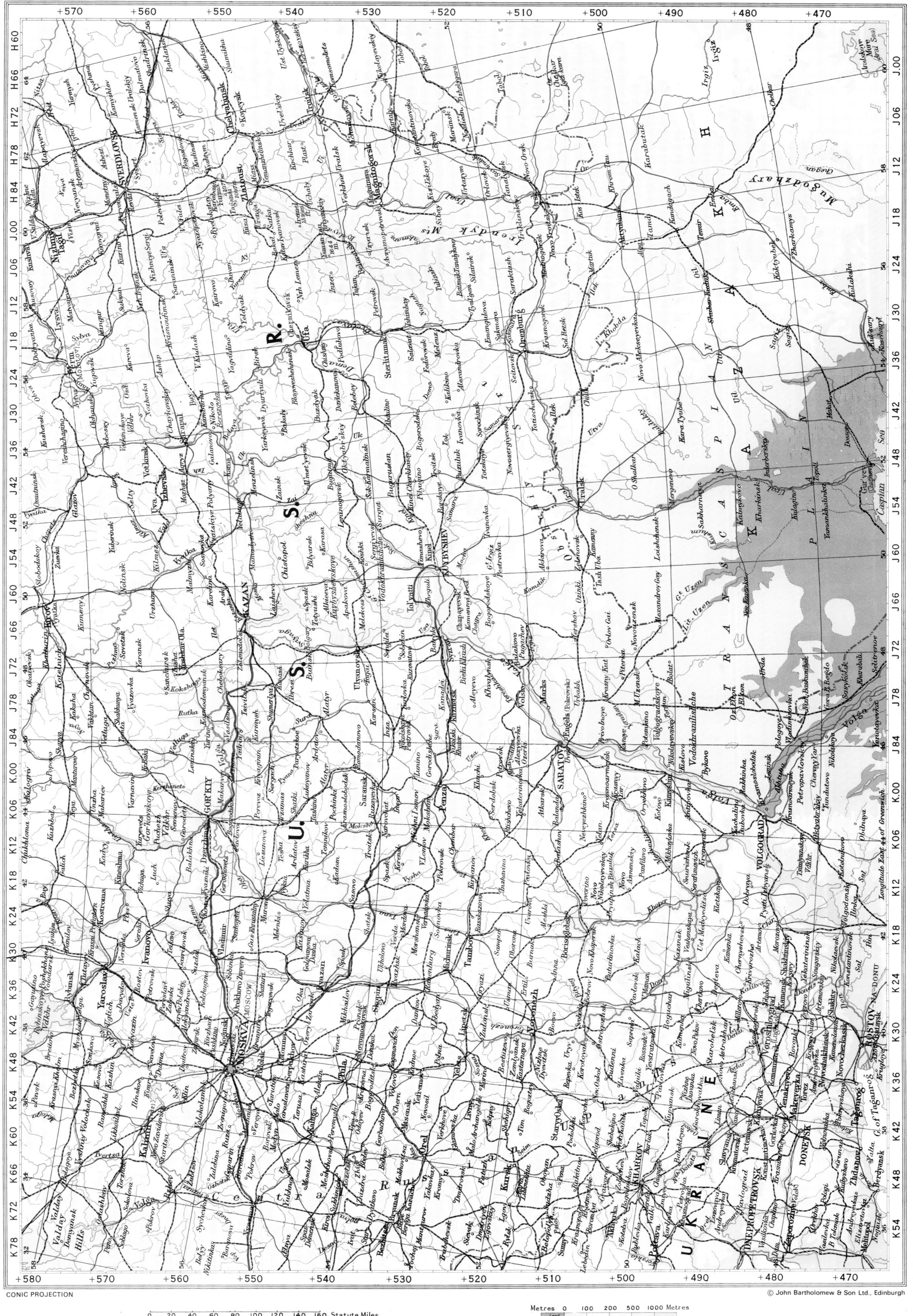
CONIC PROJECTION
© John Bartholomew & Son Ltd., Edinburgh
0 20 40 60 80 100 120 140 160 Statute Miles
0 20 40 80 120 160 200 240 Kilometres
1:6M
Metres 0 100 200 500 1000 Metres
Land Depression
Feet 0 330 660 1640 3280 Feet
Longitude East 44 of Greenwich
SVERDLOVSK
Chelyabinsk
Magnitogorsk
Zlatoust
Ufa
Orenburg
Perm
KAZAN
KUYBYSHEV
SARATOV
VOLGOGRAD
GOR'KIY
MOSKVA
Yaroslavl
Ivanovo
Kostroma
Kirov
Ul'yanovsk
Penza
Tambov
Voronezh
Kursk
KHARKOV
DONETSK
ROSTOV-NA-DONU
Tula
Orel
Kalinin
Vladimir
Ryazan
Astrakhan
Gur'yev
Caspian
Volga
Mugodzhary
Irendyk Mts
Ural
R.
S.
S.
U.
K
A
Z
K
H
S
UKRAINE

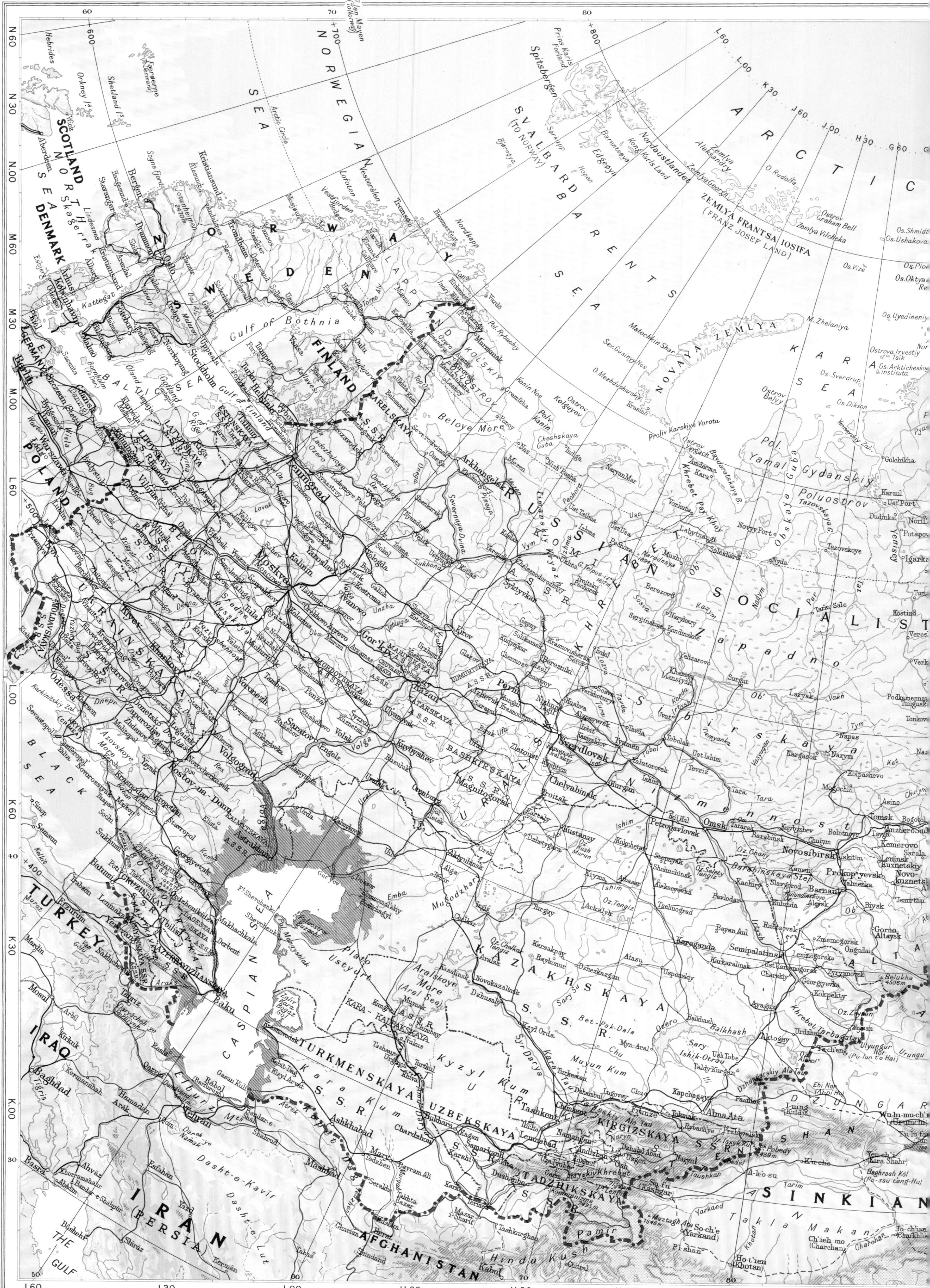

CONIC PROJECTION

Main Roads
Railways

0 100 200 300 400 500 600 Statute Miles
0 100 200 300 400 500 600 700 800 900 1000 Kilometres

1:17½

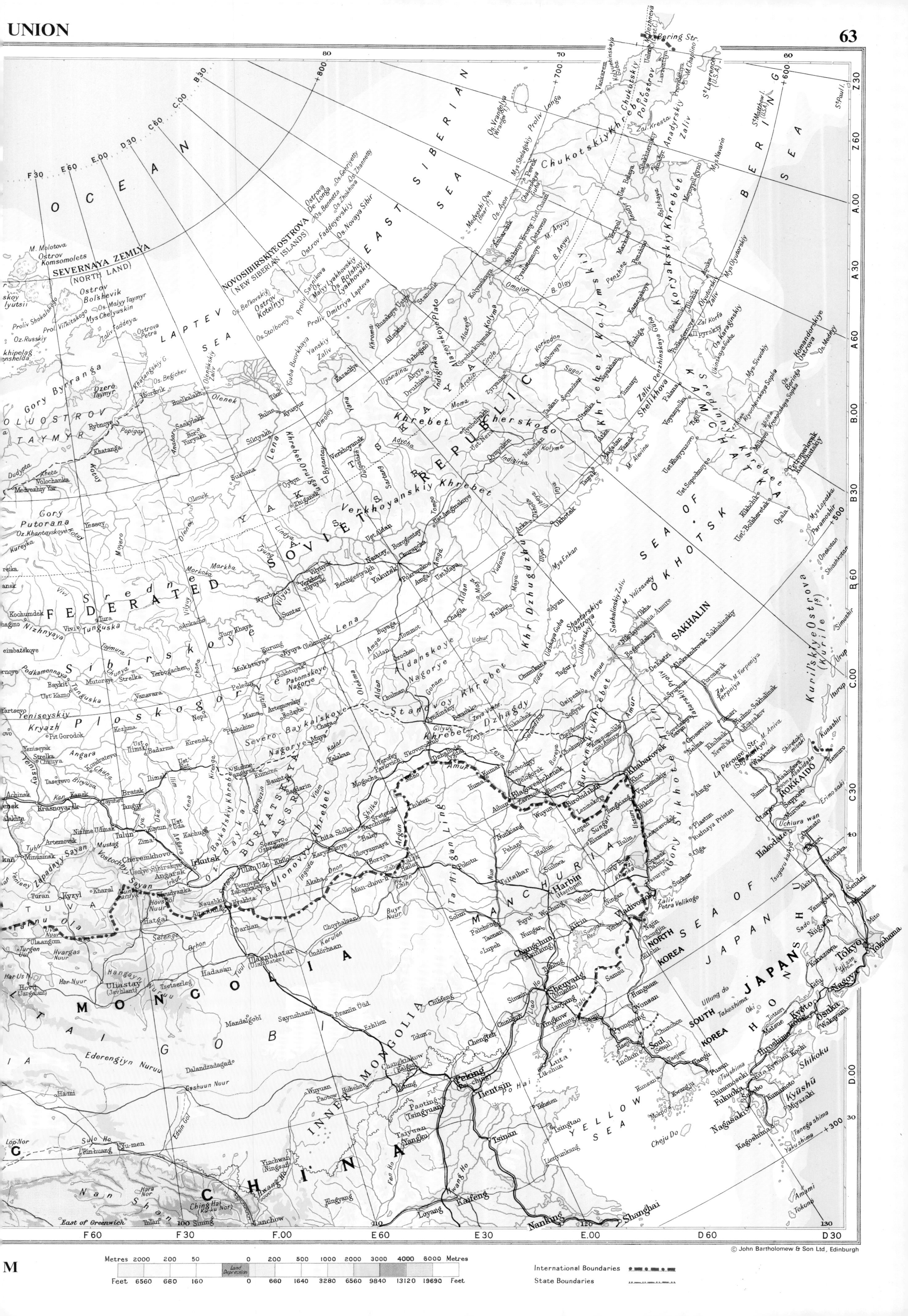
OCEAN
EAST SIBERIAN SEA
LAPTEV SEA
BERING SEA
SEA OF OKHOTSK
SEA OF JAPAN
YELLOW SEA
YAKUTSK A.S.S.R.
SOVIET REPUBLIC
FEDERATED
Sibirskoye Ploskogorye
BURYATSKAYA A.S.S.R.
MANCHURIA
MONGOLIA
INNER MONGOLIA
CHINA
GOBI
JAPAN
NORTH KOREA
SOUTH KOREA
SAKHALIN
HOKKAIDO
KAMCHATKA
SEVERNAYA ZEMLYA (NORTH LAND)
NOVOSIBIRSKIYE OSTROVA (NEW SIBERIAN ISLANDS)
Bering Str.
Verkhoyanskiy Khrebet
Khrebet Cherskogo
Stanovoy Khrebet
Yablonovyy Khrebet
Oz. Baykal
Irkutsk
Yakutsk
Khabarovsk
Vladivostok
Harbin
Peking
Tientsin
Shanghai
Nanking
Tokyo
Yokohama
Osaka
Seoul
Ulaanbaatar
Krasnoyarsk
East of Greenwich
© John Bartholomew & Son Ltd, Edinburgh
Metres 2000 200 50 0 200 500 1000 2000 3000 4000 6000 Metres
Land Depression
Feet 6560 660 160 0 660 1640 3280 6560 9840 13120 19690 Feet
International Boundaries
State Boundaries

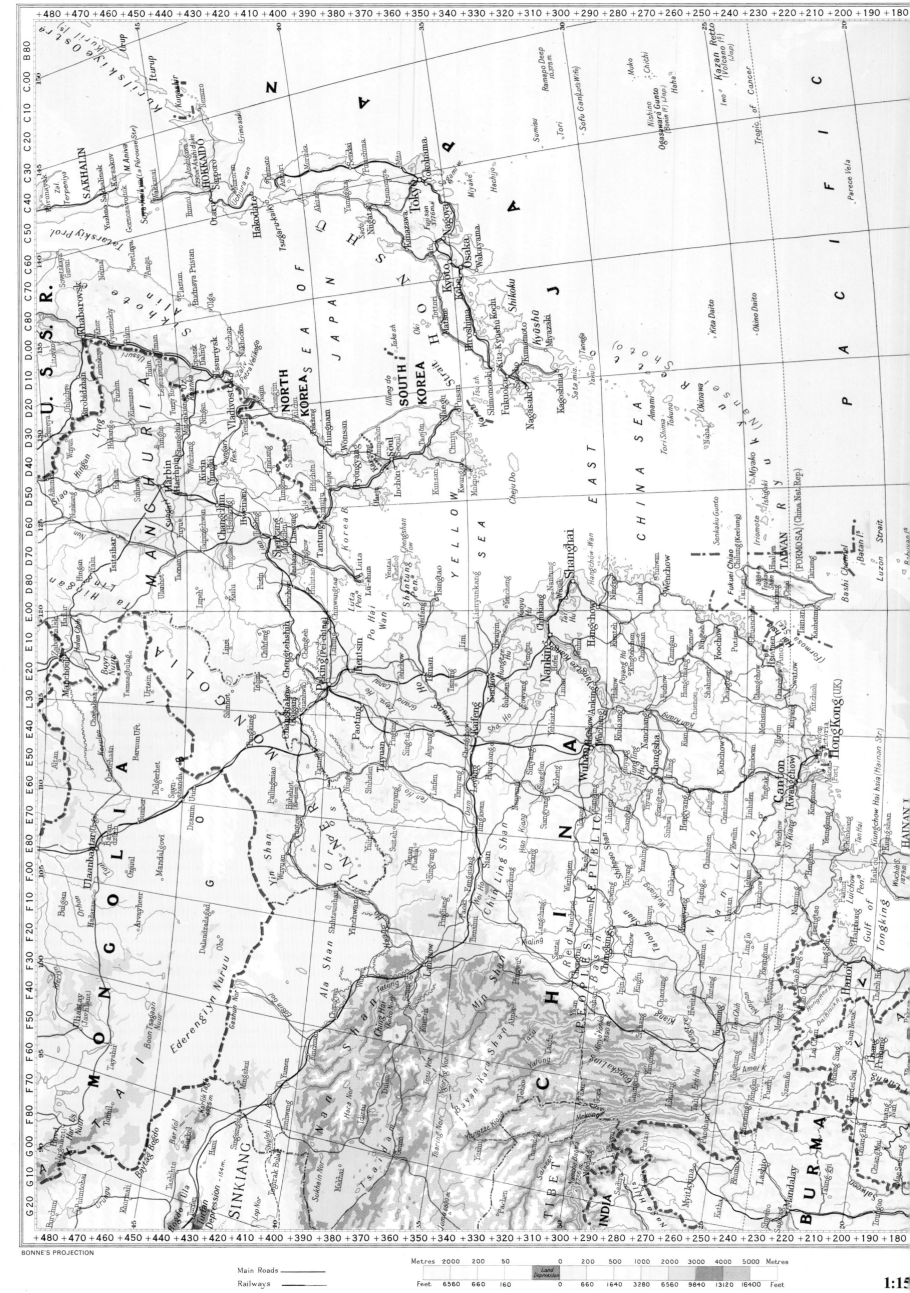

Main Roads
Railways

Metres	2000	200	50	0	200	500	1000	2000	3000	4000	5000	Metres
Feet	6560	660	160	0	660	1640	3280	6560	9840	13120	16400	Feet

Land Depression

1:15

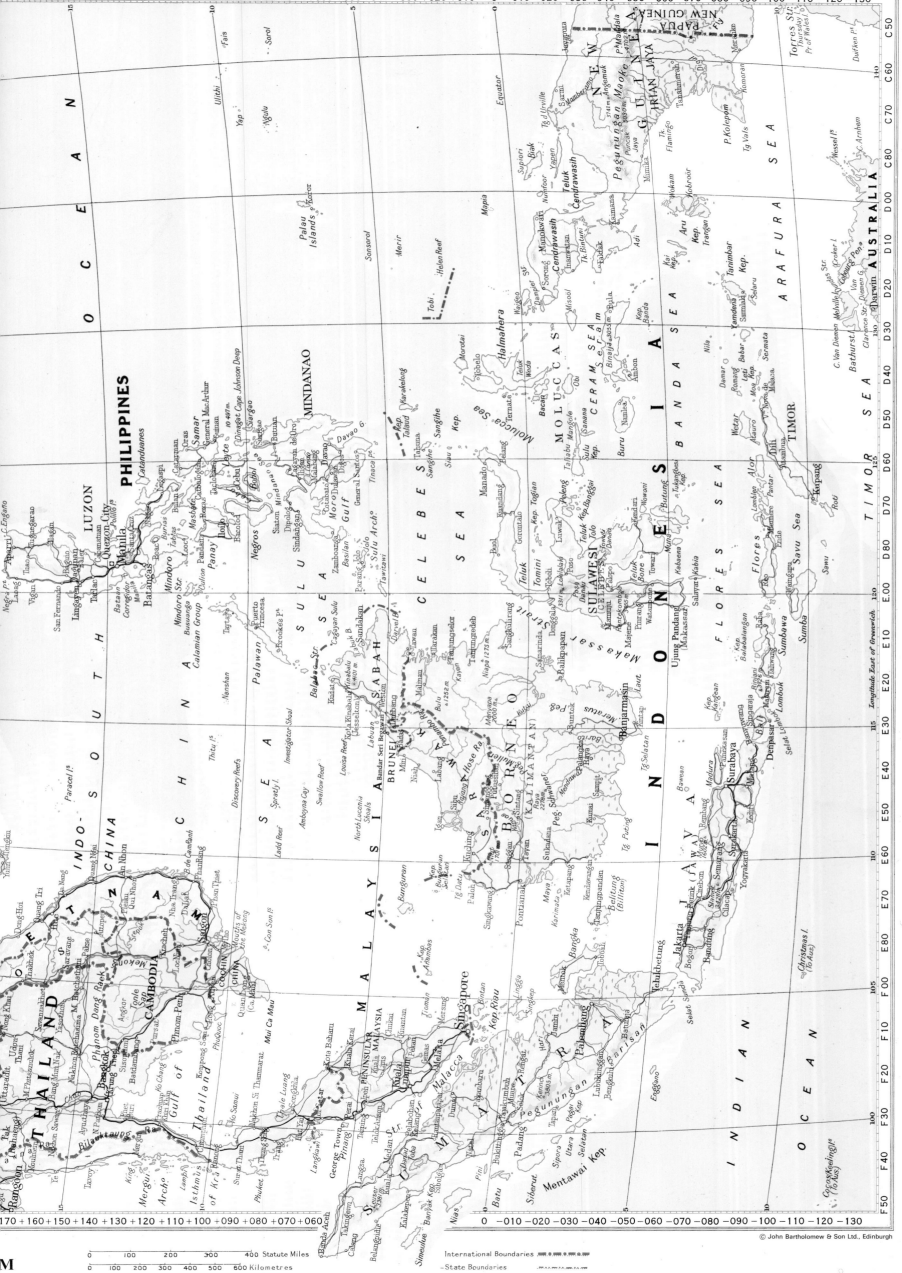
THAILAND
Bangkok
Gulf of Thailand
CAMBODIA
Phnom-Penh
VIETNAM
Saigon
INDO-CHINA
Rangoon
SOUTH CHINA SEA
OCEAN
PHILIPPINES
LUZON
Manila
Quezon City
Mindoro
Panay
Negros
Samar
Leyte
MINDANAO
Palawan
SULU SEA
CELEBES SEA
Molucca Sea
Makassar Strait
MALAYSIA
PENINSULAR MALAYSIA
Kuala Lumpur
Str. of Malacca
Singapore
SABAH
SARAWAK
BRUNEI
BORNEO (KALIMANTAN)
Pontianak
Kuching
Balikpapan
Banjarmasin
SULAWESI (CELEBES)
Manado
Ujung Pandang (Makassar)
MOLUCCAS
Halmahera
CERAM SEA
Buru
Ambon
INDONESIA
BANDA SEA
FLORES SEA
Savu Sea
ARAFURA SEA
TIMOR SEA
SUMATRA
Palembang
Padang
Mentawai Kep.
JAVA
Jakarta
Bandung
Semarang
Yogyakarta
Surabaya
Bali
Lombok
Sumbawa
Flores
Sumba
TIMOR
Kupang
NEW GUINEA
IRIAN JAYA
PAPUA NEW GUINEA
AUSTRALIA
Darwin
INDIAN OCEAN
Christmas I. (To Aus.)
Cocos (Keeling) Is (To Aus.)
Equator
Longitude East of Greenwich
0 100 200 300 400 Statute Miles
0 100 200 300 400 500 600 Kilometres
International Boundaries
State Boundaries

M

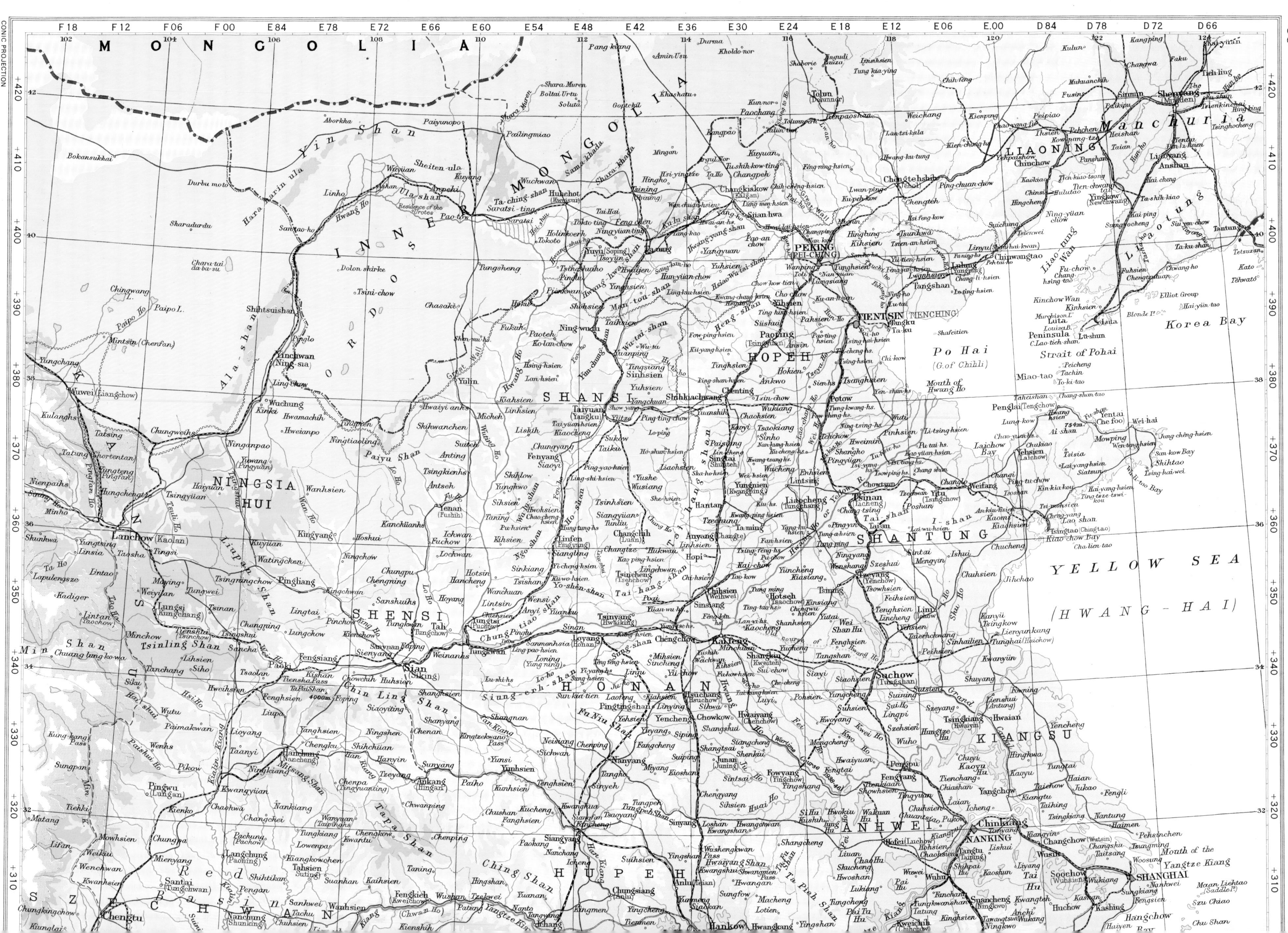

CONIC PROJECTION

Main Roads
Railways

0 20 40 60 80 100 120 140 160 180 200 220 240 Statute Miles
0 20 40 80 120 160 200 240 280 320 360 Kilometres

1:6

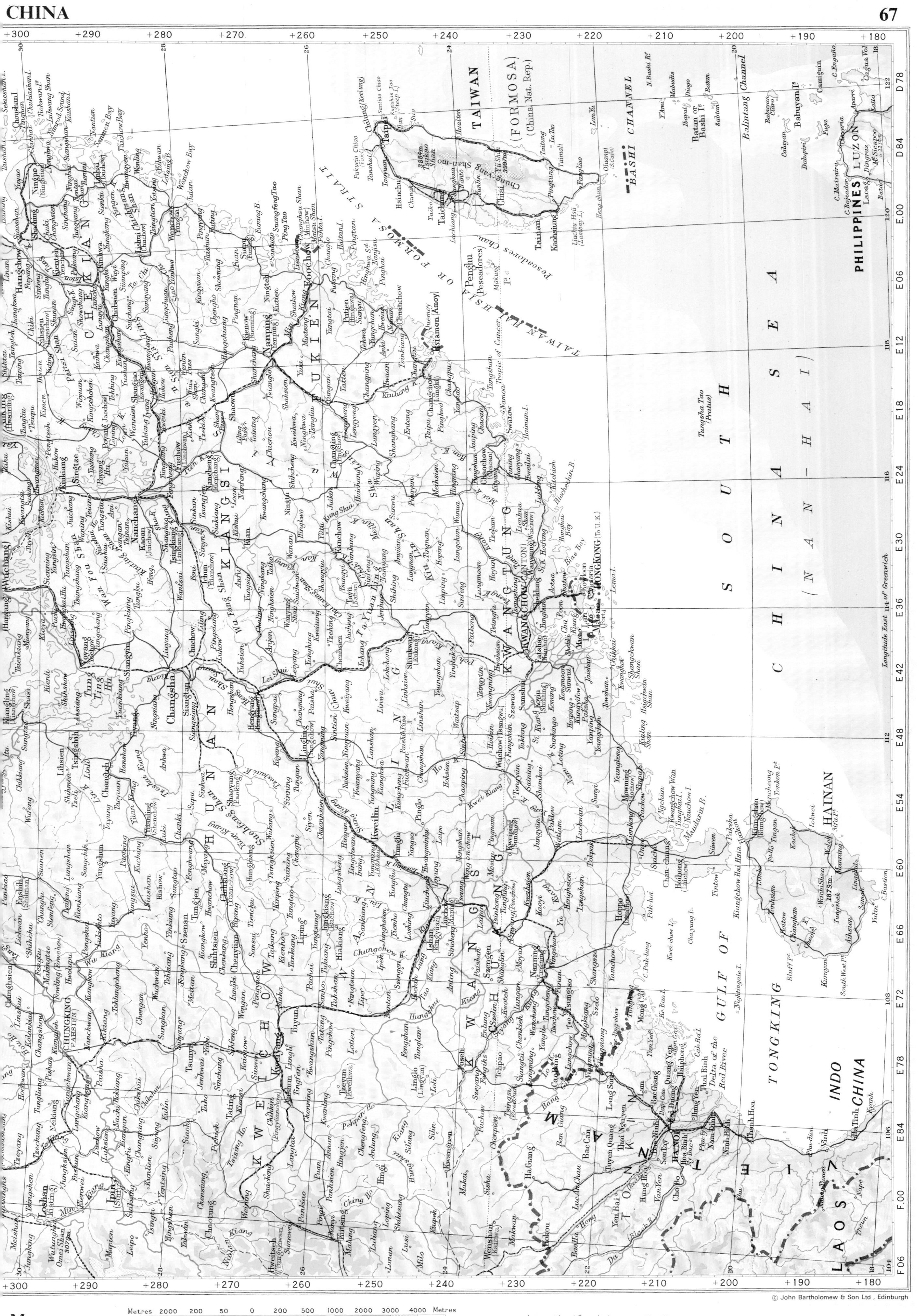
TAIWAN
(FORMOSA)
(China Nat. Rep.)
BASHI CHANNEL
Balintang Channel
PHILIPPINES
LUZON
FORMOSA STRAIT
TAIWAN HAI HSIA OR FORMOSA STRAIT
Pescadores Chan.
SOUTH CHINA SEA
(NAN - HAI)
HAINAN
GULF OF TONGKING
INDO CHINA
LAOS
KWANGTUNG
KWANGSI
FUKIEN
KIANGSI
CHEKIANG
HUNAN
KWEICHOW
TONGKING
HONGKONG
CHUNGKING
Changsha
Taipei
Foochow
Hanoi
Tropic of Cancer
Longitude East 114 of Greenwich
Metres 2000 200 50 0 200 500 1000 2000 3000 4000 Metres
Feet 6560 660 160 0 660 1640 3280 6560 9840 13120 Feet
International Boundaries
State Boundaries
M

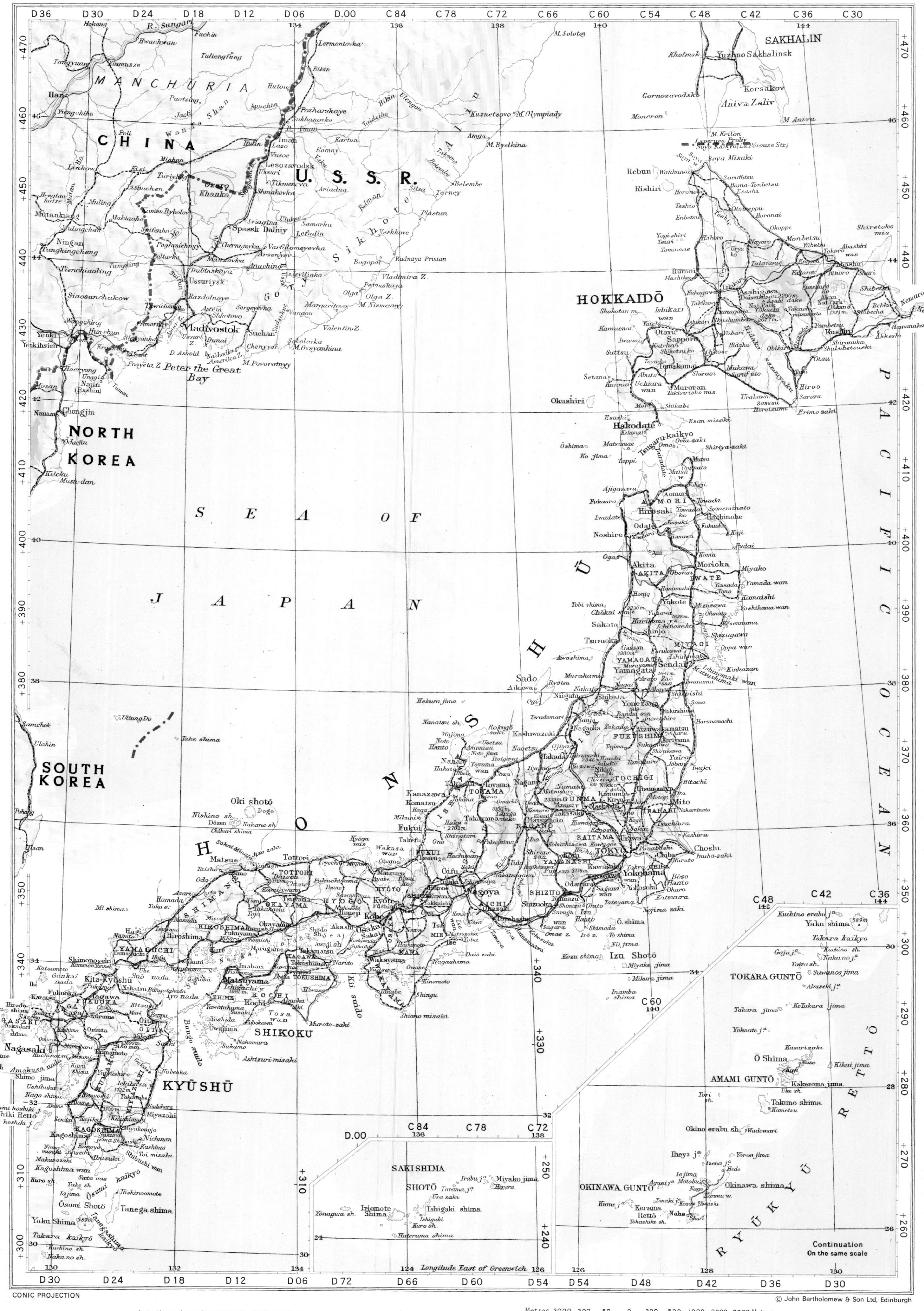

CONIC PROJECTION

© John Bartholomew & Son Ltd, Edinburgh

1:6M

0 20 40 60 80 100 120 140 160 180 Statute Miles
0 20 40 80 120 160 200 240 280 Kilometres

Metres 2000 200 50 0 200 500 1000 2000 3000 Metres
Feet 6560 660 160 0 660 1640 3280 6560 9840 Feet

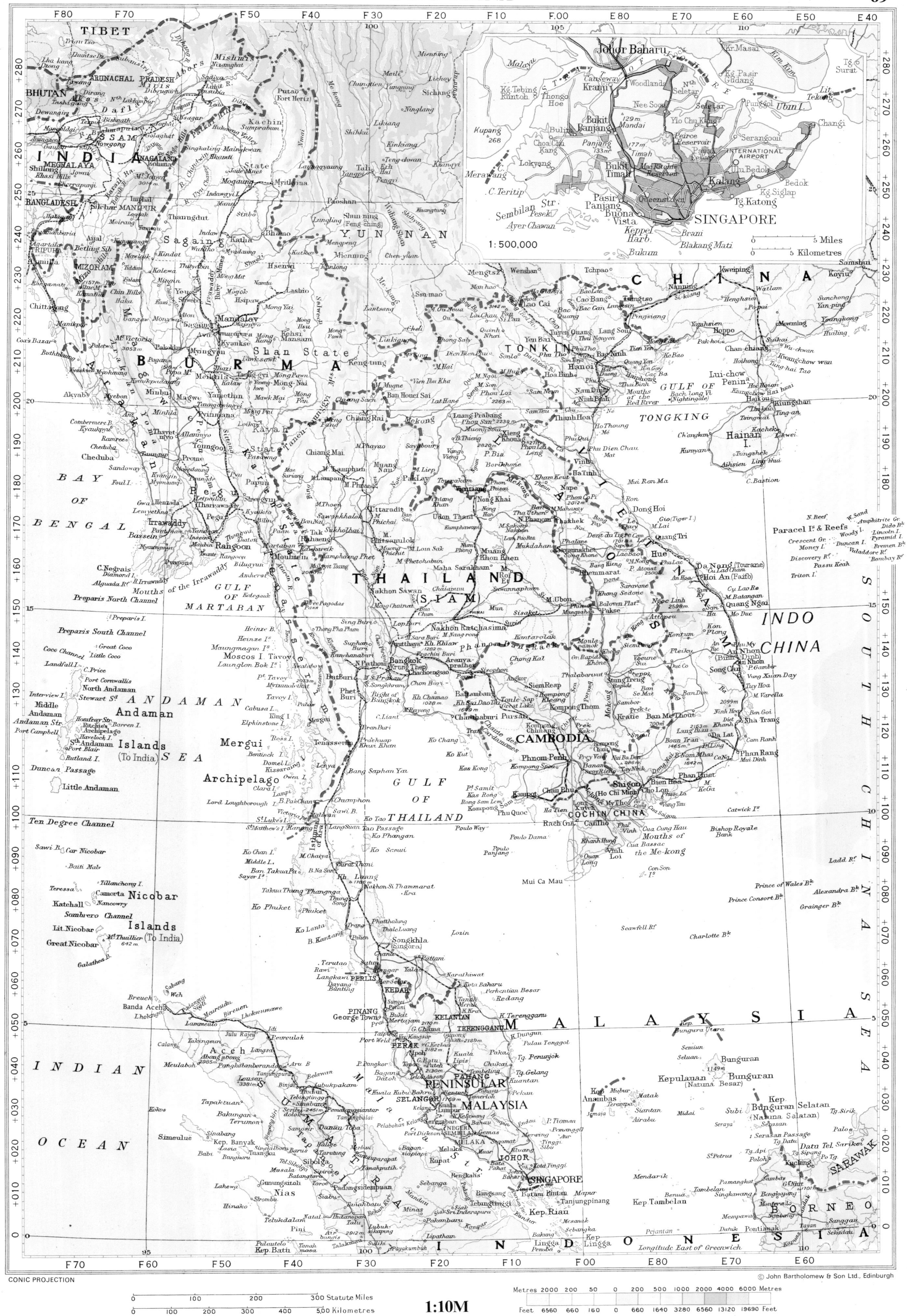

TIBET
BHUTAN
ARUNACHAL PRADESH
ASSAM
INDIA
NAGALAND
MEGHALAYA
BANGLADESH
MANIPUR
TRIPURA
MIZORAM
BURMA
Shan State
YUNNAN
CHINA
TONKIN
Hanoi
Haiphong
GULF OF TONGKING
Hainan I.
Paracel Is. & Reefs
LAOS
Vientiane
THAILAND (SIAM)
Bangkok
Mandalay
Rangoon
BAY OF BENGAL
GULF OF MARTABAN
ANDAMAN SEA
Andaman Islands (To India)
Mergui Archipelago
Nicobar Islands (To India)
CAMBODIA
Phnom Penh
Saigon (Ho Chi Minh)
COCHIN CHINA
GULF OF THAILAND
INDO CHINA
SOUTH CHINA SEA
Mouths of the Me-kong
MALAYSIA
PENINSULAR MALAYSIA
Kuala Lumpur
SINGAPORE
SUMATRA
INDIAN OCEAN
INDONESIA
BORNEO
SARAWAK
Kepulauan Bunguran (Natuna Besar)
Longitude East of Greenwich
Johor Baharu
Woodlands
Bukit Panjang
Bukit Timah
Queenstown
Changi
Serangoon
Kalang
Keppel Harb.
INTERNATIONAL AIRPORT
1:500,000
5 Miles
5 Kilometres
CONIC PROJECTION
© John Bartholomew & Son Ltd., Edinburgh
Statute Miles
Kilometres
1:10M
Metres 2000 200 50 0 200 500 1000 2000 4000 6000 Metres
Feet 6560 660 160 0 660 1640 3280 6560 13120 19690 Feet

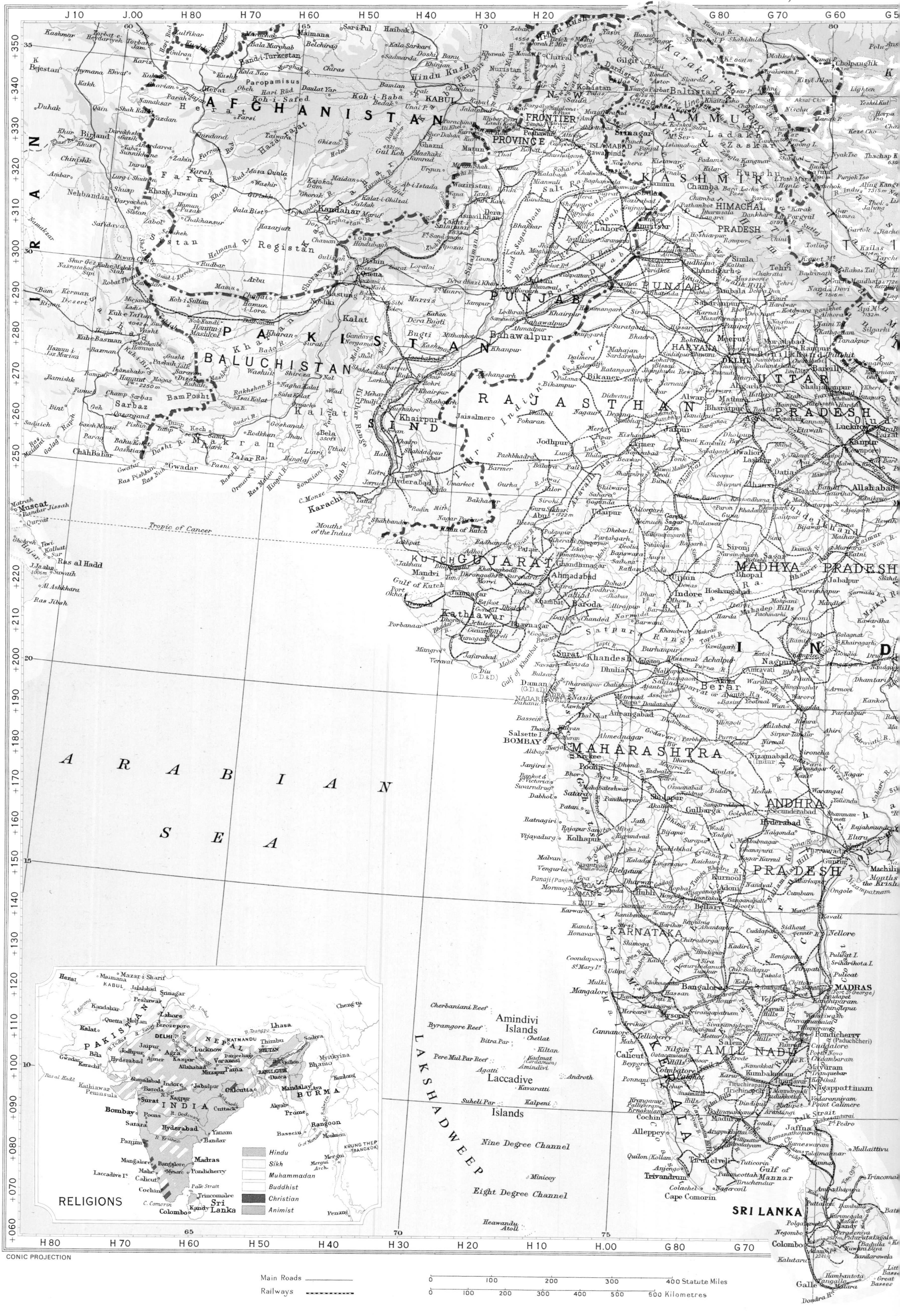

CONIC PROJECTION

RELIGIONS

- Hindu
- Sikh
- Muhammadan
- Buddhist
- Christian
- Animist

Main Roads

Railways

0 100 200 300 400 Statute Miles

0 100 200 300 400 500 600 Kilometres

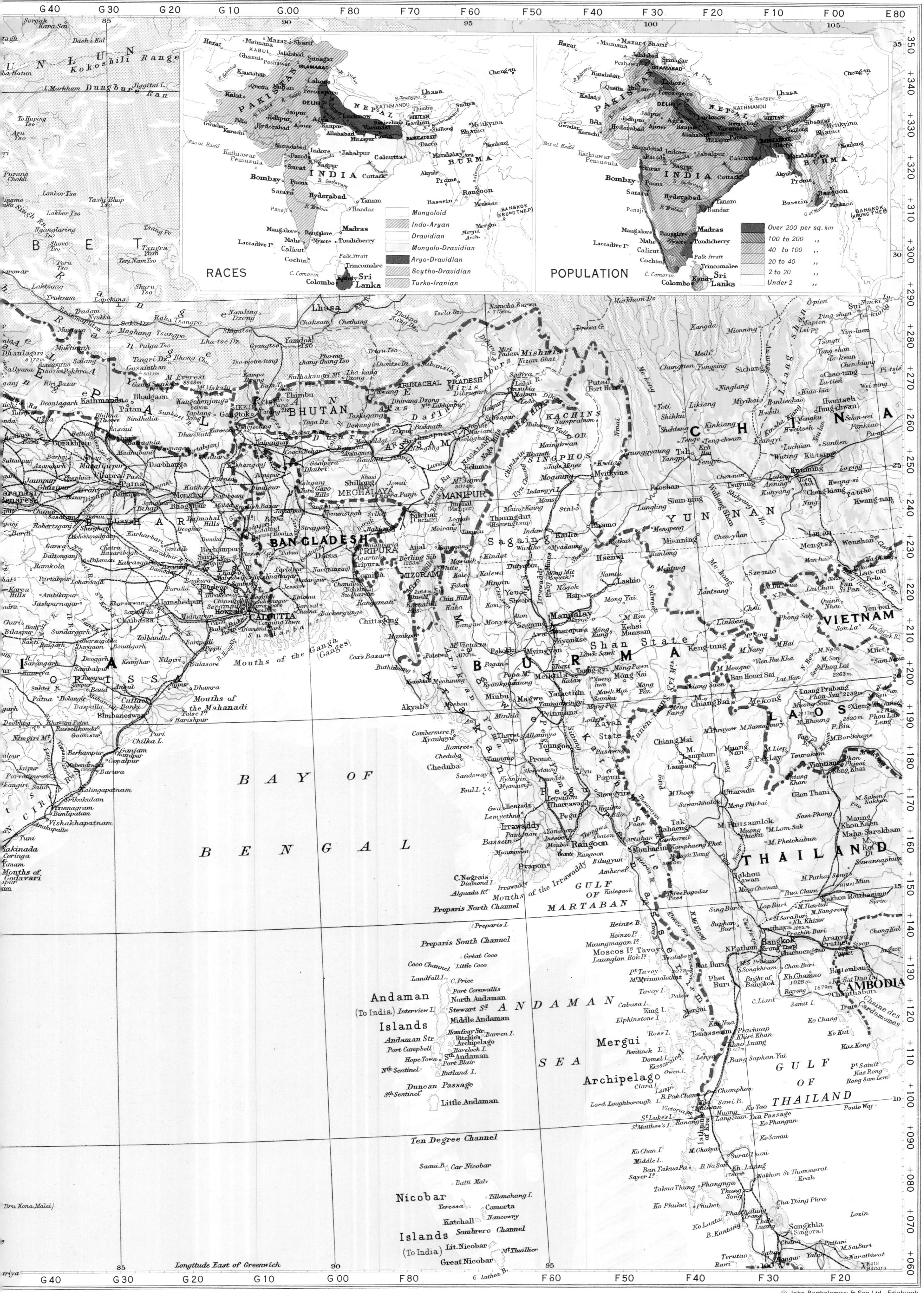

RACES

- Mongoloid
- Indo-Aryan
- Dravidian
- Mongolo-Dravidian
- Aryo-Dravidian
- Scytho-Dravidian
- Turko-Iranian

POPULATION

- Over 200 per sq. km
- 100 to 200 ,,
- 40 to 100 ,,
- 20 to 40 ,,
- 2 to 20 ,,
- Under 2 ,,

BAY OF BENGAL

ANDAMAN SEA

GULF OF MARTABAN

GULF OF THAILAND

Longitude East of Greenwich

Metres	2000	200	50	0	200	500	1000	2000	4000	6000	Metres
Feet	6560	660	160	0	660	1640	3280	6560	13120	19690	Feet

International Boundaries

State Boundaries

1:10M

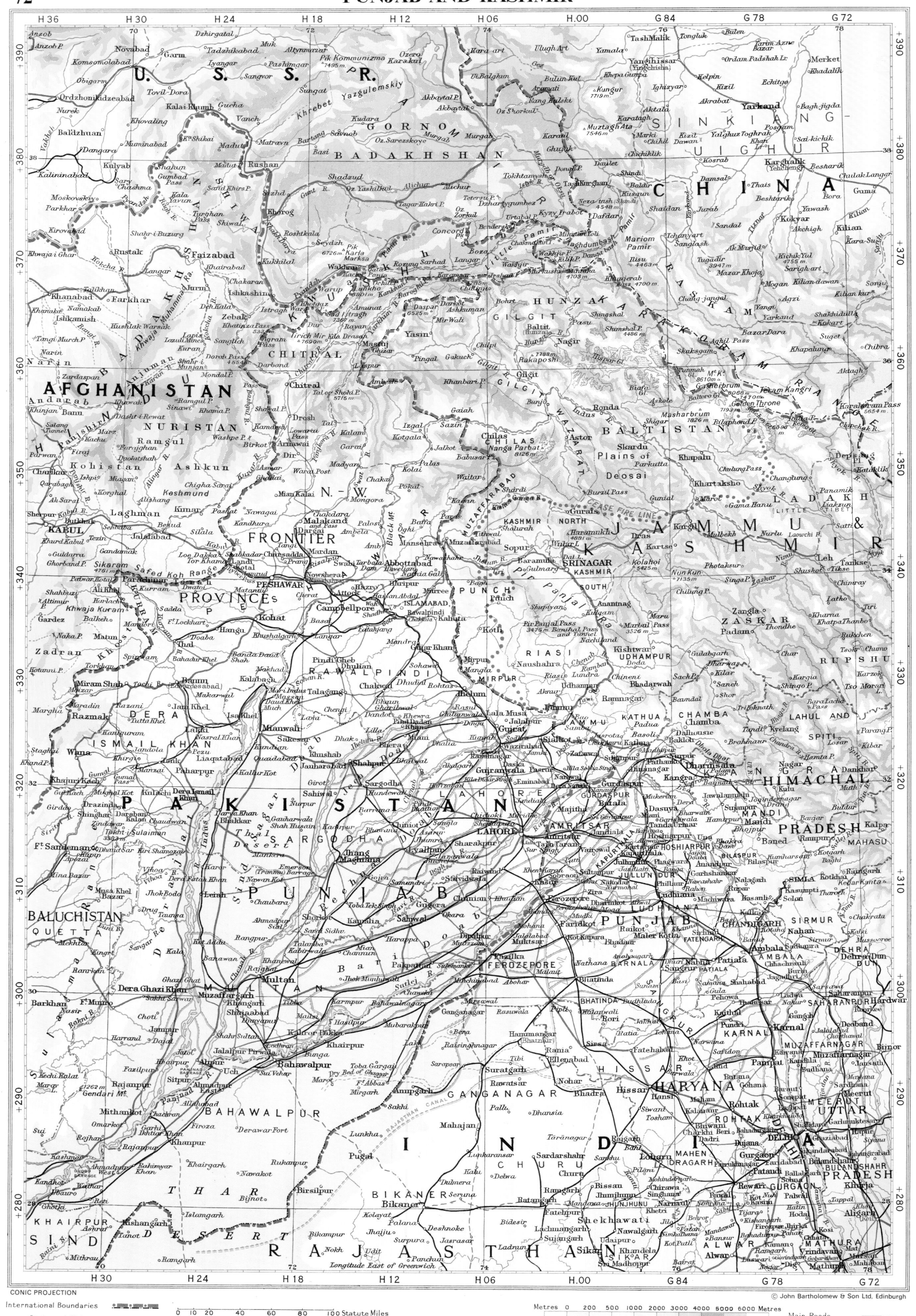

CONIC PROJECTION

International Boundaries

State and Division Boundaries

0 10 20 40 60 80 100 Statute Miles

0 10 20 40 60 80 100 120 140 160 Kilometres

1:4M

Metres 0 200 500 1000 2000 3000 4000 5000 6000 Metres

Feet 0 660 1640 3280 6560 9840 13120 16400 19690 Feet

Main Roads

Irrigation Canals

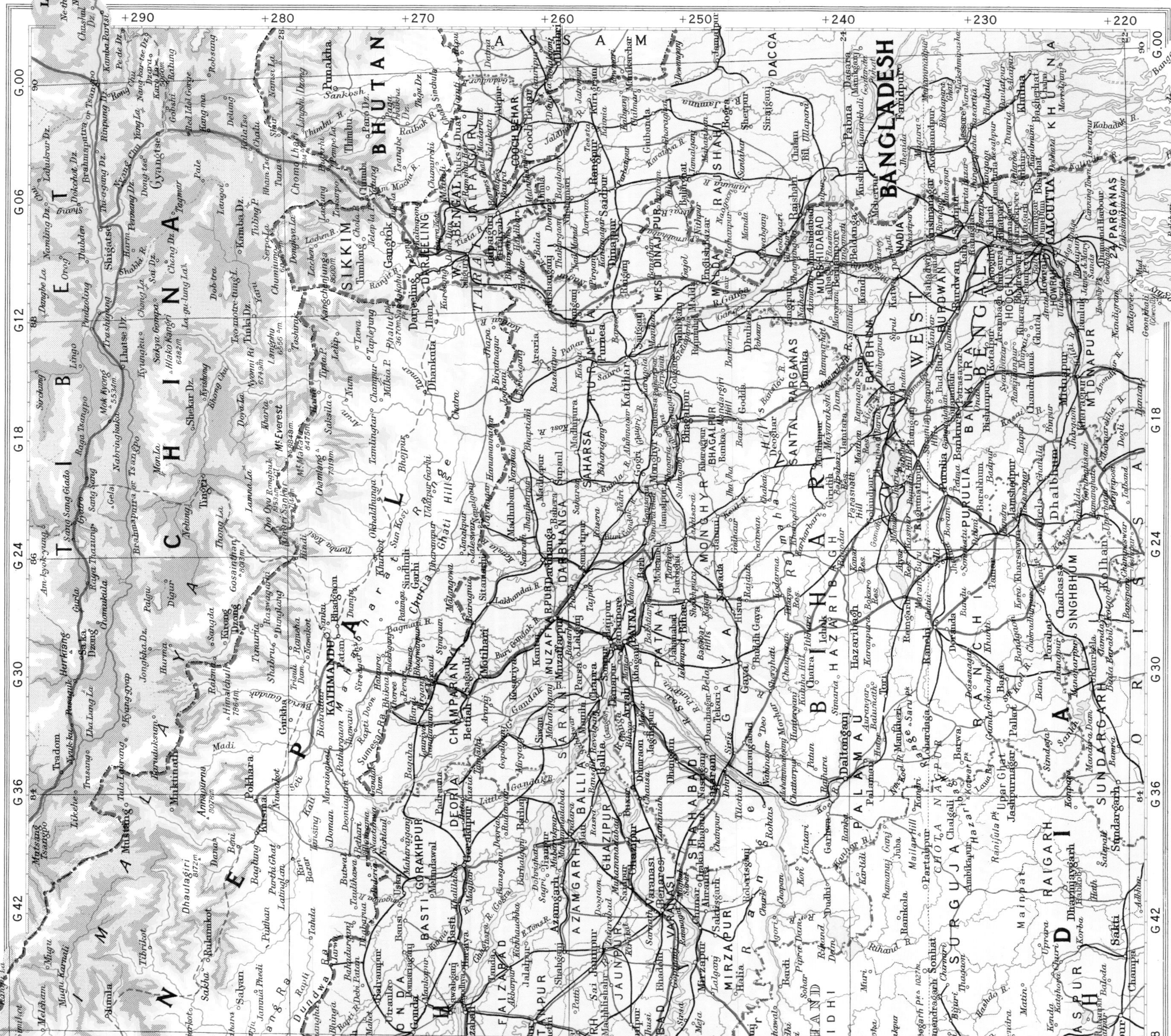

CONIC PROJECTION

© John Bartholomew & Son Ltd. Edinburgh

International Boundaries

0 10 20 40 60 80 100 Statute Miles

0 10 20 40 60 80 100 120 140 160 Kilometres

1:4M

Metres 0 200 500 1000 2000 3000 4000 5000 6000 Metres

Feet 0 660 1640 3280 6560 9840 13120 16400 19690 Feet

State and Division Boundaries

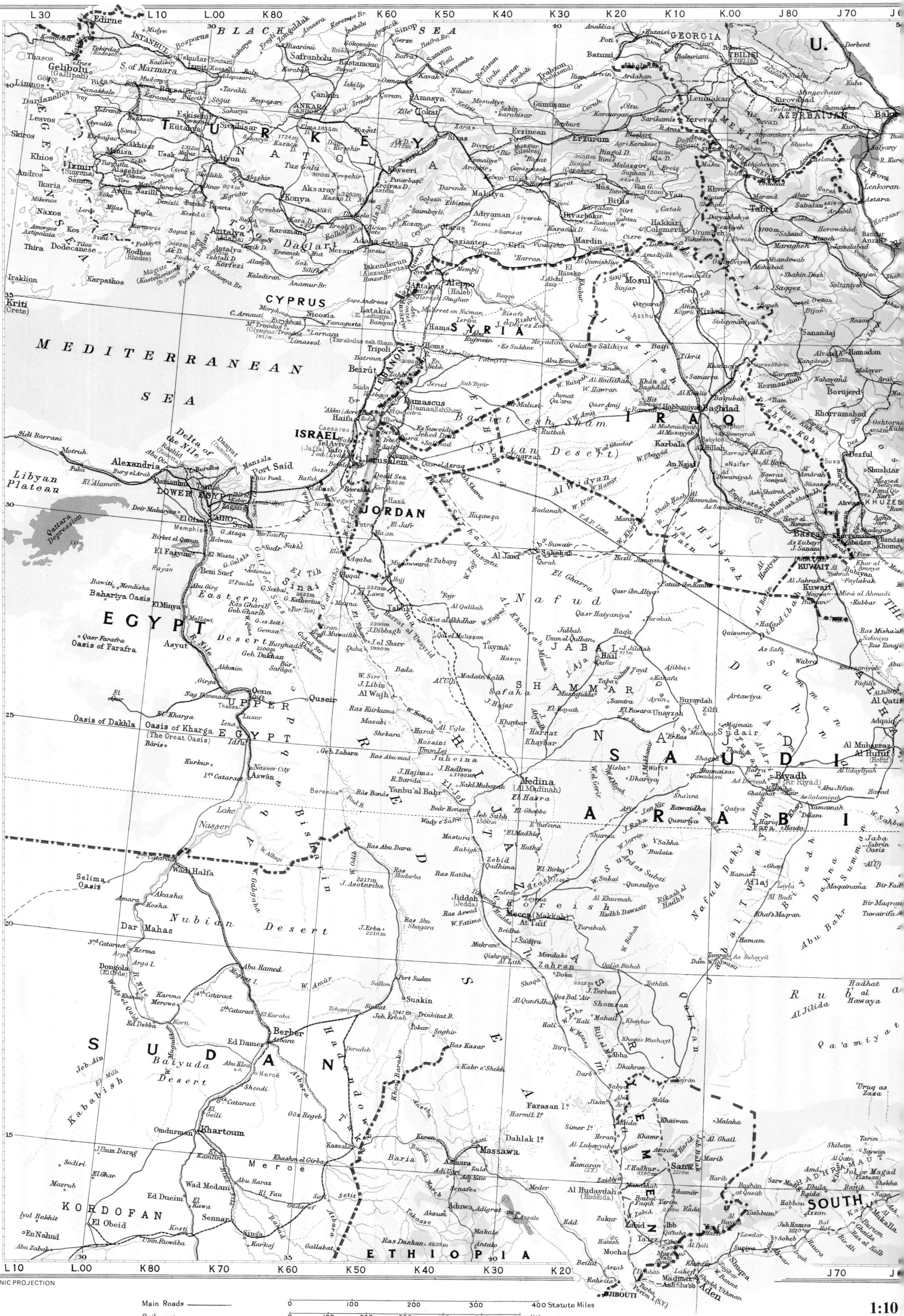

CONIC PROJECTION

Main Roads

Railways

0 100 200 300 400 Statute Miles

0 100 200 300 400 500 600 Kilometres

1:10

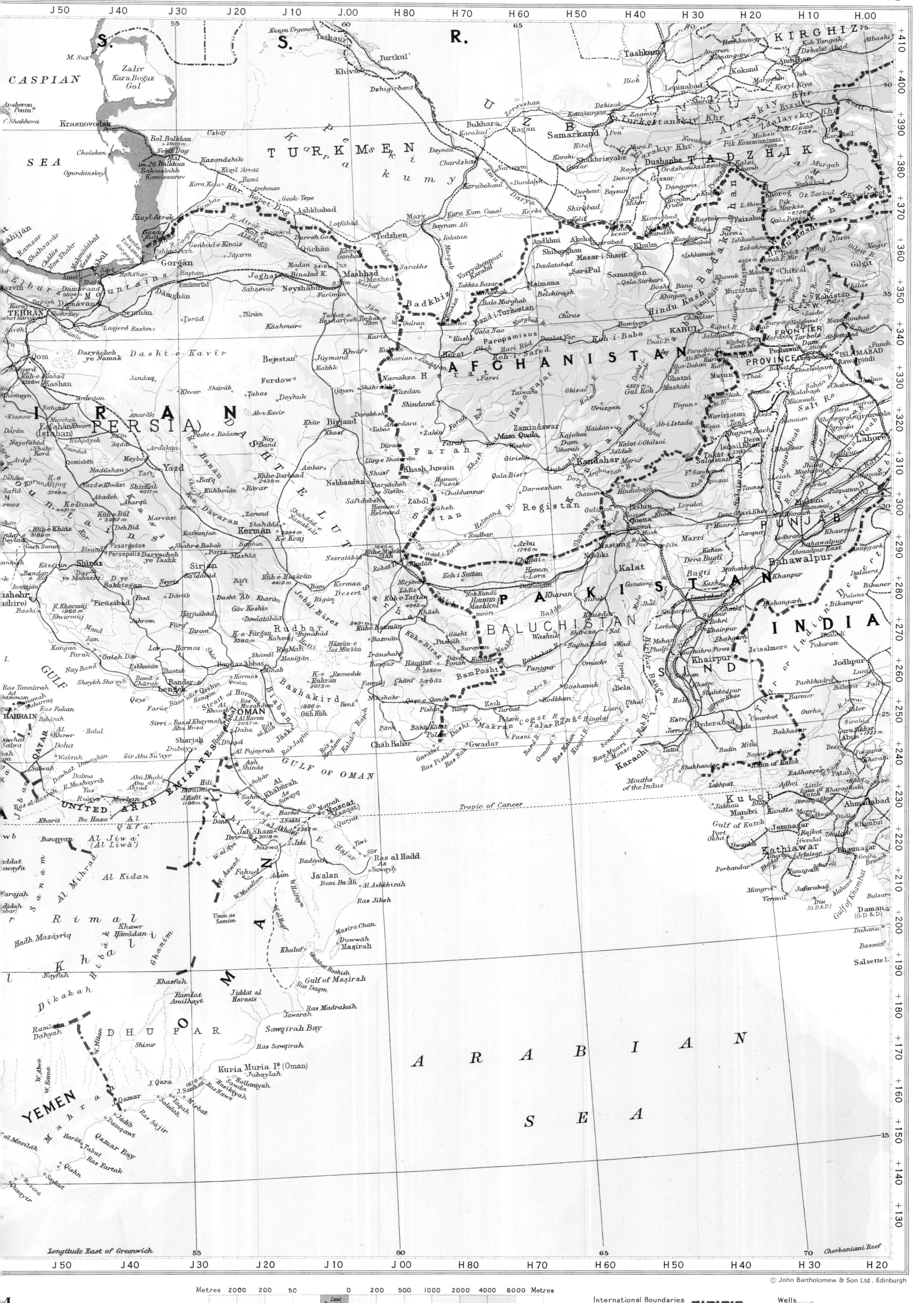

Metres	2000	200	50	0	200	500	1000	2000	4000	6000	Metres
Feet	6560	660	160	0	660	1640	3280	6560	13120	19690	Feet

Land Depression

International Boundaries

State Boundaries

Wells

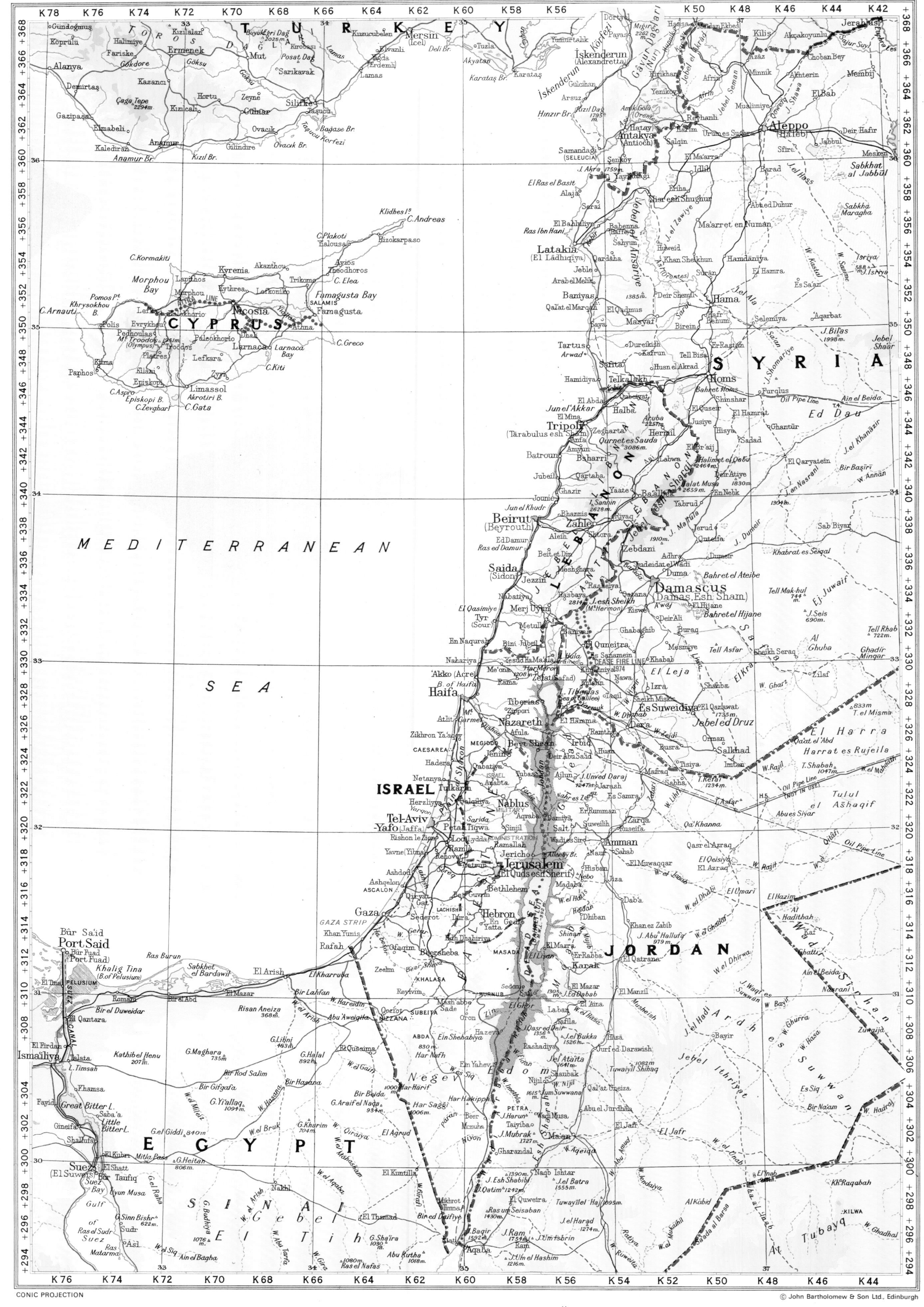
LEVANT COAST
T U R K E Y
S Y R I A
L E B A N O N
ISRAEL
J O R D A N
E G Y P T
CYPRUS
M E D I T E R R A N E A N
S E A
S I N A I
Negev
Mersin (Içel)
İskenderun (Alexandretta)
Antakya (Antioch)
Aleppo (Haleb)
Latakia (El Lādhiqīya)
Hama
Homs
Tripoli (Tārabulus esh Sham)
Beirut (Beyrouth)
Saida (Sidon)
Tyr (Sour)
Damascus (Damas, Esh Sham)
Haifa
Nazareth
Tel-Aviv -Yafo (Jaffa)
Jerusalem (El Quds esh Sherif)
Amman
Gaza
GAZA STRIP
Port Said
Ismailiya
Suez (El Suweis)
Aqaba
Nicosia
Famagusta
Larnaca
Limassol
Kyrenia
Paphos
Alanya
Anamur
Silifke
Kilis
Jerablus
Tartus
Baniyas
Zahle
Tiberias
Nablus
Hebron
Bethlehem
Jericho
Beersheba
El Arish
Rafah
Karak
Ma'an
Petra
Dead Sea
Jebel ed Druz
Es Suweidiya
Dera'a
Irbid
Zarqa
CEASE FIRE LINE
Oil Pipe Line
K78 K76 K74 K72 K70 K68 K66 K64 K62 K60 K58 K56 K54 K52 K50 K48 K46 K44 K42
CONIC PROJECTION
© John Bartholomew & Son Ltd., Edinburgh
0 10 20 30 40 50 60 70 80 Statute Miles
0 10 20 30 40 50 60 70 80 90 100 110 120 Kilometres
1:2½M
Metres 2000 200 50 0 100 200 500 1000 2000 3000 Metres
Land Depression
Feet 6560 660 160 0 330 660 1640 3280 6560 9840 Feet

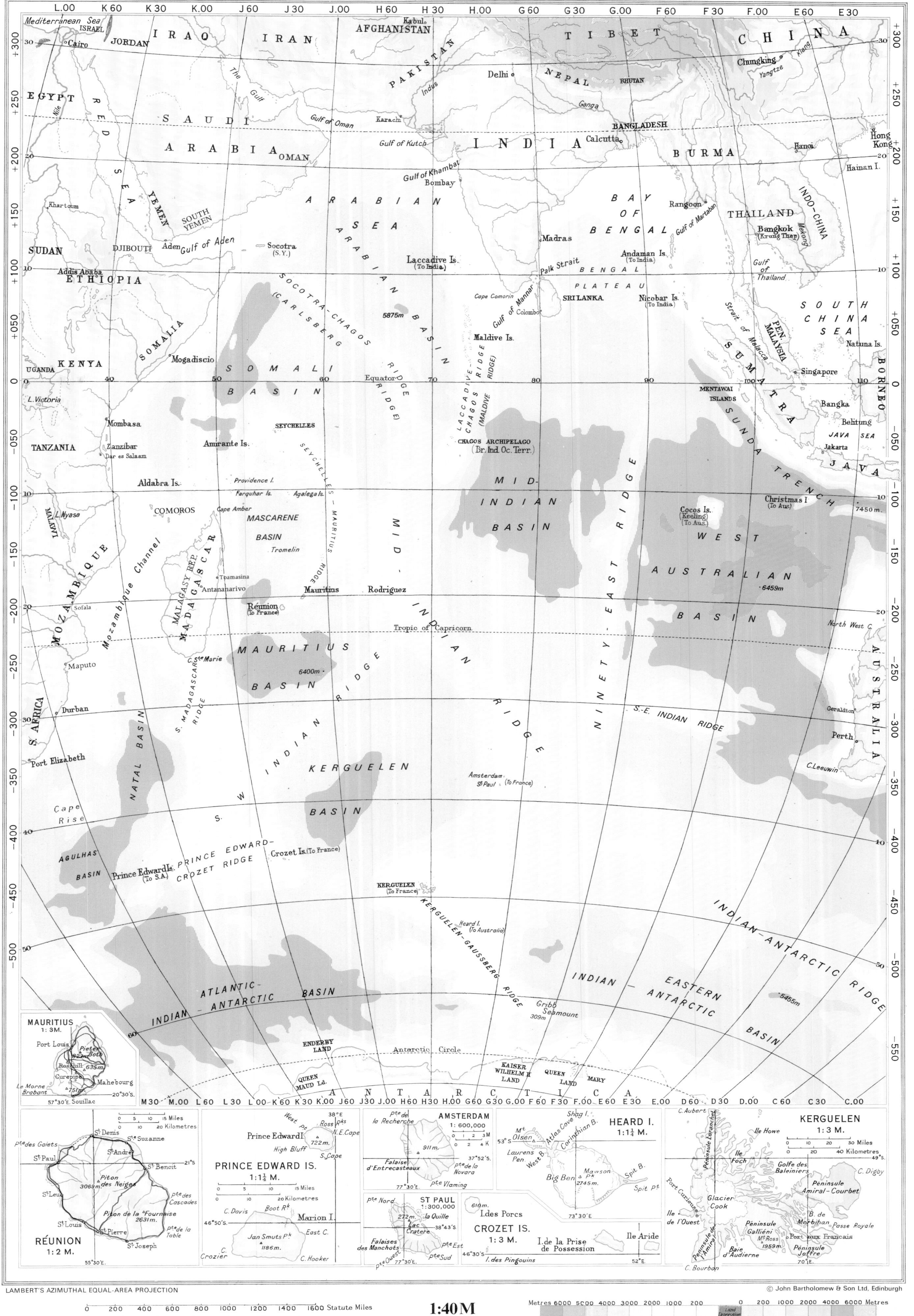

Mediterranean Sea
ISRAEL
JORDAN
IRAQ
IRAN
AFGHANISTAN
Kabul
TIBET
CHINA
Cairo
EGYPT
PAKISTAN
Delhi
NEPAL
BHUTAN
Chungking
Yangtze
SAUDI ARABIA
RED SEA
The Gulf
Indus
Ganga
Gulf of Oman
Karachi
BANGLADESH
Calcutta
Gulf of Kutch
INDIA
OMAN
BURMA
Hanoi
Hong Kong
Hainan I.
Gulf of Khambat
Bombay
YEMEN
SOUTH YEMEN
Khartoum
ARABIAN SEA
BAY OF BENGAL
Rangoon
Gulf of Martaban
THAILAND
Bangkok (Krung Thep)
INDO-CHINA
Mekong
SUDAN
DJIBOUTI
Aden
Gulf of Aden
Socotra (S.Y.)
Madras
Laccadive Is. (To India)
Andaman Is. (To India)
Palk Strait
BENGAL PLATEAU
Gulf of Thailand
Addis Ababa
ETHIOPIA
SOCOTRA-CHAGOS (CARLSBERG RIDGE)
ARABIAN BASIN
5875m
Cape Comorin
Gulf of Mannar
Colombo
SRI LANKA
Nicobar Is. (To India)
SOUTH CHINA SEA
Strait of Malacca
PEN. MALAYSIA
SUMATRA
Natuna Is.
Maldive Is.
SOMALIA
Mogadiscio
UGANDA
KENYA
SOMALI BASIN
Equator
LACCADIVE CHAGOS RIDGE (MALDIVE RIDGE)
Singapore
BORNEO
L. Victoria
MENTAWAI ISLANDS
Bangka
Mombasa
SEYCHELLES
CHAGOS ARCHIPELAGO (Br. Ind. Oc. Terr.)
Belitung
JAVA SEA
Jakarta
JAVA
TANZANIA
Zanzibar
Dar es Salaam
Amirante Is.
SUNDA TRENCH
Aldabra Is.
Providence I.
Farquhar Is.
Agalega Is.
SEYCHELLES - MAURITIUS RIDGE
MID-INDIAN BASIN
Christmas I (To Aus.)
7450m.
MALAWI
L. Nyasa
COMOROS
Cape Amber
MASCARENE BASIN
Tromelin
MID-INDIAN RIDGE
Cocos Is. (Keeling) (To Aus.)
WEST AUSTRALIAN BASIN
NINETY-EAST RIDGE
6459m
MOZAMBIQUE
Mozambique Channel
MALAGASY REP. MADAGASCAR
Toamasina
Antananarivo
Mauritius
Rodriguez
Sofala
Réunion (To France)
Tropic of Capricorn
North West C.
Maputo
C. Ste Marie
MAURITIUS BASIN
6400m
AUSTRALIA
S. MADAGASCAR RIDGE
Durban
S. AFRICA
NATAL BASIN
S.W. INDIAN RIDGE
S.-E. INDIAN RIDGE
Geraldton
Perth
Port Elizabeth
KERGUELEN BASIN
Amsterdam
St Paul (To France)
C. Leeuwin
Cape Rise
AGULHAS BASIN
Prince Edward Is. (To S.A.)
PRINCE EDWARD-CROZET RIDGE
Crozet Is. (To France)
KERGUELEN (To France)
KERGUELEN-GAUSSBERG RIDGE
Heard I. (To Australia)
INDIAN-ANTARCTIC RIDGE
INDIAN-EASTERN ANTARCTIC BASIN
5455m
ATLANTIC-INDIAN-ANTARCTIC BASIN
Gribb Seamount 309m
ENDERBY LAND
Antarctic Circle
QUEEN MAUD Ld.
KAISER WILHELM II LAND
QUEEN MARY LAND
ANTARCTICA
MAURITIUS 1: 3M.
Port Louis
Pieter Both 823m.
Rose Hill
635m
Curepipe
Mahebourg
Le Morne Brabant
751m
20°30'S.
57°30'E.
Souillac
RÉUNION 1: 2 M.
St Denis
Ste Suzanne
Pte des Galets
St Paul
Ste André
St Benoit
21°S
Piton des Neiges 3069m.
St Leu
Pte des Cascades
Piton de la Fournaise 2631m.
St Louis
St Pierre
Pte de la Table
St Joseph
55°30'E.
PRINCE EDWARD IS. 1: 1¼ M.
West Pt.
Ross Pt.
N.E. Cape
Prince Edward I.
High Bluff
722m.
S. Cape
C. Davis
Boot Rk
Marion I.
46°50'S.
East C.
Jan Smuts Pk 1186m.
C. Crozier
C. Hooker
38°E
AMSTERDAM 1: 600,000
Pte de la Recherche
911m.
37°52'S.
Falaise d'Entrecasteaux
Pte de la Novara
Pte Vlaming
77°30'E.
ST PAUL 1: 300,000
Pte Nord
272m.
Pte de la Quille
Lac Cratère
38°43'S
Falaises des Manchots
Pte Est
Pte Ouest
Pte Sud
77°30'E.
CROZET IS. 1: 3 M.
610m.
I. des Porcs
I. de la Prise de Possession
Ile Aride
46°30'S.
I. des Pingouins
52°E.
HEARD I. 1: 1¼ M.
Shag I.
Atlas Cove
Corinthian B.
Mt Olsen
53°S
Laurens Pen
West B.
Big Ben
Mawson Pk 2745m.
Spit B.
Spit Pt
73°30'E
KERGUELEN 1: 3 M.
C. Aubert
Péninsule Loranchet
Ile Howe
Ile Foch
Golfe des Baleiniers
49°S.
C. Digby
Péninsule Amiral-Courbet
Port Curieuse
Glacier Cook
Ile de l'Ouest
B. de Morbihan
Passe Royale
Péninsule Gallieni
Mt Ross 1959m.
Port aux Français
Péninsule Joffre
Péninsule de l'Amiral
Baie d'Audierne
C. Bourbon
70°E.
LAMBERT'S AZIMUTHAL EQUAL-AREA PROJECTION
© John Bartholomew & Son Ltd, Edinburgh
Statute Miles
Kilometres
1:40 M
Metres 6000 5000 4000 3000 2000 1000 200 0 200 1000 2000 4000 6000 Metres
Feet 19690 16400 13120 9840 6560 3280 660 0 660 3280 6560 13120 19690 Feet
Land Depression

AFRICA

VEGETATION

2	High Mountain Flora
3	Temperate and Mountain Forest
7	Mediterranean Forest
8	River Valley and Oasis Irrigated Areas
10	South-Eastern Sub-Tropical Forest
11	Dry Mixed Woodland and Forest
12	Tropical Rain Forest
13	Savannah and Bush Woodlands
14	Steppe Grassland
15	Hill and Plateau Grassland
16	Mediterranean and Cape, Hard Leaf (Macchia type) Vegetation
17	Halfa Grass Steppe and Semi-Desert
17A	Karroo Wax-Brush
18	Acacia Semi-Desert
18A	Thorn Bush
19	Semi-Desert
20	Waterless Desert
	Salt Swamp
	Fresh Water Swamp
	Southern Limit of Palm Trees

1:35 M.

RAINFALL JANUARY
SOUTHERN SUMMER
The Figures indicate the Rainfall in Inches

ins. mm.
16 400
12 300
8 200
4 100
2 50
1 25

RAINFALL JULY
SOUTHERN WINTER
The Figures indicate the Rainfall in Inches

LAMBERT'S ZENITHAL EQUAL-AREA PROJECTION

0 200 400 600 800 1000 Statute Miles

1:35M

0 200 400 600 800 1000 1200 1400 1600 Kilometres

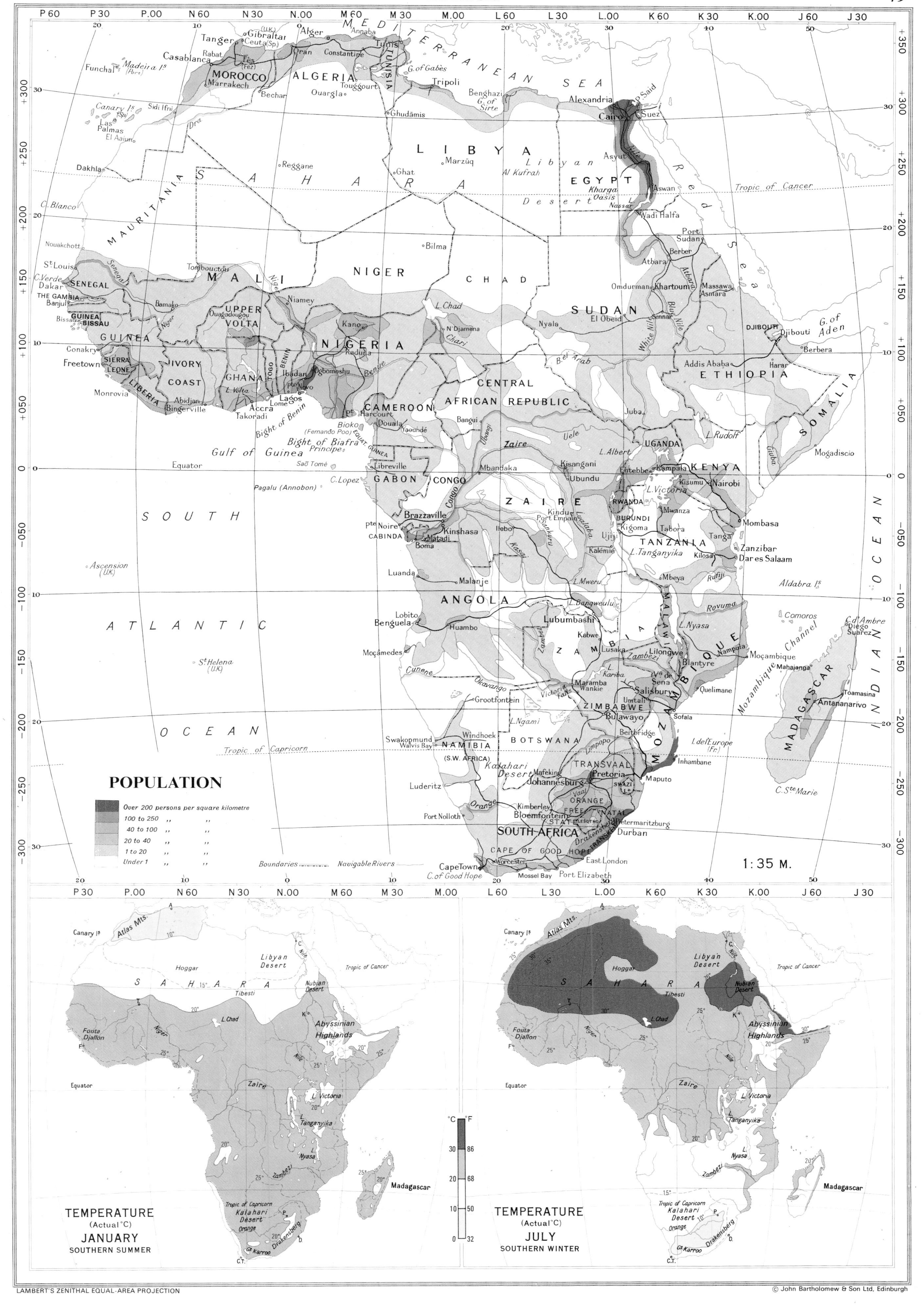

0 200 400 600 800 1000 Statute Miles **1:35M** 0 200 400 600 800 1000 1200 1400 1600 Kilometres

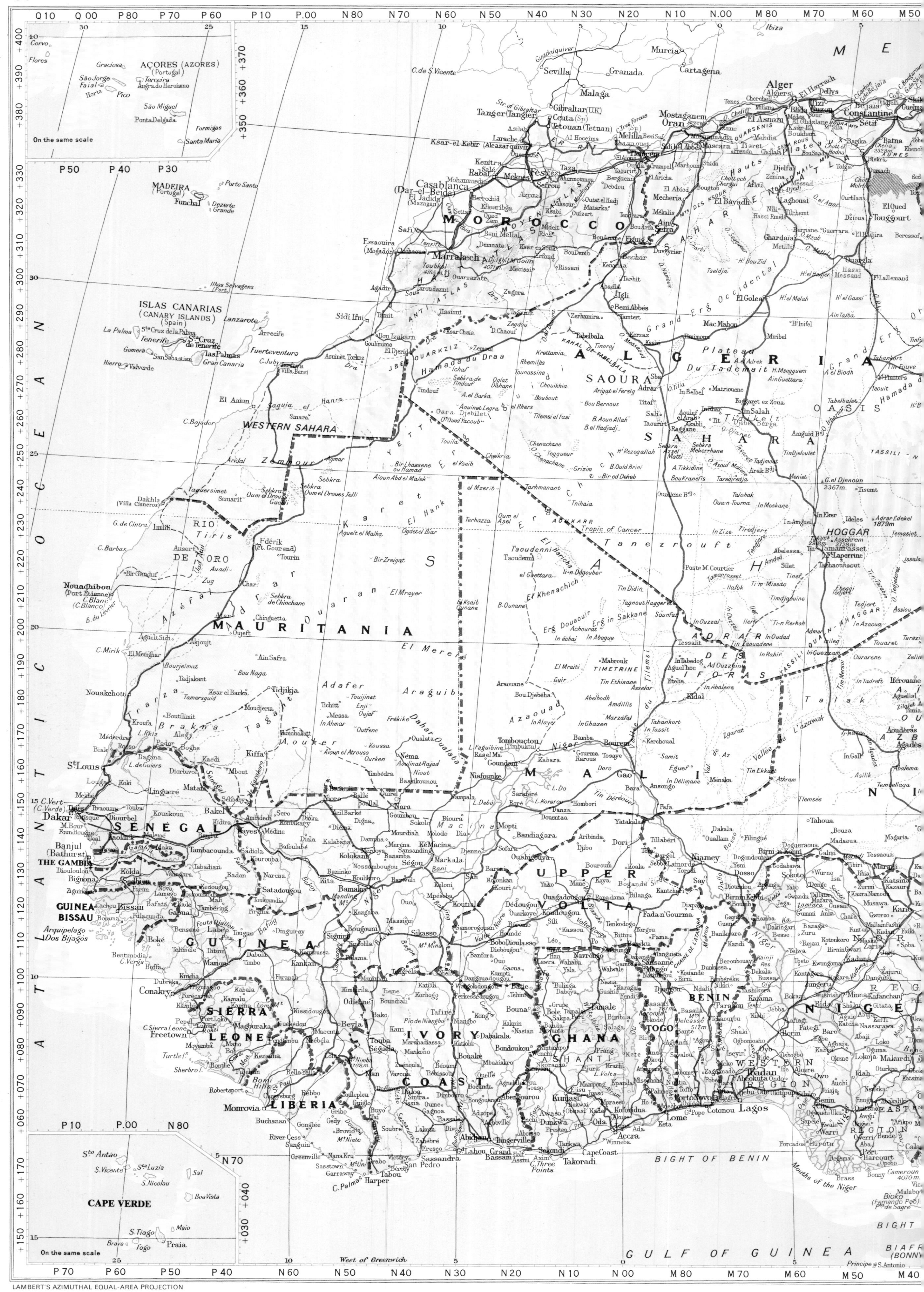
AÇORES (AZORES) (Portugal)
MADEIRA (Portugal)
ISLAS CANARIAS (CANARY ISLANDS) (Spain)
CAPE VERDE
On the same scale
MOROCCO
ALGERIA
WESTERN SAHARA
MAURITANIA
MALI
SENEGAL
THE GAMBIA
GUINEA BISSAU
GUINEA
SIERRA LEONE
LIBERIA
IVORY COAST
UPPER VOLTA
GHANA
TOGO
BENIN
NIGER
ATLANTIC OCEAN
GULF OF GUINEA
BIGHT OF BENIN
Tropic of Cancer
West of Greenwich
LAMBERT'S AZIMUTHAL EQUAL-AREA PROJECTION
Main Roads
Railways
Statute Miles
Kilometres
1:12½

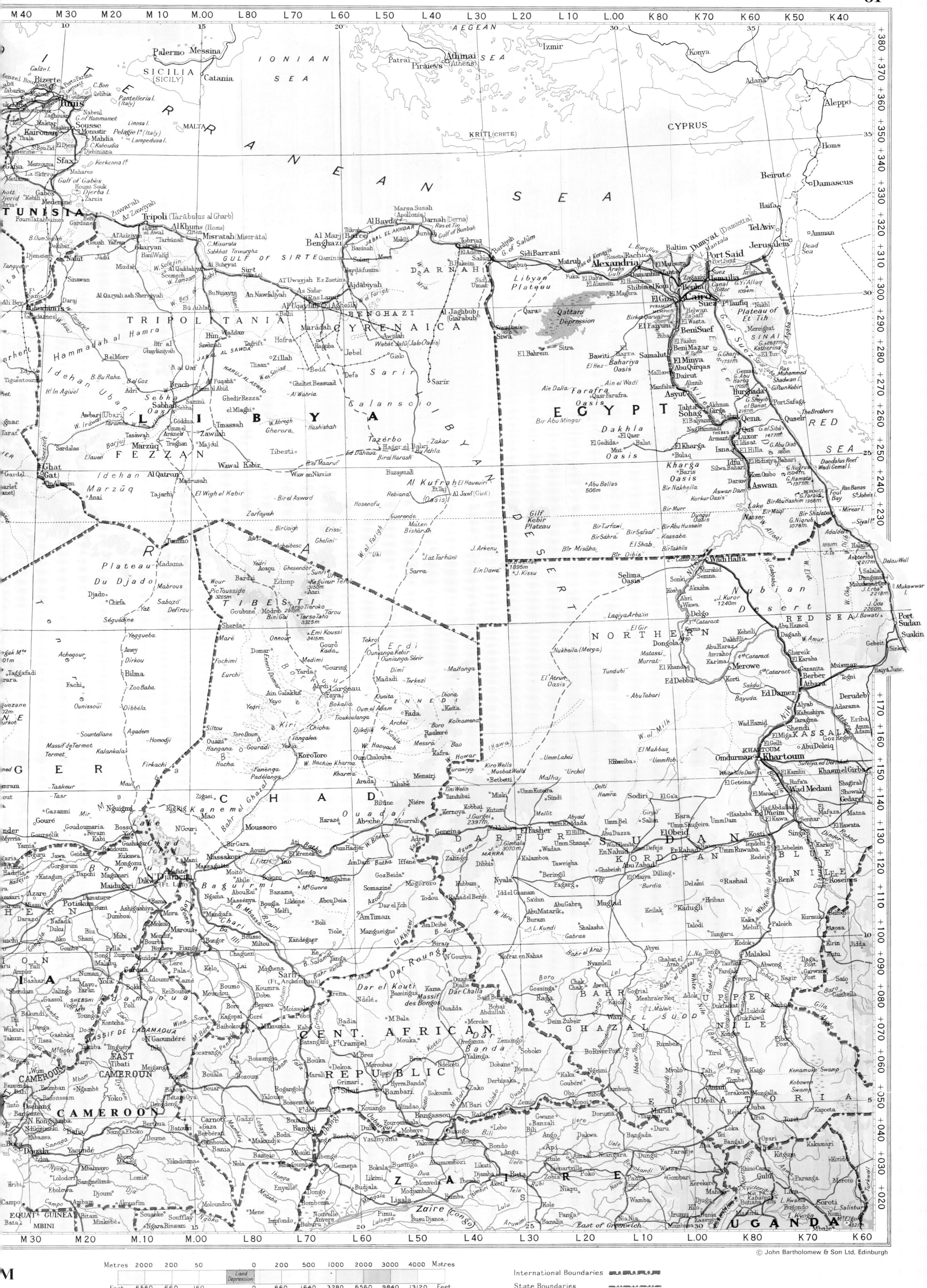

TUNISIA
Tunis
Bizerte
Sousse
Kairouan
Sfax
Gabès
Medenine
Palermo
Messina
SICILIA (SICILY)
Catania
MALTA
IONIAN SEA
AEGEAN SEA
Athinai (Athens)
Piraievs
Patrai
Izmir
Konya
Adana
Aleppo
KRITI (CRETE)
CYPRUS
Homs
Beirut
Damascus
Haifa
Tel Aviv
Jerusalem
Amman
Dead Sea
MEDITERRANEAN SEA
Tripoli (Tarābulus al Gharb)
Al Khums (Homs)
Misratah (Misrāta)
GULF OF SIRTE
Surt
Benghazi
Al Marj (Barce)
Al Bayda
Darnah (Derna)
Tubruq
Salum
Sidi Barrani
Matruh
Alexandria
Port Said
Ismailia
Suez
El Giza
Cairo
Qattara Depression
Siwa
TRIPOLITANIA
CYRENAICA
FEZZAN
LIBYA
Ghadamis (Gadames)
Hammadah al Hamra
Sabha
Marzuq
Ghat
Ajdabiyah
Al Jaghbub (Giarabub)
Al Kufrah (Oasis)
Calanscio Sarir
LIBYAN DESERT
Libyan Plateau
EGYPT
Farafra Oasis
Bahariya Oasis
Dakhla Oasis
Kharga Oasis
Asyut
Qena
Luxor
Aswan
Aswan Dam
Lake Nasser
Wadi Halfa
Hurghada
SINAI
Plateau of Et Tih
RED SEA
Gilf Kebir Plateau
Nubian Desert
Selima Oasis
Port Sudan
Suakin
Dongola
NORTHERN
Atbara
Berber
Ed Damer
Kassala
Khartoum
Omdurman
Wad Medani
El Obeid
KORDOFAN
DARFUR
El Fasher
Geneina
SUDAN
BLUE NILE
UPPER NILE
BAHR EL GHAZAL
EQUATORIA
Malakal
Wau
Juba
Kosti
Kadugli
Tibesti
Emi Koussi 3415m.
Borkou
Ennedi
Faya (Largeau)
Abeche
Ouadai
CHAD
Kanem
Lake Chad
N'Djamena (Ft. Lamy)
Baguirmi
Sarh (Ft. Archambault)
Maiduguri
Plateau du Djado
Bilma
Ténéré
Agadem
NIGER
CAMEROUN
CAMEROON
Garoua
Ngaoundéré
Douala
Yaoundé
Massif de l'Adamaoua
CENT. AFRICAN REPUBLIC
Bangui
Bambari
Bangassou
Fort Crampel
Fort Sibut
Berbérati
Carnot
ZAIRE
Zaire (Congo)
Lisala
Buta
Isiro
Bunia
UGANDA
Gulu
Lira
Soroti
Lake Albert
EQUAT.L GUINEA
MBINI
Bata
Metres 2000 200 50 0 200 500 1000 2000 3000 4000 Metres
Feet 6560 660 160 0 660 1640 3280 6560 9840 13120 Feet
Land Depression
International Boundaries
State Boundaries

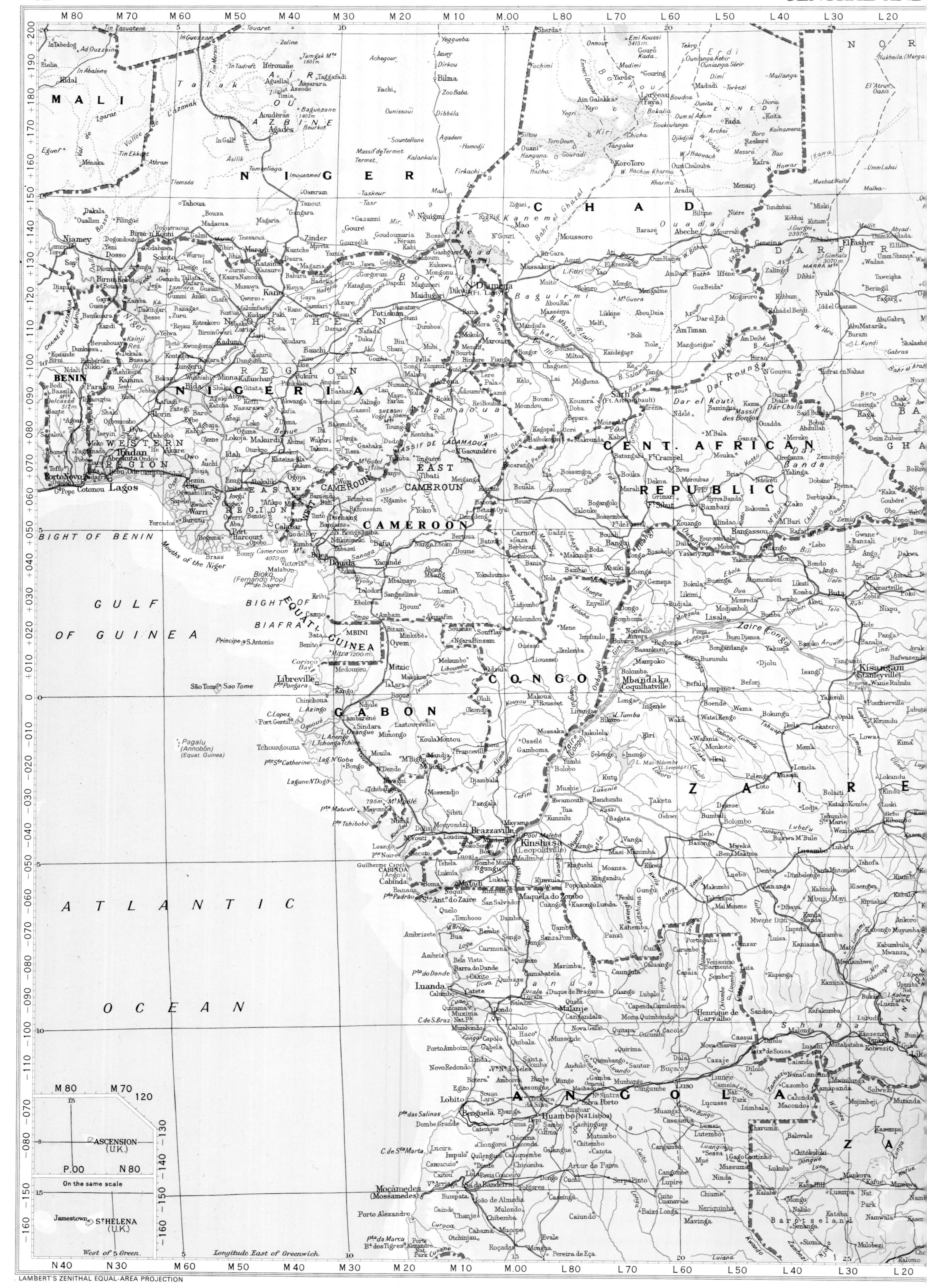

Main Roads
Railways

0 50 100 200 300 400 500 Statute Miles

0 50 100 200 300 400 500 600 700 800 Kilometres

1:12

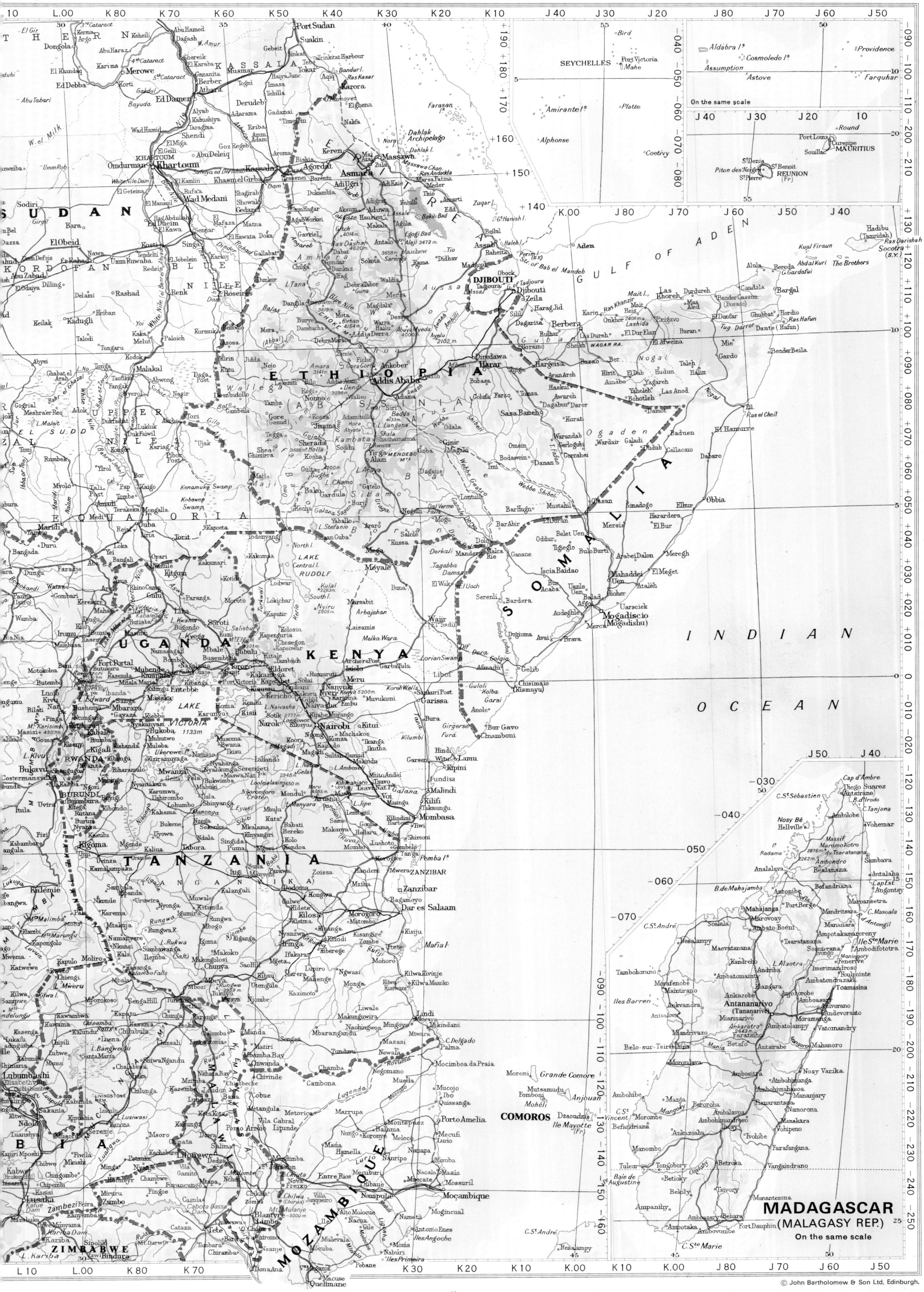

SEYCHELLES

On the same scale

MAURITIUS

REUNION (Fr)

COMOROS

MADAGASCAR (MALAGASY REP.)

On the same scale

Metres	2000	200	50	Land Depression	0	200	500	1000	2000	3000	4000
Feet	6560	660	160		0	660	1640	3280	6560	9840	13120

International Boundaries

State Boundaries

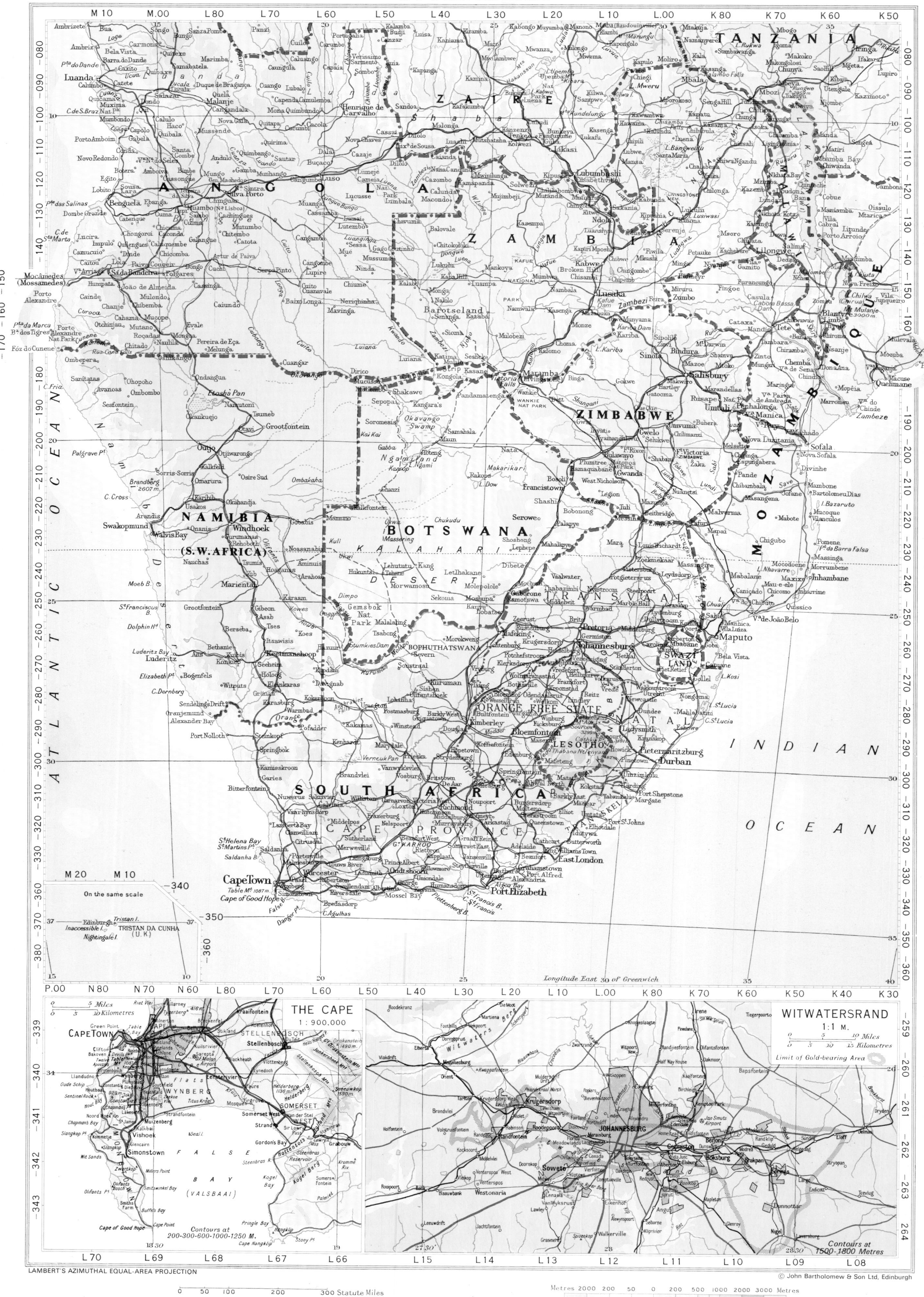

LAMBERT'S AZIMUTHAL EQUAL-AREA PROJECTION

© John Bartholomew & Son Ltd, Edinburgh

0 50 100 200 300 Statute Miles
0 50 100 200 300 400 500 Kilometres

1:12½M

Metres 2000 200 50 0 200 500 1000 2000 3000 Metres
Feet 6560 660 160 0 660 1640 3280 6560 9840 Feet

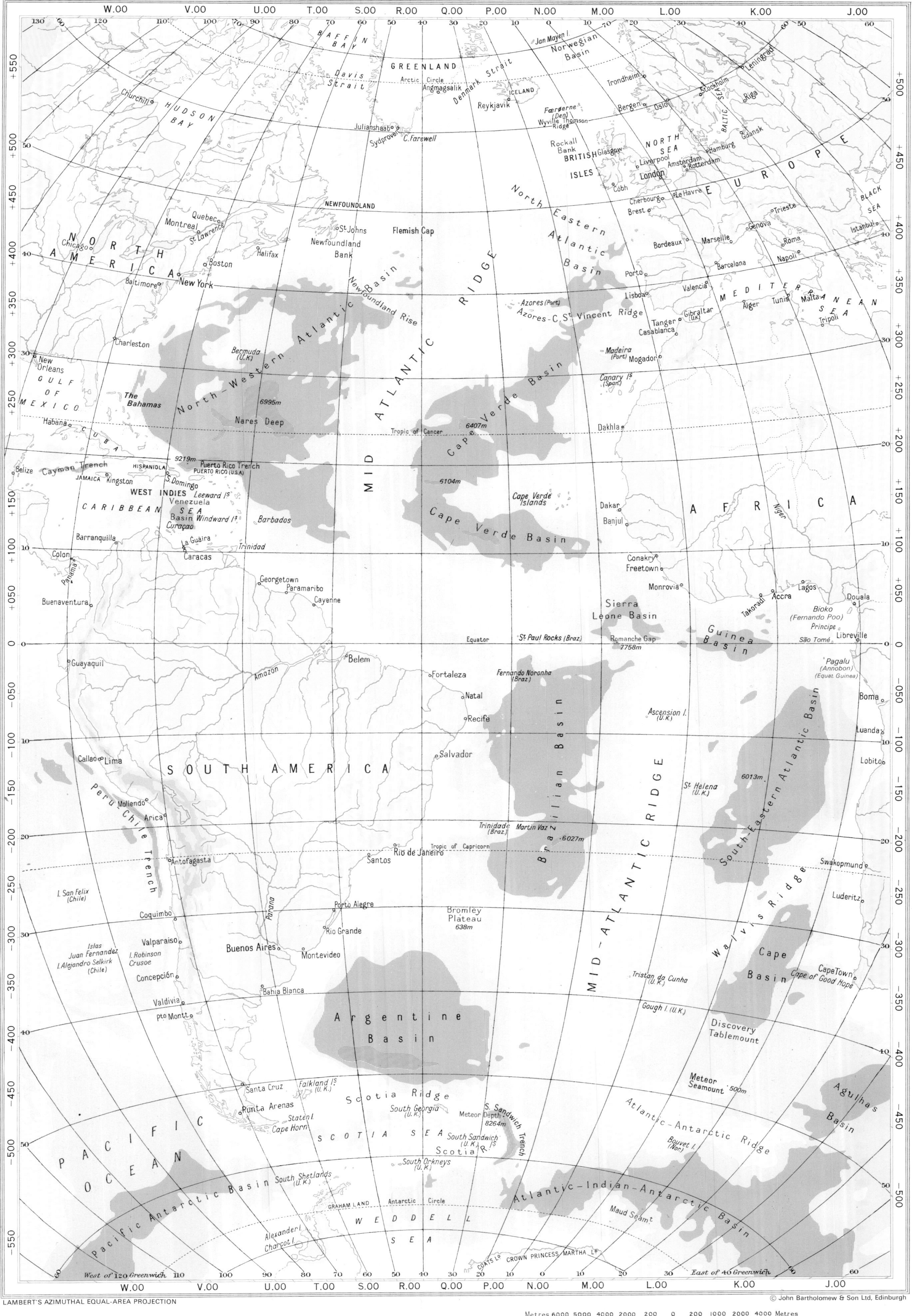
BAFFIN BAY
GREENLAND
Davis Strait
Arctic Circle
Angmagsalik
Denmark Strait
ICELAND
Reykjavik
Jan Mayen I.
Norwegian Basin
Trondheim
Leningrad
Stockholm
Riga
Bergen
Oslo
BALTIC SEA
Gdansk
Churchill
HUDSON BAY
Julianshaab
Sydprøven
C. Farewell
Færøerne (Den)
Wyville Thomson Ridge
Rockall Bank
BRITISH ISLES
Glasgow
NORTH SEA
Hamburg
Liverpool
Amsterdam
Rotterdam
London
Cobh
Cherbourg
Le Havre
Brest
EUROPE
BLACK SEA
Trieste
Istanbul
Quebec
Montreal
St Lawrence
NEWFOUNDLAND
St Johns
Flemish Cap
Newfoundland Bank
Halifax
NORTH AMERICA
Chicago
Boston
New York
Baltimore
North Eastern Atlantic Basin
Genova
Marseille
Roma
Bordeaux
Napoli
Barcelona
Porto
Lisboa
Valencia
MEDITERRANEAN SEA
Alger
Tunis
Malta
Tripoli
Newfoundland Basin
Newfoundland Rise
MID ATLANTIC RIDGE
Azores (Port)
Azores-C. St Vincent Ridge
Tanger
Gibraltar (UK)
Casablanca
Charleston
Bermuda (U.K.)
North-Western Atlantic Basin
Madeira (Port)
Mogador
Canary Is (Span)
New Orleans
GULF OF MEXICO
The Bahamas
6995m
Nares Deep
Cape Verde Basin
Habana
CUBA
Tropic of Cancer
6407m
Dakhla
Belize
Cayman Trench
HISPANIOLA
9219m
Puerto Rico Trench
PUERTO RICO (USA)
JAMAICA
Kingston
S. Domingo
WEST INDIES
Leeward Is
6104m
Cape Verde Islands
Dakar
Banjul
AFRICA
Niger
Venezuela Basin
CARIBBEAN SEA
Windward Is
Curaçao
Barbados
Cape Verde Basin
Barranquilla
La Guaira
Caracas
Trinidad
Colon
Panama
Conakry
Freetown
Georgetown
Paramaribo
Cayenne
Monrovia
Takoradi
Accra
Lagos
Douala
Buenaventura
Sierra Leone Basin
Bioko (Fernando Poo)
Principe
Equator
St Paul Rocks (Braz)
Romanche Gap
7758m
Guinea Basin
São Tomé
Libreville
Guayaquil
Belem
Amazon
Pagalu (Annobon) (Equat. Guinea)
Fortaleza
Fernando Noronha (Braz)
Natal
Recife
Boma
Ascension I. (U.K.)
Brazilian Basin
South-Eastern Atlantic Basin
Luanda
Callao
Lima
Salvador
Lobito
SOUTH AMERICA
MID-ATLANTIC RIDGE
6013m
St Helena (U.K.)
Peru Chile Trench
Mollendo
Arica
Trinidade (Braz)
Martin Vaz
6027m
Tropic of Capricorn
Rio de Janeiro
Santos
Antofagasta
Swakopmund
Walvis Ridge
I. San Felix (Chile)
Luderitz
Parana
Porto Alegre
Bromley Plateau
638m
Coquimbo
Rio Grande
Valparaiso
Islas Juan Fernandez
I. Robinson Crusoe
I. Alejandro Selkirk (Chile)
Buenos Aires
Montevideo
Cape Basin
Cape Town
Cape of Good Hope
Concepción
Tristan da Cunha (U.K.)
Bahia Blanca
Valdivia
Gough I. (U.K.)
Pto Montt
Argentine Basin
Discovery Tablemount
Meteor Seamount
500m
Santa Cruz
Falkland Is (U.K.)
Scotia Ridge
Agulhas Basin
Punta Arenas
South Georgia (U.K.)
Meteor Depth
S. Sandwich Trench
8264m
Staten I.
Cape Horn
SCOTIA SEA
South Sandwich Is (U.K.)
Scotia R.
Atlantic-Antarctic Ridge
Bouvet I. (Nor)
PACIFIC OCEAN
South Orkneys (U.K.)
South Shetlands (U.K.)
Pacific Antarctic Basin
Atlantic-Indian-Antarctic Basin
GRAHAM LAND
Antarctic Circle
Maud Seamt
WEDDELL SEA
Alexander I.
Charcot I.
COATS Ld
CROWN PRINCESS MARTHA Ld
West of 120 Greenwich
East of 40 Greenwich
W.00
V.00
U.00
T.00
S.00
R.00
Q.00
P.00
N.00
M.00
L.00
K.00
J.00
© John Bartholomew & Son Ltd, Edinburgh
LAMBERT'S AZIMUTHAL EQUAL-AREA PROJECTION
0 200 400 600 800 1000 Statute Miles
0 400 800 1200 1600 Kilometres
1:48M
Metres 6000 5000 4000 2000 200 0 200 1000 2000 4000 Metres
Feet 19690 16400 13120 6560 660 0 660 3280 6560 13120 Feet

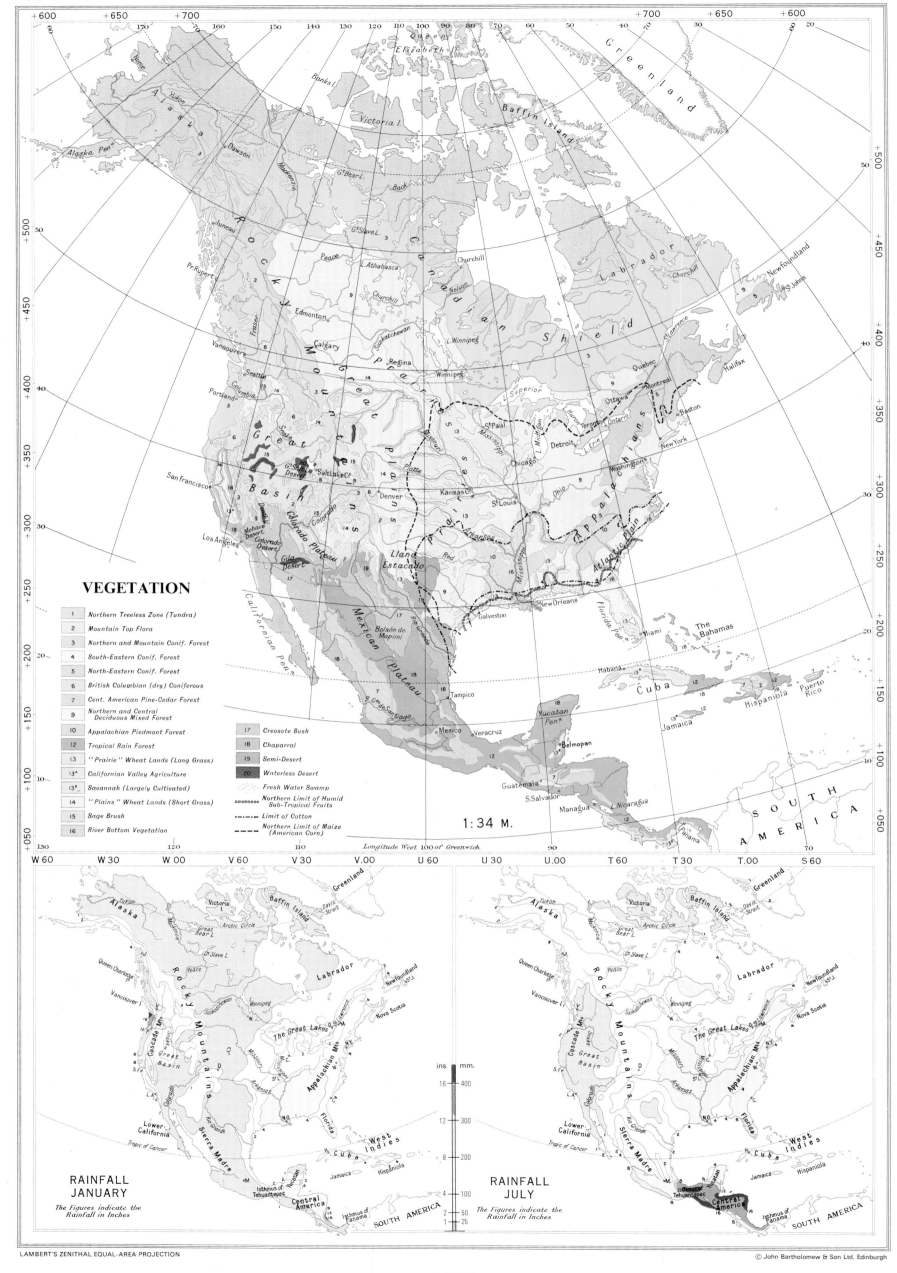

LAMBERT'S ZENITHAL EQUAL-AREA PROJECTION

0 200 400 600 800 Statute Miles **1:34M** 0 200 400 600 800 1000 1200 Kilometres

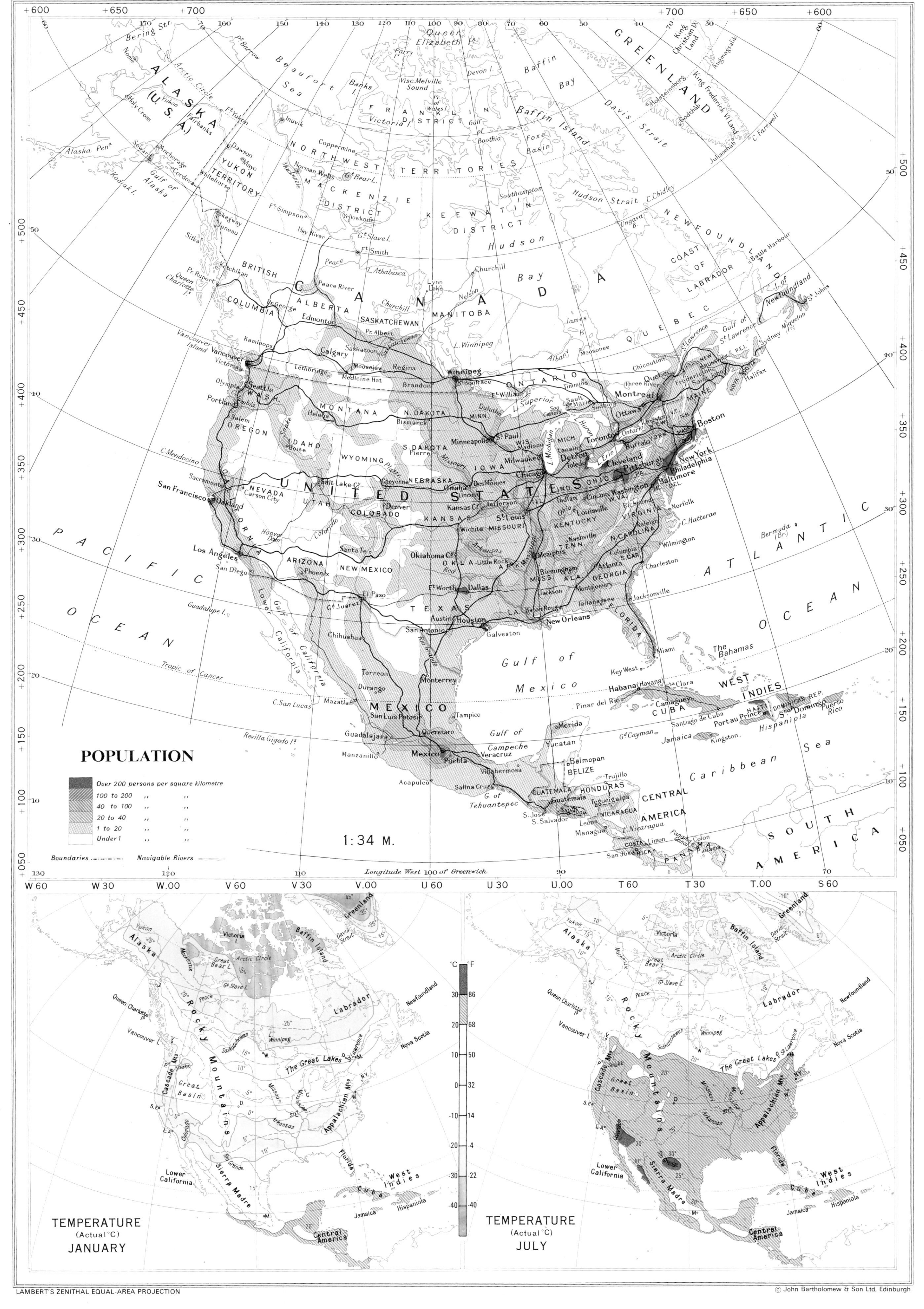
POPULATION
Over 200 persons per square kilometre
100 to 200
40 to 100
20 to 40
1 to 20
Under 1
Boundaries
Navigable Rivers
1:34 M.
Longitude West 100 of Greenwich
PACIFIC OCEAN
ATLANTIC OCEAN
CANADA
UNITED STATES
MEXICO
GREENLAND
ALASKA (U.S.A.)
WEST INDIES
CENTRAL AMERICA
SOUTH AMERICA
Gulf of Mexico
Caribbean Sea
Hudson Bay
TEMPERATURE (Actual °C) JANUARY
TEMPERATURE (Actual °C) JULY
LAMBERT'S ZENITHAL EQUAL-AREA PROJECTION
© John Bartholomew & Son Ltd, Edinburgh
1:34M
0 200 400 600 800 Statute Miles
0 200 400 600 800 1000 1200 Kilometres

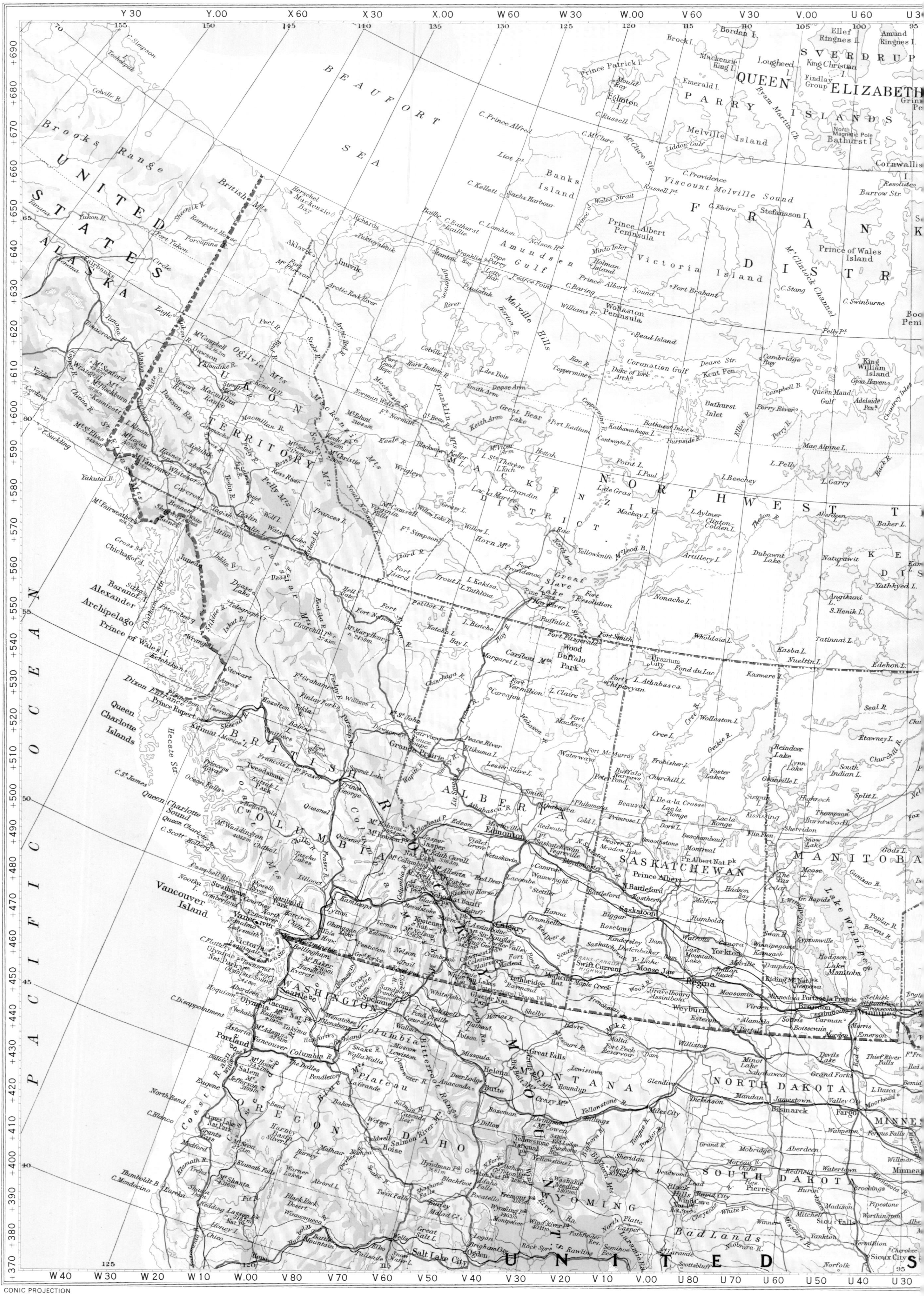

Y 30 Y.00 X 60 X 30 X.00 W 60 W 30 W.00 V 60 V 30 V.00 U 60 U 30

W 40 W 30 W 20 W 10 W.00 V 80 V 70 V 60 V 50 V 40 V 30 V 20 V 10 V.00 U 80 U 70 U 60 U 50 U 40 U 30

CONIC PROJECTION

Main Roads

Railways

0 50 100 200 300 400 500 Statute Miles

0 50 100 200 300 400 500 600 700 800 Kilometres

1:12½

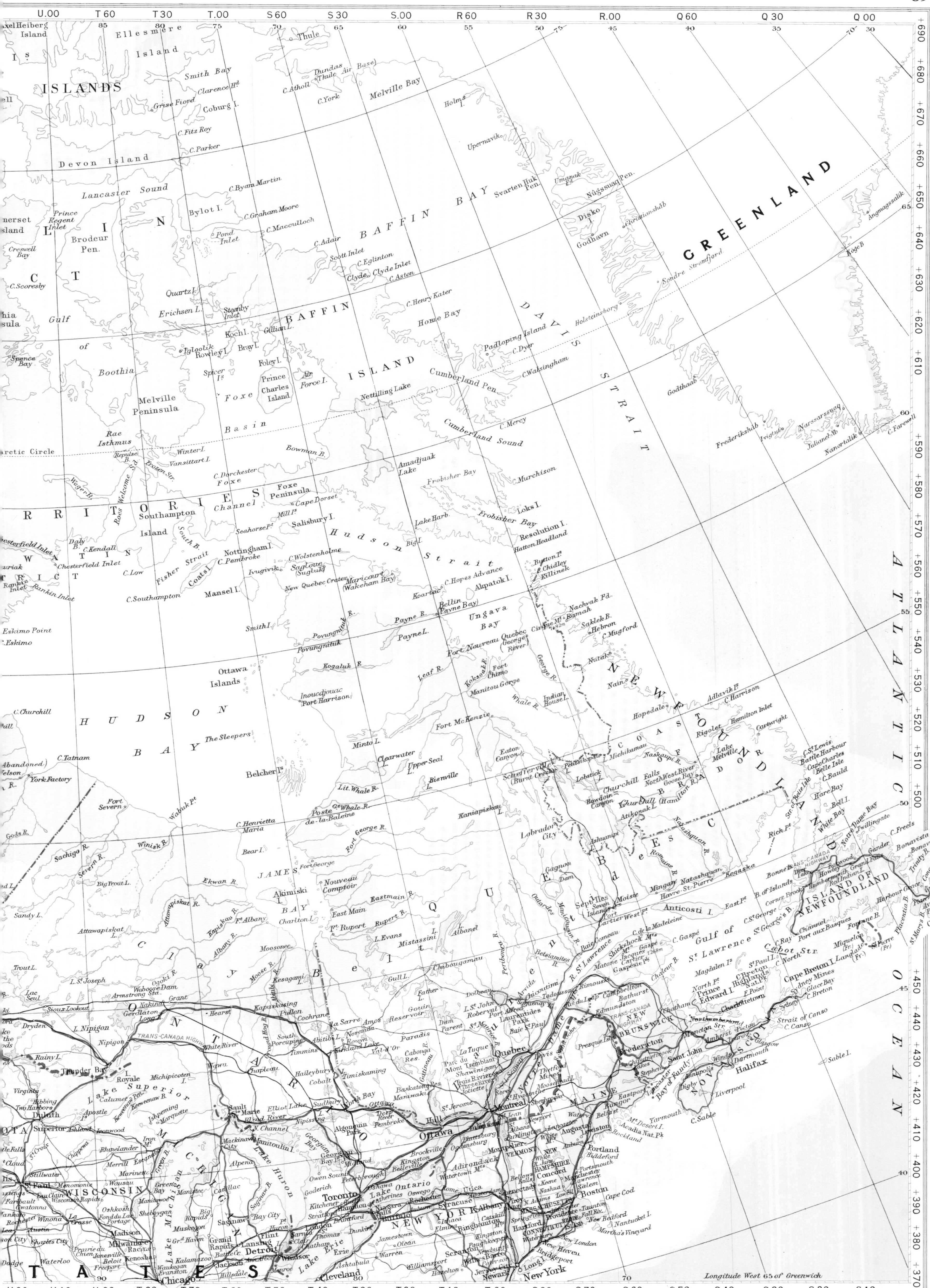

GREENLAND

BAFFIN BAY

DAVIS STRAIT

HUDSON BAY

ATLANTIC OCEAN

Longitude West 65 of Greenwich

Metres	2000	200	50	0	200	500	1000	2000	3000	4000	Metres
Feet	6560	660	160	0	660	1640	3280	6560	9840	13120	Feet

International Boundaries

Province Boundaries

M

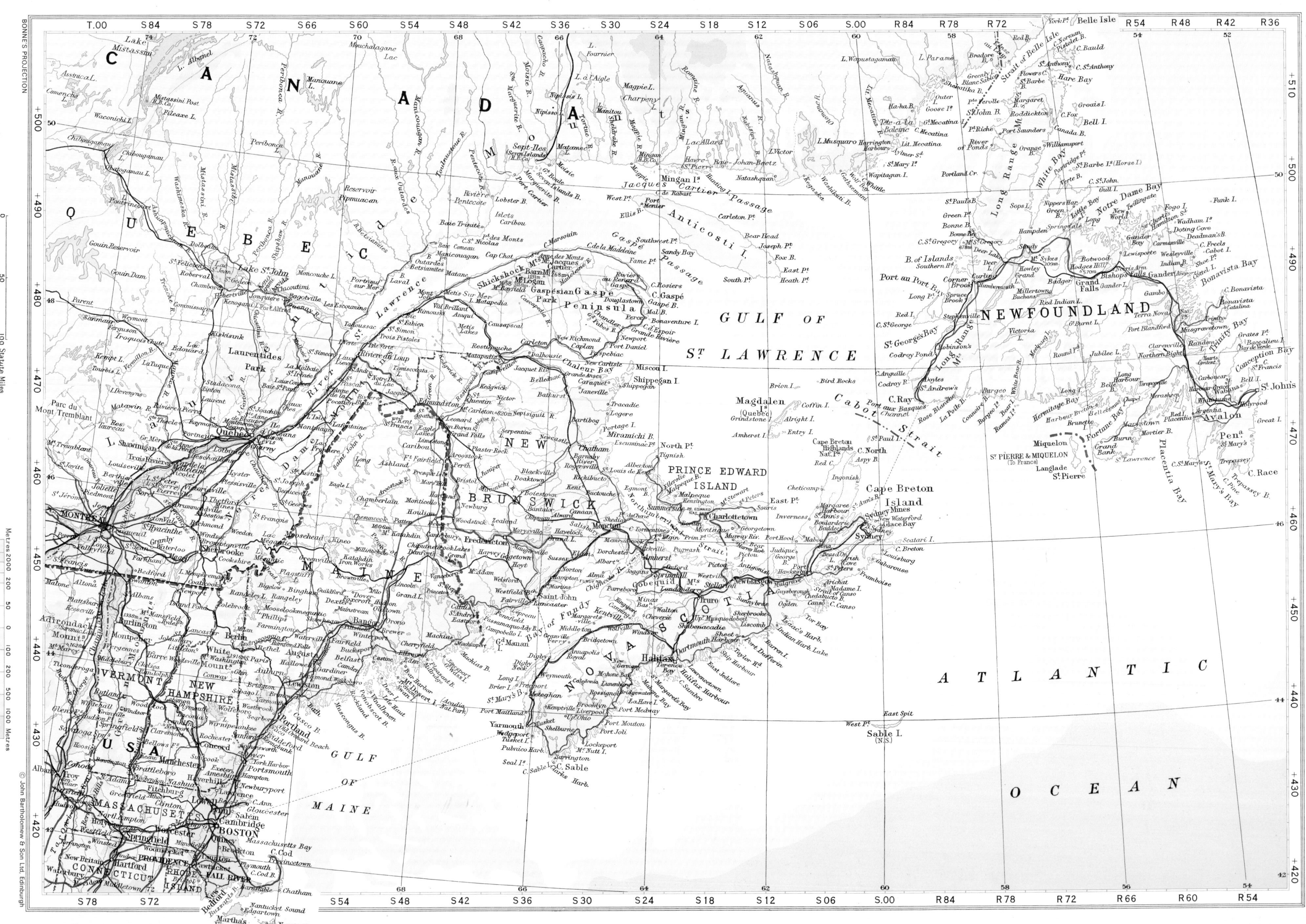

BONNE'S PROJECTION

0 50 100 Statute Miles
0 50 100 150 Kilometres

1:5M

Metres 2000 200 50 0 100 200 500 1000 Metres
Feet 6560 660 160 0 330 660 1640 3280 Feet

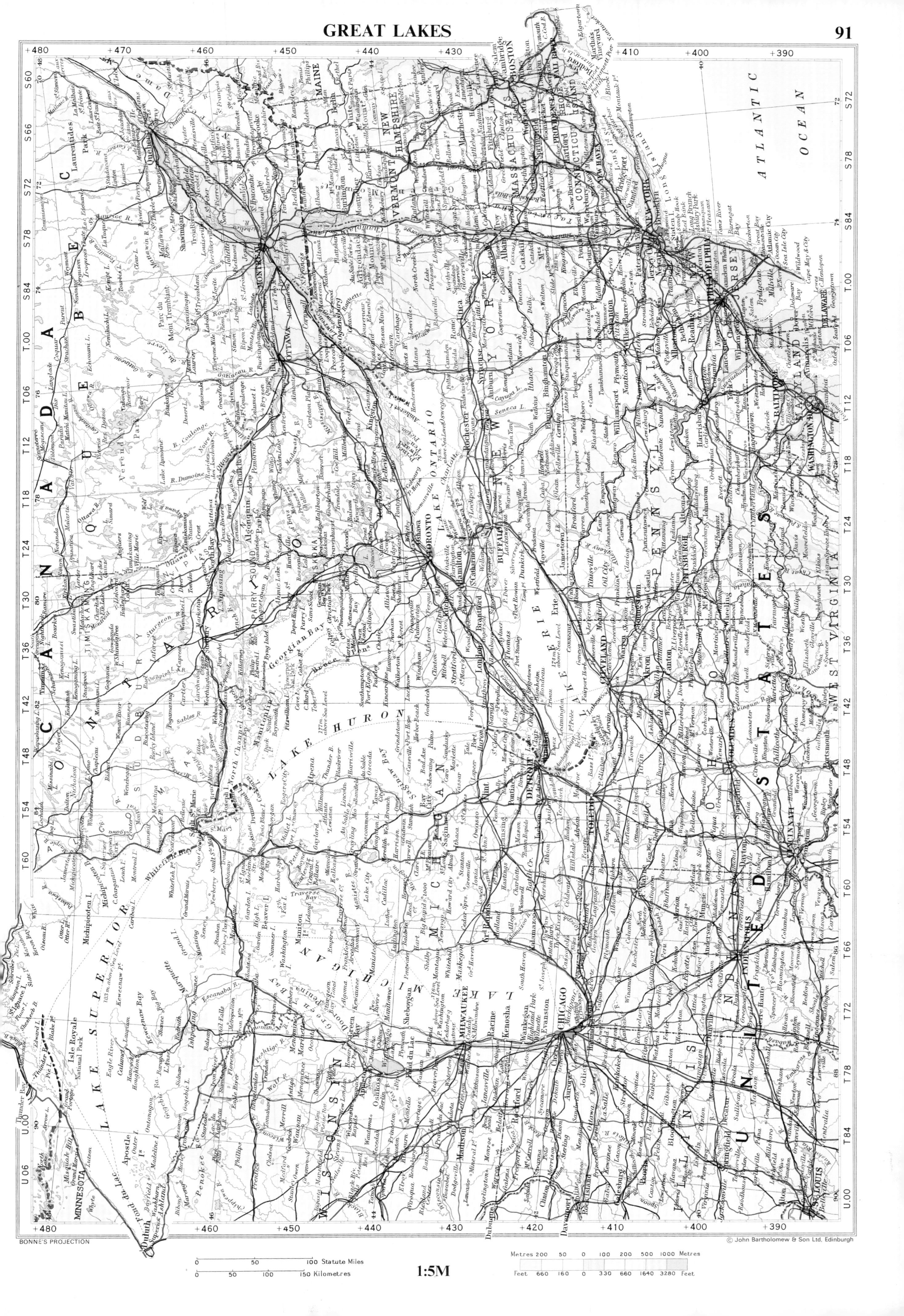
LAKE SUPERIOR
LAKE HURON
LAKE MICHIGAN
LAKE ERIE
LAKE ONTARIO
Georgian Bay
ATLANTIC
OCEAN
C A N A D A
O N T A R I O
Q U E B E C
U N I T E D   S T A T E S
MAINE
NEW HAMPSHIRE
VERMONT
MASSACHUSETTS
RHODE ISLAND
CONNECTICUT
NEW YORK
NEW JERSEY
PENNSYLVANIA
DELAWARE
MARYLAND
WEST VIRGINIA
OHIO
INDIANA
ILLINOIS
MICHIGAN
WISCONSIN
MINNESOTA
MONTREAL
OTTAWA
TORONTO
BOSTON
PHILADELPHIA
BALTIMORE
WASHINGTON
PITTSBURGH
CLEVELAND
BUFFALO
DETROIT
TOLEDO
COLUMBUS
CINCINNATI
INDIANAPOLIS
CHICAGO
MILWAUKEE
ST LOUIS
Quebec
Long Island
Isle Royale National Park
BONNE'S PROJECTION
© John Bartholomew & Son Ltd. Edinburgh
0 50 100 Statute Miles
0 50 100 150 Kilometres
1:5M
Metres 200 50 0 100 200 500 1000 Metres
Feet 660 160 0 330 660 1640 3280 Feet

PACIFIC COAST

BONNE'S PROJECTION

Metres 2000 200 50 0 100 200 500 1000 2000 3000 4000 Metres

Land Depression

Feet 6560 660 160 0 330 660 1640 3280 6560 9840 13120 Feet

1:5M

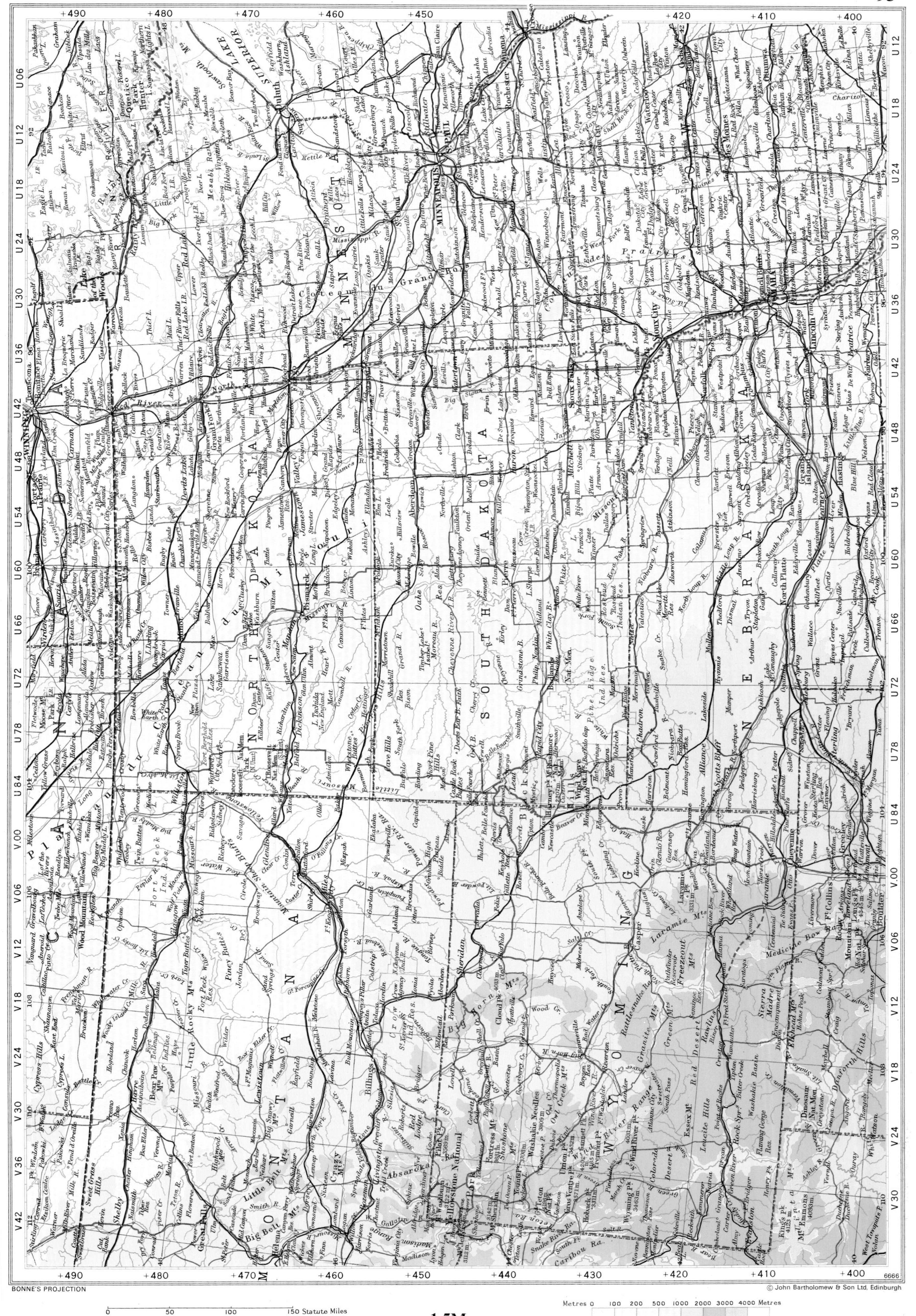

MINNESOTA
NORTH DAKOTA
SOUTH DAKOTA
NEBRASKA
IOWA
MONTANA
WYOMING
LAKE SUPERIOR
BONNE'S PROJECTION
© John Bartholomew & Son Ltd, Edinburgh
0 50 100 150 Statute Miles
0 50 100 150 200 250 Kilometres
1:5M
Metres 0 100 200 500 1000 2000 3000 4000 Metres
Feet 0 330 660 1640 3280 6560 9840 13120 Feet

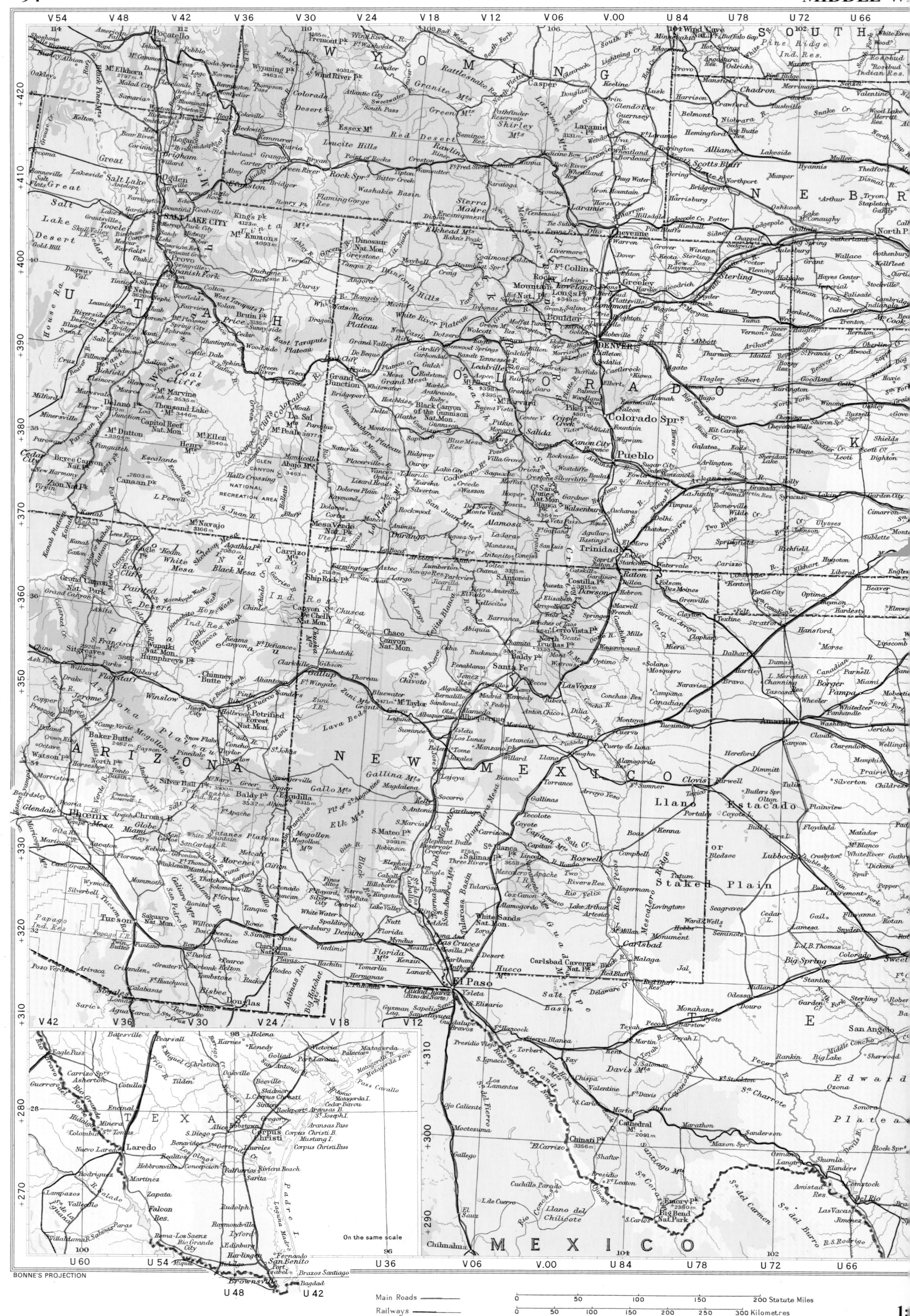
WYOMING
UTAH
COLORADO
ARIZONA
NEW MEXICO
NEBRASKA
SOUTH
TEXAS
MEXICO
Llano Estacado
Staked Plain
Great Salt Lake Desert
Salt Lake
SALT LAKE CITY
Ogden
Provo
Cheyenne
Laramie
Casper
Rawlins
Rock Sprs
DENVER
Boulder
Colorado Sprs
Pueblo
Trinidad
Grand Junction
Durango
Santa Fe
Albuquerque
Las Vegas
Gallup
Flagstaff
Phoenix
Tucson
El Paso
Las Cruces
Roswell
Carlsbad
Amarillo
Lubbock
Clovis
Laredo
Corpus Christi
Brownsville
San Angelo
Big Spring
Odessa
Midland
Alliance
Scotts Bluff
Sterling
Greeley
Fort Collins
Raton
Alamosa
Leadville
Aspen
Gunnison
Montrose
Glen Canyon National Recreation Area
Mesa Verde Nat. Pk.
Grand Canyon Nat. Park
Zion Nat. Pk.
Rocky Mountain Nat. Pk.
Big Bend Nat. Park
White Sands Nat. Mon.
Carlsbad Caverns Nat. Pk.
On the same scale
BONNE'S PROJECTION
Main Roads
Railways
0 50 100 150 200 Statute Miles
0 50 100 150 200 250 300 Kilometres

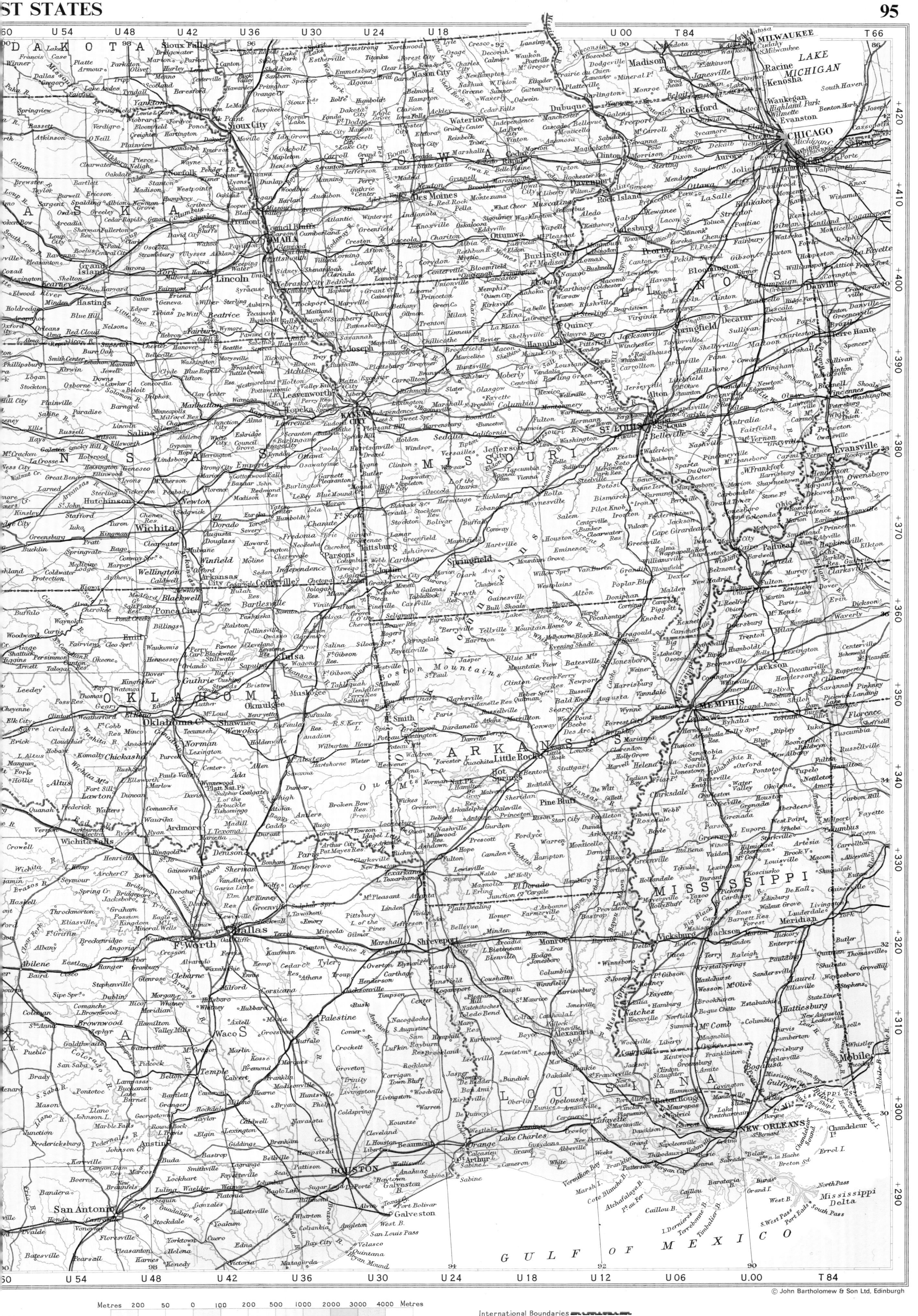

Metres 200 50 0 100 200 500 1000 2000 3000 4000 Metres

Feet 660 160 0 330 660 1640 3280 6560 9840 13120 Feet

International Boundaries

State Boundaries

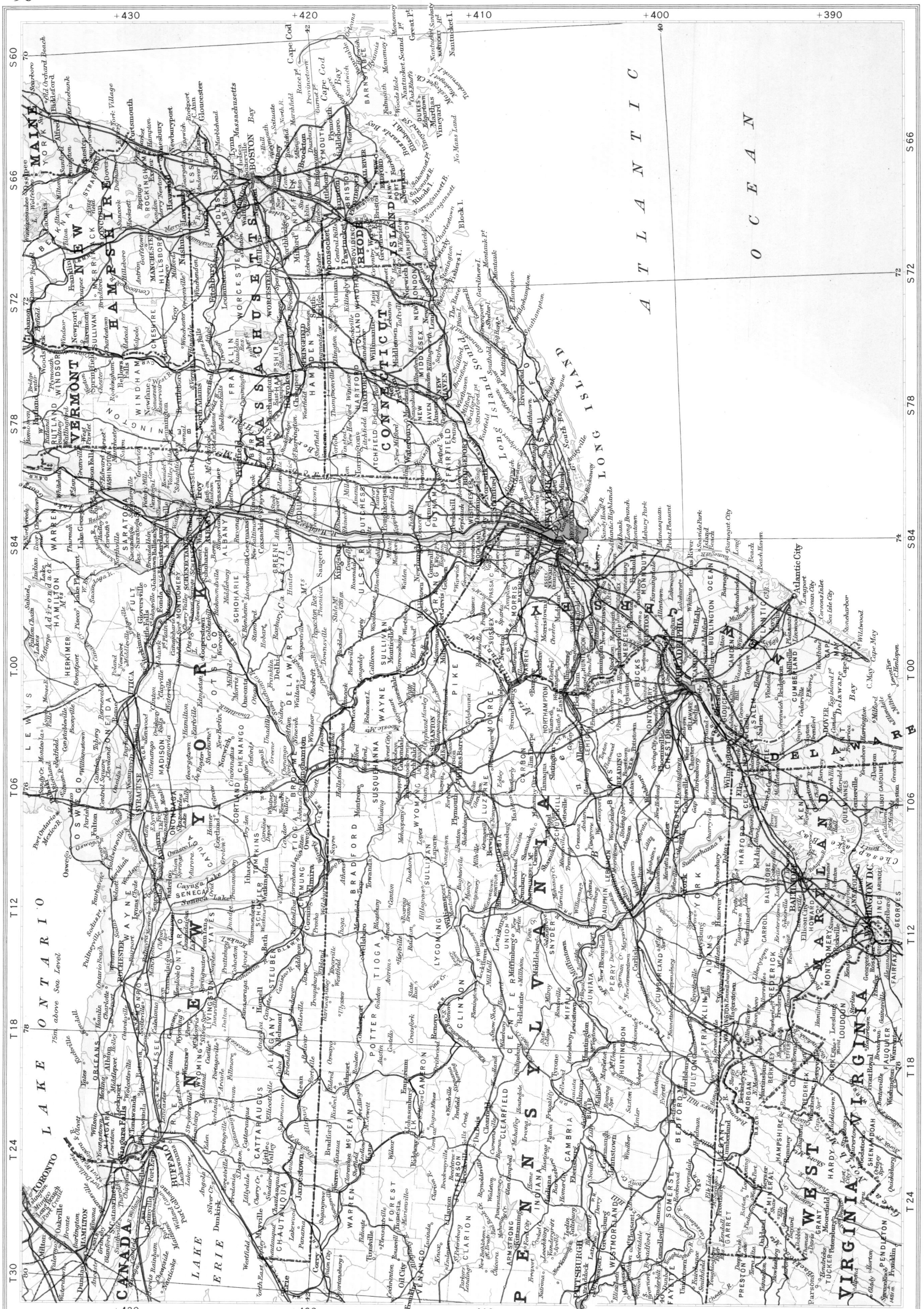

+430 +420 +410 +400 +390

S60 S66 S72 S78 S84 T00 T06 T12 T18 T24 T30

ATLANTIC OCEAN

CONIC PROJECTION

0 10 20 40 60 Statute Miles

0 10 20 40 60 80 100 Kilometres

1:2½M

Metres 200 100 50 0 100 200 500 1000 Metres

Feet 660 330 160 0 330 660 1640 3280 Feet

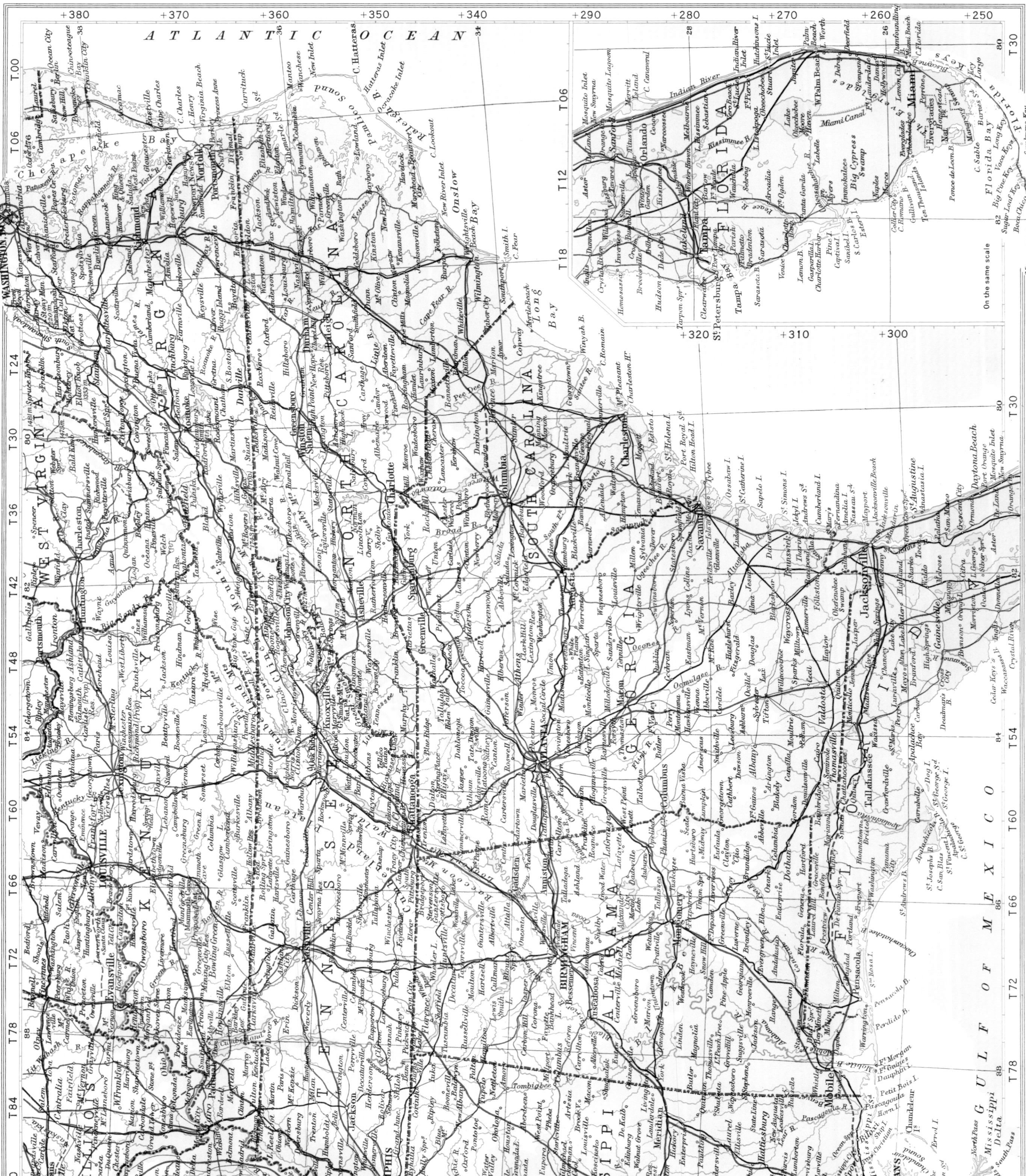

BONNE'S PROJECTION

0 50 100 Statute Miles

0 50 100 150 Kilometres

1:5M

Metres 200 50 0 100 200 500 1000 Metres

Feet 660 160 0 330 660 1640 3280 Feet

On the same scale

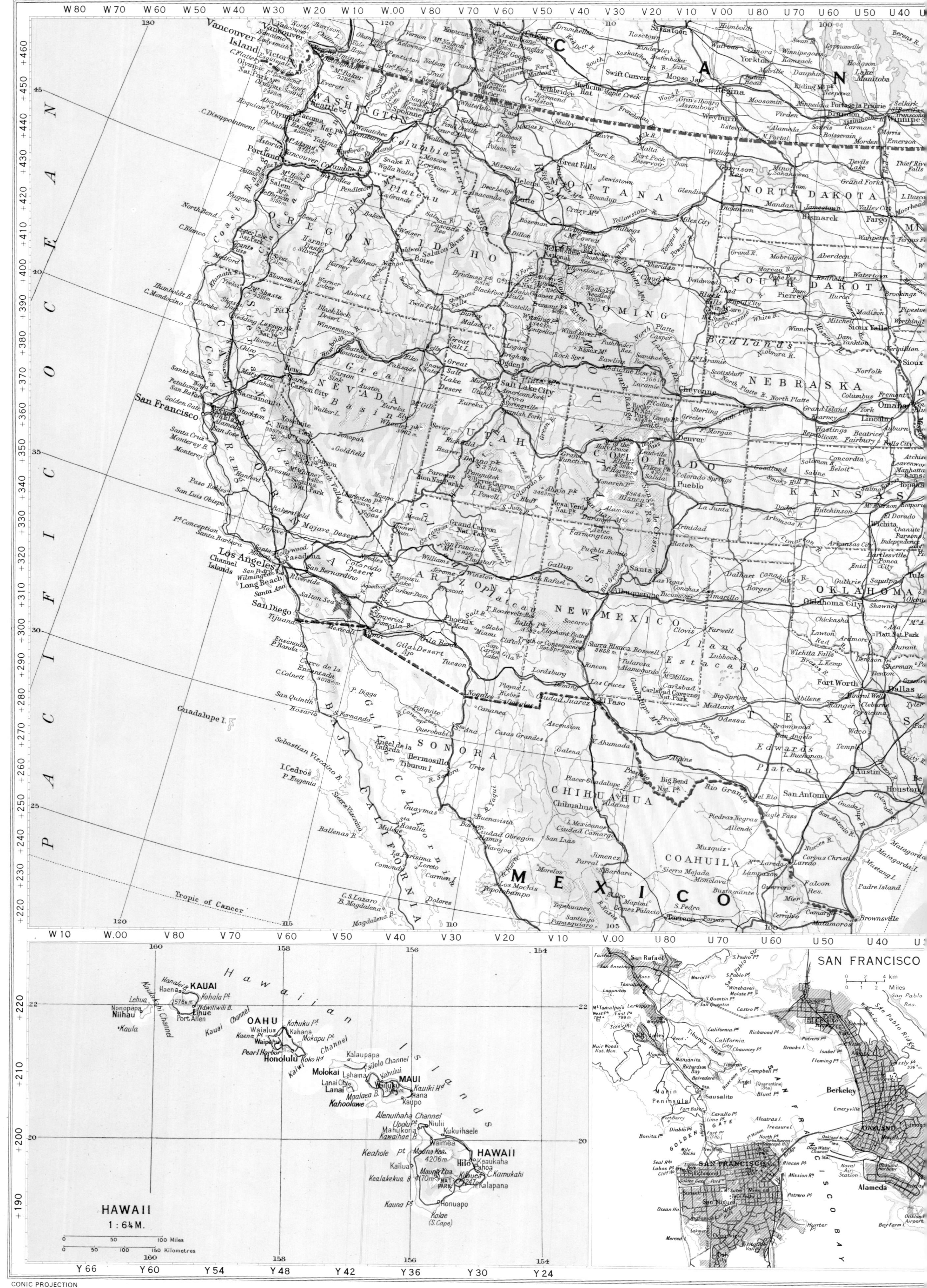

CONIC PROJECTION

Main Roads
Railways

0 50 100 200 300 400 500 Statute Miles
0 50 100 200 300 400 500 600 700 800 Kilometres

1:12½

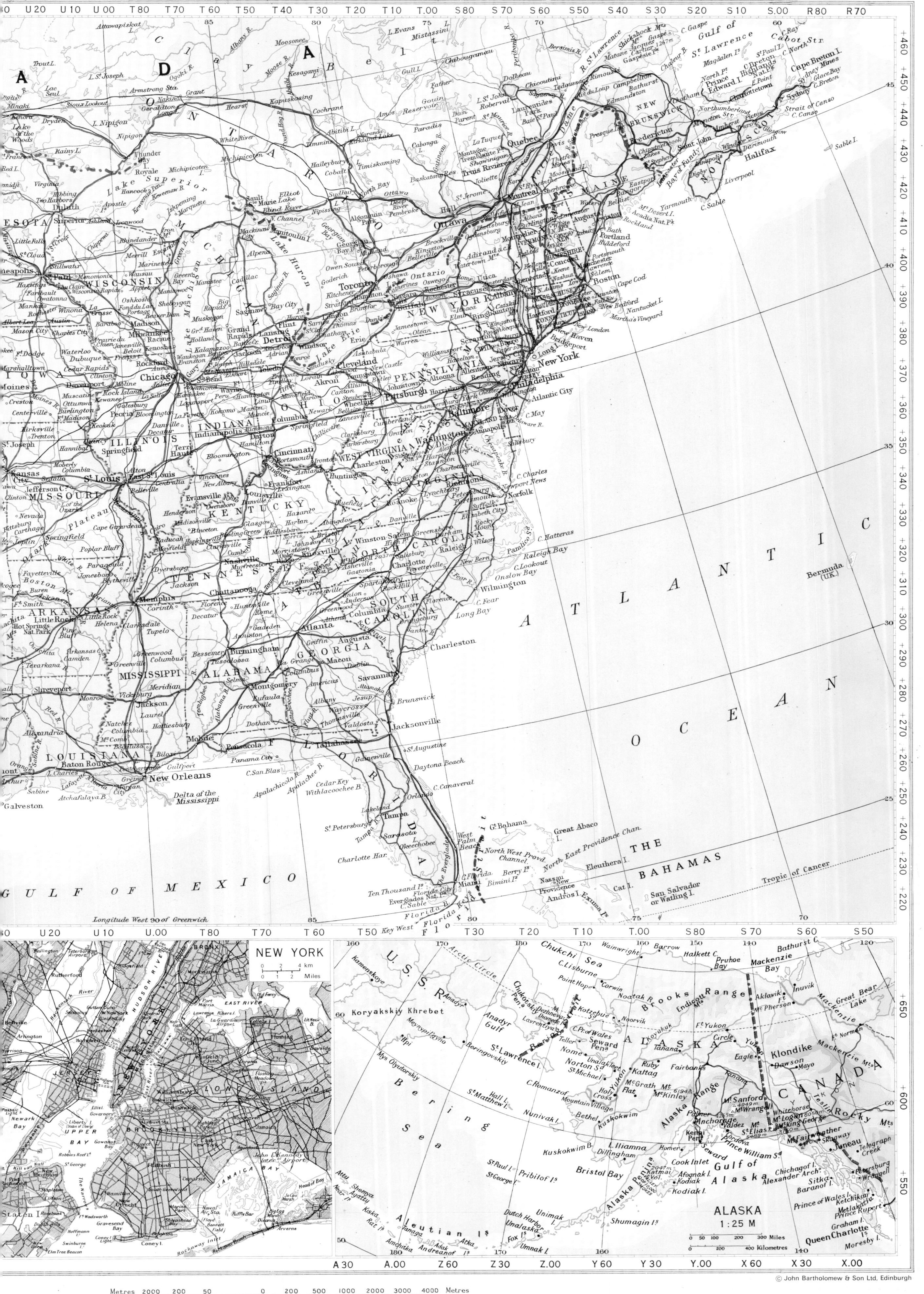
A T L A N T I C
O C E A N
G U L F O F M E X I C O
THE BAHAMAS
Tropic of Cancer
Gulf of St Lawrence
NEW YORK
PENNSYLVANIA
WEST VIRGINIA
VIRGINIA
NORTH CAROLINA
SOUTH CAROLINA
GEORGIA
FLORIDA
ALABAMA
MISSISSIPPI
LOUISIANA
ARKANSAS
TENNESSEE
KENTUCKY
OHIO
INDIANA
ILLINOIS
MISSOURI
IOWA
WISCONSIN
MICHIGAN
MAINE
NEW BRUNSWICK
NOVA SCOTIA
Lake Superior
Lake Huron
Lake Michigan
Lake Erie
Ontario
New York
Philadelphia
Baltimore
Washington
Boston
Montreal
Ottawa
Quebec
Toronto
Detroit
Chicago
Cleveland
Pittsburgh
St Louis
Memphis
Atlanta
New Orleans
Jacksonville
Charleston
Norfolk
Halifax
Bermuda (UK)
Longitude West 90 of Greenwich
NEW YORK
0 2 4 km
0 1 2 Miles
BRONX
HUDSON RIVER
EAST RIVER
MANHATTAN
JERSEY CITY
BROOKLYN
LONG ISLAND
UPPER BAY
JAMAICA BAY
Staten I.
Newark Bay
U. S. S. R.
Koryakskiy Khrebet
Chukchi Sea
Arctic Circle
Bering Sea
Brooks Range
ALASKA
CANADA
Klondike
Gulf of Alaska
Bristol Bay
Aleutian Is
Alaska Range
Mt McKinley
Anchorage
Fairbanks
Juneau
ALASKA
1:25 M
0 50 100 200 300 Miles
0 100 200 400 Kilometres
© John Bartholomew & Son Ltd, Edinburgh
Metres 2000 200 50 0 200 500 1000 2000 3000 4000 Metres
Land Depression
Feet 6560 660 160 0 660 1640 3280 6560 9840 13120 Feet
International Boundaries
State Boundaries
M

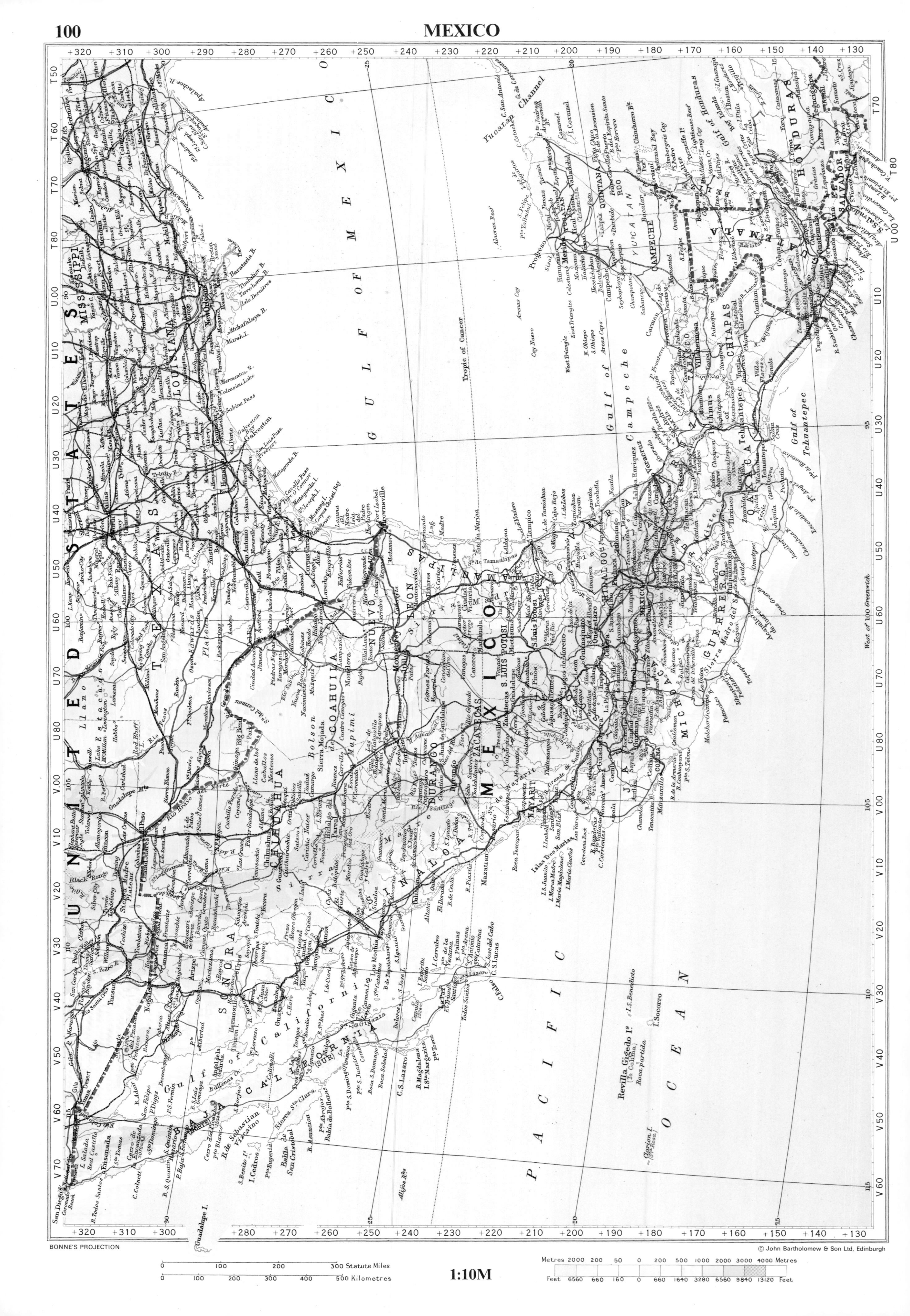

BONNE'S PROJECTION
© John Bartholomew & Son Ltd, Edinburgh
0 100 200 300 Statute Miles
0 100 200 300 400 500 Kilometres
1:10M
Metres 2000 200 50 0 200 500 1000 2000 3000 4000 Metres
Feet 6560 660 160 0 660 1640 3280 6560 9840 13120 Feet

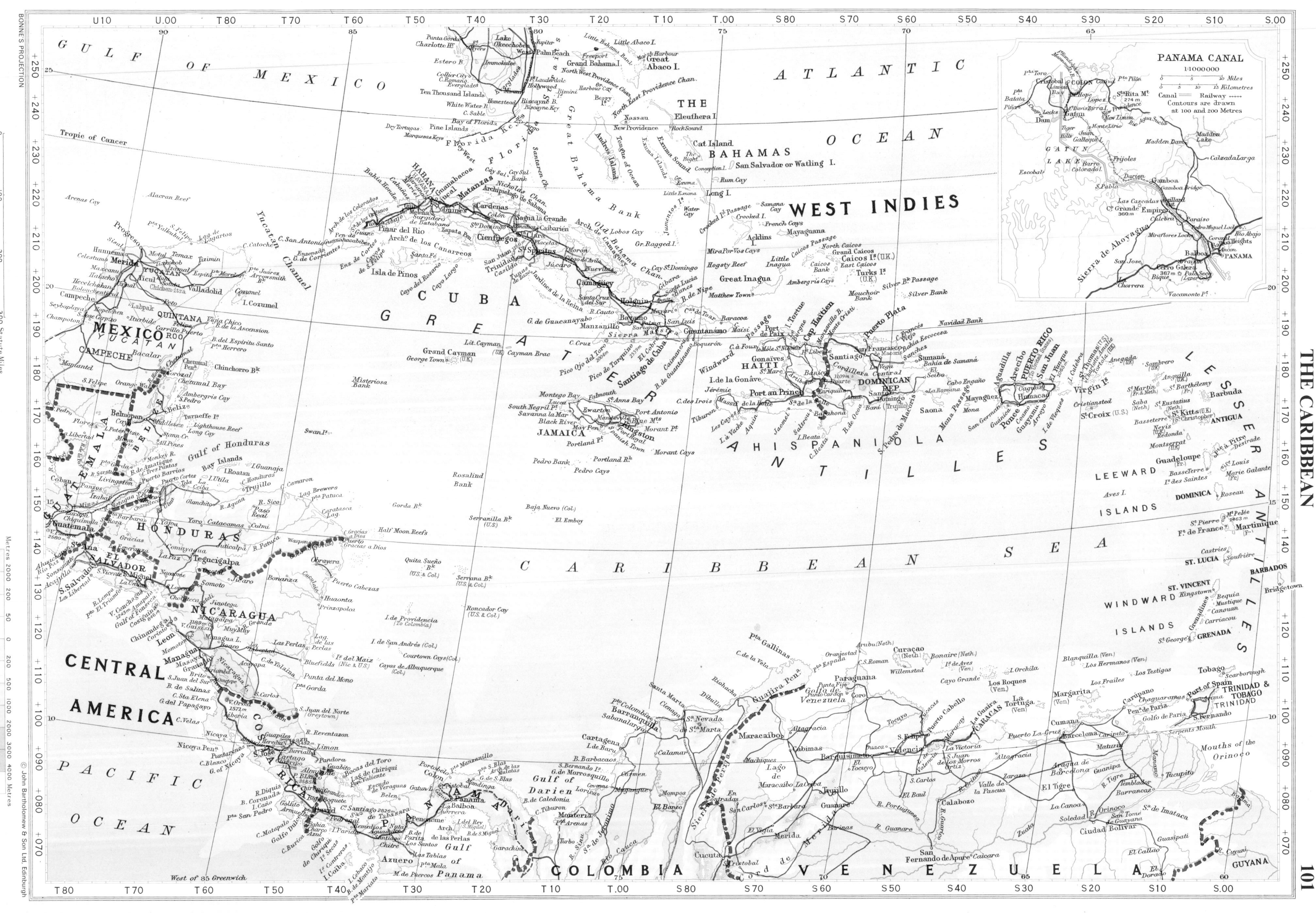
PANAMA CANAL
1:1000000
Canal — Railway
Contours are drawn at 100 and 200 Metres
ATLANTIC OCEAN
WEST INDIES
THE BAHAMAS
GULF OF MEXICO
CARIBBEAN SEA
LESSER ANTILLES
GREATER ANTILLES
LEEWARD ISLANDS
WINDWARD ISLANDS
HISPANIOLA
CUBA
JAMAICA
HAITI
DOMINICAN REP.
PUERTO RICO
VENEZUELA
COLOMBIA
GUYANA
TRINIDAD & TOBAGO
CENTRAL AMERICA
MEXICO
HONDURAS
NICARAGUA
COSTA RICA
PANAMA
EL SALVADOR
GUATEMALA
PACIFIC OCEAN
HABANA
Tropic of Cancer
West of 85 Greenwich
BONNE'S PROJECTION
© John Bartholomew & Son Ltd, Edinburgh
0 100 200 300 Statute Miles
0 100 200 300 400 500 Kilometres
1:10M
Metres 2000 200 50 0 200 500 1000 2000 3000 4000 Metres
Feet 6560 660 160 0 660 1640 3280 6560 9840 13120 Feet

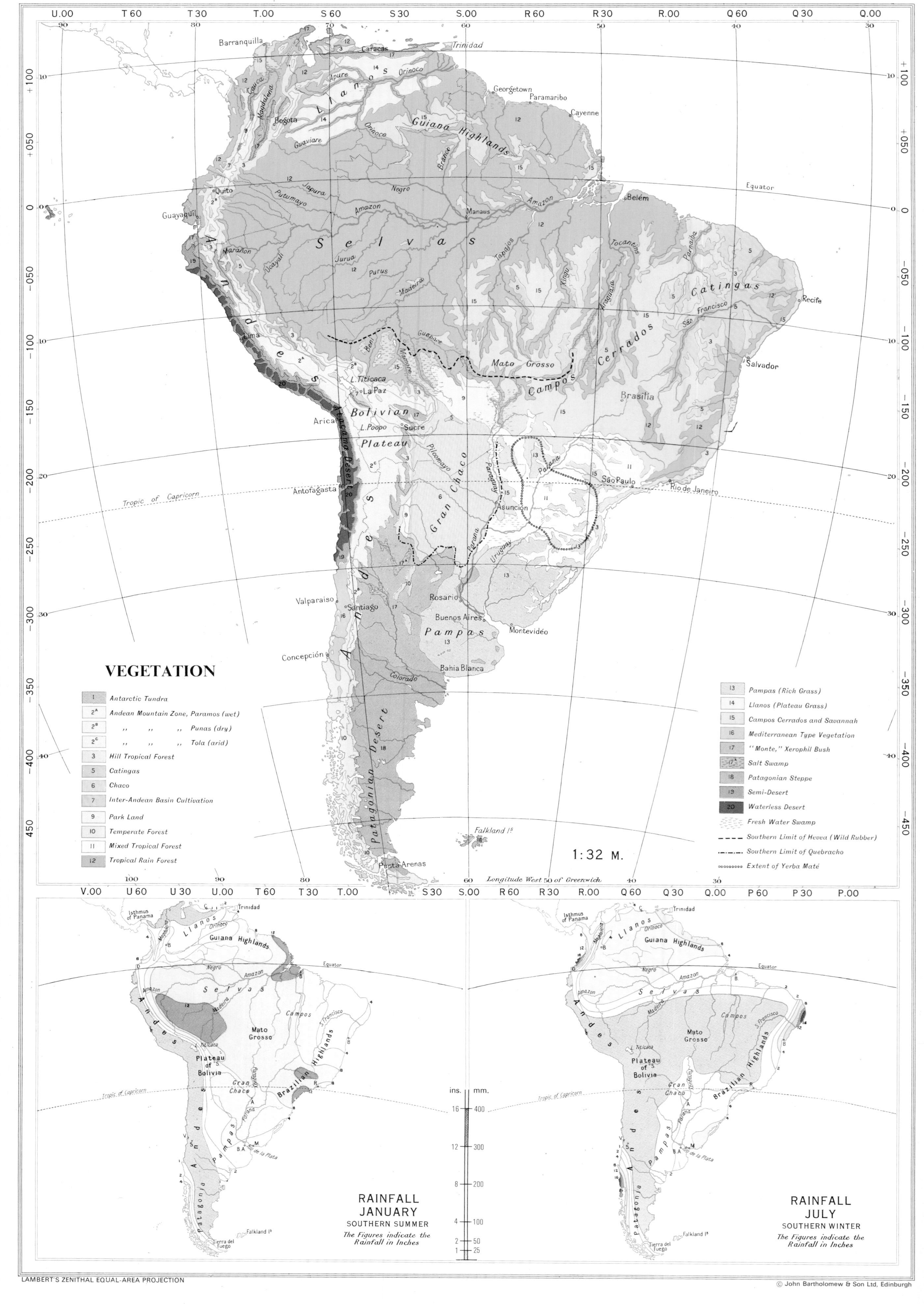

0 200 400 600 800 Statute Miles **1:32M** 0 200 400 600 800 1000 1200 Kilometres

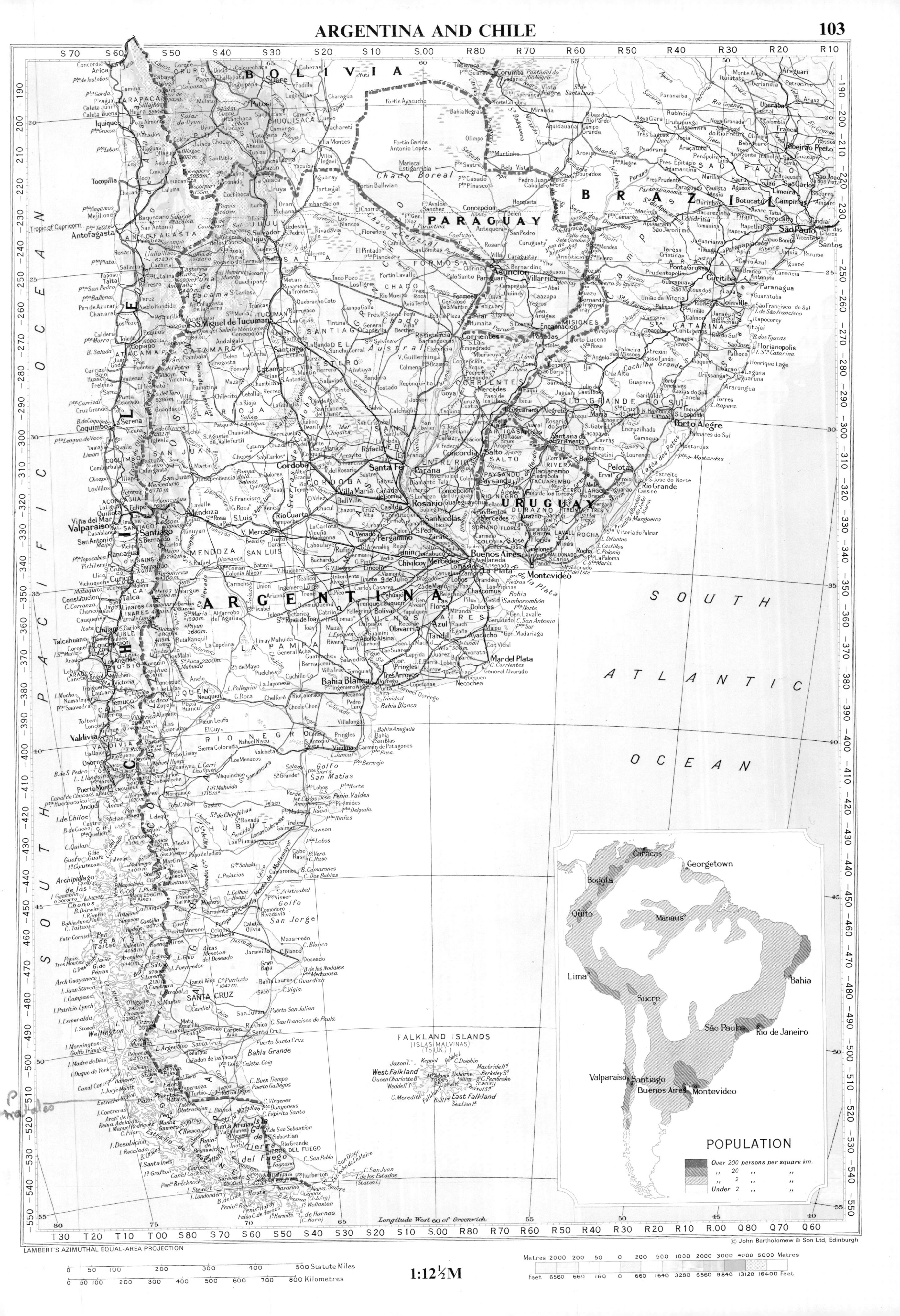
BOLIVIA
PARAGUAY
BRAZIL
ARGENTINA
URUGUAY
CHILE
PACIFIC OCEAN
SOUTH ATLANTIC OCEAN
Tropic of Capricorn
FALKLAND ISLANDS
(ISLAS MALVINAS)
(To U.K.)
West Falkland
East Falkland
Buenos Aires
Montevideo
Santiago
Valparaiso
Asuncion
La Plata
Cordoba
Rosario
Mendoza
Bahia Blanca
Mar del Plata
Antofagasta
Concepcion
Valdivia
Puerto Montt
Punta Arenas
São Paulo
Porto Alegre
Curitiba
Longitude West 60 of Greenwich
POPULATION
Over 200 persons per square km.
" 20 " "
" 2 " "
Under 2 " "
Caracas
Georgetown
Bogota
Quito
Manaus
Lima
Bahia
Sucre
São Paulo
Rio de Janeiro
Valparaiso
Santiago
Buenos Aires
Montevideo
LAMBERT'S AZIMUTHAL EQUAL-AREA PROJECTION
1:12½M
0 50 100 200 300 400 500 Statute Miles
0 50 100 200 300 400 500 600 700 800 Kilometres
Metres 2000 200 50 0 200 500 1000 2000 3000 4000 5000 Metres
Feet 6560 660 160 0 660 1640 3280 6560 9840 13120 16400 Feet
© John Bartholomew & Son Ltd, Edinburgh

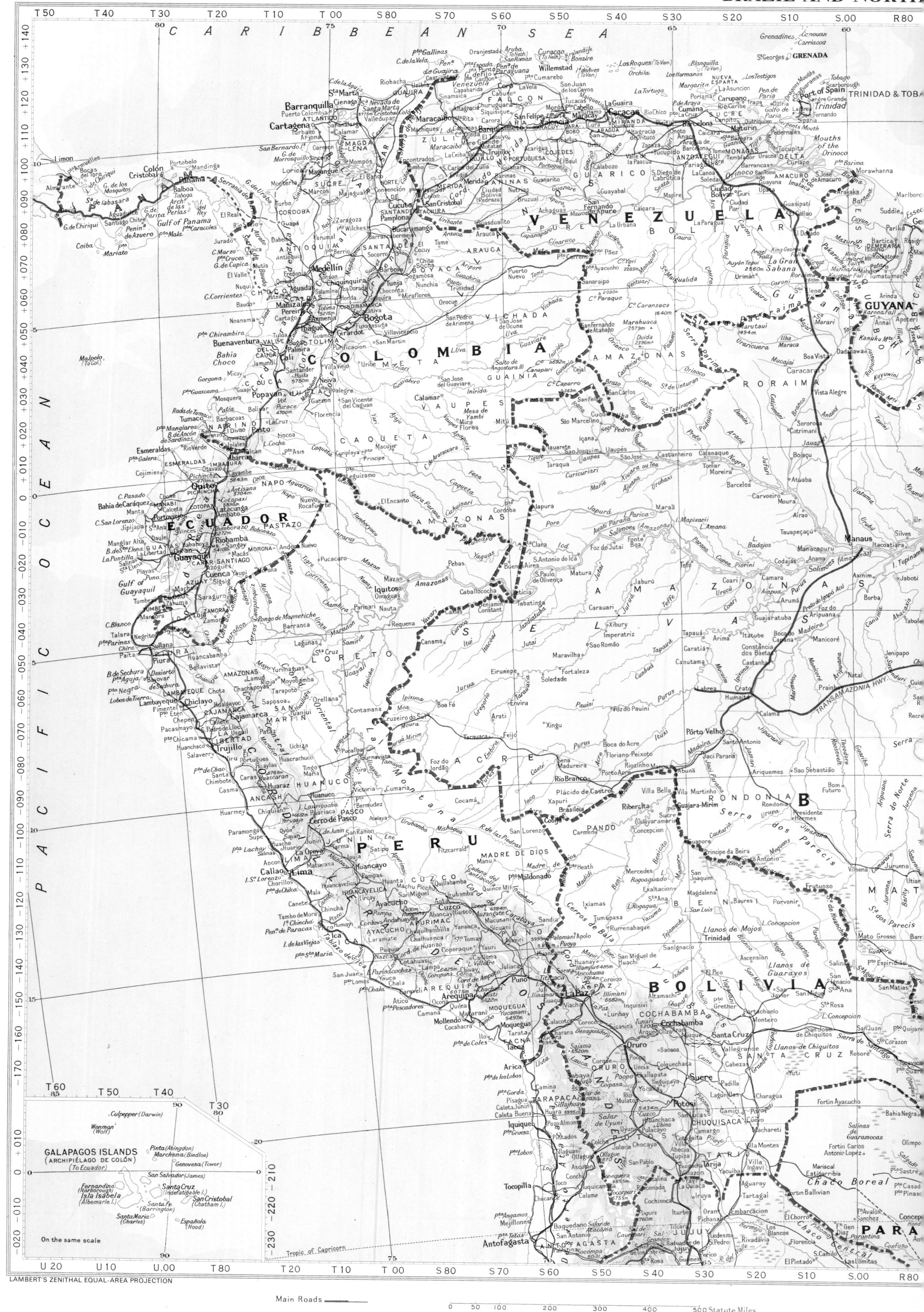
C A R I B B E A N S E A
P A C I F I C O C E A N
COLOMBIA
VENEZUELA
ECUADOR
PERU
BOLIVIA
GUYANA
TRINIDAD & TOBA
GRENADA
PANAMA
A M A Z O N A S
RORAIMA
RONDONIA
ACRE
GALAPAGOS ISLANDS
(ARCHIPIÉLAGO DE COLÓN)
(To Ecuador)
On the same scale
Bogota
Caracas
Quito
Lima
La Paz
Manaus
Barranquilla
Cartagena
Medellín
Cali
Guayaquil
Iquitos
Callao
Arequipa
Cuzco
Cochabamba
Santa Cruz
Sucre
Potosi
Oruro
Antofagasta
Arica
Iquique
Tocopilla
Maracaibo
Valencia
Barquisimeto
Ciudad Bolívar
Porto Velho
Rio Branco
Tropic of Capricorn
LAMBERT'S ZENITHAL EQUAL-AREA PROJECTION
Main Roads
Railways
0 50 100 200 300 400 500 Statute Miles
0 50 100 200 300 400 500 600 700 800 Kilometres
1:12½

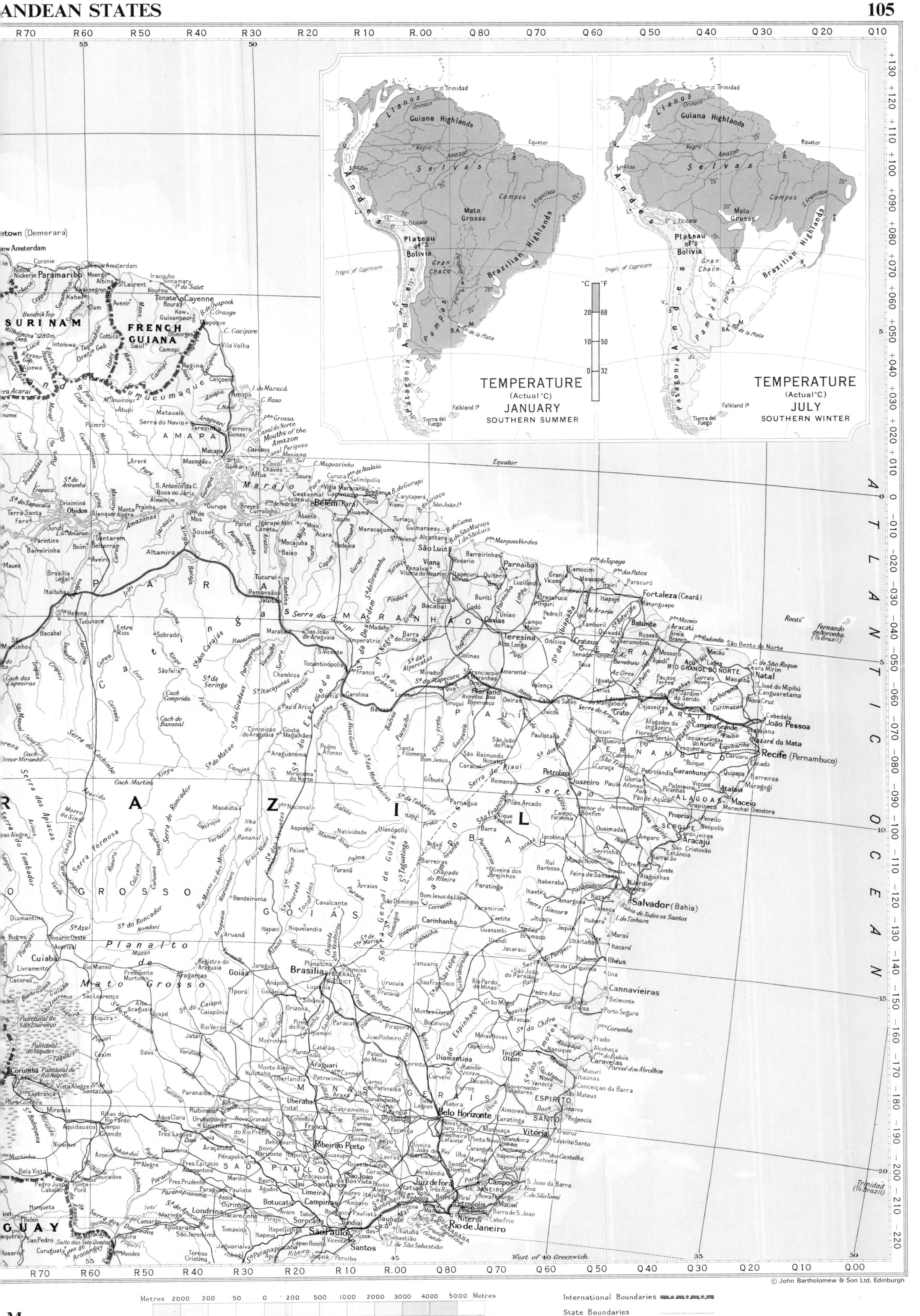
TEMPERATURE
(Actual °C)
JANUARY
SOUTHERN SUMMER
TEMPERATURE
(Actual °C)
JULY
SOUTHERN WINTER
°C °F
20 68
10 50
0 32
Trinidad
Llanos
Orinoco
Guiana Highlands
Equator
Negro
Amazon
Selvas
Campos
S. Francisco
Mato Grosso
Brazilian Highlands
L. Titicaca
Plateau of Bolivia
Gran Chaco
Tropic of Capricorn
Pampas
Andes
Patagonia
Falkland Is
Tierra del Fuego
ATLANTIC OCEAN
SURINAM
FRENCH GUIANA
AMAPÁ
PARÁ
MARANHÃO
PIAUÍ
CEARÁ
RIO GRANDE DO NORTE
PARAÍBA
PERNAMBUCO
ALAGOAS
SERGIPE
BAHIA
GOIÁS
MATO GROSSO
MINAS GERAIS
ESPÍRITO SANTO
SÃO PAULO
BRAZIL
Paramaribo
Cayenne
Macapá
Belém (Pará)
São Luís
Fortaleza (Ceará)
Natal
João Pessoa
Recife (Pernambuco)
Maceió
Aracaju
Salvador (Bahia)
Teresina
Brasília
Goiás
Belo Horizonte
Vitória
Rio de Janeiro
Niterói
São Paulo
Santos
Campinas
Cuiabá
Corumbá
Santarém
Óbidos
Marajó
Mouths of the Amazon
Planalto de Mato Grosso
Rocas
Fernando de Noronha (To Brazil)
Trinidad (To Brazil)
West of 40 Greenwich
© John Bartholomew & Son Ltd, Edinburgh
Metres 2000 200 50 0 200 500 1000 2000 3000 4000 5000 Metres
Feet 6560 660 160 0 660 1640 3280 6560 9840 13120 16400 Feet
International Boundaries
State Boundaries

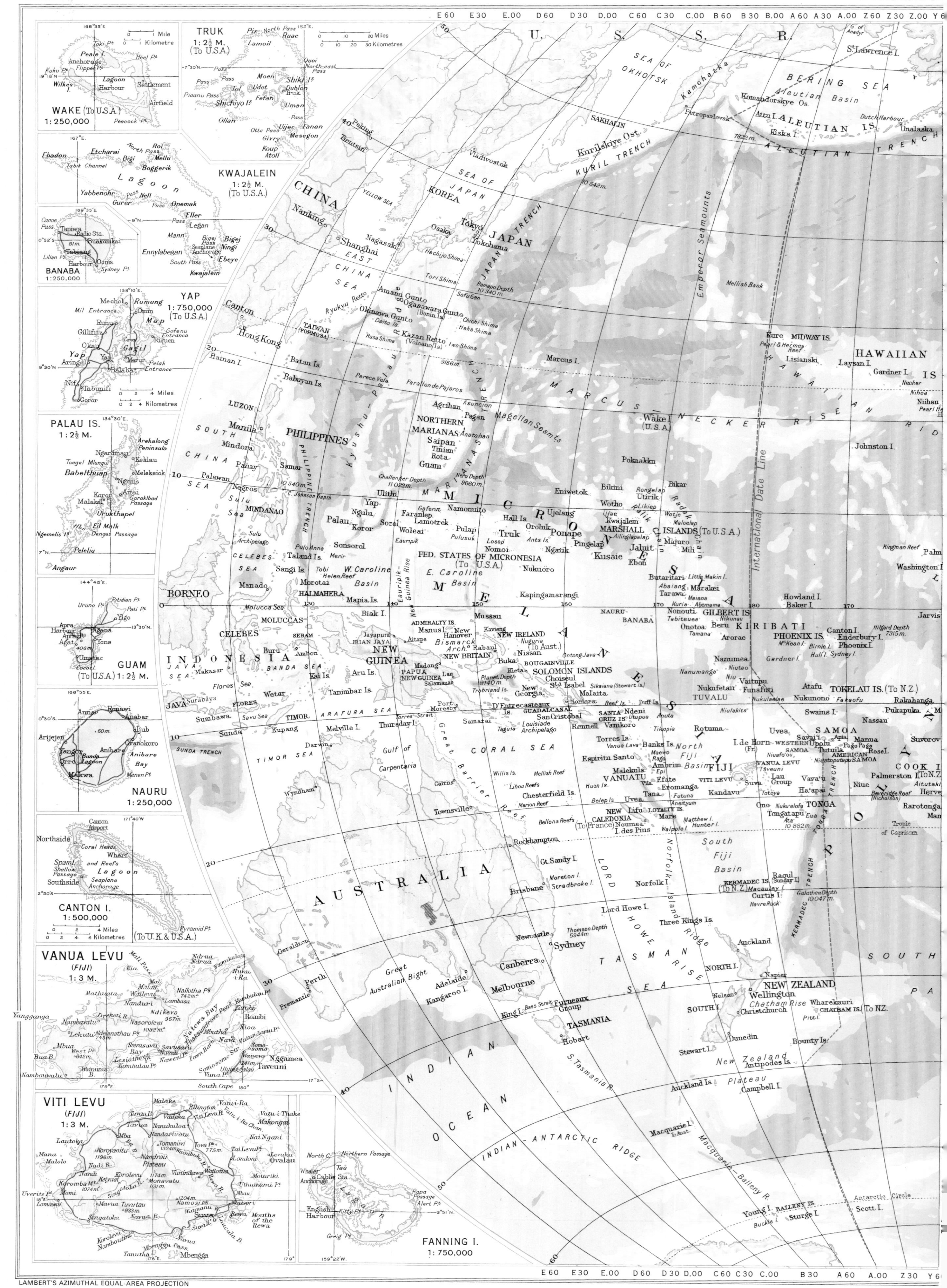

0 100 200 400 600 800 1000 1200 1400 1600 Statute Miles
0 200 400 800 1200 1600 2000 2400 Kilometres

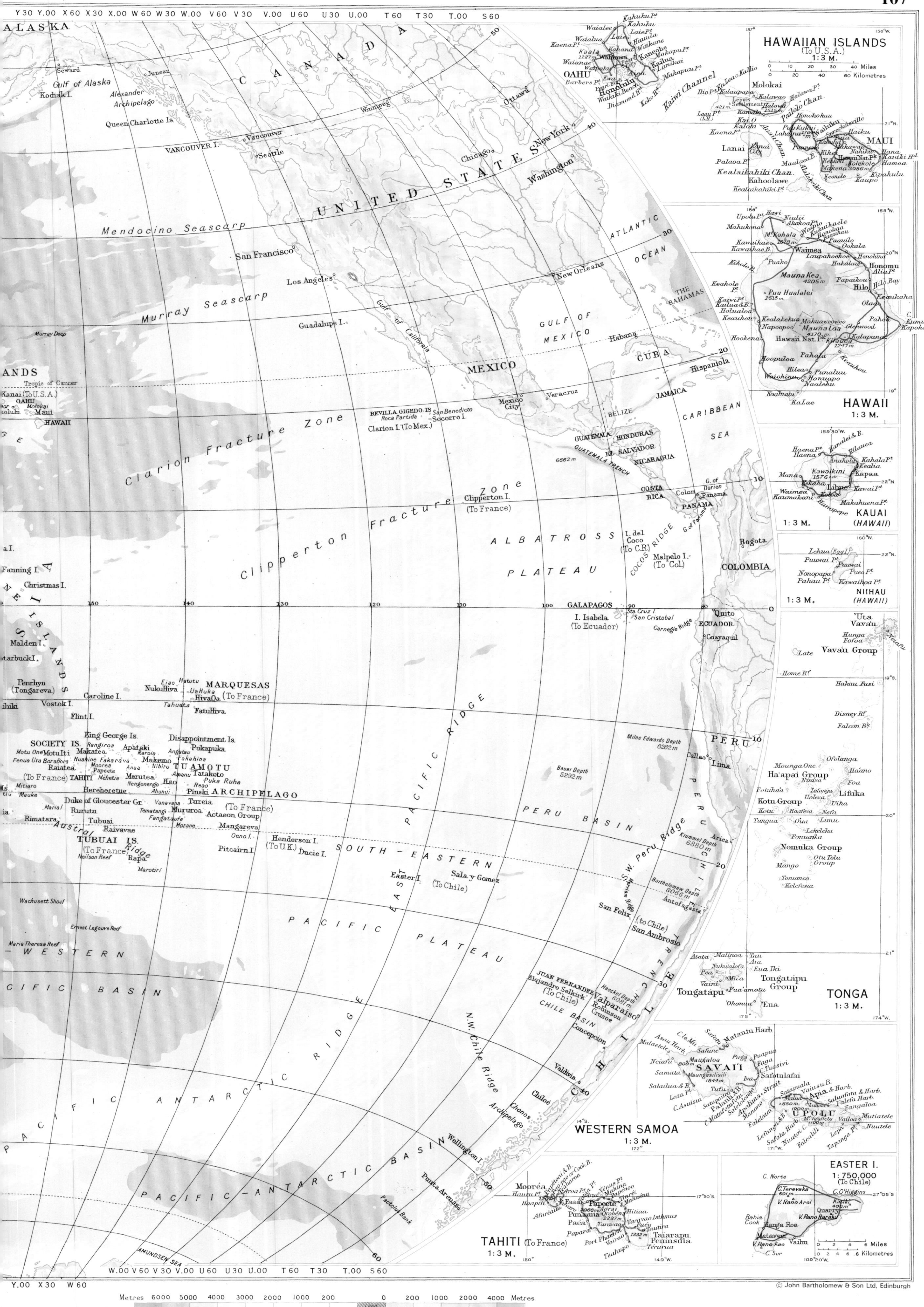
ALASKA
CANADA
UNITED STATES
Gulf of Alaska
Kodiak I.
Alexander Archipelago
Queen Charlotte Is.
VANCOUVER I.
Vancouver
Seattle
Winnipeg
Ottawa
Chicago
New York
Washington
Mendocino Seascarp
San Francisco
Los Angeles
Murray Seascarp
Murray Deep
Guadalupe I.
Gulf of California
ATLANTIC OCEAN
New Orleans
THE BAHAMAS
GULF OF MEXICO
Habana
CUBA
Hispaniola
MEXICO
Veracruz
Mexico City
JAMAICA
BELIZE
CARIBBEAN SEA
GUATEMALA
HONDURAS
EL SALVADOR
NICARAGUA
GUATEMALA TRENCH
COSTA RICA
PANAMA
Colon
G. of Darien
G. of Panama
REVILLA GIGEDO IS
Roca Partida
San Benedicto
Socorro I.
Clarion I. (To Mex.)
Clarion Fracture Zone
Tropic of Cancer
Kanai (To U.S.A.)
OAHU
Molokai
Maui
HAWAII
Clipperton Fracture Zone
Clipperton I. (To France)
ALBATROSS PLATEAU
I. del Coco (To C.R.)
COCOS RIDGE
Malpelo I. (To Col.)
Bogota
COLOMBIA
Fanning I.
Christmas I.
GALAPAGOS
Sta Cruz I.
San Cristobal
I. Isabela (To Ecuador)
Carnegie Ridge
Quito
ECUADOR
Guayaquil
Malden I.
Starbuck I.
Penrhyn (Tongareva)
Vostok I.
Caroline I.
Flint I.
MARQUESAS
Nukuhiva
Hivaoa (To France)
Fatuhiva
SOCIETY IS.
TAHITI
Raiatea
(To France)
King George Is.
Apataki
Disappointment Is.
Pukapuka
Makatea
Mukemo
TUAMOTU ARCHIPELAGO
Tatakoto
Marutea
Hao
Hereheretue
Pinaki
Tureia
Duke of Gloucester Gr.
Mururoa
(To France)
Actaeon Group
Rimatara
Rurutu
Tubuai
Raivavae
TUBUAI IS.
(To France)
Austral Ridge
Rapa
Mangareva
Oeno I.
Henderson I. (To U.K.)
Ducie I.
Pitcairn I.
PERU
Callao
Lima
Milne Edwards Depth 6262 m
Bauer Depth 5292 m
PERU BASIN
SOUTH-EASTERN PACIFIC PLATEAU
EAST PACIFIC RIDGE
Easter I.
Sala y Gomez (To Chile)
S.W. Peru Ridge
PERU-CHILE TRENCH
Arica
Krummel Depth 6880 m
Bartholomew Depth 8066 m
Antofagasta
San Felix
San Ambrosio (to Chile)
Wachusett Shoal
Ernest Legouve Reef
Maria Theresa Reef
JUAN FERNANDEZ
Alejandro Selkirk (To Chile)
Robinson Crusoe
Valparaiso
Haeckel Depth 6081 m
CHILE BASIN
Concepcion
N.W. Chile Ridge
Valdivia
Chiloe
Chonos Archipelago
Wellington I.
Punta Arenas
Pactolus Bank
PACIFIC-ANTARCTIC RIDGE
PACIFIC-ANTARCTIC BASIN
AMUNDSEN SEA
HAWAIIAN ISLANDS (To U.S.A.) 1:3 M.
OAHU
Honolulu
Kaiwi Channel
Molokai
Maui
Lanai
Kahoolawe
HAWAII 1:3 M.
Mauna Kea 4205 m
Mauna Loa 4170 m
Hilo
KAUAI (HAWAII) 1:3 M.
NIIHAU (HAWAII) 1:3 M.
Vava'u Group
Ha'apai Group
Nomuka Group
Tongatapu Group
TONGA 1:3 M.
WESTERN SAMOA 1:3 M.
SAVAI'I
UPOLU
Apia
TAHITI (To France) 1:3 M.
Papeete
Taiarapu Peninsula
EASTER I. 1:750,000 (To Chile)
Hanga Roa
Metres 6000 5000 4000 3000 2000 1000 200 0 200 1000 2000 4000 Metres
Land Depression
Feet 19690 16400 13120 9840 6560 3280 660 0 660 3280 6560 13120 Feet
© John Bartholomew & Son Ltd, Edinburgh

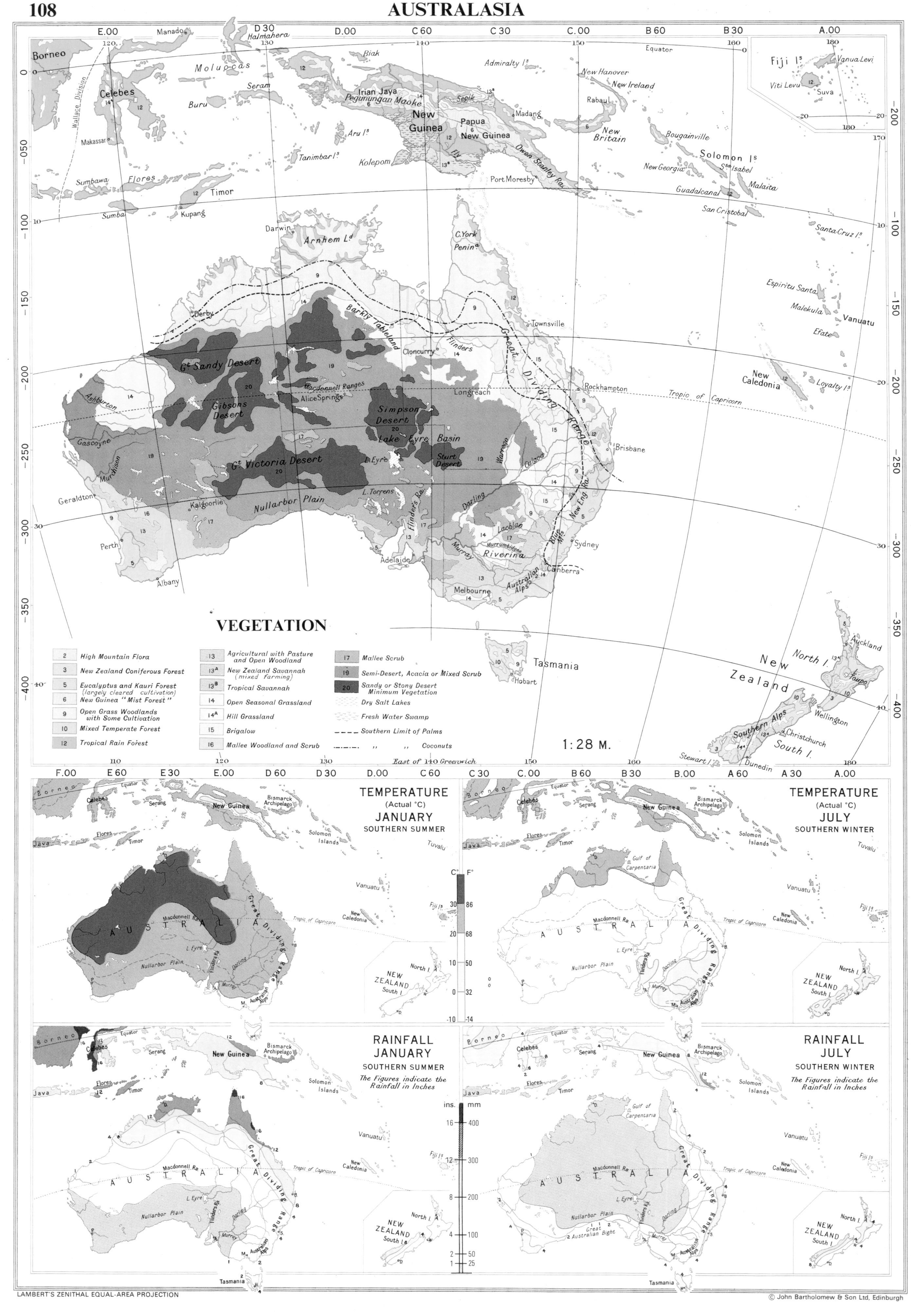

0 200 400 600 800 Statute Miles **1:28M** 0 200 400 600 800 1000 1200 Kilometres

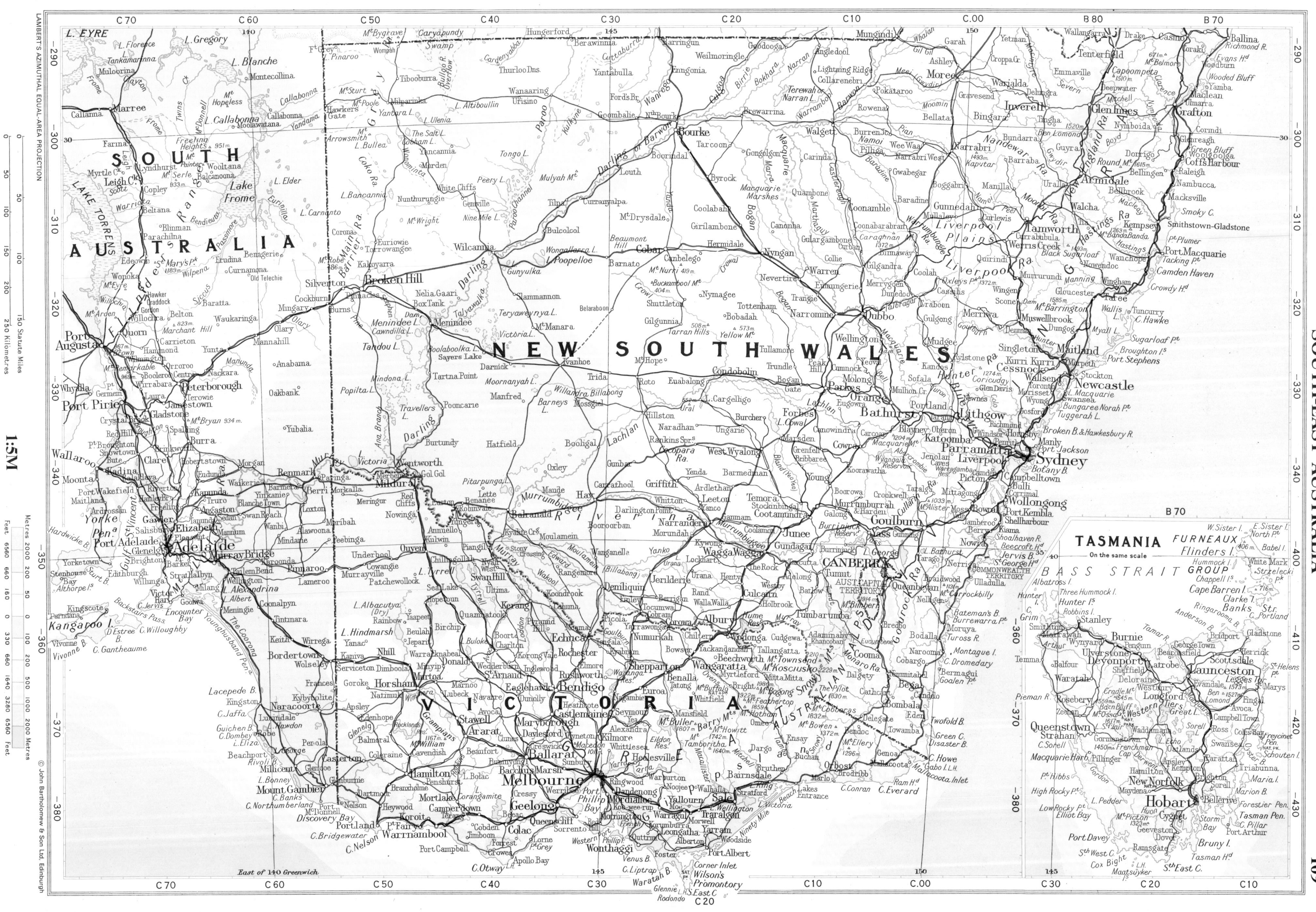
NEW SOUTH WALES
VICTORIA
SOUTH AUSTRALIA
AUSTRALIAN CAPITAL TERRITORY
TASMANIA
On the same scale
BASS STRAIT
FURNEAUX GROUP
LAKE TORRENS
Sydney
Melbourne
Adelaide
Canberra
Hobart
Newcastle
Wollongong
Geelong
Ballarat
Bendigo
Launceston
Broken Hill
LAMBERT'S AZIMUTHAL EQUAL-AREA PROJECTION
© John Bartholomew & Son Ltd. Edinburgh
0 50 100 150 Statute Miles
0 50 100 150 200 250 Kilometres
1:5M
Metres 2000 200 50 0 100 200 500 1000 2000 Metres
Feet 6560 660 160 0 330 660 1640 3280 6560 Feet

FLORES SEA

JAVA

TIMOR SEA

Joseph Bonaparte Gulf

Kimberley Plateau

Great Sandy Desert

Gibson Desert

WESTERN AUSTRALIA

Great Victoria Desert

Nullarbor Plain

Great Australian Bight

Tropic of Capricorn

INDIAN OCEAN

Perth · Fremantle · Geraldton · Carnarvon · Port Hedland · Broome · Derby · Wyndham · Kalgoorlie · Coolgardie · Esperance · Albany · Bunbury · Darwin · Katherine · Kupang · Dili · Denpasar · Surabaya · Semarang · Bandung

POPULATION

Over 500 persons per square mile
,, 50 ,, ,,
,, 5 ,, ,,
Under 5 ,, ,,

Darwin · Townsville · Cloncurry · Alice Springs · Brisbane · Kalgoorlie · Perth · Adelaide · Sydney · Canberra · Melbourne · Hobart

Longitude East 130 of Greenwich

BONNE'S PROJECTION

Main Roads

Railways

Artesian Basins

0 50 100 200 300 400 500 Statute Miles

0 50 100 200 300 400 500 600 700 800 Kilometres

1:12

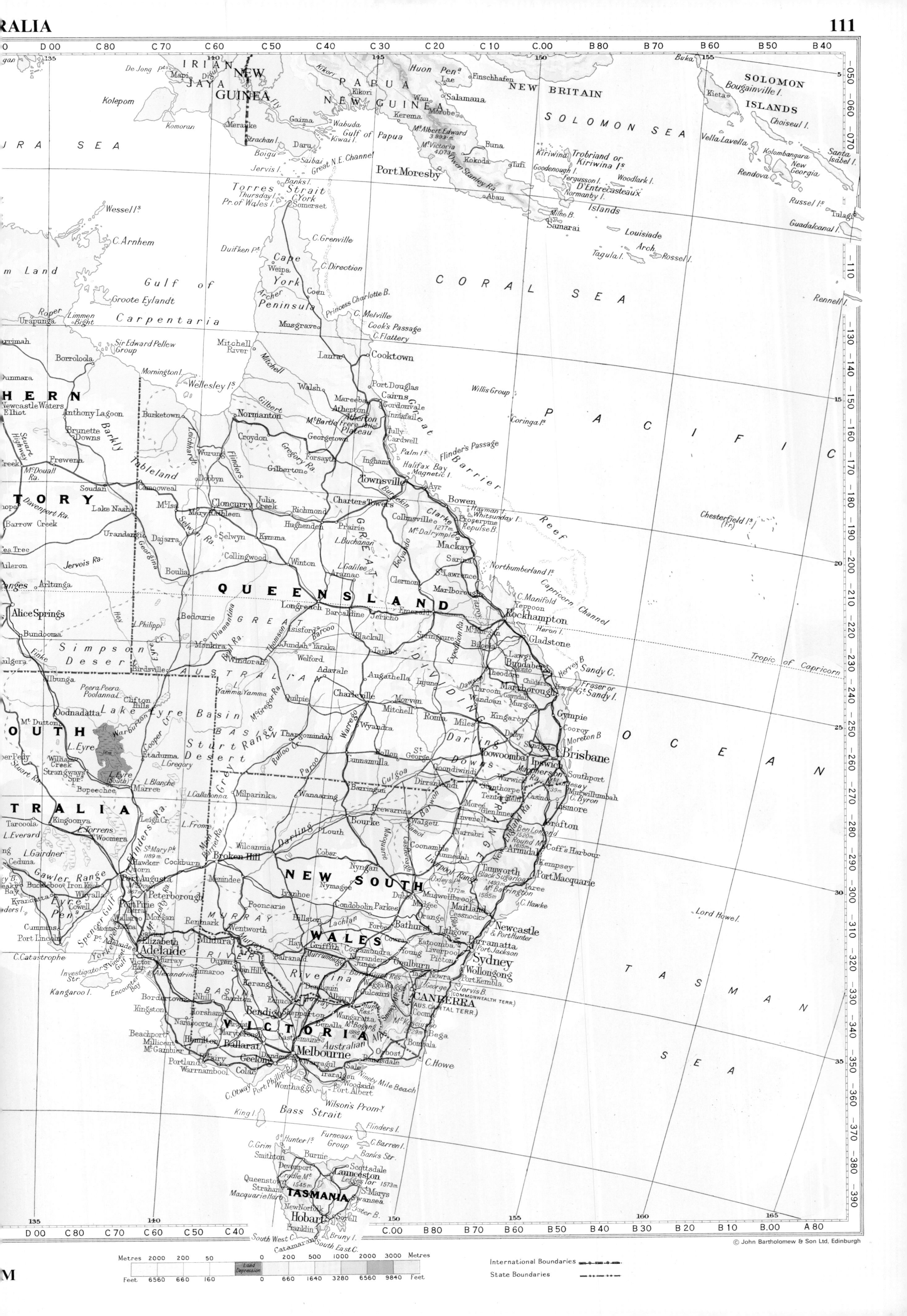
IRIAN JAYA
NEW GUINEA
PAPUA NEW GUINEA
NEW BRITAIN
SOLOMON ISLANDS
Bougainville I.
Choiseul I.
SOLOMON SEA
Port Moresby
Torres Strait
Trobriand or Kiriwina Is
D'Entrecasteaux Islands
Louisiade Arch.
Gulf of Carpentaria
Cape York Peninsula
CORAL SEA
PACIFIC OCEAN
Great Barrier Reef
Tropic of Capricorn
QUEENSLAND
GREAT DIVIDING RANGE
Cooktown
Cairns
Townsville
Mackay
Rockhampton
Gladstone
Bundaberg
Brisbane
Toowoomba
Alice Springs
Simpson Desert
Lake Eyre Basin
Sturt Desert
L. Eyre
SOUTH AUSTRALIA
NEW SOUTH WALES
Broken Hill
Bourke
Tamworth
Newcastle
Sydney
Wollongong
CANBERRA
Adelaide
Port Augusta
Mildura
MURRAY RIVER BASIN
Riverina
VICTORIA
Bendigo
Ballarat
Geelong
Melbourne
Australian Alps
Bass Strait
King I.
Furneaux Group
TASMANIA
Launceston
Hobart
TASMAN SEA
Lord Howe I.
Metres 2000 200 50 0 200 500 1000 2000 3000 Metres
Land Depression
Feet 6560 660 160 0 660 1640 3280 6560 9840 Feet
International Boundaries
State Boundaries
© John Bartholomew & Son Ltd, Edinburgh

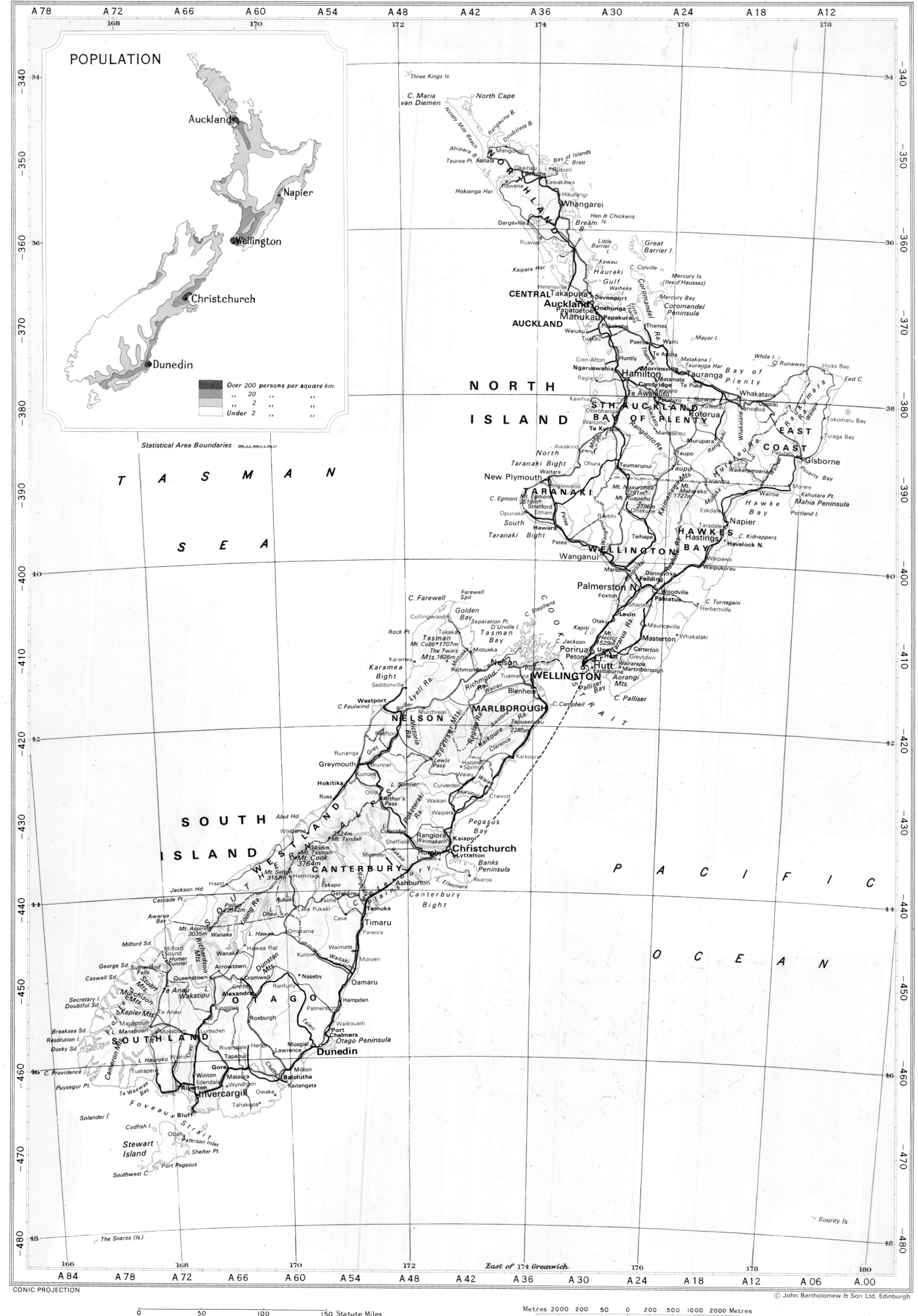

0 50 100 150 Statute Miles

0 50 100 150 200 250 Kilometres

1:5M

Metres 2000 200 50 0 200 500 1000 2000 Metres

Feet 6560 660 160 0 660 1640 3280 6560 Feet

GENERAL INDEX

For explanatory notes on the use of Index see page 1 of Atlas.

LIST OF ABBREVIATIONS

Afghan., Afghanistan.
Afr., Africa.
Ala., Alabama.
Alta., Alberta.
Alg., Algeria.
Antarc., Antarctica.
Arch., Archipelago.
Argent., Argentina.
Ariz., Arizona.
Ark., Arkansas.
Aust., Australia.
B, Bay, Bahia.
B.C., British Columbia.
Belg., Belgium, Belgian.
Bol., Bolivia.
Bots., Botswana.
Bulg., Bulgaria.
C., Cape, Cabo.
Cal., California.
Can., Canal.
Car., Carolina.
Cel., Celebes.
Cent., Central.
Chan., Channel.
Co., County.
Col., Colony.
Colo., Colorado.
Colomb., Colombia.
Conn., Connecticut.
Cord., Cordillera.
Cr., Creek.
Czech., Czechoslovakia.
Del., Delaware.
Den., Denmark.
Dep., Department.
Des., Desert.
Dist., District.
Div., Division.
Dom., Dominican, Dominion.
E., East, Eastern.
Ecua., Ecuador.
Eiln., Eilanden.
Eng., England.
Equat., Equatorial.
Ethio., Ethiopia.
Fd., Fjord.
Fla., Florida.
Fr., French, France.
G., Gulf.
Ga., Georgia.
Geb., Gebirge.
Ger., Germany.
G.F., Goldfield.
Gt., Great.
Guat., Guatemala.
Harb., Harbour.
Hd., Head.
Hisp., Hispaniola.
Hond., Honduras.
Hung., Hungary.
I., Is., Island, Islands.
Ia., Iowa.
Ida., Idaho.
Ill., Illinois.
Ind., Indiana.
Indon., Indonesia.
It., Italian, Italy.
Iv. Cst., Ivory Coast.
Jap., Japan.
Kan., Kansas.
Ky., Kentucky.
L., Lake, Loch, Lough, Lago
La., Louisiana.
Lab., Labrador.
Ld., Land.
Leb., Lebanon.
Lit., Little.
Lith., Lithuania.
Lr., Lower.
Madag., Madagascar.
Man., Manitoba.
Mass., Massachusetts.
Maur., Mauritania.
Md., Maryland.
Me., Maine.
Mex., Mexico.
Mich., Michigan.
Minn., Minnesota.
Miss., Mississippi.
Mo., Missouri.
Mong., Mongolia.
Mont., Montana.
Mozamb., Mozambique.
Mt., Mte., Mount, Mont, Monte.
N., North, Northern, New.
N.B., New Brunswick.
N.C., North Carolina.
N. Dak., North Dakota.
Neb., Nebraska.
Nev., Nevada.
Nfd., Newfoundland.
N.H., New Hampshire.
N.I., Netherlands Indies.
Nic., Nicaragua.
N. Ire., Northern Ireland.
N.J., New Jersey.
N. Mex., New Mexico.
N.S., Nova Scotia.
N.S.W., New South Wales.
N.-W. Terr., North-West Territories.
N.Y., New York.
N.Z., New Zealand.
O., Ohio.
Oc., Ocean.
O.F.S., Orange Free State.
Okla., Oklahoma.
Ont., Ontario.
Ore., Oregon.
Oz., Ozero.
Pa., Pennsylvania.
Pac., Pacific.
Pak., Pakistan.
Pan., Panama.
Para., Paraguay.
P.E.I., Prince Edward Island.
Pen., Peninsula.
Phil., Philippines.
Pk., Peak, Park.
Plat., Plateau.
Port., Portuguese, Portugal.
Prot., Protectorate.
Prov., Province.
Pt., Point.
Pto., Puerto.
Qnsld., Queensland.
Que., Quebec.
R., River, Rio.
Ra., Range.
Reg., Region.
Rep., Republic.
Res., Reservoir.
Rhod., Rhodesia.
R.I., Rhode Island.
Rom., Romania.
Russ., Russia.
S., South, Southern.
Sa., Serra, Sierra.
Sard., Sardinia.
Sask., Saskatchewan.
S.C., South Carolina.
Scot., Scotland.
Sd., Sound.
S. Dak., South Dakota.
Set., Settlement.
Sol., Solomon.
Som., Somaliland.
Sp., Spanish, Spain.
St., Ste., Sta., Saint, Sainte, Santa.
Str., Strait.
Swed., Sweden.
Switz., Switzerland.
Tanz., Tanzania.
Tenn., Tennessee.
Terr., Territory.
Tex., Texas.
Trans., Transvaal.
U.A.E., United Arab Emirates.
Ukr., Ukraine.
Up., Upper.
U.S.A., United State of America.
U.S.S.R., Union of Soviet Socialist Reps.
Ut., Utah.
Va., Virginia.
Val., Valley.
Venez., Venezuela.
Vict., Victoria.
Vol., Volcano.
Vt., Vermont.
W., West, Western.
Wash., Washington.
W.I., West Indies.
Wis., Wisconsin.
Wyo., Wyoming.
Yugosl., Yugoslavia.

Aachen, W. Germany M53+507 48
Aagerbate, Syria K45+350 76
Aalen, W. Germany M30+488 48
Aalsmeer, Netherlands M62+523 44
Aalst (Alost), Belgium M66+509 44
Aalten, Netherlands M51+519 44
Aarau, Switzerland M42+474 45
Aarberg, Switzerland M46+470 45
Aarburg, Switzerland M43+473 45
Aardenburg, Netherlands M69+513 44
Aare, R., Switzerland M44+472 45
Aargau, canton, Switzerland M41+474 45
Aba, Zaire K88+036 83
Abacaxis, Brazil R82-040 104
Abaco I., Gt., Bahamas, The T13+263 101
Abaco I., Lit., Bahamas, The T17+268 101
Abadan, Iran J70+303 74
Abadeh, Iran J44+312 75
Abaete, Brazil R23-016 105
Abajo Mts., Utah V27+378 94
Abajo Pk., Utah V27+376 98
Abakan, U.S.S.R. F83+537 63
Abancay, Peru S78-137 104
Abarqu, Iran J40+311 75
Abashiri, Japan C34+440 68
Abashiri Bay, Japan C32+442 68
Abau, Papua New Guinea C09-102 111
Abaya L., Ethiopia K42+062 83
Abbasabad, Iran J52+366 75
Abbeville, France M79+501 54
Abbeville, Georgia T50+320 97
Abbeville, Louisiana U12+300 95
Abbeyfeale, Ireland, Rep. N56+524 43
Abbeyleix, Ireland, Rep. N44+529 43
Abbot Ice Shelf, Antarctica T80-730 27
Abbottabad, Pakistan H11+342 72
Abdul Aziz, Jebel, Syria K30+365 74
Abdulino, U.S.S.R. J35+537 61
Abeche, Chad L56+138 81
Abeele, Belgium M74+508 44
Abelessa, Algeria M62+226 80
Abengourou, Ivory Coast N22+068 80
Abeokuta, Nigeria M70+072 80
Aberaeron, Wales N26+522 38
Aberdare, Wales N21+517 38
Aberdeen, Mississippi T81+338 97
Aberdeen, Montana V14+450 93
Aberdeen, S. Dakota U51+455 93
Aberdeen, Washington W23+470 92
Aberdeen, Scotland N12+571 40
Aberdeen L., N.-W. Terr. U55+645 88
Aberfeldy, Scotland N23+566 41
Aberfoyle, Scotland N26+562 41
Abergavenny, Wales N18+518 38
Aberystwyth, Wales N24+524 38
Abha, Saudi Arabia K12+181 74
Abidjan, Benin N24+054 80
Ab-i-Istada L., Afghanistan H42+325 75
Abilene, Kansas U44+389 95
Abilene, Texas U58+324 95
Abingdon, Virginia T42+367 97
Abington, Massachusetts S65+421 96
Abisko, Sweden L66+683 46
Abitibi L., Ontario T28+488 89
Abitibi R., Ontario T40+500 89
Abomey, Benin M78+072 80
Aboyne, Scotland N17+571 40
Abqaiq, Saudi Arabia J61+262 74
Abrantes, Portugal N49+395 52
Abrets, les, France M57+456 54
Abrud, Romania L42+469 58
Abruzzi, dep., Italy M07+420 56
Abtenau, Austria M10+475 48
Abu, India H14+246 70
Abu Deleiq, Sudan K68+158 81
Abu Dhabi, U.A.E. J33+245 75
Abu ed Duhur, Syria K48+357 76
Abu el Jirdhan, Jordan K55+303 76
Abu Jifan, Saudi Arabia J73+246 74
Abu Kemal, Syria K24+345 74
Abul Abyadh I., U.A.E. J38+243 75
Abu Mombasi, Zaire L46+034 82
Abuna, Brazil S32-098 104
Abu Qurqas, Egypt K86+278 81
Abuya Myeda, mt., Ethiopia K30+106 83
Abu Zabad, Sudan L04+122 81
Abyei, Sudan L08+096 81
Abyy, U.S.S.R. C30+685 63
Åbyn, Sweden L52+650 46
Acajutla, El Salvador T88+136 101
Acambaro, Mexico U64+200 100
Acaponeta, Mexico V02+225 100
Acapulco, Mexico U59+168 100
Acara & R., Brazil R20-022 105
Acarigua, Venezuela S55+095 104
Acatlan, Mexico U49+182 100
Accomac, Virginia T04+377 97
Accra, Ghana N02+056 80
Accrington, England N14+538 37
Achaguas, Venezuela S49+075 104
Achao, Chile S81-424 103
Achill & I., Ireland, Rep. N60+539 42
Achinsk, U.S.S.R. F86+564 63
Achray, Ontario T17+459 91
Acklins, I., Bahamas, The S84+225 101
Aconcagua, mt., Argentina S60-325 103
Acores, Is., Atlantic Ocean P70+390 80
Acoyapa, Nicaragua T61+120 101
Acre & B., Israel K60+329 76
Actaeon Group, Tuamotu Archipelago X05-228 107
Acton Vale, Quebec S75+457 91
Ada, Minnesota U39+473 93
Ada, Oklahoma U40+348 95
Adair, C., N.-W. Territories S68+713 89
Adairville, Kentucky T71+367 97
Adak, I., Aleutian Is. Z70+514 99
Adalia. See Antalya
Adam, Oman J15+223 75
Adama, Ethiopia K34+084 83
Adamello, mt., Italy M27+462 56
Adammaby, New S. Wales C08-360 109
Adams, New York T06+438 91
Adam's Bridge, India-Sri Lanka G63+091 70
Adams, Mt., Washington W09+462 92
Adams, Pk., Sri Lanka G58+069 70
Adana, Turkey K58+370 74
Ada-Pazari, Turkey K88+408 74
Adare, Ireland, Rep. N53+525 43
Adare, C., Antarctica A55-710 27
Addis Ababa, Ethiopia K38+090 83
Addis Derra, Ethiopia K38+102 83
Addison, New York T13+421 96
Adelaer, C., Greenland Q65+610 26
Adelaide, Cape Province L22-328 84
Adelaide, S. Australia C69-350 109
Adelaide, I., Antarctica S50-670 27
Adelaide Pen., N.-W. Terr. U45+674 88
Adelboden, Switzerland M45+465 45
Adelie Ld., Antarctica C60-680 27
Adelong, New South Wales C12-354 109
Ademuz, Spain N08+401 53
Aden, Yemen, South K00+127 74
Aden, G. of, Africa-Arabia J60+130 30
Adh Dhahiriya, Jordan K60+314 76
Adhoi, India H27+234 70
Adhra, Syria K51+336 76
Adi, I., New Guinea D08-042 65
Adi Kaie, Ethiopia K34+146 83
Adilabad, India G67+197 70
Adirondack Mts., New York S84+444 91
Adi Ugri, Ethiopia K38+148 83
Admiralty G., W. Australia D54-142 110
Admiralty Is., Pacific Ocean C15-023 106
Adolfo Alsina, Argentina S16-371 103
Adoni, India G76+156 70
Adoumre, Cameroon M08+092 81
Adour R., France N08+434 55
Adra, Spain N19+367 52
Adraj, Saudi Arabia J55+201 75
Adrano, Sicily M01+376 57
Adrar, Algeria N02+276 80
Adria, Italy M18+451 56
Adrian, Michigan T55+419 91
Adriatic Sea, Italy L84+425 56
Aduwa, Ethiopia K36+140 83
Aegean Sea, Greece L30+385 59
Aegina, I., Greece L39+377 59
Aeltre, Belgium M69+511 44
Ærøskøbing, Denmark M27+549 47
Aerschot, Belgium M61+510 44
Aesch, Switzerland M44+475 45
Afferden, Netherlands M54+516 44
Affua, Brazil R31-004 105
Afghanistan, Asia H60+340 75
Afif, Saudi Arabia K12+239 74
Afogados de Ingazeira, Brazil Q46-078 105
Afognak I., Alaska Y20+582 99
Afrin, Syria K49+365 76
Afula, Israel K58+326 76
Afyon, Turkey K87+387 74
Agab Workei, Ethiopia K48+136 83
Agadès, Niger M42+168 80
Agadir, Morocco N58+304 80
Agartala, India F82+239 71
Agathla Pk., Arizona V32+368 94
Agattu, I., Aleutian Is. A40+518 99
Agawa, Ontario T57+476 91
Agde, France M69+433 55
Agen, France M86+442 55
Aghda, Iran J38+325 75
Agiabampo, Mexico V25+264 100
Agira, Sicily M03+376 57
Agno, Switzerland M37+460 45
Agordat, Ethiopia K42+154 83
Agra, India G72+272 73
Agram. See Zagreb
Agrigento, Sicily M08+373 57
Agrihan, I., Mariana Is. C25+180 106
Agrinion, Greece L52+387 59
Agropoli, Italy M00+404 57
Agua Clara, Brazil R47-204 105
Aguadas, Colombia T03+056 104
Aguadilla, Puerto Rico S42+185 101
Aguadulce, Panama T33+082 101
Agua Limpa, Brazil R26-042 105
Agua Prieta, Mexico V27+312 100
Aguaray, Argentina S22-222 103
Aguascalientes, Mexico U74+218 100
Agudo, Spain N29+390 52
Agudos, Brazil R24-224 105
Aguilar, Spain N28+375 52
Aguilar de Campôs, Spain N26+428 52
Aguilas, Spain N10+374 53
Aguirre, B., Argentina S35-550 103
Agulhas C., Cape Province L60-348 84
Agusta, W. Australia E29-340 110
Ahar, Iran J77+385 74
Ahmadnegar, India H01+191 70
Ahmadpur East, Pakistan H23+291 72
Ahmadabad, India H14+230 70
Ahraura, India G42+250 73
Ahtopol, Bulgaria L13+421 58
Ahuachapan, El Salvador T89+140 101
Ahualulco, Mexico U85+207 100
Ahus, Sweden M04+559 47
Ahvaz, Iran J67+313 74
Ahvenanmaa, Finland L60+603 47
Ahwar, Yemen, South J80+135 74
Aigle, Switzerland M48+463 45
Aihunkiu, China D45+489 64
Aijal, India F73+239 71
Aikawa, Japan C71+380 68
Ailsa Craig, I., Scotland N31+552 41
Aim, U.S.S.R. D06+588 63
Ain, dep., France M56+461 54
Ain Gallaka, Chad L70+180 81
Ain Safra, Mauritania N72+194 80
Ainsworth, Nebraska U60+426 95
Aintree, England N18+535 37
Aira, Ethiopia K58+090 83
Airdrie, Scotland N24+558 41
Aire, France N02+437 55
Aire R., England N07+537 37
Airolo, Switzerland M38+465 45
Aishihik L., Yukon X12+612 88
Aisne, dep., France M68+495 54
Aitkin, Minnesota U22+465 93
Aiun, El, Morocco N80+270 80
Aix, France M57+435 55
Aix, Mt., Washington W07+469 92
Aix-la-Chapelle. See Aachen
Aiyina, I., Greece L39+377 59
Aiyion, Greece L48+383 59
Aizpute, Latvia L50+567 47
Aizuwakamatsu, Japan C60+375 68
Ajaccio & G. d', Corsica M38+419 57
Ajaigarh, India G58+249 73
Ajanta, India G85+205 70
Ajanta Ra. See Sahiadriparvat
Ajibba, Saudi Arabia K04+273 74
Ajigasawa, Japan C58+408 68
Ajlun, Jordan K56+323 76
Ajmer, India H02+263 70
Ajodhya, (Ayodhya), India G46+267 73
Ajoewa, Surinam R72+026 105
Akalkot, India G83+176 70
Akan Nat. Park, Japan C36+435 68
Akanthou, Cyprus K67+354 76
Akaoka, Japan D08+335 68
Akarnania and Aitolia, Greece L51+388 59
Akaroa, New Zealand A42-437 112
Akashi, Japan D00+347 68
Akbarpur, India G60+263 73
Akcha, Afghanistan H53+369 75
Akhdhar, Jebel, Oman J14+232 75
Akhisar, Turkey L13+389 74
Akhterine, Syria K46+365 76
Akhtyrka, Ukraine K61+504 60
Akimiski I., N.-W. Terr. T38+532 89
Akita, Japan C59+397 68
Akkrum, Netherlands M55+530 44
Aklavik, N.-W. Territories W86+689 88
Ako, Nigeria M26+104 82
Akola, India G77+207 70
Akpatok I., North-West Territories S49+603 89
Akra, Jebel el, Turkey K54+359 74
Akron, Colorado U80+402 94
Akron, Ohio T39+411 91
Akrotiri Pen., Crete L35+356 59
Aksaray, Turkey K66+383 74
Aksehir, Turkey K82+383 74

Aksha, *U.S.S.R.* E40+503 **63**
Aksı, *Estonia* L20+585 **47**
Akti, *Greece* L35+403 **59**
Aktyubinsk, *Kazakh.* J17+504 **62**
Akure, *Nigeria* M58+072 **80**
Akureyri, *Iceland* P19+657 **46**
Akyab, *Burma* F73+202 **71**
Alabama, state, *U.S.A.* T70+326 **99**
Alabama R., *Alabama* T74+313 **99**
Alaejos, *Spain* N31+413 **52**
Alagoa de Baixo, *Brazil* Q44–082 **105**
Alagoas, *Brazil* Q35–096 **105**
Alagoinhas, *Brazil* Q50–122 **105**
Alagon, *Spain* N07+417 **53**
Alaja, *Syria* K55+358 **76**
Alajuela, *Costa Rica* T55+100 **101**
Alakurtii, *U.S.S.R.* K85+672 **62**
Alakpa, *Nigeria* M64+086 **82**
Al' Ala, *Saudi Arabia* K41+267 **74**
Alameda, *California* W14+377 **92**
Alameda, *Saskatchewan* U74+496 **88**
Alamogordo, *New Mexico* V06+330 **94**
Alamogorda Res., *New Mex.* U87+346 **94**
Alamos, *Mexico* V24+271 **100**
Alamosa, *Colorado* V06+374 **94**
Åland, *See* Ahvenanmeri
Ålands Hav, *Sweden-Finland* L64+600 **47**
Alapaevsk, *U.S.S.R.* H80+578 **61**
Alasehir, *Turkey* L09+384 **74**
Ala Shan, *China* F10+394 **64**
Al Ashkharah, *Oman* J03+219 **75**
Alaska, state, *U.S.A.* Y00+630 **99**
Alaska, G. of, *Alaska* X60+586 **99**
Alaska Pen., *Alaska* Y60+560 **99**
Alaska Ra., *Alaska* Y25+610 **99**
Alaska Highway, *Alaska-Can.* X38+632 **88**
Alatyr, *U.S.S.R.* J80+548 **61**
Alavus, *Finland* L38+626 **46**
Alawoona, *S. Australia* C57–348 **109**
Al 'Ayn, *Oman* J31+196 **75**
Alaysky Khrebet, *Kirgiz* H20+400 **62**
Alazeiskoye Plat., *U.S.S.R.* C10+680 **63**
Albacete, *Spain* N11+390 **53**
Alba de Tormes, *Spain* N33+408 **52**
Albaida, *Spain* N03+389 **53**
Alba Iulia, *Romania* L39+461 **58**
Albanel L., *Quebec* S78+511 **90**
Albania, *S. Europe* L60+410 **51**
Albany, *Alabama* T70+342 **99**
Albany, *Georgia* T55+315 **97**
Albany, *Kentucky* T61+367 **97**
Albany, *Missouri* U26+403 **95**
Albany, *New York* S83+426 **91**
Albany, *Oregon* W19+446 **92**
Albany, *W. Australia* E13–350 **110**
Albany R., *Ontario* T52+514 **89**
Albarracin, *Spain* N09+405 **53**
Al Bayda', *Libya* L49+326 **81**
Albemarle Sd., *N. Carolina* T08+360 **97**
Albergaria a-Velha, *Portugal* N50+407 **52**
Alberique, *Spain* N03+391 **53**
Albert, *New Brunswick* S28+457 **90**
Albert L., *Zaire* K86+014 **83**
Albert, Mt., *Quebec* S37+489 **90**
Alberta, prov., *Canada* - **88**
Alberta Mt., *Alberta* V75+526 **88**
Albert Edward, Mt., *Papua New Guinea* C18–084 **111**
Albert Lea, *Minnesota* U20+437 **93**
Alberton, *Prince Edward I.* S24+468 **90**
Alberton, *Victoria* C20–386 **109**
Albertville, *France* M52+457 **54**
Albi, *France* M77+439 **55**
Albia, *Iowa* U17+410 **95**
Albina, *Surinam* R56+054 **105**
Albion, *Michigan* T59+423 **91**
Albion, *New York* T19+432 **91**
Albocácer, *Spain* N00+403 **53**
Alborg, *Denmark* M30+570 **47**
Albufeira, *Portugal* N49+371 **52**
Albufera de Mexcaltitlan, *Mex.* V04+220 **100**
Albuñol, *Spain* N19+368 **52**
Albuquerque, *New Mexico* V10+350 **94**
Alburquerque, *Spain* N42+392 **52**
Albury, *New South Wales* C19–360 **109**
Alcacer do Sal, *Portugal,* N51+384 **52**
Alcala de Chisvert, *Spain* M99+403 **53**
Alcala de Henares, *Spain* N20+405 **52**
Alcamo, *Sicily* M12+380 **57**
Alcañices, *Spain* N38+417 **52**
Alcañiz, *Spain* N01+410 **53**
Alcantara, *Brazil* Q87–024 **105**
Alcantara, *Spain* N41+397 **52**
Alcantarilla, *Spain* N07+380 **53**
Alcaraz, *Spain* N15+387 **53**
Alcázar de San Juan, *Spain* N19+394 **52**
Alcazarquivir, (Ksar-el-Kebir,) *Morocco* N36+350 **80**
Alcira, *Spain* N03+391 **53**
Alcobaca, *Portugal* N54+395 **52**
Alcolea del Pinar, *Spain* N15+410 **53**
Alcoutim, *Portugal* N45+375 **52**
Alcoy, *Spain* N03+387 **53**
Aldabra Is., *Indian Ocean* J76–093 **77**
Aldama, *Chihuahua, Mexico* V06+288 **100**
Aldama, *Tamaulipas, Mexico* U49+229 **100**
Aldan & R., *U.S.S.R.* D58+588 **63**
Aldeburgh, *England* M80+522 **39**
Aldeia Cumare, *Brazil* R34–109 **105**
Alderney, I., *Channel Is.* N13+497 **54**
Aldershot, *England* N05+512 **39**
Al Dola, *Yemen, South* J85 + 146 **74**
Aledo, *Illinois* U04+412 **95**
Alegrete, *Brazil* R65–298 **103**
Aleih, *Lebanon* K56+338 **76**
Alejandro Selkirk, I., *Chile* T35–338 **107**
Aleksandrov, *U.S.S.R.* K38+564 **60**
Aleksandrovsk Sakhalinskiy, *U.S.S.R.* C46+510 **63**
Aleksandry Zemlya, *Arctic Oc.* K00+808 **62**
Alekseyeka, *Kazakh.* H25+520 **62**
Alemquer, *Brazil* R59–019 **105**
Alençon, *France* M89+484 **54**
Alenquer, *Portugal* N54+390 **52**
Aleppo, *Syria* K47+362 **76**
Ales, *France* M65+441 **55**
Aleshki, *U.S.S.R.* K19+516 **61**
Alessandria, *Italy* M38+449 **56**
Ålesund, *Norway* M53+625 **46**
Aletschhorn, mt., *Switzerland* M42+465 **45**
Aleutian Is., *Bering Sea* A00+512 **99**
Aleutian Ra., *Alaska* Y40+580 **26**
Alexander Arch., *Alaska* X05+575 **99**
Alexander I., *Antarctica* S60–700 **27**
Alexandra, *New Zealand* A63–452 **112**
Alexandra, *Victoria* C26–372 **109**
Alexandretta. *See* Iskenderun
Alexandria, *Egypt* L00+310 **81**
Alexandria, *Louisiana* U14+312 **95**
Alexandria, *Minnesota* U32+459 **93**
Alexandria, *Ontario* S88+453 **91**
Alexandria, *Virginia* T13+388 **96**
Alexandrina, L., *S. Aust.* C65–355 **109**
Alexandroúpolis, *Greece* L25+408 **59**
Alexveeka, *U.S.S.R.* J82+522 **61**
Aleysk, *U.S.S.R.* G44+525 **62**
Al Falluja, *Iraq* K07+334 **74**
Alfaro, *Spain* N11+422 **53**
Alfred, *Maine* S64+435 **96**
Alfredo Chaves, *Brazil* R40–290 **103**
Alga, *Kazakh* J16+498 **62**
Ålgård, *Norway* M55+588 **47**
Algauer Alpen, *Austria, etc.* M29+474 **48**
Algeciras, *Spain* N33+361 **52**
Algeria, *N.-W. Africa* M70+280 **80**
Al Ghail, *Yemen* K00+161 **74**
Alghero, *Sardinia* M40+405 **57**
Algiers (El Djezair), *Algeria* M72+366 **55**
Algoa B., *Cape Province* L24–338 **84**
Algoma, *Ontario* T47+462 **91**
Algoma, *Wisconsin* T75+446 **91**
Algona, *Iowa* U26+430 **95**
Algonquin Park, *Ontario* T22+456 **91**
Alguada Reef, *Burma* F65+158 **71**
Alhama de Granada, *Spain* N24+370 **52**
Al Harsha, *Saudi Arabia* J52+196 **75**
Al Hauta, *Yemen, South* J70 + 159 **74**
Al Hillah, *Iraq* K03+325 **74**
Alia, *Sicily* M08+378 **57**
Aliabad, *Iran* J50+366 **75**
Aliaga, *Spain* N04+407 **53**
Alibag, *India* H13+187 **70**
Alicante, *Spain* N03+384 **53**
Alice, *Texas* U48+278 **94**
Alice Springs, *N. Terr., Aust.* D06–237 **111**
Aliceville, *Alabama* T80+331 **95**
Alicudi, I., *Italy* M04+386 **57**
Aliganj, *India* G65+275 **73**
Aligarh, *India* G73+278 **72**
Ali Khel, *Afghanistan* H32+340 **75**
Alimnia, I., *Greece* L13+363 **59**
Aling Kangri, *Tibet* G55+328 **70**
Alingsås, *Sweden* M15+579 **47**
Alipur Duar, *India* G02+265 **73**
Alipur, *Pakistan* H24+294 **72**
Alipura, *India* G64+252 **73**
Alirajpur, *India* H03+222 **70**
Alivérion, *Greece* L36+385 **59**
Al Jesab, *Saudi Arabia* J86+150 **74**
Aljustrel, *Portugal* N49+379 **52**
Alken, *Belgium* M58+509 **44**
Al Khubba, *Saudi Arabia* J45+222 **75**
Alkmar, *Netherlands* M61+526 **44**
Allahabad, *India* G49+254 **73**
Allanmyo, *Burma* F58+194 **71**
Allard, *Montana* U88+470 **93**
Allariz, *Spain* N47+422 **52**
Allata, *Ethiopia* K38+066 **83**
Allaykha, *U.S.S.R.* C15+708 **63**
Alle, *Belgium* M60+498 **44**
Allegan, *Michigan* T65+426 **91**
Allegheny Mts., *U.S.A.* T41+370 **99**
Allegheny R., *Penn., etc.* T23+420 **96**
Allen, Bog of, *Ireland, Rep.* N43+534 **43**
Allen L., *Ireland, Rep.* N48+541 **42**
Allenby Bridge, *Jordan* K57+319 **76**
Allende, *Mexico* V03+268 **100**
Allentown, *Pennsylvania* T03+406 **96**
Alleppey, *India* G82+096 **70**
Alliance, *Nebraska* U77+422 **94**
Alliance, *Ohio* T37+409 **91**
Allier, dep. *France* M73+464 **54**
Allier, R., *France* M69+453 **54**
Alliston, *Ontario* T29+442 **91**
Alloa, *Scotland* N23+561 **41**
All Pines, *Belize* T80+168 **101**
Allumette I., *Quebec* T12+458 **91**
Alma, *Michigan* T58+434 **91**
Alma, *New Brunswick* S29+456 **90**
Alma Ata, *Kazakh.* G78+431 **62**
Almaden, *Spain* N29+388 **52**
Almagro, *Spain* N22+389 **52**
Almansa, *Spain* N07+389 **53**
Al Mat, *Iraq.* K28+330 **74**
Almazán, *Spain* N15+415 **53**
Almeirim, *Brazil* R45–015 **105**
Almeirim, *Portugal* N52+392 **52**
Almelo, *Netherlands* M50+524 **44**
Almeria & Gulf, *Spain* N09+369 **53**
Al'met'yevsk, *U.S.S.R.* J60+547 **61**
Almirante, *Panama* T44+094 **101**
Almiropótamos, *Greece* L35+383 **59**
Almiros, *Greece* L43+392 **59**
Almodôvar, *Portugal* N48+375 **52**
Almodóvar, *Spain* N25+388 **52**
Almond R., *Scotland* N21+564 **41**
Almont, *N. Dakota* U69+467 **93**
Almonte, *Ontario* T07+452 **91**
Almora, *India* G62+296 **73**
Almorox, *Spain* N26+402 **52**
Almudebar, *Spain* N04+421 **53**
Almunia de Doña Godina, la, *Spain* N08+415 **53**
Al Musayyib, *Iraq* K04+329 **74**
Al Muwaila, *Saudi Arabia* K57+277 **74**
Alness, *Scotland* N26+577 **40**
Alnwick, *England* N10+554 **37**
Alocén, *Spain* N17+405 **53**
Aloja, *Latvia* L31+578 **47**
Alon, *Burma* F59+221 **71**
Alón. *See* Iliodhrómia, I.
Alor, I., *Indonesia* D60–084 **65**
Alora, *Spain* N28+368 **52**
Alor Setar, *Malaysia* F28+062 **69**
Alost, *Belgium* M66+509 **44**
Aloysius, Mt., *W. Australia* D43–260 **110**
Alpena, *Michigan* T51+451 **91**
Alpes-Maritimes, dep., *Fr.* M48+438 **55**
Alphen, *Netherlands* M62+521 **44**
Alpine, *Texas* U83+304 **98**
Alps, mts., *Cent. Europe* M42+460 **50**
Al Qatrun, *Libya* M02+250 **81**
Al Qayyara, *Iraq* K11+359 **74**
Al Qunfidhah, *Saudi Arabia* K23+192 **74**
Al Qurnah, *Iraq* J75+310 **74**
Als, I., *Denmark* M30+549 **47**
Al Selaïl, *Saudi Arabia* K00+194 **74**
Alsten, *Norway* M15+660 **46**
Alston, *England* N15+548 **37**
Alsunga, *Latvia* L51+570 **47**
Alta Gracia, *Argentina* S26–316 **103**
Altagracia, *Venezuela* S69+107 **104**
Altagracia de Orituco, *Venez.* S38+099 **104**
Altai, Mts., *Central Asia* G20+505 **62**
Altamachi, *Bolivia* S38–167 **104**
Altamaha R., *Georgia* T43+318 **99**
Altamira, *Brazil* R44–032 **105**
Altamura, *Italy* L80+408 **57**
Altan Bulag, *Mongolia* E81+503 **63**
Altar, *Mexico* V40+307 **100**
Altata, *Mexico* V18+246 **100**
Altdorf, *Switzerland* M38+469 **45**
Altea, *Spain* N00+386 **53**
Altenburg, *E. Germany* M16+510 **48**
Altin Kopru, *Iraq* K05+358 **74**
Altmark, *E. Germany* M21+527 **48**
Alto Molocue, *Mozambique* K44-156 **83**
Alton, *Illinois* U01+390 **95**
Alton, *Missouri* U09+367 **97**
Altona, *Germany* M30+535 **48**
Altona, *New York* S82+449 **91**
Altoona, *Pennsylvania* T21+405 **96**
Altrincham, *England* N14+534 **37**
Alstätten, *Switzerland* M33+474 **45**
Alturas, *California* W03+415 **92**
Altus, *Oklahoma* U56+346 **95**
Altyn Tagh, *China* G30+380 **30**
Al Ugla, *Saudi Arabia* K43+258 **74**
Al 'Uj, *Saudi Arabia* J66+228 **74**
Alūksne, *Latvia* L18+574 **47**
Alula, *Somalia* J56+118 **83**
Alumine, *Argentina* S66–392 **103**
Alupka, *U.S.S.R.* K65+444 **60**
Alushta, *U.S.S.R.* K63+446 **60**
Alva, *Oklahoma* U52+368 **95**
Alvarado, *Mexico* U35+188 **100**
Alvear, *Argentina* S22–352 **103**
Ålvesta, *Sweden* M03+569 **47**
Alvho, *Sweden* M01+615 **47**
Alvin, *Texas* U32+294 **95**
Alvito, *Portugal* N48+383 **52**
Alvord, L., *Oregon* V82+424 **92**
Alwar, *India* G81+275 **72**
Alward, *New Brunswick* S33+462 **90**
Alyab, *Sudan* K68+172 **81**
Alyth, *Scotland* N19+566 **41**
Alytus, *Lithuania* L36+544 **47**
Amadeus L., *N. Terr., Aust.* D25–246 **110**
Amadi, *Sudan* K88+056 **81**
Amadiyah, *Iraq* K10+371 **74**
Amadjuak, *N.-W. Territories* S75+641 **89**
Amadjuak L., *N.-W. Terr.* S65+648 **89**
Amakusa Nada, *Japan* D32+325 **68**
Amål, *Sweden* M14+591 **47**
Amalfi, *Italy* M03+407 **57**
Amalias, *Greece* L52+378 **59**
Amami Gunto, *Japan* D34+283 **68**
Amanalco, *Mexico* U60+192 **100**
Amantea, *Italy* L84+392 **57**
Amapa, *Brazil* R34+020 **105**
Amapala, *Honduras* T76+133 **101**
Amarah, *Iraq* J77+320 **74**
Amarante, *Brazil* Q77–063 **105**
Amarapura, *Burma* F53+218 **71**
Amaravti, *India* G73+210 **70**
Amargosa, *Brazil* Q59–130 **105**
Amarillo, *Texas* U68+352 **94**
Amarracão, *Brazil* Q70–030 **105**
Amasra, *Turkey* K74+418 **74**
Amasya, *Turkey* K55+406 **74**
Amatique, G. de, *Guatemala* T82+160 **100**
Amatitlan, *Guatemala* U04+145 **100**
Amazon, Mths. of the, *Brazil* R30+006 **105**
Amazonas, R., *Brazil* R53–020 **105**
Amb, *Pakistan* H12+343 **72**
Ambala, *India* G79+304 **72**
Ambam, *Cameroon* M22+024 **82**
Ambar, *Iran* J06+318 **75**
Ambarchik, *U.S.S.R.* B15+697 **63**
Ambato, *Ecuador* T22–013 **104**
Ambato Boéni, *Madagascar* J80–164 **83**
Amberg, *Germany* M18+494 **48**
Ambergris Cay, *Bahamas, The* S70 + 212 **101**
Ambergris Cay, *Belize* T78+180 **101**
Ambérieu, *France* M58+460 **54**
Ambert, *France* M68+455 **54**
Ambikapur, *India* G41+231 **73**
Ambilobe, *Madagascar* J66–132 **83**
Ambleside, *England* N18+544 **37**
Amblève, *Belgium* M53+504 **44**
Ambohimahasoa, *Madagascar* J78–212 **83**
Ambon, I., *Indonesia* D41–037 **65**
Ambositra, *Madagascar* J76–206 **83**
Ambrim, I., *Vanuatu* A67+169 **106**
Ambriz, *Angola* M10–080 **82**
Ambrizete, *Angola* M12–074 **82**
Amchitka, I., *Aleutian Is.* A05+508 **99**
Amd, *Yemen, South* J72 + 154 **74**
Amderma, *U.S.S.R.* H82+698 **62**
Ameca, *Mexico* U85+205 **100**
Ameland I., *Netherlands* M55+534 **44**
Amelia, *Italy* M16+426 **56**
Amelia, *Virginia* T18+374 **97**
American Falls, *Utah* V47+428 **94**
American Fork, *Utah* V41+404 **94**
Americus, *Georgia* T56+320 **99**
Amerongen, *Netherlands* M57+520 **44**
Amersfoort, *Netherlands* M58+522 **44**
Amersham, *England* N04+517 **39**
Ames, *Iowa* U22+420 **95**
Amesbury, *Massachusetts* S65+429 **96**
Amethi, *India* G49+262 **73**
Amfiklia, *Greece* L44+387 **59**
Amfilokhia, *Greece* L53+389 **59**
Amga & R., *U.S.S.R.* D18+610 **63**
Amgu, *U.S.S.R.* C74+457 **63**
Amherst, *Burma* F45+160 **71**
Amherst, *Massachusetts* S75+424 **96**
Amherst, *Nova Scotia* S25+458 **90**
Amherst I., *Ontario* T10+441 **91**
Amherstburg, *Ontario* T49+422 **91**
Amiens, *France* M76+499 **54**
Amik Lake, *Ontario* T28+456 **91**
Amindivi I., *Indian Oc.* H14+110 **70**
Amingaon, *India* F79+263 **71**
Aminuis, *Namibia* L64+236 **84**
Amirante Is., *Indian Ocean* J40–060 **77**
Amla, *Saudi Arabia* K11+206 **74**
Amlah, *Saudi Arabia* J89+173 **74**
Amlwch, *Wales* N26+534 **38**
Amm Adam, *Sudan* K54+164 **81**
Amman, *Jordan* K54+319 **76**
Ammanford, *Wales* N24+518 **38**
Amol, *Iran* J46+364 **75**
Amorgós, I., *Greece* L24+372 **59**
Amos, *Quebec* T18+488 **89**
Amoy. *See* Hsiamen.
Amparo, *Brazil* R10–225 **105**
Amqui, *Quebec* S44+485 **90**
Amraho, *Sudan* K78+186 **81**
Amran, *Yemen* K06+157 **74**
Amreli, *India* H23+214 **70**
Amriswil, *Switzerland* M34+475 **45**
Amritsar, *India* H01+316 **72**
Amroha, *India* G69+289 **73**
Amstelveen, *Netherlands* M61+523 **44**
Amsterdam, *Netherlands* M60+524 **44**
Amsterdam, *New York* S85+429 **96**
Amsterdam, I., *Indian Ocean* G75–380 **77**
Am Timan, *Chad* L60+110 **81**
Amu Darya, *Turkmen* H75+400 **62**
Amund Ringnes I., *North-West Territories* U45+782 **88**
Amundsen G., *N.-W. Terr.* W10+706 **88**
Amundsen Sea, *Antarctica* V20–720 **27**
Amur, R., *U.S.S.R. - China* D60+528 **63**
Amyun, *Lebanon* K55+343 **76**
An, *Burma* F66+198 **71**
Anabama, *S. Australia* C59–328 **109**
Anabta, *Jordan* K59+323 **76**
Anaconda, *Montana* V48+461 **92**
Anadarko, *Oklahoma* U48+350 **95**
Anadyr & R., *U.S.S.R.* A15+645 **63**
Anadyrskiy Zaliv, *U.S.S.R.* Z80+640 **63**
Anáfi. I., *Greece* L25+364 **59**
Anah, *Iraq* K18+345 **74**
Anai, *Libya* M20+240 **81**
Anaimalai Hills, *India* G80+106 **70**
Anaiza, *Saudi Arabia* K05+262 **74**
Anakapalle, *India* G42+177 **71**
Analalava, *Madagascar* J74–148 **83**
Anama, *Brazil* S08–035 **104**
Anambas Kep., *Indonesia* E84+030 **65**
Anamizu, *Japan* C78+372 **68**
Anamosa, *Iowa* U08+422 **95**
Anandpur, *India* G81+312 **72**
Anantapur, *India* G74+146 **70**
Anar, *Iran* J28+309 **75**
Anarak, *Iran* J38+333 **75**
Anardarra, *Afghanistan* H80+328 **75**
Añatolia, *Turkey* K80+390 **74**
Anatuya, *Argentina* S17–284 **103**
Anchorage, *Alaska* Y00+612 **99**
Anchuras, *Spain* N29+395 **52**
Ancohuma, mt., *Bolivia* S51–160 **104**
Ancon, *Peru* T14–118 **104**
Ancona, *Italy* M09+435 **56**
Ancud, *Chile* S82–418 **103**
And Fd., *Norway* L83+692 **46**
Andacolla, *Argentina* S64–371 **103**
Andalgala, *Argentina* S38–275 **103**
Andalsnes, *Norway* M44+626 **46**
Andaman Is. and Sea, *Bay of Bengal* F65+124 **71**
Andeer, *Switzerland* M33+466 **45**
Andelfingen, *Switzerland* M38+476 **45**
Andenne, *Belgium* M59+505 **44**
Andermatt, *Switzerland* M38+466 **45**
Anderson, *Indiana* T64+401 **91**
Anderson, *S. Carolina* T46+345 **97**
Anderson R., *N.-W. Terr.* W40+684 **88**
Andes, Cord. de los, *South America* S70–429 **103**
Andevoranto, *Madagascar* J66–189 **83**
Andhra Pradesh, *India* G70+167 **70**
Andikithira, I., *Greece* L40+358 **59**
Andimilos, I., *Greece* L35+368 **59**
Andiparos, I., *Greece* L30+370 **59**
Andizhan, *Uzbek* H15+409 **62**
Andkhui, *Afghanistan* H59+369 **75**
Andoas Nuevo, *Ecuador* T11–023 **104**
Andorra & rep., *Pyrenees* M81+425 **53**
Andover, *England* N09+512 **39**
Andover, *Massachusetts* S67+427 **96**
Andover, *S. Dakota* U47+454 **93**
Andøya, *Norway* L86+691 **46**
Andrade, *Mozambique* K60-186 **84**
Andreanof Is., *Aleutian Is.* Z73+513 **99**
Andreas, C., *Cyprus* K62+357 **76**
Andreyevka, *Ukraine* K57+488 **60**
Andria, *Italy* L83+412 **57**
Andriba, *Madagascar* J73–176 **83**
Andritsaina, *Greece* L49+375 **59**
Andros I., *Bahamas, The* T18 + 244 **101**
Andros, I., *Greece* L31+378 **59**
Androscoggin R., *Maine* S66+444 **90**
Anegada, B., *Argentina* S10–402 **103**
Anegada, I., *Virgin Is.* S26+188 **101**
Aneiza, Jebel, *Iraq* K34+322 **74**
Anelo, *Argentina* S53–383 **103**
Aneta, *N. Dakota* U48+477 **93**
Aney, *Niger* M14+192 **81**
Angalé, *Cent. Afr. Rep.* L54+098 **81**
Angangueo, *Mexico* U62+195 **100**
Angaston, *S. Australia* C66–345 **109**
Angel Fall, *Venezuela* S15+056 **104**
Angel de la Guarda, I., *Mex.* V50+292 **100**
Angelholm, *Sweden* M13+562 **47**
Angemuk, mt., *New Guinea* C70+036 **65**
Angers, *France* N04+475 **54**
Angikuni L., *N.-W. Terr.* U60+628 **88**
Angkor, *Cambodia* F06+134 **69**
Angledool, *New S. Wales* C12–291 **109**
Anglesey, I., *Wales* N27+533 **38**
Angliers, *Quebec* T25+475 **91**
Angmagssalik, *Greenland* Q55+660 **26**
Angol, *Chile* S76–379 **103**
Angola, *New York* T24+426 **96**
Angola, *W. Africa* L76–100 **82**
Angora. *See* Ankara
Angoulême, *France* M89+456 **54**
Angoumois, prov., *France* M89+459 **54**
Angra, *Brazil* Q86–229 **105**

Anguilla, I., *Leeward Is.* S18+183 **101**
Angul, *India* G30+208 **71**

Anhalt, *Germany* M18+517 **48**
Anholt, I., *Denmark* M20+567 **47**
Anhwei, prov., *China* E18+320 **66**
Animas Ra., *New Mexico* V22+316 **94**
Anina, *Romania* L49+451 **58**
Anita, *Montana* V18+459 **93**
Anjengo, *India* G80+087 **70**
Anjou, prov., *France* N03+473 **54**
Anjouan I., *Comoro Is.* K04-122 **83**
Anjozorobe, *Madagascar* J74-184 **83**
Ankacho, *U.S.S.R.* E72+632 **63**
Ankang, *China* E65+327 **66**
Ankara, *Turkey* K73+399 **74**
Anking (Hwaining), *China* E17+305 **67**
Ankober, *Ethiopia* K30+094 **83**
Ankwo, *China* E28+384 **66**
Anlier, *Belgium* M56+498 **44**
Anlu, *China* E37+313 **66**
Anlu. *See* Chungsiang
Ann C., *Antarctica* J55-660 **27**
Ann, C., *Massachusetts* S63+427 **96**
Anna, *Illinois* T85+374 **97**
Anna, *U.S.S.R.* K27+514 **61**
Annai, *Guyana* R85+039 **104**
An Najaf, *Iraq* K04+320 **74**
Annam, *Vietnam* E80+174 **69**
Annan & R., *Scotland* N20+550 **41**
Annapolis, *Brazil* R24-164 **105**
Annapolis, *Maryland* T09+390 **96**
Annapolis, *Nova Scotia* S33+447 **90**
Annapurna, Mt., *Nepal* G38+285 **71**
Ann Arbor, *Michigan* T52+423 **91**
An Nasiriyah, *Iraq* J84+311 **74**
Annecy & L. d', *France* M53+459 **54**
Anniston, *Alabama* T65+336 **97**
Annobon I., *See* Pagalu
Annonay, *France* M62+452 **55**
Annuello, *Victoria* C43-348 **109**
An Numas, *Saudi Arabia* K16+193 **74**
Anoka, *Minnesota* U22+452 **93**
Anole, *Somalia* K18-008 **83**
Ano Viannos, *Crete* L27+350 **59**
Anpehi, *China* E65+410 **66**
Ansariya, Jebel el, *Syria* K53+356 **76**
Ansbach, *W. Germany* M27+493 **48**
Anshan, *China* D75+412 **64**
Anshun, *China* E84+263 **67**
Ansi, *China* F54+407 **64**
Ansin, *China* E25+389 **66**
Anson B., *N. Terr., Aust.* D29-134 **110**
Ansongo, *Mali* M88+156 **80**
Ansonia, *Connecticut* S78+413 **96**
Anstruther, *Scotland* N16+562 **41**
Anta, *Peru* S74-134 **104**
Antakya (Antioch), *Turkey* K53+362 **76**
Antalo, *Ethiopia* K32+132 **83**
Antalya, *Turkey* K86+369 **74**
Antalya, G. of, *Turkey* K84+367 **74**
Antarctic Peninsula, S25-660 **27**
Antelope I., *Utah* V43+410 **94**
Antequera, *Paraguay* R73-240 **103**
Antequera, *Spain* N27+370 **52**
Anthony, *Kansas* U48+371 **95**
Anthony Lagoon, *N.T., Aust.* C87-178 **111**
Antibes, *France* M47+436 **55**
Anticosti I., *Quebec* S18+495 **90**
Antigo, *Wisconsin* T85+451 **91**
Antigonish, *Nova Scotia* S12+456 **90**
Antigua, I., *Leeward Is.* S10+170 **101**
Antilhue, *Chile* S78-398 **103**
Antilla, *Cuba* T05+209 **101**
Antilles, Greater, *West Indies* - **101**
Antilles, Lesser, *West Indies* - **101**
Antioquia, *Colombia* T05+064 **104**
Antipodes Is., *Pacific Ocean* A04-500 **106**
Antivari. *See* Bar
Antlers, *Oklahoma* U34+343 **95**
Antofagasta, *Chile* S62-235 **103**
Antofagasta de la S., *Arg.* S44-261 **103**
Antofalla, mt., *Argentina* S48-256 **103**
Antoing, *Belgium* M69+506 **44**
Antongil, B. d', *Madagascar* J60-158 **83**
Antonito, *Colorado* V06+370 **94**
Antrain, *France* N09+485 **54**
Antrim & co., *N. Ireland* N37+547 **42**
Antrim Hills, *N. Ireland* N36+550 **42**
Antsirabe, *Madagascar* J78-198 **83**
Antsirana, *Madagascar* J64-124 **83**
Antsla, *Estonia* L20+578 **47**
Antung, *China* *See* Tantung
Antwerp. *See* Antwerpen
Antwerpen, & prov., *Belg.* M63+512 **44**
Anupgarh, *India* H11+292 **72**
Anupshahr, *India* G71+283 **73**
Anuradhapura, *Sri Lanka* G58+084 **70**
Anvers. *See* Antwerpen
Anyang, *China* E33+361 **66**
Anyi, *China* E54+351 **66**
Anykščiai, *Lithuania* L29+556 **47**
Anzhero Sudzhensh, *U.S.S.R.* G21+560 **62**
Aomori, *Japan* C56+408 **68**
Aonla, *India* G65+283 **73**
Aosta, *Italy* M46+457 **56**
Aouderas, *Niger* M40+176 **80**
Aouni, *Chad* L80+130 **81**
Apakova, *U.S.S.R.* J61+545 **61**
Apalachee B., *Florida* T54+300 **97**
Apalachicola & B., *Florida* T60+297 **97**
Aparri, *Philippines* D80+183 **65**
Apataki, I., *Tuamotu Arch.* X70-150 **107**
Apatin, *Yugoslavia* L66+457 **58**
Ape, *Latvia* L19+575 **47**
Apeldoorn, *Netherlands* M54+522 **44**
Apennines, mts., *Italy* M18+440 **50**
Api, mt., *Nepal* G54+300 **73**
Apiai, *Brazil* R23-244 **103**
Apodi, *Brazil* Q47-055 **105**
Apollo Bay, *Victoria* C38-388 **109**
Apolo, *Bolivia* S51-146 **104**
Apostle Is., *Wisconsin* U02+470 **91**
Apostoles, *Argentina* R65-278 **103**
Apoteri, *Guyana* R82+040 **104**
Apozai, *Pakistan* H34+312 **70**
Appalachian Mts., *U.S.A.* T54+346 **99**
Appenzell & canton, *Switz.* M34+473 **45**
Appleby, *England* N15+546 **37**
Applecross, *Scotland* N35+574 **40**
Appleton, *Wisconsin* T81+443 **91**
Appleton City, *Missouri* U24+382 **95**
Approuague, *Fr. Guiana* R41+042 **105**
Apsley, *Tasmania* C17-424 **109**
Apsley, *Victoria* C53-370 **109**
Apt, *France* M58+439 **55**
Apuhi, *Brazil* R88-052 **104**
Aqaba, *Jordan* K60+295 **76**
Aqiq, *Sudan* K40+180 **83**
Aqraba, *Jordan* K58+321 **76**
Aqua, *Mexico* V06+296 **100**
Aquidauana, *Brazil* R65-205 **105**
Aquila, L', *Italy* M10+424 **56**
Aquin, *Haiti* S80+182 **101**
Arabia, pen., *S.W. Asia* **74**
Arabian Sea, *S. Asia* H60+150 **30**
Aracaju, *Brazil* Q43-109 **105**
Aracati, *Brazil* Q47-046 **105**
Arad, *Romania* L52+462 **58**
Arada, *Chad* L56+150 **81**
Arafura Sea, *Indonesia* D00-094 **65**
Aragua de Barcelona, *Venez.* S29+094 **104**
Araguaia, R., *Brazil* R24-070 **105**
Araguari, *Brazil* R19-187 **105**
Arak, *Iran* J62+341 **74**
Arakaka, *Guyana* S00+078 **104**
Arakan, *Burma* F60+200 **71**
Arakan Yoma, *Burma* F66+205 **71**
Araks, R., *Iran* J78+390 **62**
Aralsk, *Kazakh* H80+468 **62**
Aralskoye More (Aral Sea), *Kazakh-Uzbek* J00+450 **62**
Aramac, *Queensland* C28-225 **111**
Arambagh, *India* G13+229 **73**
Aran I., *Ireland, Rep.* N51+550 **42**
Aran Is., *Ireland, Rep.* N58+531 **43**
Aranda de Duero, *Spain* N22+417 **52**
Arani, *Bolivia* S34-175 **104**
Aranjuez, *Spain* N22+400 **52**
Aran Mawddwy, *Wales* N22+528 **38**
Aransas B., *Texas* U42+280 **94**
Araouane, *Mali* N22+186 **80**
Arapiraca, *Brazil* Q41-048 **105**
Arapey, *Uruguay* R75-309 **103**
Arapkir, *Turkey* K40+390 **74**
Arapuni, *New Zealand* A28-380 **112**
Ararangua, *Brazil* R27-289 **103**
Ararat, *Victoria* C42-373 **109**
Ararat, mt., *Turkey* K04+398 **74**
Araria, *India* G15+262 **73**
Arassuahy, *Brazil* Q72-169 **105**
Araty, *Brazil* S64-079 **104**
Arauca, *Colombia* S64+070 **104**
Arauco, *Chile* S80-372 **103**
Aravalli Ra., *India* H10+254 **70**
Araxa, *Brazil* R12-196 **105**
Arbatax, *Sardinia* M31+399 **57**
Arbil, *Iraq* K06+363 **74**
Arboga, *Sweden* L85+594 **47**
Arbois, *France* M56+469 **54**
Arbon, *Switzerland* M33+475 **45**
Arbroath, *Scotland* N16+566 **41**
Arcade, *New York* T21+425 **91**
Arcadia, *Michigan* T67+445 **91**
Arcadia, *Wisconsin* U07+442 **93**
Arcen, *Netherlands* M53+515 **44**
Archbald, *Pennsylvania* T04+415 **96**
Archidona, *Spain* N26+371 **52**
Arcot, *India* G64+129 **70**
Arctic Ocean - **26**
Arctic Red River, *N.-W. Terr.* W80+672 **88**
Ardabil, *Iran* J71+383 **74**
Ardahan, *Turkey* K14+412 **74**
Ardakan, *Iran* J35+324 **75**
Årdal, *Norway* M43+612 **47**
Ardal, *Iran* J55+321 **75**
Ardara, *Ireland, Rep.* N51+548 **42**
Ardatov, *U.S.S.R.* K11+552 **61**
Ardèche, dep., *France* M64+446 **55**
Ardee, *Ireland, Rep.* N39+539 **42**
Arden, Forest of, *England* N11+523 **37**
Ardennes, dep., *France* M61+496 **54**
Ardennes Mts., *Belg., etc.* M57+499 **44**
Arderin, *Ireland, Rep.* N46+530 **43**
Ardez, *Switzerland* M29+468 **45**
Ardgay, *Scotland* N26+579 **40**
Ardglass, *N. Ireland* N34+543 **42**
Ardino, *Bulgaria* L29+416 **58**
Ardistan, *Iran* J46+335 **75**
Ardlethan, *New S. Wales* C19-344 **109**
Ardmore, *Oklahoma* U41+342 **95**
Ardmore B., *Ireland, Rep.* N46+519 **43**
Ardrishaig, *Scotland* N33+560 **41**
Ardrossan, *Scotland* N29+556 **41**
Ardrossan, *S. Australia* C73-344 **109**
Ardud, *Romania* L43+476 **49**
Arecibo, *Puerto Rico* S40+185 **101**
Areia, *Brazil* Q58-133 **105**
Areia Branco, *Brazil* Q43-050 **105**
Areião, *Brazil* R26-044 **105**
Arenales, *Argentina* S09-343 **103**
Arenales, mt., *Chile* S80-471 **103**
Arenas de San Pedro, *Spain* N31+402 **52**
Arendal, *Norway* M37+584 **47**
Arenys de Mar, *Spain* M75+416 **53**
Arequipa, *Peru* S70-163 **104**
Arèvalo, *Spain* N28+410 **52**
Arezzo, *Italy* M19+434 **56**
Argentan, *France* N00+487 **54**
Argentat, *France* M78+451 **55**
Argentina, rep., *S. America* **103**
Argentino, L., *Argentina* S75-503 **103**
Argent-sur-Sauldre, *France* M75+475 **54**
Argo, *Sudan* K88+192 **81**
Argolis, G of, *Greece* L42+372 **59**
Argonne, *France* M60+493 **54**
Argos, *Greece* L44+376 **59**
Arguedas, *Spain* N10+424 **53**
Argun, R., *U.S.S.R.-China* E04+510 **63**
Argungu, *Nigeria* M62+128 **80**
Argyll, co., *See* Strathclyde
Århus, *Denmark* M29+561 **47**
Ariake Wan, *Japan* D23+313 **68**
Ariano Irpino, *Italy* M00+412 **57**
Arica, *Chile* S62-186 **103**
Arica, *Colombia* S70-021 **104**
Ariège, dep., *France* M80+430 **55**
Arikemes, *Brazil* S19-099 **104**
Arilje, *Yugoslavia* L59+437 **58**
Arima, *Brazil* S22-057 **104**
Arinda, *Guyana* R82+047 **104**
Aripuana, *Brazil* S02-052 **104**
Arisaig & Sd. of, *Scotland* N35+568 **41**
Arivechi, *Mexico* V24+290 **100**
Ariza, *Spain* N13+413 **53**
Arizona, *Argentina* S32-356 **103**
Arizona, state, *U.S.A.* V50+347 **98**
Arizona Plat., *Arizona* V36+446 **94**
Arizpe, *Mexico* V30+304 **100**
Arka, *Yemen, South* J76+136 **74**
Arka, *U.S.S.R.* C48+601 **63**
Arkabutla Res., *Mississippi* U01+348 **95**
Arkadelphia, *Arkansas* U18+342 **95**
Arkadhia, *Greece* L46+374 **59**
Arkaig L., *Scotland* N31+570 **40**
Arkansas, state, *U.S.A.* U20+350 **99**
Arkansas R., *Arkansas, etc.* U20+354 **99**
Arkansas City, *Arkansas* U07+336 **97**
Arkansas City, *Kansas* U42+370 **95**
Arkhangelsk, *U.S.S.R.* K25+647 **62**
Arklow, *Ireland, Rep.* N37+528 **43**
Arkoi, I., *Greece* L19+374 **59**
Arles, *France* M62+437 **55**
Arlon, *Belgium* M55+497 **44**
Arltunga, *N. Terr., Aust.* D02-232 **111**
Armagh & co., *N. Ireland* N40+543 **42**
Armenia, *Colombia* T04+048 **104**
Armenia, *U.S.S.R.* K05+405 **74**
Armentieres, *France* M73+507 **54**
Armidale, *New S. Wales* B81-305 **109**
Arminna, *Egypt* K80+222 **81**
Armirós, B of, *Crete* L34+354 **59**
Armisticio, *Paraguay* R57-249 **103**
Armori, *India* G60+205 **70**
Armstrong, *Ontario* T83+502 **89**
Armyanskaya, rep., *U.S.S.R.* K00+400 **62**
Arnaudville, *Louisiana* U11+304 **97**
Arnauti, C., *Cyprus* K76+351 **76**
Arnawai, *Pakistan* H20+353 **72**
Arnhem, *Netherlands* M55+520 **44**
Arnhem, C., *N. Terr., Aust.* C78-122 **111**
Arnhem Ld., *N. Terr., Aust.* D10-130 **110**
Arnissa, *Greece* L49+408 **59**
Arnöy, *Norway* L56+701 **46**
Arnprior, *Ontario* T08+454 **91**
Arnsberg, *W. Germany* M42+514 **48**
Arnstadt, *E. Germany* M24+508 **48**
Arolla, *Switzerland* M45+460 **45**
Aroostook, *New Brunswick* S46+468 **90**
Arorae, I., *Kiribati* A20-030 **106**
Arosa, *Switzerland* M32+468 **45**
Arouelli, *Chad* L44+186 **81**
Aroya, *Colorado* U79+338 **94**
Arrah, *India* G32+255 **73**
Arran I., *Scotland* N31+556 **41**
Arras, *France* M73+503 **54**
Arrayas, *Brazil* R11-131 **105**
Arroba, *Spain* N27+391 **52**
Arromanches, *France* N05+493 **54**
Arronches, *Portugal* N44+391 **52**
Arrow L., *Ireland, Rep.* N50+541 **42**
Arrowsmith, Mt., *N.S.W.* C51-301 **109**
Arrowtown, *New Zealand* A67-449 **112**
Arroyo, *Puerto Rico* S35+180 **101**
 Års, *Denmark* M33+568 **47**
Arsk, *U.S.S.R.* J60+561 **61**
Arta, *Greece* L54+392 **59**
Artawiya, *Saudi Arabia* J88+266 **74**
Artemovsk, *U.S.S.R.* F68+545 **63**
Artemovsk, *Ukraine* K42+486 **60**
Artemovski, *U.S.S.R.* E32+582 **63**
Artemovski, *U.S.S.R.* H79+573 **61**
Artenay, *France* M79+481 **54**
Artesia, *New Mexico* U86+328 **94**
Artibonite, R., *Haiti* S74+190 **101**
Artigas, *Uruguay* R69-304 **103**
Artillery L., N.-W. Terr. V17+636 **88**
Artois, prov., *France* M76+503 **54**
Artvin, *Turkey* K20+412 **74**
Aru, *Zaire* K84+028 **83**
Aruanã, *Brazil* R36-148 **105**
Aru Kep., *Indonesia* D04-063 **65**
Arumã, *Brazil* S13-046 **104**
Arundel, *England* N04+508 **39**
Arundel, *Quebec* S88+460 **91**
Aruppukkottai, *India* G72+095 **70**
Arusha, *Tanzania* K50-034 **83**
Aru Tso, *Tibet* G46+339 **71**
Arvada, *Wyoming* V07+446 **93**
Arvida, *Quebec* S67+484 **90**
Arvika, *Sweden* M14+597 **47**
Arvilla, *N. Dakota* U45+479 **93**
Arzamas, *U.S.S.R.* K07+554 **61**
Arzeu, *Algeria* N02+358 **80**
Arzua, *Spain* N49+429 **52**
As, *Belgium* M57+510 **44**
Aš, *Czechoslovakia* M17+502 **48**
Asahigawa, *Japan* C46+437 **68**
Asansol, *India* G18+237 **73**
Åsarna, *Sweden* M04+627 **46**
Asbestos, *Quebec* S70+458 **91**
Asbury Park, *New Jersey* S84+402 **96**
Ascension, *Bolivia* S19-156 **104**
Ascension, B. de la, *Mexico* T74+196 **100**
Ascension I., *Atlantic Ocean* N87-080 **85**
Aschaffenburg, *W. Germany* M35+499 **48**
Ascoli, *Italy* M09+428 **56**
Ascona, *Switzerland* M37+462 **45**
Ascot, *England* N04+514 **39**
Ascotan, *Chile* S50-215 **103**
Aseda, *Sweden* L88+572 **47**
Åsele, *Sweden* L76+641 **46**
Åsen, *Sweden* M07+613 **47**
Asenovgrad, *Bulgaria* L31+420 **58**
Ashburton, *England* N23+505 **38**
Ashburton, *New Zealand* A49-439 **112**
Ashburton, R., *W. Aust.* E20-230 **110**
Ashdod, *Israel* K62+318 **76**
Asheboro, *N. Carolina* T29+357 **97**
Asheville, *N. Carolina* T45+356 **97**
Ash Fork, *Arizona* V45+352 **94**
Ashkhabad, *Turkmen* J10+380 **62**
Ashland, *Kansas* U58+372 **95**
Ashland, *Kentucky* T46+385 **97**
Ashland, *Maine* S51+466 **90**
Ashland, *Montana* V08+456 **93**
Ashland, *Ohio* T44+409 **91**
Ashland, *Oregon* W16+422 **92**
Ashland, *Pennsylvania* T08+408 **96**
Ashland, *Virginia* T15+376 **97**
Ashland, *Wisconsin* U09+466 **93**
Ashland City, *Tennessee* T72+363 **97**
Ashley, *New S. Wales* C01-292 **109**
Ashley, *N. Dakota* U56+461 **93**
Ashraf, *Iran* J39+367 **75**
Ash Shihr, *Yemen, South* J62+148 **74**
Ashtabula, *Ohio* T35+418 **91**
Ashton-under-Lyne, *England* N12+535 **37**
Ashton, *Idaho* V40+441 **93**
Ashuanipi L., *Labrador* S37+528 **89**
Ashuradeh, *Iran* J37+369 **75**
Ashville, *Alabama* T67+338 **97**
Asinara, I. & G. di, *Sardinia* M39+409 **57**
Asino, *U.S.S.R.* G24+570 **62**
Asir, *Saudi Arabia* K20+203 **74**
Askeaton, *Ireland, Rep.* N54+526 **43**
Askersund, *Sweden* M01+589 **47**
Askvoll, *Norway* M59+614 **47**
Aslandus, *Iran* J76+394 **74**
Asmara, *Ethiopia* K36+152 **83**
Aspern, *Austria* L81+483 **49**
Aspiring, Mt., *New Zealand* A68-444 **112**
Aspres-sur-Buech, *France* M56+445 **55**
Assab, *Ethiopia* K14+130 **83**
As Sabya, *Yemen* K14+172 **74**
As Safa, *Saudi Arabia* J80+277 **74**
Assam, *India* F70+255 **71**
As Sauda, *Yemen* K07+160 **74**
Assaye, *India* G84+203 **70**
Asse, *Belgium* M65+509 **44**
Assen, *Netherlands* M52+530 **44**
Asshur, *Iraq* K14+356 **74**
Assiniboia, *Saskatchewan* V05+496 **88**
Assiniboine, Mt., *Alberta* V63+507 **88**
Assiniboine R., *Manitoba* U50+498 **88**
Assinica L., *Quebec* T01+504 **90**
Assu & R., *Brazil* Q41-056 **105**
Assumar, *Portugal* N44+391 **52**
Assynt L., *Scotland* N30+582 **40**
Asten, *Netherlands* M56+514 **44**
Asti, *Italy* M41+449 **56**
Astipálaia, I., *Greece* L22+366 **59**
Aston, C., *N.-W. Territories* S44+700 **89**
Astor, *Kashmir* H01+353 **72**
Astorga, *Spain* N36+425 **52**
Astoria, *Oregon* W23+462 **92**
Astrakhan, *U.S.S.R.* J73+463 **62**
Åsträsk, *Sweden* L60+646 **46**
Astros, *Greece* L44+374 **59**
Astudillo, *Spain* N26+422 **52**
Asuncion, *Paraguay* R76-252 **103**
Aswân, *Egypt* K72+238 **81**
Asyût, *Egypt* K82+270 **81**
Atacama, Des., *Chile* S56-200 **103**
Atakpame, *Togo* M84+076 **80**
Atalaia, *Brazil* Q36-094 **105**
Atalándi, *Greece* L42+387 **59**
Atambua, *Timor I., Indon.* D62-090 **65**
Atar, *Mauritania* N78+206 **80**
Atara, *Yemen* J89+145 **74**
Ataran, R., *Burma* F42+160 **71**
Atbara, *Sudan* K66+178 **81**
Atbasar, *Kasakh.* H39+518 **62**
Atchafalaya B., *Louisiana* U08+294 **95**
Atchison, *Kansas* U31+396 **95**
Ateca, *Spain* N11+413 **53**
Ath, *Belgium* M67+506 **44**
Athabasca, *Alberta* V49+549 **88**
Athabasca, L., *Alta.-Sask.* V30+592 **88**
Athabasca R., *Alberta* V65+544 **88**
Athboy, *Ireland, Rep.* N41+536 **42**
Athenry, *Ireland, Rep.* N52+533 **43**
Athens. *See* Athinai
Athens, *Georgia* T51+339 **97**
Athens, *Tennessee* T57+354 **97**
Atherton Plat., *Queensland* C30-176 **111**
Athinai, *Greece* L38+380 **59**
Athleague, *Ireland, Rep.* N49+535 **43**
Athlone, *Ireland, Rep.* N48+534 **43**
Athna, *Cyprus* K67+350 **76**
Athol, *Massachusetts* S73+426 **96**
Athol, *New Zealand* A68-455 **112**
Atholl, Forest of, *Scotland* N24+568 **41**
Athy, *Ireland, Rep.* N42+530 **43**
Atico, *Peru* S82-162 **104**
Atienza, *Spain* N18+412 **52**
Atikonak L., *Labrador* S27+528 **89**
Atka, *U.S.S.R.* B80+607 **63**
Atka, I., *Aleutian Is.* Z55+519 **99**
Atkarsk, *U.S.S.R.* K00+518 **61**
Atlanta, *Georgia* T56+337 **97**
Atlanta, *Michigan* T55+450 **91**
Atlantic, *Iowa* U30+414 **95**
Atlantic City, *New Jersey* S86+394 **96**
Atlin, *British Columbia* W81+597 **88**
Atlit, *Israel* K60+327 **76**
Atoka, *Oklahoma* U36+344 **95**
Atrauli, *India* G70+280 **73**
At Tā'if, *Saudi Arabia* K28+211 **74**
Attalla, *Alabama* T66+340 **97**
Attawapiskat, L. & R., *Ont.* T78+520 **89**
Attica, *Indiana* T73+403 **95**
Attica, *New York* T20+428 **96**
Attiki, *Greece* L41+382 **59**
Attleboro, *Massachusetts* S68+419 **96**
Attleborough, *England* M84+525 **39**
Attock, *Pakistan* H16+339 **72**
Attu, I., *Aleutian Is.* A40+524 **99**
Atukesi, *Japan* C31+430 **68**
Atupi, *Brazil* R55+014 **105**
Aube, dep., *France* M64+482 **54**
Aubel, *Belgium* M55+507 **44**
Aubenas, *France* M63+446 **55**
Aubonne, *Switzerland* M52+465 **45**
Auburn, *Alabama* T63+326 **97**
Auburn, *Indiana* T60+414 **91**
Auburn, *Maine* S61+441 **90**
Auburn, *Nebraska* U35+404 **95**
Auburn, *New York* T10+429 **96**
Aubusson, *France* M77+459 **54**
Auce, *Latvia* L43+564 **47**
Auch, *France* M86+437 **55**
Auchterarder, *Scotland* N22+563 **41**
Auckland, *New Zealand* A31-369 **112**
Auckland Is., *Pacific Ocean* A85-550 **106**
Aude, dep., *France* M75+431 **55**
Audegle, *Somalia* K02+018 **83**
Audenarde, *Belgium* M68+508 **44**
Audierne, B. d', *France* N27+479 **54**
Audubon, *Iowa* U30+416 **95**
Aughnacloy, *N. Ireland* N42+544 **42**
Aughrim, Ireland, Rep. N38+528 **43**
Augsburg, *W. Germany* M25+484 **48**
Augusta, *Arkansas* U08+353 **97**

Augusta, *Georgia* T42+334 **97**
Augusta, *Kansas* U42+377 **95**
Augusta, *Kentucky* T54+387 **97**
Augusta, *Maine* S59+444 **90**
Augusta, *Sicily* L89+372 **57**
Augusta, *Wisconsin* U07+447 **91**
Augustów, *Poland* L43+538 **49**
Augustus, Mt., *W. Australia* E12-246 **110**
Auletta, *Italy* L87+406 **57**
Aumale, *Algeria* M68+360 **80**
Aunis, prov., *France* N08+461 **54**
Aura, *Finland* L44+606 **47**
Auraiya, *India* G63+264 **73**
Aurangabad, *India* G33+247 **73**
Aurangabad, *India* G88+199 **70**
Auray, *France* N18+477 **54**
Aurillac, *France* M76+449 **55**
Aurora, *Illinois* T80+418 **91**
Aurora, *Ontario* T27+440 **91**
Aus, *Namibia* L82-266 **84**
Au Sable, *Michigan* T50+445 **91**
Au Sable Forks, *New York* S82+445 **91**
Austin, *Minnesota* U18+437 **93**
Austin, *Nevada* V73+395 **92**
Austin, *Texas* U46+303 **95**
Austin, L., *W. Australia* E12-276 **110**
Austral Is., *Pacific Oc.* Y00-250 **107**
Australia, *Australasia* **110-111**
Australian Alps, *Vic.-N.S.W.* C10-368 **109**
Australian Capital Terr.
Australia C06-355 **109**
Austria, *Central Europe* M06+474 **50**
Autlan, *Mexico* U87+197 **100**
Autun, *France* M64+470 **54**
Auvergne, prov., *France* M72+454 **55**
Auxerre, *France* M69+478 **54**
Aux Sources, Mt.,
Lesotho L06-288 **84**
Ava, *Burma* F54+218 **71**
Avallon, *France* M66+475 **54**
Avalon Pen., *Newfoundland* R52+473 **90**
Avanoas, *Namibia* M12-184 **84**
Avare, *Brazil* R24-231 **105**
Avaviken, *Sweden* L68+656 **46**
Aveiro, *Brazil* R60-034 **105**
Aveiro, *Portugal* N52+406 **52**
Avelgem, *Belgium* M69+508 **44**
Avellanada, *Argentina* R80-347 **103**
Avellino, *Italy* M01+409 **57**
Avenir, *French Guiana* R53+048 **105**
Averoy, *Norway* M45+630 **46**
Aversa, *Italy* M05+410 **57**
Avesnes, *France* M66+501 **54**
Avesta, *Sweden* L83+601 **47**
Aveyron, dep., *France* M73+441 **55**
Avezzano, *Italy* M09+419 **57**
Avia Teria, *Argentina* S04-266 **103**
Aviemore, *Scotland* N23+572 **40**
Avigliano, *Italy* L86+408 **57**
Avignon, *France* M61+440 **55**
Avila, *Spain* N28+406 **52**
Aviz, *Portugal* N47+391 **52**
Avoca, *Iowa* U32+414 **95**
Avoca, *Tasmania* C14-418 **109**
Avoca, *Victoria* C39-371 **109**
Avola, *Sicily* L89+369 **57**
Avon, co., *England* N15+515 **38**
Avon R., *England* N10+523 **37**
Avon R., *Scotland* N20+574 **40**
Avranches, *France* N08+487 **54**
Awaji Shima, *Japan* D00+344 **68**
Awakino, *New Zealand* A32-387 **112**
Awe L., *Scotland* N32+563 **41**
Awjilah, *Libya* L52+292 **81**
Awusa L., *Ethiopia* K40+070 **83**
Axat, *France* M77+428 **55**
Axel, *Netherlands* M67+513 **44**
Axel Heiberg, *North-West*
Territories U15+790 **89**
Axminster, *England* N18+508 **38**
Ayabaca, *Peru* T28-046 **104**
Ayacucho, *Argentina* R82-371 **103**
Ayacucho, *Peru* S85-132 **104**
Ayaguz, *Kazakh* G59+480 **62**
Ayakhta, *U.S.S.R.* F66+593 **63**
Ayamonte, *Spain* N44+372 **52**
Ayan, *U.S.S.R.* C70+563 **63**
Ayancik, *Turkey* K61+419 **74**
Ayaviri, *Peru* S64-147 **104**
Aydin, *Turkey* L13+379 **74**
Ayerbe, *Spain* N04+423 **53**
Ayia, *Greece* L43+397 **59**
Ayion Oros, *Greece* L35+403 **59**
Ayios Evstratios, *Greece* L30+395 **59**
Aylesbury, *England* N05+518 **39**
Aylmer, *Ontario* T36+428 **91**
Aylmer, L., *N.-W. Territories* V20+643 **88**
Aylsham, *England* M82+528 **39**
Aylwin, *Quebec* T06+460 **91**
Aymores, *Brazil* Q67-196 **105**
Ayon Ostrov, *U.S.S.R.* A65+700 **63**
Ayora, *Spain* N06+390 **53**
Ayr, *Queensland* C15-195 **111**
Ayr & R., *Scotland* N28+555 **41**
Ayun, *Saudi Arabia* K08+265 **74**
Ayutla, *Guatemala* U13+147 **100**
Ayutla, *Mexico* U55+169 **100**
Ayutthaya, *Thailand* F27+144 **69**
Ayvalik, *Turkey* L20+394 **74**
Aywaille, *Belgium* M56+505 **44**
Azaila, *Spain* N03+413 **53**
Azamgarh, *India* G41+261 **73**
Azare, *Nigeria* M28+116 **81**
Azaz, *Syria* K48+366 **76**
Azerbaydzhanskaya, rep.,
U.S.S.R. J80+410 **62**
Azi, *Latvia* L27+563 **47**
Azogues, *Ecuador* T23+026 **104**
Azores Is. *See* Açores Is.
Azov, Sea of, *U.S.S.R.* K48+460 **60**
Azpeitia, *Spain* N14+432 **53**
Aztec, *New Mexico* V15+367 **98**
Azua, *Dominican Rep.* S64+184 **101**
Azuaga, *Spain* N34+382 **52**
Azul, *Argentina* R89-367 **103**
Azzan, *South Yemen* J74+144 **74**
Az Zubayr, *Iraq* J74+304 **74**
Baabda, *Lebanon* K57+338 **76**
Baalbek, *Lebanon* K53+340 **76**
Baarle Nassau, *Netherlands* M60+514 **44**
Baarn, *Netherlands* M58+522 **44**
Babahoya, *Ecuador* T26-018 **104**
Babar, I., *Indonesia* D32-080 **65**
Babati, *Tanzania* K56-042 **83**
Babel I., *Tasmania* C11-399 **109**
Bab el Mandeb, *Red Sea* K10+120 **30**
Babenna, *Syria* K54+356 **76**
Babine L., *Brit. Columbia* W38+550 **88**
Babispe, *Mexico* V23+305 **100**
Babol, *Iran* J44+366 **75**
Babura, *Nigeria* M40+126 **82**
Babuyan Is., *Philippines* D80+192 **64**
Babylon, *Iraq* K03+326 **74**
Bacabal, *Brazil* R69-053 **105**
Bacadehuachi, *Mexico* V24+298 **100**
Bacalar, *Mexico* T81+187 **100**
Bacan, I., *Indonesia* D45+006 **65**
Bacău, *Romania* L18+465 **58**
Bacchus Marsh, *Victoria* C33-377 **109**
Bacerac, *Mexico* V23+303 **100**
Bach long Vi, I., *Vietnam* E74+202 **69**
Back R., *N.-W. Territories* U40+660 **88**
Backbone Mts., *W. Va.-Md.* T27+393 **96**
Bäckefors, *Sweden* M17+588 **47**
Backergunge, *Bangladesh* F88+224 **71**
Backstairs Pass., *S. Aust.* C72-357 **109**
Bac-Ninh, *Vietnam* E83+212 **69**
Bacoachi, *Mexico* V40+296 **100**
Bacoachic, *Mexico* V28+309 **100**
Bacolod, *Philippines* D72+106 **65**
Bacup, *England* N13+537 **37**
Bada, *Saudi Arabia* K48+269 **74**
Badajoz, *Brazil* R17-026 **105**
Badajoz, *Spain* N41+389 **52**
Badalona, *Spain* M77+415 **53**
Badarma, *U.S.S.R.* F15+578 **63**
Badas, *Brunei* E33+046 **65**
Bad Axe, *Michigan* T48+438 **91**
Bad Ems, *W. Germany* M44+503 **48**
Baden, *W. Germany* M43+480 **48**
Baden, *Switzerland* M40+475 **45**
Baden-Baden, *W.Germany* M40+487 **48**
Badin, *Pakistan* H36+246 **70**
Badiya, *Oman* J09+225 **75**
Bad Kissingen, *W. Germany* M29+502 **48**
Bad Lands, *Nebraska, etc.* U80+426 **98**
Badnur, *India* G72+218 **70**
Badon, *Senegal* N74+128 **80**
Badrinath, *India* G63+308 **70**
Baduen, *Somalia* J74+070 **83**
Badulla, *Sri Lanka* G53+070 **70**
Baena, *Spain* N26+376 **52**
Baerle-Duc, *Belgium* M60+514 **44**
Baetas, *Brazil* S14-061 **104**
Baffin B., *N.-W. Territories* S30+714 **89**
Baffin I., *N.-W. Territories* S60+680 **89**
Bafia, *Cameroon* M24+046 **81**
Bafoulabe, *Mali* N64+136 **80**
Bafq, *Iran* J28+316 **75**
Bafra, *Turkey* K54+415 **74**
Baft, *Iran* J21+291 **75**
Bagata, *Zaire* L72-038 **82**
Bage, *Brazil* R54-312 **103**
Bagenalstown. *See* Muine Bheag
Baghdad, *Iraq* K04+334 **74**
Bagherhat, *Bangladesh* G01+227 **73**
Baghin, *Iran* J19+302 **75**
Baghpat, *India* G76+290 **72**
Baginbum Hd., *Ireland, Rep.* N41+522 **43**
Bagley, *Minnesota* U32+475 **93**
Bagnell, *Missouri* U16+382 **97**
Bagnols-sur-Ceze, *France* M62+442 **55**
Bagotville, *Quebec* S65+484 **90**
Baguio, *Philippines* D86+165 **65**
Bahaar-i-Gaz, *Iran* J37+368 **75**
Bahadurgarh, *India* G79+287 **72**
Bahama I., Grand, *Bahamas, The* T20+266 **101**
Bahamas, The, *West Indies* T10+250 **101**
Bahawalpur, *Pakistan* H19+294 **72**
Baheri, *India* G63+287 **73**
Bahia. *See* Salvador
Bahia Blanca, *Argentina* S13-386 **103**
Bahia de Caráquez, *Ecuador* T33-007 **104**
Bahia Laura, *Argentina* S39-483 **103**
Bahia Negra, *Paraguay* R79-202 **103**
Bahia Solano, *Colombia* T14+063 **104**
Bahra, *Saudi Arabia* K33+214 **74**
Bahraich, *India* G50+276 **73**
Bahrain, *The Gulf* J57+261 **75**
Bahret el Ateibe, *Syria* K50+335 **76**
Bahret el Hijane, *Syria* K50+333 **76**
Bahret Homs, *Syria* K51+346 **76**
Bahu Kalat, *Iran* H81+257 **75**
Bahus, *Brazil* R48-184 **105**
Baiao, *Brazil* R26-028 **105**
Baibokoum, *Chad* L86+078 **81**
Baiburt, *Turkey* K30+403 **74**
Baidaratskaya B., *U.S.S.R.* H60+700 **62**
Baie St Paul, *Quebec* S63+474 **91**
Baie Verte, *New Brunswick* S25+460 **90**
Baiji, *Iraq* K09+350 **74**
Baikit, *U.S.S.R.* F51+617 **63**
Baikonur, *Kazakh* H53+479 **62**
Baile-Atha-Cliath. *See* Dublin
Bailen, *Spain* N21+381 **52**
Baillie, *N.-W. Territories* W50+706 **88**
Baimak Tanalykovo, *U.S.S.R.* J14+526 **61**
Bainbridge, *Georgia* T57+309 **97**
Bairnsdale, *Victoria* C14-378 **109**
Baitral Faqih, *Yemen* K10+146 **74**
Baitik Bogdo, *China* F80+450 **64**
Baixo Longa, *Angola* L66-164 **84**
Baja, *Hungary* L66+462 **58**
Baja California, state, *Mexico* V60+300 **100**
Baján, *Mexico* U68+265 **100**
Bajmok, *Yugoslavia* L64+460 **58**
Bakaly, *U.S.S.R.* J37+552 **61**
Bakel, *Senegal* N74+148 **80**
Baker, *Montana* U86+463 **93**
Baker, *Oregon* V77+448 **92**
Baker I., *Pacific Ocean* Z70+004 **106**
Baker L., *N.-W. Territories* U40+644 **88**
Baker, Mt., *Washington* W10+483 **98**
Baker Butte, *Arizona* V38+344 **94**
Bakersfield, *California* V84+354 **92**
Bakhasar, *India* H23+247 **70**
Baklansk, *U.S.S.R.* H64+558 **61**
Bakloh, *India* G85+325 **72**
Bako, *Ethiopia* K50+058 **83**
Bakonyerdo, *Hungary* L72+473 **49**
Baku, *Azerbaydzhan* J60+405 **62**
Bala, *Wales* N22+529 **38**
Balabac Str., *Philippines* E20+076 **65**
Balagnat, *India* G58+220 **70**
Balakhta, *U.S.S.R.* F79+552 **63**
Balaklava, *U.S.S.R.* K68+445 **60**
Balaklava, *S. Australia* C70-342 **109**
Bala Murghab, *Afghanistan* H70+356 **75**
Balancan, *Mexico* U10+178 **100**
Balaquer, *Spain* M83+418 **53**
Balashov, *U.S.S.R.* K11+515 **61**
Balasore, *India* G18+215 **71**
Balat, *Egypt* L04+256 **81**
Balaton, L., *Hungary* L74+469 **49**
Balazote, *Spain* N13+389 **53**
Balboa, *Panama* T27+090 **101**
Balbriggan, *Ireland, Rep.* N37+536 **42**
Balcarce, *Argentina* R80-379 **103**
Balchik, *Bulgaria* L11+434 **58**
Balclutha, *New Zealand* A62-463 **112**
Bald Knob, *Arkansas* U10+353 **95**
Bald Knob, *W. Virginia* T30+384 **97**
Baldwin, *Illinois* U02+382 **97**
Baldwin, *Michigan* T65+439 **91**
Baldwinsville, *New York* T08+431 **96**
Baldy Pk., *Arizona* V28+340 **98**
Baldy Pk., *New Mexico* V04+358 **94**
Baleares, Is., *Medit. Sea* M72+395 **53**
Balearic Is. *See* Baleares
Balen, *Belgium* M59+512 **44**
Baler, *Philippines* D81+158 **65**
Balestrand, *Norway* M51+612 **47**
Baley, *U.S.S.R.* E20+517 **63**
Balfour, *N. Dakota* U63+479 **93**
Balfour, *Tasmania* C30-413 **109**
Bali, I., *Indonesia* E30-084 **65**
Balikesir, *Turkey* L13+397 **74**
Balikpapan, *Borneo* E19-012 **65**
Balk, *Netherlands* M57+529 **44**
Balkh, *Afghanistan* H49+368 **75**
Balkhash & Oz., *Kazakh* H00+469 **62**
Ballabgarh, *India* G76+283 **72**
Ballachulish, *Scotland* N31+567 **41**
Ballaghaderreen, *Ireland, Rep.* N51+539 **42**
Ballantrae, *Scotland* N30+551 **41**
Ballara, *Queensland* C60-210 **111**
Ballarat, *Victoria* C37-376 **109**
Ballater, *Scotland* N18+570 **40**
Ballé, *Mali* N52+154 **80**
Ballenas, B. de, *Mexico* V50+268 **100**
Ballenas Channel, *Mexico* V52+292 **100**
Balleny Is., *Antarctica* B10-670 **27**
Ballia, *India* G35+257 **73**
Ballina, *Ireland, Rep.* N55+541 **42**
Ballina, *New S. Wales* B69-289 **109**
Ballinasloe, *Ireland, Rep.* N49+533 **43**
Ballindine, *Ireland, Rep.* N54+537 **42**
Ballingarry, *Ireland, Rep.* N53+525 **43**
Ballinluig, *Scotland* N22+566 **41**
Ballinrobe, *Ireland, Rep.* N55+536 **42**
Ballinskelligs B., *Ireland, Rep.* N62+518 **43**
Ballston Spa, *New York* S83+430 **96**
Ballybay, *Ireland, Rep.* N41+541 **42**
Ballybofey, *Ireland, Rep.* N47+548 **42**
Ballybunion, *Ireland, Rep.* N56+525 **43**
Ballycastle, *Ireland, Rep.* N56+543 **42**
Ballycastle, *N. Ireland* N37+552 **42**
Ballyclare, *N. Ireland* N36+547 **42**
Ballyconnell, *Ireland, Rep.* N45+541 **42**
Ballycotton B., *Ireland, Rep.* N47+518 **43**
Ballyduff, *Ireland, Rep.* N48+521 **43**
Ballygar, *Ireland, Rep.* N50+535 **43**
Ballygawley, *N. Ireland* N42+545 **42**
Ballyhaise, *Ireland, Rep.* N44+540 **42**
Ballyhaunis, *Ireland, Rep.* N53+538 **42**
Ballyhoura Hills, *Ireland, Rep.* N51+523 **43**
Ballyjamesduff, *Ireland, Rep.* N43+539 **42**
Ballymahon, *Ireland, Rep.* N47+534 **43**
Ballymena, *N. Ireland* N37+549 **42**
Ballymoney, *N. Ireland* N39+551 **42**
Ballymote, *Ireland, Rep.* N51+541 **42**
Ballynahinch, *N. Ireland* N35+544 **42**
Ballyquintin Pt., *N. Ireland* N33+543 **42**
Ballyragget, *Ireland, Rep.* N44+528 **43**
Ballyshannon, *Ireland, Rep.* N49+545 **42**
Ballyvaghan, *Ireland, Rep.* N55+531 **43**
Balmoral, *Victoria* C49-372 **109**
Balombo, *Angola* M00-124 **82**
Balotra, *India* H16+258 **70**
Balrampur, *India* G47+274 **73**
Balranald, *New S. Wales* C39-346 **109**
Balsam, L., *Ontario* T23+446 **91**
Balta, *Ukraine* L02+479 **60**
Baltanas, *Spain* N26+419 **52**
Baltic Sea, *N.-W. Europe* **47**
Baltim, *Egypt* K84+316 **81**
Baltimore, *Ireland, Rep.* N56+515 **43**
Baltimore, *Maryland* T10+393 **91**
Baltingglass, *Ireland, Rep.* N40+529 **43**
Baltistan, *Kashmir* G84+354 **72**
Baltiysk, *U.S.S.R.* L60+547 **47**
Baluchistan, *Pakistan* H60+275 **70**
Balurghat, *India* G07+252 **73**
Bam, *Iran* J10+290 **75**
Bama, *Nigeria* M08+116 **81**
Bamako, *Mali* N48+126 **80**
Bambari, *Cent. Afr. Rep.* L56+056 **81**
Bamberg, *W. Germany* M25+499 **48**
Bamenda, *Cameroon* M30+058 **81**
Bamfield, *Michigan* T53+446 **91**
Bamian, *Afghanistan* H43+348 **75**
Bampton, *England* N21+510 **38**
Bampur, *Iran* H87+272 **75**
Bam Tso, *Tibet* G04+281 **71**
Banaras, *India* G42+254 **73**
Banat, *Romania* L50+455 **58**
Banayyan, *Saudi Arabia* J53+232 **75**
Banbridge, *N. Ireland* N38+544 **42**
Banbury, *England* N08+521 **39**
Ban Chamai, *Thailand* F32+082 **69**
Banchory, *Scotland* N15+570 **40**
Bancroft, *Ontario* T17+450 **91**
Banda, *India* G58+255 **73**
Banda Atjeh, *Sumatra* F59+056 **65**
Banda Sea, *Indonesia* D50-055 **65**
Banda Banda, Mt., *N.S.W.* B76-312 **109**
Bandar. *See* Machilipatnam
Bandar Abbas, *Iran* J22+272 **75**
Bandarawela, *Sri Lanka* G54+068 **70**
Bandar e Deylam, *Iran* J59+302 **75**
Bandar e Lengeh, *Iran* J31+266 **75**
Bandar e Rig, *Iran* J56+295 **75**
Bandar e Shapur, *Iran* J64+304 **74**
Bandar Jissah, *Oman* J08+235 **75**
Bandar Shah, *Iran* J36+370 **75**
Bandera, *Argentina* S13-289 **103**
Banderas, B., *Mexico* V03+206 **100**
Bandiagara, *Mali* N22+140 **80**
Bandikui, *India* G81+269 **70**
Bandin Tologoi, *China* F07+412 **64**
Band-i-Qir, *Iran* J66+316 **74**
Bandirma, *Turkey* L12+404 **74**
Bandol, *France* M56+431 **55**
Bandon & R., *Ireland, Rep.* N52+517 **43**
Bandundu, *Zaire* L76-034 **82**
Bandung, *Java* E75-068 **65**
Baned, *India* G78+315 **72**
Banes, *Cuba* T05+210 **101**
Bañeza, la, *Spain* N35+422 **52**
Banff, *Scotland* N15+577 **40**
Banff & Park, *Alberta* V63+510 **88**
Bangada, *Congo* L12+040 **83**
Bangalore, *India* G74+131 **70**
Bangassou, *Cent. Afr. Rep.* L42+048 **81**
Bangka, I., *Indonesia* E84-022 **65**
Bangkok, (Krung Thep),
Thailand G27+138 **69**
Bangkok, Bight of, *Thailand* F28+131 **69**
Bangladesh, *S. Asia* G05+246 **71**
Bang Mun Nak, *Thailand* F28+160 **65**
Bangor, *Maine* S53+448 **90**
Bangor, *N. Ireland* N34+546 **42**
Bangor, *Pennsylvania* T02+408 **96**
Bangor, *Wales* N25+532 **38**
Bang Saphan Yai, *Thailand* F33+113 **69**
Bangui, *Cent. Afr. Rep.* L68+044 **81**
Bangweulu L., *Zambia* L02-112 **83**
Ban Houei Sai, *Laos* F27+203 **69**
Bania, *Cent. Afr. Rep.* L84+040 **82**
Bani Bu 'Ali, *Oman* J05+221 **75**
Banica, *Dominican Rep.* S69+190 **101**
Baniyas, *Syria* K54+352 **76**
Baniyas, *Syria* K56+332 **76**
Banja Luka, *Yugoslavia* L77+448 **56**
Banjarmasin, *Indonesia* E32-034 **65**
Ban Jaruga, *Yugoslavia* L79+454 **56**
Banjul, *The Gambia* P10+134 **80**
Banka, *India* G18+249 **73**
Banki, *India* G26+203 **71**
Bankipore, *India* G29+256 **73**
Banks I., *N.-W. Territories* W00+730 **88**
Banks I., *Queensland* C46-102 **111**
Banks Is., *Pacific Ocean* A72-145 **106**
Banks Pen., *New Zealand* A40-437 **112**
Banks Str., *Tasmania* C12-406 **109**
Bankura, *India* G17+232 **73**
Bann R., *Ireland, Rep.* N39+525 **43**
Bann R., *N. Ireland* N37+544 **42**
Banningville. *See* Bandundu
Bannockburn, *Scotland* N24+561 **41**
Bannu, *Pakistan* H26+330 **72**
Bañolas, *Spain* M73+421 **53**
Baños de Montemayor, *Spain* N35+403 **52**
Ban-pot, *Thailand* F31+160 **69**
Bansda, *India* H09+208 **70**
Bansi, *India* G43+272 **73**
Banswara, *India* H03+236 **70**
Bantalor, *New Brunswick* S38+463 **90**
Ban Thakham, *Thailand* F34+089 **69**
Bantry & B., *Ireland, Rep.* N57+517 **43**
Banu, *Afghanistan* H34+356 **75**
Banur, *India* G80+305 **72**
Banyak Kep., *Indonesia* F46+022 **65**
Banyo, *Cameroon* M20+068 **81**
Banyuwang, *Java* E34-082 **65**
Banzare Coast, *Antarctica* D65-660 **27**
Banzyville, *See* Yasanyama
Bapaume, *France* M73+501 **54**
Baquedano, *Chile* S58-230 **103**
Ba'quba, *Iraq* K02+337 **74**
Bar, *Yugoslavia* L65+421 **58**
Bara, *Sudan* K88+138 **81**
Barabanki, *India* G53+270 **73**
Barabinsk, *U.S.S.R.* G70+553 **62**
Baraboo, *Wisconsin* T89+435 **91**
Baracoa, *Cuba* S87+203 **101**
Barada, *Syria* K47+359 **76**
Baradine & R., *N.S.W.* C06-309 **109**
Barahona, *Dominican Rep.* S66+182 **101**
Barahona, *Spain* N16+413 **53**
Barail Ra., *India* F70+252 **71**
Baraimi, *U.A.E.* J26+243 **75**
Barak R., *India* F70+250 **71**
Baramula, *Kashmir* H04+342 **72**
Baranagar, *India* G09+227 **73**
Baranof I., *Alaska* X00+570 **99**
Baranovichi, *U.S.S.R.* L23+532 **60**
Baranôw, *Poland* L51+505 **49**
Baraque Michel, *Belgium* M53+505 **44**
Barataria B., *Louisiana* U00+292 **95**
Baratta, *S. Australia* C65-320 **109**
Baraunda, *India* G57+250 **73**
Baraut, *India* G76+291 **72**
Barbacena, *Brazil* Q83-212 **105**
Barbacoas, *Colombia* T19+016 **104**
Barbadillo del Mercada, *Spain* N20+421 **52**
Barbados, I., *Windward Is.* R88+132 **101**
Barbastro, *Spain* M89+420 **53**
Barbezieux, *France* N01+455 **54**
Barbuda, I., *Leeward Is.* S10+177 **101**
Barca d'Alva, *Portugal* N41+410 **52**
Barcaldine, *Queensland* C28-234 **111**
Barcarrota, *Spain* N41+385 **52**
Barce. *See* Marj, el
Barcellona Pozza di Gotto,
Sicily L89+382 **57**
Barcellos, *Brazil* S18-010 **104**
Barcelona, *Spain* M76+414 **53**
Barcelona, *Venezuela* S27+101 **104**
Barcelonnette, *France* M50+444 **55**
Barcelos, *Portugal* N52+415 **52**
Barco de Avila, el, *Spain* N33+404 **52**
Barcoo, R., *Queensland* C34-242 **111**
Bardera, *Somalia* K15+022 **83**
Bardi, *India* G45+245 **73**
Bardia, *Libya* L30+318 **81**
Bardsey, I., *Wales* N29+528 **38**
Bardstown, *Kentucky* T63+378 **97**
Bareilly, *India* G63+284 **73**
Barents Sea, *Arctic Ocean* K30+750 **62**
Barentsøya, I., *Arctic Ocean* L50+785 **62**
Barfurush. *See* Babol
Bargal, *Somalia* J54+112 **83**
Barh, *India* G26+255 **73**

Index

Barhaj, *India* G37+263 **73**
Bar Harbor, *Maine* S49+444 **90**
Bari, *India* G74+267 **73**
Bari, *Italy* L79+411 **57**
Bari Doab, *Pakistan* H12+304 **72**
Barinas, *Venezuela* S61+086 **104**
Baring, C., *N.-W. Territories* V72+700 **88**
Baringa, *Zaire* L56+008 **82**
Barisal, *Bangladesh* F88+227 **71**
Barisan, Pegunungar, *Sum.* F25-014 **65**
Barito, R., *Indonesia* E32-028 **65**
Barkah, *Oman* J12+238 **75**
Barkald, *Norway* M24+620 **47**
Barkhan, *Pakistan* H33+299 **72**
Barkly Tableland, *Australia* C70-192 **111**
Bârlad, *Romania* L14+462 **58**
Bar le Duc, *France* M60+488 **54**
Barlee, L., *W. Australia* E03-290 **110**
Barlee Ra., *W. Australia* E20-236 **110**
Barletta, *Italy* L83+413 **57**
Barmedman, *New S. Wales* C15-341 **109**
Barmer, *India* H21+257 **70**
Barmera, *S. Australia* C57-342 **109**
Barmouth, *Wales* N24+527 **38**
Barnaby River, *N.B.* S33+469 **90**
Barnard Castle, *England* N11+545 **37**
Barnato, *New S. Wales* C30-316 **109**
Barnaul, *U.S.S.R.* G33+535 **62**
Barn Bluff, *Tasmania* C25-417 **109**
Barne Inlet, *Antarctica* B30-800 **27**
Barnegat B., *New Jersey* S85+398 **91**
Barnesville, *Minnesota* U39+466 **93**
Barneveld, *Netherlands* M56+521 **44**
Barnsley, *England* N09+536 **37**
Barnstable, *Massachusetts* S62+417 **96**
Barnstaple, *England* N24+511 **38**
Baroda, *India* H10+222 **70**
Barotseland, *Zambia* L41-160 **84**
Baroyeca, *Mexico* V24+279 **100**
Barpeta, *India* F84+263 **71**
Barquinha, *Portugal* N51+394 **52**
Barquisimeto, *Venezuela* S56+100 **104**
Barra, *Saudi Arabia* J85+249 **74**
Barra Hd., *Scotland* N45+568 **41**
Barra, I., *Scotland* N45+570 **40**
Barra, Sd. of, *Scotland* N44+571 **40**
Barraba, *New S. Wales* B87-304 **109**
Barrackpore, *India* G10+228 **73**
Barracon, *Argentina* R52-263 **103**
Barra de Tonala, *Mexico* U23+160 **100**
Barra do Corda, *Brazil* R01-055 **105**
Barra do Pirai, *Brazil* Q83-224 **105**
Barra do Rio Doce, *Brazil* Q59-196 **105**
Barra do Rio Grande, *Brazil* Q80-111 **105**
Barra dos Bugres, *Brazil* R73-150 **104**
Barra Mansa, *Brazil* Q85-224 **105**
Barran, *Somalia* J68+102 **83**
Barranca, *Peru* T10-048 **104**
Barranca Bermeja, *Colombia* S83+071 **104**
Barrancas, *Venezuela* S13+088 **104**
Barrancos, *Portugal* N42+382 **52**
Barranqueras, *Argentina* R84-276 **103**
Barranquilla, *Colombia* S89+109 **104**
Barre, *Vermont* S75+442 **91**
Barreiras, *Brazil* R00-122 **105**
Barreirinha, *Brazil* R72-029 **105**
Barreirinhas, *Brazil* Q77-026 **105**
Barreiro, *Portugal* N54+387 **52**
Barreiros, *Brazil* Q31-087 **105**
Barreme, *France* M52+440 **55**
Barrie, *Ontario* T28+444 **91**
Barrier I., Great, *N.Z.* A27-360 **112**
Barrier I., Little, *N.Z.* A29-362 **112**
Barrington, Mt., *N.S.W.* B82-321 **109**
Barringun, *New S. Wales* C26-290 **109**
Barron, *Wisconsin* U11+454 **93**
Barrow, *Argentina* S02-382 **103**
Barrow-in-Furness, *England* N19+541 **37**
Barrow R., *Ireland, Rep.* N42+524 **43**
Barrow Str., *N.-W. Terr.* U45+736 **88**
Barrow Creek, *N. T., Aust.* D08-214 **111**
Barry, *Wales* N20+514 **38**
Barry Mts., *Victoria* C20-372 **109**
Barsi, *India* G85+182 **70**
Bar-sur-Aube, *France* M62+482 **54**
Bar-sur-Seine, *France* M64+481 **54**
Bartibog, *New Brunswick* S34+473 **90**
Bartica, *Guyana* R82+063 **104**
Bartle Frere Mt., *Queensland* C35-176 **111**
Bartlesville, *Oklahoma* U36+367 **95**
Baruva, *India* G32+190 **71**
Barvaux, *Belgium* M57+503 **44**
Barwa, *India* G34+232 **73**
Barwani, *India* H01+220 **70**
Barwon, R., *New S. Wales* C26-302 **109**
Basel (Basle), *Switzerland* M44+476 **45**
Baselland, canton, *Switz.* M43+474 **45**
Bashi, *Iran* J53+286 **75**
Bashi Chan., *Phil.-Taiwan* D80+215 **67**
Bashkirskaya, aut. rep., *U.S.S.R.* J30+550 **62**
Basia, *India* G30+229 **73**
Basilan, I., *Philippines* D77+066 **65**
Basilicata, reg., *Italy* L83+405 **57**
Basingstoke, *England* N07+513 **39**
Baskatong L., *Quebec* T05+468 **91**
Båsmo, *Norway* M06+663 **46**
Basongo, *Zaire* L58-044 **82**
Basra, *Iraq* J73+305 **74**
Bas-Rhin, dep., *France* M42+486 **54**
Bass Str., *Vict.-Tasm.* C30-395 **111**
Bassac, *Laos* E85+149 **69**
Bassein, *Burma* F61+168 **71**
Bassein, *India* H13+196 **70**
Basses, Gt. & Lit., *Sri Lanka* G50+061 **70**
Basses-Alpes. *See* Alpes-de-Haute Provence
Basses-Pyrénées. *See* Pyrénées Atlantiques,
Basse Terre, *Leeward Is.* S09+160 **101**
Bassevelde, *Belgium* M68+512 **44**
Båstad, *Sweden* M13+564 **47**
Bastak, *Iran* J33+272 **75**
Basti, *India* G43+268 **73**
Bastia, *Corsica* M33+427 **56**
Bastogne, *Belgium* M56+500 **44**
Bastrop, *Louisiana* U11+328 **95**
Basura, *Mexico* V43+311 **100**
Basutoland. *See* Lesotho
Bata, *Equatorial Guinea* M32+018 **82**
Bataan, *Philippines* D88+147 **65**
Batabano, *Cuba* T43+227 **101**
Batacosa, *Mexico* V24+278 **100**
Batala, *India* G89+318 **72**
Batalha, *Portugal* N53+397 **52**
Batan Is., *Philippines* D78+210 **64**
Batangas, *Philippines* D84+137 **65**
Batavia, *Argentina* S35-348 **103**
Batavia, *See* Jakarta
Batavia, *New York* T19+430 **96**
Bataysk, *U.S.S.R.* K31+471 **61**
Batchawana, *Ontario* T55+472 **91**
Batchelor, *N. Terr., Aust.* D24-131 **110**
Batdambang, *Cambodia* F11+130 **69**
Bateman's B., *New S. Wales* B89-358 **109**
Batenburg, *Netherlands* M56+518 **44**
Batesburg, *S. Carolina* T39+339 **97**
Batesville, *Arkansas* U10+358 **95**
Batesville, *Mississippi* U00+344 **97**
Bath, *England* N14+514 **38**
Bath, *Maine* S59+439 **90**
Bath, *New York* T14+423 **96**
Bathgate, *Scotland* N22+559 **41**
Bathurst. *See* Banjul
Bathurst, *New Brunswick* S34+476 **90**
Bathurst, *New S. Wales* C03-334 **109**
Bathurst Inl., *N.-W. Terr.* V15+670 **88**
Bathurst I., *N. Terr., Aust.* D28-116 **110**
Bathurst I., *N.-W. Terr.* U60+756 **88**
Batie, *Upper Volta* N18+098 **80**
Batiscan, *Quebec* S74+465 **91**
Batlow, *New South Wales* C12-355 **109**
Batna, *Algeria* M52+356 **80**
Baton Rouge, *Louisiana* U07+304 **95**
Batopilas, *Mexico* V14+270 **100**
Batraki, *U.S.S.R.* J68+532 **61**
Batroun, *Lebanon* K56+342 **76**
Batticaloa, *Sri Lanka* G50+077 **70**
Battice, *Belgium* M55+506 **44**
Battih, *Saudi Arabia* J67+150 **74**
Battle Creek, *Michigan* T61+424 **91**
Battleford, *Saskatchewan* V20+529 **88**
Battleford, N., *Saskatchewan* V20+530 **88**
Battle Harbour, *Labrador* R65+526 **89**
Battle Mountain, *Nevada* V72+406 **92**
Batu, *Indonesia* F40-005 **65**
Batumi, *U.S.S.R.* K20+418 **62**
Baturaja, *Sumatra* F05-040 **65**
Baturi, *Mexico* V23+258 **100**
Baturite, *Brazil* Q54-044 **105**
Bauchi, *Nigeria* M32+104 **81**
Baud, *India* G34+208 **71**
Baudette, *Minnesota* U28+488 **93**
Baudo, *Colombia* T13+052 **104**
Baudouinville. *See* Moba
Bauge, *France* M88+475 **54**
Baunt, *U.S.S.R.* E40+553 **63**
Baures, *Bolivia* S22-137 **104**
Bauru, *Brazil* R24-221 **105**
Bauska, *Latvia* L35+564 **47**
Bautzen, *E. Germany* M03+512 **48**
Bawal, *India* G80+281 **72**
Bawean, I., *Indonesia* E44-058 **65**
Bawiti, *Egypt* L08+282 **81**
Bawku, *Ghana* N00+110 **80**
Bawtry, *England* N06+534 **37**
Bay Is., *Honduras* T68+164 **101**
Bayamo, *Cuba* T11+204 **101**
Bayana, *India* G77+269 **73**
Bayan Aul, *Kazakh* G86+507 **62**
Bayan Dzurikhe, *Mongolia* E76+477 **64**
Bayanga, *Cent. Afr. Rep.* L84+054 **81**
Bayan Kara Shan, *China* F30+335 **64**
Bayan Tumen, *Mongolia* E34+480 **64**
Bayazit, *Turkey* K08+396 **74**
Bay City, *Michigan* T53+436 **91**
Bay City, *Texas* U36+290 **95**
Bayern, *W. Germany* M18+490 **48**
Bayeux, *France* N05+493 **54**
Bayir, *Jordan* K50+308 **76**
Baykal, Oz, *Russia* E80+533 **63**
Bay Minette, *Alabama* T77+308 **97**
Bayona, *Spain* N53+421 **52**
Bayonne, *France* N09+435 **55**
Bayou Bodcau Res., *La.-Ark.* U20+329 **95**
Bayovar, *Peru* T36-058 **104**
Bayram Ali, *Turkmen* H77+375 **62**
Bayreuth, *W. Germany* M21+499 **48**
Bayrischer Wald, *W. Germany* M12+490 **48**
Bays, L. of, *Ontario* T24+453 **91**
Baza, Sa. de, *Spain* N08+375 **53**
Bazar Musa Khel, *Pakistan* H31+309 **72**
Bazaruto, I., *Mozambique* K58-218 **84**
Bazas, *France* N01+444 **55**
Bazias, *Romania* L52+448 **58**
Bazman, *Iran* J00+278 **75**
Beach, *N. Dakota* U84+470 **93**
Beachport, *S. Australia* C60-374 **109**
Beachy Hd., *England* M89+508 **39**
Beacon, *New York* S84+415 **96**
Beaconsfield, *Tasmania* C20-412 **109**
Beal Ra., *Queensland* C52-250 **111**
Beaminster, *England* N17+508 **38**
Bear Is. *See* Medvezhi Osa.
Bear L. & R., *Ida.-Ut.* V38+420 **94**
Beardmore Gl., *Antarctica* A70-850 **27**
Bearn, prov., *France* N03+432 **55**
Bear Paw Mts., *Montana* V26+483 **93**
Beata, I., *Dominican Rep.* S69+175 **101**
Beatenberg, *Switzerland* M43+467 **45**
Beatrice, *Nebraska* U40+403 **95**
Beattock, *Scotland* N21+553 **41**
Beattyville, *Kentucky* T52+376 **97**
Beauceville, *Quebec* S64+462 **91**
Beaufort, *S. Carolina* T34+325 **97**
Beaufort, *Victoria* C40-374 **109**
Beaufort Basin, *Arctic Oc.* Y30+750 **26**
Beaufort Sea, *Arctic Ocean* W60+720 **26**
Beaufort West, *Cape Prov.* L44-324 **84**
Beaugency, *France* M80+478 **54**
Beauly & Firth, *Scotland* N27+575 **40**
Beaumaris, *Wales* N25+533 **38**
Beaumont, *Belgium* M65+502 **44**
Beaumont, *France* M76+491 **54**
Beaumont, *New Zealand* A62-458 **112**
Beaumont, *Texas* U25+302 **95**
Beaune, *France* M61+470 **54**
Beauport, *Quebec* S67+469 **91**
Beauraing, *Belgium* M60+501 **44**
Beauvais, *France* M78+494 **54**
Beauvoir-sur-Mer, *France* N12+469 **54**
Beaver, *Oklahoma* U64+368 **94**
Beaver, *Utah* V46+383 **94**
Beaver I., *Michigan* T63+457 **91**
Beaver R., *Saskatchewan* V25+542 **88**
Beaver Dam, *Wisconsin* T83+435 **91**
Beaver Falls, *Pennsylvania* T32+408 **91**
Beaverhead Mts., *Idaho* V53+454 **92**
Beawar, *India* H04+261 **70**
Beazley, *Argentina* S40-337 **103**
Bebedouro, *Brazil* R21-209 **105**
Becerrea, *Spain* N43+429 **52**
Bechuanaland. *See* Botswana
Becleau, *Romania* L35+472 **49**
Beda, *Yemen* J84+142 **74**
Bedak, *Afghanistan* H44+345 **75**
Bedar, *Spain* N12+372 **53**
Beddgelert, *Wales* N25+530 **38**
Bedford, *Pennsylvania* T21+400 **96**
Bedford, *Quebec* S78+451 **91**
Bedford, *Virginia* T27+373 **97**
Bedford & co., *England* N03+521 **39**
Bedretto, *Switzerland* M39+465 **45**
Bedr Honein, *Saudi Arabia* K38+237 **74**
Beduval, *Saskatchewan* V16+552 **88**
Bedzin, *Poland* L66+504 **49**
Beeac, *Victoria* C48-382 **109**
Beebe, *Arkansas* U11+351 **97**
Beechey, L., *N.-W. Terr.* V10+653 **88**
Beechworth, *Victoria* C20-364 **109**
Beecroft Hd., *N.S.W.* B85-350 **109**
Beek, *Netherlands* M54+518 **44**
Beek, *Netherlands* M55+509 **44**
Beekbergen, *Netherlands* M54+522 **44**
Beenoskee, *Ireland, Rep.* N60+522 **43**
Beerlegem, *Belgium* M68+509 **44**
Beernem, *Belgium* M70+511 **44**
Beers, *Netherlands* M55+517 **44**
Beersheba, *Israel* K61+312 **76**
Beeville, *Texas* U46+284 **94**
Befale, *Zaire* L54+004 **82**
Befandriana, *Madagascar* J68-154 **83**
Bega, *New South Wales* C01-367 **109**
Behbehan, *Iran* J57+306 **75**
Beho, *Belgium* M54+502 **44**
Beidha, *Saudi Arabia* K30+208 **74**
Beilen, *Netherlands* M51+529 **44**
Beilul, *Ethiopia* K16+130 **83**
Beinwil, *Switzerland* M41+473 **45**
Beira, *Mozambique* K60-198 **84**
Beirût (Beyrouth), *Lebanon* K57+339 **76**
Beisan, *Israel* K57+325 **76**
Beitbridge, *Zimbabwe* L00-222 **84**
Beit-et-Din, *Lebanon* K56+337 **76**
Beit Guvrin, *Israel* K60+316 **76**
Beius, *Romania* L46+467 **58**
Beja, *Portugal* N47+380 **52**
Béjar, *Spain* N35+404 **52**
Bejestan, *Iran* J11+346 **75**
Bejucal, *Cuba* T44+230 **101**
Békéscsaba, *Hungary* L54+467 **49**
Bela, *Pakistan* H52+261 **70**
Bela, *India* G47+259 **73**
Belair, *Louisiana* T89+298 **97**
Belang, *Celebes* D61+010 **65**
Belangpidie, *Sumatra* F50+038 **65**
Belaya Tserkov, *Ukraine* K89+498 **60**
Belcher Is., *N.-W. Terr.* T25+560 **89**
Belchirag, *Afghanistan* H58+358 **75**
Belchite, *Spain* N04+413 **53**
Belcoo, *Ireland, Rep.* N47+543 **42**
Beldanga, *India* G10+240 **73**
Belebey, *U.S.S.R.* J35+541 **61**
Belém (Pará), *Brazil* R21-014 **105**
Belem, *Mexico* V32+278 **96**
Belen, *Argentina* S42-278 **103**
Belen, *New Mexico* V11+346 **94**
Belen, *Panama* T35+090 **101**
Belfast, *Maine* S54+444 **90**
Belfast & L., *N. Ireland* N35+546 **42**
Belfeld, *Netherlands* M53+513 **44**
Belfield, *N. Dakota* U79+469 **93**
Belford, *England* N11+556 **37**
Belfort, *France* M49+476 **54**
Belgaum, *India* H02+159 **70**
Belgium, *Europe* M63+507 **50**
Belgorod, *U.S.S.R.* K51+507 **60**
Belgorod Onestrovskiy, *Ukr.* K88+462 **60**
Belgrade. *See* Beograd
Belgrano, *Argentina* R82-358 **103**
Belin, *France* N05+445 **55**
Belitung, I., *Indonesia* E72-029 **65**
Belize, *Belize* T80+176 **101**
Belize, *Central America* T84+170 **101**
Bell I., *Newfoundland* R63+507 **90**
Bellac, *France* M84+461 **54**
Bella Coola, *Brit. Columbia* W40+521 **88**
Bellaire, *Michigan* T61+450 **91**
Bellaire, *Ohio* T35+400 **91**
Bellary, *India* G78+152 **70**
Bellavista, *Peru* T22-056 **104**
Bellbrook, *New S. Wales* B75-308 **109**
Belledune, *New Brunswick* S35+478 **90**
Bellefontaine, *Ohio* T53+404 **91**
Bellefonte, *Pennsylvania* T17+409 **96**
Belle Fourche, *S. Dakota* U83+447 **93**
Belle Ile, *France* N19+473 **54**
Belle Isle, *New Brunswick* S34+457 **90**
Belle Isle, *Newfoundland* R62+518 **90**
Belle Isle, Str. of, *Nfd., etc.* R72+513 **90**
Belleme, *France* M87+484 **54**
Belle Plain, *Iowa* U14+418 **95**
Bellerive, *Tasmania* C16-429 **109**
Belleville, *France* M62+461 **54**
Belleville, *Kansas* U46+398 **95**
Belleville, *Illinois* U00+386 **95**
Belleville, *Ontario* T14+422 **91**
Bellevue, *Iowa* U03+423 **95**
Bellevue, *Ontario* T55+467 **91**
Belley, *France* M56+458 **54**
Belle Yella, *Liberia* N60+076 **80**
Bellinger, *New S. Wales* B74-304 **109**
Bellingham, *England* N13+551 **37**
Bellingham, *Washington* W14+485 **98**
Bellingshausen Sea, *Antarc.* T60-670 **27**
Bellinzona, *Switzerland* M36+462 **45**
Bellows Falls, *Vermont* S75+431 **96**
Belluno, *Italy* M16+462 **56**
Bell Ville, *Argentina* S16-325 **103**
Belmez, *Spain* N32+383 **52**
Belmond, *Iowa* U22+429 **95**
Belmont, *Missouri* T85+367 **97**
Belmont, *New York* T18+422 **96**
Belmont L., *Pennsylvania* T03+418 **96**
Belmonte, *Brazil* S47-058 **104**
Belmonte, *Brazil* Q54-158 **105**
Belmonte, *Portugal* N44+404 **52**
Belmullet, *Ireland, Rep.* N60+542 **42**
Belo Horizonte, *Brazil* Q84-200 **105**
Beloit, *Kansas* U48+394 **95**
Beloit, *Wisconsin* T84+425 **95**
Belomorsk, *Karelskaya* K61+645 **62**
Belorado, *Spain* N19+424 **52**
Beloretsk, *U.S.S.R.* J10+540 **61**
Belorusskaya S.S.R. *See* Byelorussia
Belostok. *See* Bialystok
Beloye Oz., *U.S.S.R.* K44+602 **60**
Beloyo More, *U.S.S.R.* K30+658 **62**
Belp, *Switzerland* M45+469 **45**
Belt, Lille, *Denmark* M31+553 **47**
Belt, Store, *Denmark* M24+555 **47**
Beltana, *S. Australia* C70-308 **109**
Belterra, *Brazil* R60-026 **105**
Belton, *S. Australia* C68-322 **109**
Belturbet, *Ireland, Rep.* N45+541 **42**
Belvedere Marittimo, *Italy* L85+396 **57**
Belver, *Portugal* N48+395 **52**
Belvidere, *Illinois* T83+422 **95**
Belvidere, *New Jersey* T01+408 **96**
Belyy, Os., *U.S.S.R.* H30+730 **62**
Bemidji, *Minnesota* U30+474 **93**
Benagerie, *S. Australia* C58-315 **109**
Ben Alder, *Scotland* N27+568 **41**
Benalla, *Victoria* C24-365 **109**
Benapol, *India* G07+230 **73**
Benares, *See* Varanasi
Benavente, *Spain* N34+420 **52**
Benbecula, I., *Scotland* N44+574 **40**
Benbury, *Ireland, Rep.* N59+536 **42**
Ben Cruachan, *Scotland* N31+564 **41**
Bencubbin, *W. Australia* E11-308 **110**
Bend, *Oregon* W08+441 **92**
Ben Dearg, *Scotland* N30+578 **40**
Bendery, *Moldavia* L03+469 **60**
Bendigo, *Victoria* C34-368 **109**
Bendoc, *Victoria* C07-371 **109**
Benevento, *Italy* M01+412 **57**
Bengal, B. of, *India, etc.* G00+180 **71**
Bengal, East, *Bangladesh* G03+240 **73**
Bengal, West, *India* G14+235 **73**
Ben Gardane, *Tunisia* M24+330 **81**
Benghazi, *Libya* L60+320 **81**
Benguela, *Angola* M10-126 **82**
Benha, *Egypt* K82+304 **81**
Ben Hope, *Scotland* N28+584 **40**
Beni, R., *Bolivia* S43-130 **104**
Beni-Abbès, *Algeria* N14+302 **80**
Benicarlo, *Spain* M88+404 **53**
Benin, rep., *W. Africa* M80+098 **80**
Benin, Bight of, *W. Africa* M80+050 **80**
Benin City, *Nigeria* M56+064 **80**
Beni Saf, *Algeria* N08+354 **80**
Beni Suef, *Egypt* K84+290 **81**
Benito, *Rio Muni* M32+014 **82**
Benjamin Constant, *Brazil* S61-044 **104**
Benkelman, *Nebraska* U70-400 **95**
Benkovac, *Yugoslavia* L87+441 **56**
Ben Lawers, *Scotland* N25+565 **41**
Ben Ledi, *Scotland* N26+563 **41**
Ben Lomond, *N.S.W.* B80-301 **109**
Ben Lomond, *Scotland* N28+562 **41**
Ben Lomond, *Tasmania* C15-416 **109**
Ben Macdhui, *Scotland* N22+571 **40**
Ben More, *Scotland* N27+564 **41**
Ben More Assynt, *Scotland* N29+581 **40**
Bennett, *Brit. Columbia* X00+599 **88**
Bennettsville, *S. Carolina* T28+346 **97**
Ben Nevis, *Scotland* N30+568 **41**
Bennington, *Vermont* S79+429 **96**
Benson, *Arizona* V32+320 **94**
Benson, *Minnesota* U34+453 **93**
Benson Mines, *New York* T00+442 **91**
Bentinck's I., *Burma* F42+117 **71**
Benton, *Arkansas* U16+345 **97**
Benton Harbor, *Michigan* T69+421 **91**
Benue R., *Nigeria* M40+080 **80**
Ben Vorlich, *Scotland* N25+563 **41**
Benwee Hd., *Ireland, Rep.* N59+543 **42**
Ben Wyvis, *Scotland* N27+577 **40**
Beograd, *Yugoslavia* L57+448 **58**
Beppu, *Japan* D21+332 **68**
Berar, *India* G74+205 **70**
Berat, *Albania* L60+407 **59**
Berawinnia, *New S. Wales* C33-290 **109**
Berber, *Sudan* K66+180 **81**
Berbera, *Somalia* K00+104 **83**
Berberati, *Cent. Afr. Rep.* L86+044 **81**
Berdichev, *Ukraine* L09+498 **60**
Berdigyastyakh, *U.S.S.R.* D46+623 **63**
Berdyansk, *Ukraine* K50+468 **60**
Bere Regis, *England* N13+507 **39**
Beresford, *S. Dakota* U42+430 **93**
Beresti, *Romania* L13+461 **58**
Berezniki, *U.S.S.R.* J20+594 **62**
Berezovo, *U.S.S.R.* H60+641 **62**
Berg, *Norway* L77+695 **46**
Berga, *Spain* M79+421 **53**
Bergamo, *Italy* M32+457 **56**
Bergen, *E. Germany* M10+544 **48**
Bergen, *Norway* M58+604 **47**
Bergen, *W. Germany* M31+528 **48**
Bergen-op-Zoom, *Neth.* M64+515 **44**
Bergerac, *France* M87+449 **55**
Bergisch Gladbach, *W. Germany* M46+510 **48**
Bergün, *Switzerland* M32+466 **45**
Berhampur, *India* G10+241 **73**
Berhampur, *India* G31+192 **71**
Beri, *India* G80+287 **72**
Bering, *U.S.S.R.* Z62+648 **63**
Beringen, *Belgium* M59+510 **44**
Bering Sea, *Asia-America* A00+590 **99**
Bering Str., *Asia-America* Z30+652 **99**
Berislavl, *Ukraine* K69+468 **60**
Berjeik, *Netherlands* M58+513 **44**
Berkåk, *Norway* M30+629 **46**
Berkeley, *California* W14+379 **92**
Berkley, *Virginia* T08+368 **97**
Berkovitsa, *Bulgaria* L42+433 **58**
Berkshire (Berks), co., *Eng.* N08+515 **39**
Berkshire Hills, *Massachusets* S79+423 **96**
Berlin, *Germany* M10+525 **48**
Berlin, *New Hampshire* S67+445 **91**
Berlin, *Wisconsin* T83+440 **91**
Bermagui, *N.S.W.* C00-364 **109**

Bermillo de Savago, Spain N37+414 52
Bermudas, Is., Atlantic Oc. S30+320 99
Bern & canton, Switzerland M45+469 45
Bernalillo, New Mexico V10+353 94
Bernasconi, Argentina S23-379 103
Bernay, France M86+492 54
Bernburg, E. Germany M20+518 48
Berne. See Bern
Berneau, Belgium M56+507 44
Berneck, Switzerland M32+474 45
Berner Alpen, Switzerland M46+463 45
Bernina, Passo del, Switz. M30+464 45
Beromunster. See Munster
Berri, S. Australia C57-343 109
Berri, prov., France M76+471 54
Berriedale, Scotland N21+582 40
Berrigan, New S. Wales C25-357 109
Berry, New South Wales B86-348 109
Berry Is., Bahamas, The T18+256 101
Berryville, Virginia T18+391 96
Bersillies, Belgium M65+503 44
Berthierville, Quebec S79+461 91
Berthold, N. Dakota U71+483 93
Bertoua, Cameroon M08+046 81
Bertraghboy B., Ireland, Rep. N59+534 43
Bertrix, Belgium M59+499 44
Beru, I., Kiribati A23-018 106
Berwick, Pennsylvania T08+411 96

Berwick-upon-Tweed, Eng. N12+558 37
Berwyn Mts., Wales N20+529 38
Berzee, Belgium M64+503 44
Bescançon, France M54+473 54
Beskidy Zachodnie, mts.,
Central Europe L54+495 49
Besni, Turkey K43+378 74
Bessala, Congo L86-026 82
Bessemer, Alabama T72+334 97
Best, Netherlands M58+515 44
Betanzos, Spain N49+434 52
Betbetti, Sudan L34+152 81
Bethanie, Namibia L76-264 84
Bethany, Missouri U24+403 95
Bethel, Maine S65+444 90
Bethlehem, O.F.S. L10-284 84
Bethlehem, Israel K59+317 76
Bethlehem, Pennsylvania T02+406 96
Betling Sib., India F75+238 71
Betsiamites, Quebec S52+490 90
Betsiamites R., Quebec S58+493 90
Bettiah, India G32+268 73
Beugen, Netherlands M54+517 44
Beulah, Victoria C46-360 109
Beveland, Noord, I.,
Netherlands M67+516 44
Beveland, Zuid, I.,
Netherlands M66+515 44
Beveren, Belgium M65+512 44
Beverley, England N02+538 37
Beverlo, Belgium M59+511 44
Beverly, Massachusetts S65+426 96
Beverst, Belgium M57+509 44
Bewdley, England N14+524 38
Bex, Switzerland M48+463 45
Beyla, Guinea N52+088 80
Beypazari, Turkey K79+402 74
Beypore, India G85+113 70
Beysehir, Turkey K80+376 74
Bezdán, Yugoslavia L67+458 58
Bezhitsa, U.S.S.R. K64+533 60
Beziers, France M71+434 55
Bezwada, India G56+165 70
Bhabua, India G38+250 73
Bhadarwah, Kashmir G85+329 72
Bhadaur, India G88+305 72
Bhadaura, India G76+248 73
Bhadohi, India G44+254 73
Bhadra, India G89+291 72
Bhadreswar, India G10+228 73
Bhagalpur, India G18+252 73
Bhakkar, Pakistan H23+317 72
Bhamo, Burma F46+242 71
Bhandara, India G62+211 70
Bhannis, Lebanon K56+339 76
Bhanrer Ra., India G63+234 73
Bharatpur, India G75+272 73
Bhatgaon, Nepal G27+276 73
Bhatinda, India H00+302 72
Bhatnair, India H04+295 72
Bhatpara, India G09+229 73
Bhavnagar, India H17+216 70
Bhawani Patna, India G40+200 71
Bhera, Pakistan H12+325 72
Bhilwara, India H02+254 70
Bhima R., India G82+172 70
Bhind, India G67+265 73
Bhir (Bir), India G85+190 70
Bhiwani, India G83+288 72
Bhojpur, India G35+255 73
Bhong Chu, R., Tibet G17+286 71
Bhopal, India G75+233 73
Bhuj, India H32+232 70
Bhusawal, India G85+210 70
Bhutan, S. Asia G00+270 71
Biafra, Bight of, W. Africa M38+026 80
Biak, I., New Guinea C84-010 65
Białogard, Poland L84+540 49
Białowieza, Poland L37+527 49
Białystok, Poland L41+531 49
Biarritz, France N09+435 55
Biasca, Switzerland M36+464 45
Biderach, Germany M32+481 48
Bibon, Wisconsin U07+464 91
Bic, Quebec S52+484 90
Bicknell, Indiana T74+388 91
Bida, Nigeria M54+092 80
Bidar, India G74+179 70
Biddeford, Maine S63+435 96
Bideford & B., England N25+510 38
Bidon, Algeria M84+222 80
Biel, Switzerland M47+471 45
Bielefeld, Germany M39+520 48
Bieler See, Switzerland M47+471 45
Bielopole, Ukraine K64+512 60
Bielsk, Poland L41+528 49
Bienne. See Biel
Bière, Switzerland M52+466 45
Bietschhorn, mt., Switz. M43+464 45
Big I., N.-W. Territories S63+620 89
Big L., Arkansas U01+357 95
Biga, Turkey L16+404 74
Big Bell, W. Australia E13-272 110
Big Belt Mts., Montana V40+468 93
Big Bend Nat. Pk., Texas U80+292 94
Big Blue R., Kan.-Neb. U40+400 95
Bigelow, Maine S63+451 90
Biggar, Saskatchewan V18+518 88
Biggar, Scotland N21+556 41
Biggleswade, England N02+521 39
Big Hatchet Mts., New Mex. V20+316 94
Bighorn Mts., Wyoming V15+444 98
Bighorn R., Montana, etc. V19+450 98
Bignona, Senegal P08+128 80
Big Rapids, Michigan T63+437 91
Big Salmon R., Yukon W80+612 88
Big Sandy R., Kentucky, etc. T45+380 93
Big Spring, Texas U68+322 94
Bigtimber, Montana V30+458 93
Big Trout L., Ontario T88+540 89
Bihac, Yugoslavia L85+448 56
Bihar, India G26+252 73
Bihar, India G30+248 71
Biharamulo, Tanzania K82-026 83
Bihorului, Mti, Romania L45+464 58
Bijagos, Arqui. Dos.,
Guinea-Bissau P04+114 80
Bijapur, India G85+168 70
Bijar, Iran J74+359 74
Bijawar, India G63+246 73
Bijeljina, Yugoslavia L65+448 58
Bijnabad, Iran J12+280 75
Bijnor, India G71+294 72
Bikaner, India H10+280 72
Bikin, U.S.S.R. D04+467 63
Bikini, I., Marshall Is. A85+120 106
Bilaspur, India G79+312 72
Bilaspur, India G47+220 73
Bilauktaung Ra.,
Burma-Thailand F38+145 65
Bilbao, Spain N18+433 52
Bileća, Yugoslavia L70+429 58
Bilecik, Turkey L00+402 74
Bilé Karpaty, Czechoslovakia L74+490 49
Bilimbaevski, U.S.S.R. J02+568 61
Bilin, Burma F47+173 71
Bilisht, Albania L54+406 59
Bilkis, Iran J15+371 75
Billabong, R. See Moulamein
Billeroo, S. Australia C60-312 109
Billings, Montana V21+458 93
Billiton, I. See Belitung.
Bilma, Niger m12+184 81
Bilo Goro, Yugoslavia L78+458 56
Biloxi, Mississippi T84+304 95
Bilsi, India G67+282 73
Bilta, Norway L50+693 46
Bilthoven, Netherlands M59+t21 44
Bilugyun, I., Burma F45+164 71
Bilyarsk, U.S.S.R. J58+550 61
Bilzen, Belgium M55+509 44
Bimbe, Angola L84-120 82
Bimberi, Mt., New S. Wales C08-356 109
Bimlipatam, India G39+178 71
Binaiya, mt., Ceram I., Indon. D34-032 65
Binche, Belgium M65+504 44
Bindki, India G56+261 73
Bindura, Zimbabwe K82-172 84
Binefar, Spain M88+418 53
Bingara, New South Wales B86-299 109
Bingen, W. Germany M43+500 48
Bingerville, Ivory Coast N24+054 80
Bingham, England N06+529 37
Bingham, Maine S59+451 90
Bingham Canyon, Utah V43+406 94
Binghamton, New York T06+422 96
Bingiri, Zaire L28-054 82
Bingol, Turkey K28+390 74
Binh Dinh (An Nhon),
Vietnam E65+139 69
Binn, Switzerland M41+464 45
Binnaway, New S. Wales C06-315 109
Bint, Iran J03+263 75
Bintan, I.,
Riau Arch., Indonesia F02+011 65
Bintuni, Tk., New Guinea D12-024 65
Bir Ali, Yemen, South J70+140 74
Birao, Japan C40+423 68
Birchip, Victoria C43-360 109
Birchwood, New Zealand A73-459 112
Birdsboro, Pennsylvania T05+403 96
Birdsville, Queensland C64-278 111
Birdum,
N. Terr., Australia D11-156 110
Birecik, Turkey K42+371 74
Birein, Syria K50+350 76
Bir Fadhil, Saudi Arabia J61+222 74
Bir Gara, Chad L84+132 81
Birhan, mt., Ethiopia K42+108 83
Birjand, Iran J04+328 75
Birkao, Somalia K20-012 83
Birkenhead, England N18+534 37
Bir Malusi, Iraq K30+335 74
Bir Maqran, Saudi Arabia J61+217 74
Birmingham, Alabama T71+335 93
Birmingham, England N11+525 37
Birmingham, Michigan T49+426 91
Birney, Montana V10+452 93
Birni-n-Kebbi, Nigeria M64+122 80
Birni-n' Konni, Niger M58+136 80
Birobidzhan, U.S.S.R. D12+488 63
Birq, Saudi Arabia K21+181 74
Birr, Ireland, Rep. N47+531 43
Birrie, R., New South Wales C18-294 109
Birsilpur, India H16+282 72
Birsk, U.S.S.R. J28+554 61
Birzhay, Lithuania L31+562 47
Bisalpur, India G61+283 73
Bisauli, India G66+283 73
Bisbee, Arizona V29+314 94
Bisbee, N. Dakota U56+486 93
Biscay, B. of, France-Spain N24+460 50
Bischofszell, Switzerland M34+475 45
Biscoe, B., Antartica Y00-770 27
Biscoe, I., Antartica S40-660 27
Biscotasing, Ontario T43+472 91
Bisha, Saudi Arabia K09+201 74
Bishnath, India F71+266 71
Bishnupur, India G16+230 73
Bishop Mt., Wyoming V24+410 93
Bishop Auckland, England N10+547 37
Bishop's Falls, Nfd. R63+490 90
Bishops Stortford, England M89+519 39
Bishri, Jebel el, Syria K36+354 74
Bisisthal, Switzerland M37+469 45
Biskia, Ethiopia K46+154 83
Bismarck, N. Dakota U65+468 93
Bismarck Arch., Pacific Oc. C00-050 106
Bismarck C., Greenland P25+770 26
Bison, S. Dakota U75+455 93
Bissau, India G89+282 72
Bissau, Guinea-Bissau P04+118 80
Bissett, Ontario T18+462 91
Bistcho, L., Alberta V85+598 88
Bithur, India G58+266 73
Bitlis, Turkey K18+385 74
Bitola, Yugoslavia L52+411 58
Bitterfeld, E. Germany M16+516 48
Bitter Root Mts., Idaho V64+469 92
Bivio, Switzerland M32+465 45
Biwa Ko, Japan C84+352 68
Biysk, U.S.S.R. G27+526 62
Bizerte, Tunisia M32+372 81
Bjelóvar, Yugoslavia L79+459 56
Björkö, Sweden L66+599 47
Bjorli, Norway M41+623 46
Björna, Sweden L68+636 46
Bjørnør, Norway M29+642 46
Bjørnøya, I., Barents Sea L63+743 62
Black Hd., Ireland, Rep. N55+532 43
Black Hills, S. Dakota U85+442 98
Black Isle, Scotland N25+576 40
Black Mt., Pakistan H13+345 72
Black Mts., Arizona V57+358 92
Black Mts., Wales N19+519 38
Black Ra., New Mexico V17+330 94
Black R., Arkansas, etc. U08+360 95
Black Sea, Europe-Asia K60+440 30
Blackall, Queensland C27-242 111
Blackburn, England N15+537 37
Blackdown Hills, England N19+509 38
Blackfoot, Idaho V44+432 92
Blackpool, England N18+538 37
Blackriver, Michigan T50+448 91
Black River Falls, Wisconsin U05+443 91
Black Rock, Arkansas U07+361 97
Black Rock Des., Nevada V84+412 92
Blacksod B., Ireland, Rep. N61+541 42
Black Sugar Loaf, mt.,
New South Wales B81-314 109
Blackville, New Brunswick S35+467 90
Blackville, S. Carolina T38+333 97
Black Volta R., Ghana N14+094 80
Blackwater, Ireland, Rep. N38+524 43
Blackwater L., N.-W. Terr. W28+644 88
Blackwater Res., Scotland N29+567 41
Blackwater R.,
Cork, etc. Ireland, Rep. N47+520 43
Blackwater R.,
Meath, Ireland, Rep. N40+537 42
Blackwater R., N. Ireland N40+545 42
Blackwell, Oklahoma U44+368 95
Blaenavon, Wales N19+518 38
Blagoveshchensk, U.S.S.R. D44+504 63
Blagoveshchensk, U.S.S.R. J24+550 61
Blagoevgrad, Bulgaria L42+420 58
Blair, Nebraska U37+416 95
Blair Atholl, Scotland N23+568 41
Blairgowrie, Scotland N20+566 41
Blairmore, Alberta V56+496 88
Blaj, Romania L36+462 58
Blanc, C., Mauritania P12+208 80
Blanc, le, France M83+466 54
Blanc, Mt., France-Italy M48+458 54
Blanca, B., Argentina S10-394 103
Blanca Pk., Colorado V03+378 98
Blanca, Sierra, New Mexico V05+332 94
Blanche, L., S. Australia C62-292 109
Blanche Town, S. Australia C62-343 109
Blanchewater, S. Australia C63-295 109
Blanco, C., Oregon W28+428 92
Blanco Pico, Costa Rica T50+095 101
Bland, Virginia T37+371 97
Blandford, England N13+509 39
Blanes, Spain M73+417 53
Blaney Park, Michigan T65+462 91
Blangy, France M80+499 54
Blankenberge, Belgium M71+513 44
Blantyre-Limbe, Malawi K60-158 83
Blaregnies, Belgium M67+504 44
Blasket Sd., Ireland, Rep. N63+521 43
Blaton, Belgium M68+505 44
Blaye, France N04+451 55
Blayney, New South Wales C04-336 109
Blazowa, Poland L47+499 49
Blenheim, New Zealand A36-415 112
Blenheim, Ontario T42+424 91
Blessington, Ireland, Rep. N39+532 43
Blida, Algeria M72+364 80
Blind River, Ontario T48+462 91
Blinman, S. Australia C68-311 109
Blitta, Togo M84+084 80
Blitzen, Mt., Nevada V68+414 92
Block I., Rhode Island S70+412 96
Bloemfontein, O.F.S. L22-290 84
Blois, France M82+476 54
Blokzijl, Netherlands M54+527 44
Bloody Foreland,
Ireland, Rep. N50+552 42
Bloomfield, Iowa U14+408 95
Bloomington, Illinois T84+407 95
Bloomsburg, Pennsylvania T09+410 96
Blossburg, Pennsylvania T12+417 96
Blount Springs, Alabama T70+340 97
Blue Mt., India F72+227 71
Blue Mts., Jamaica T10+180 101
Blue Mts., New S. Wales B88-334 109
Blue Mts., Oregon V81+450 92
Blue Mts., Pennsylvania T04+407 96
Blue Earth, Minnesota U25+437 93
Bluefield, W. Virginia T37+373 97
Bluefields, Nicaragua T53+120 101
Blue Lake, Michigan T60+448 91
Blue Ridge, mts., U.S.A. T48+350 99
Blue Stack Mts.,
Ireland, Rep. N49+547 42
Bluff, New Zealand A70-466 112
Bluff, Utah V28+371 98
Bluff Knoll, W. Australia E15-344 110
Blumenau, Brazil R25-270 103
Blyth, England N09+551 37
Blytheville, Arkansas U00+359 95
Blyukherovsk, U.S.S.R. D70+552 63
Bo, Sierra Leone N70+082 80
Boac, Philippines D79+134 65
Boaco, Nicaragua T65+124 101
Boafé, Brazil S71-072 104
Boardman, N. Carolina T24+345 97
Boat of Garten, Scotland N22+572 40
Boa Vista, Brazil Q59-088 105
Boa Vista, Brazil S03+027 104
Boa Vista Tocantins, Brazil R15-064 105
Bobadah, New S. Wales C20-323 109
Bobi, Paraguay R67-269 103
Bobo Dioulasso, Upper Volta N26+112 80
Bobolice, Poland L81+539 49
Bobrov, U.S.S.R. K30+510 61
Bobruysk, Byelorussia L05+532 60
Bocas del Toro, Panama T43+094 101
Bocca do Curua, Brazil R56-054 105
Bocca do Tauary, Brazil S69-082 104
Bochnia, Poland L57+500 49
Bocholt, Belgium M57+512 44
Bocholt, W. Germany M50+519 48
Bochum, W. Germany M47+515 48
Bocota, Mozambique K70-228 84
Bodola, Zaire L48+018 82
Bodalla, New South Wales C00-361 109
Bodaybo, U.S.S.R. E34+578 63
Boden, Sweden L50+658 46
Boden See, Switzerland-
Germany M33+476 45
Boderg L., Ireland, Rep. N48+539 42
Bodmin & Moors, England N28+505 38
Bodø, Norway M04+672 46
Boela, Ceram I., Indonesia D27-032 65
Boende, Congo L56-004 82
Boentok, Borneo E31-016 65
Boeol, Celebes D82+011 65
Boertange, Netherlands M47+530 44
Bofin L., Ireland, Rep. N48+538 42
Bogalusa, Louisiana T89+308 95
Bogan, R., New S. Wales C18-312 109
Bogandé, Upper Volta N00+128 80
Bogan Gate, New S. Wales C14-331 109
Bogbonga, Zaire L64+014 82
Bogdarin, U.S.S.R. E39+544 63
Bogdo Ula, China G02+434 64
Boggabri, New South Wales C00-307 109
Boggeragh Mts.,
Ireland, Rep. N54+520 43
Boghari. See Ksar El Boukhari
Boghor Regis, England N04+508 39
Bogong, Mt., Victoria C16-367 109
Bogor, Java, Indonesia E80-065 65
Bogorodskoye, U.S.S.R. J67+524 61
Bogorodskoye, U.S.S.R. C57+525 63
Bogota, Colombia S83+046 104
Bogotol, U.S.S.R. G03+561 62
Bogra, Bangladesh G04+249 73
Bohemia, Czechoslovakia M06+496 48
Böhmer Wald, Germany-
Czechoslovakia M12+492 48
Bohol, I., Philippines D64+100 65
Boiestown, New Brunswick S38+465 90
Boigu, I., Papua
New Guinea C47-093 111
Boim, Brazil R61-027 105
Bois, L. des, N.-W. Terr. W17+668 88
Bois Blanc I., Michigan T57+458 91
Boisé, Idaho V68+436 92
Boise City, Oklahoma U75+368 94
Bois-le-Duc. See 'sHertogenbosch
Boissevain, Manitoba U60+493 88
Boké, Guinea N86+110 80
Bokhara, R., New S. Wales C16-294 109
Bokki, Cameroon M10+088 81
Bokn Fd., Norway M58+591 47
Bokoro, Chad L76+122 81
Bolan, Pakistan H42+295 70
Bolan Pass, Pakistan H46+296 70
Bolangir, India G38+206 71
Bolbee, France M87+496 54
Bole, Ghana N14+090 80
Bölebyn, Sweden L52+654 46
Bolgrad, Ukraine L08+457 60
Bolintin, Romania L25+444 58
Bolivar, Argentina S07-362 105
Bolivar, Colombia T11+018 104
Bolivar, Missouri U20+376 95
Bolivia, rep., S. America — 104
Bollstabruk, Sweden L74+630 46
Bolmen, L., Sweden M08+569 47
Bolobo, Zaire L82-022 82
Bologna, Italy M22+445 56
Bologoye, U.S.S.R. K66+578 60
Bolotnoye, U.S.S.R. G34+554 62
Bolsena, L. di, Italy M19+426 56
Bolshevik, Ostrov, U.S.S.R. F10+787 63
Bolshoy Lyakhovskiy, Ostrov,
U.S.S.R. C45+735 63
Boltaña, Spain N00+425 53
Bolton, England N15+536 37
Bolu, Turkey K82+408 74
Bolus Hd., Ireland, Rep. N62+518 43
Bolzano, Italy M22+465 56
Bomal, Belgium M57+504 44
Bomba, Gulf of, Libya L40+322 81
Bombala, New S. Wales C04-369 109
Bombarral, Portugal N55+393 52
Bombay, India H13+190 70
Bomfim, Brazil Q61-104 105
Bomfim, Brazil R22-166 105
Bomhus, Sweden L77+606 47
Bom Jardin, Brazil S63-067 104
Bom Jesus do Gurgueia,
Brazil Q86-092 105
Bømlo, I., Norway M59+597 47
Bomnak, U.S.S.R. D36+547 63
Bomoseen, L., Vermont S79+437 96
Bonaduz, Switzerland M33+468 45
Bonaire, I., Neth. Antilles S49+122 94
Bonar Bridge, Scotland N26+579 40
Bonaventure I., Quebec S25+485 90
Bonavista, Newfoundland R49+482 90
Bonavista B., Newfoundland R48+489 90
Bondo, Zaire L36+038 82
Bône ('Annaba), Algeria M44+368 81
Bone, G. of, Celebes D86-035 65
Bo'ness, Scotland N21+560 41
Bongor, Chad L88+104 81
Bonham, Texas U37+336 95
Bonifacio & B. de, Corsica M35+414 57
Bonn, W. Germany M48+507 48
Bonne Bay, Newfoundland R78+496 90

Bonne Terre, Missouri U04+379 97
Bonneval, France M82+482 54
Bonneville Salt Flats, Utah V54+410 94
Bonney, L., S. Aust. C58-376 109
Bonnie Rock, W. Australia E09-304 110
Bonny, France M73+475 54
Bonny, Nigeria M46+044 80
Book Plat., Colorado V20+397 94
Boolaboolka L., N.S.W. C40-326 109
Booleroo Centre, S. Australia C70-329 109
Booligal, New S. Wales C31-339 109
Boom, Belgium M64+511 44
Boone, Iowa U23+422 95
Boone, N. Carolina T40+362 97
Booneville, Mississippi T82+346 97
Boon Tsagan Nur, Mongolia F36+456 64
Boonville, Missouri U16+390 95
Boonville, New York T02+435 96
Boorindal, New S. Wales C23-304 109
Booroorban, New S. Wales C32-348 109
Boorowa, New S. Wales C08-344 109
Boort, Victoria C38-360 109
Boothia, G. of, N.-W. Terr. T70+700 89
Boothia Pen., N.-W. Terr. U20+706 89
Bootle, England N20+543 37
Bootle, England N18+534 37
Boqueron, Cuba T01+200 101
Boquete, Panama T45+088 101
Boramo, Somalia K10+100 83
Borås, Sweden M12+577 47
Borazjan, Iran J53+292 75
Borba, Brazil R88-044 104
Bordeaux, France N04+448 55
Borders, reg., Scotland N16+555 41
Bordertown, S. Australia C55-363 109
Borga, Sweden M00+648 46
Borge Fjell, Norway M08+653 46
Borger, Netherlands M49+529 44
Borger, Texas U68+357 94
Borgholm, Sweden L80+569 47
Borgne, Haiti S75+198 101
Borisoglebsk, U. S.S.R. K17+514 61
Borisov, Byelorussia L09+551 60
Bo River Post, Sudan L12+068 81
Borja, Spain N09+418 53
Borjas Blancas, Spain M83+415 53
Borkum I., W. Germany M49+536 48
Borlänge, Sweden L88+605 47
Borneo, Indonesia — 65
Bornholm, I., Denmark M00+551 47
Bor Nor, China E14+476 64
Borodino, U.S.S.R. K56+554 60
Borogontsy, U.S.S.R. D20+626 63
Borovë, Albania L57+397 59
Borovichi, U.S.S.R. K67+586 60
Borris, Ireland, Rep. N41+526 43
Borrisoleigh, Ireland, Rep. N48+527 43
Borroloola, N. Terr., Aust. C81-161 111
Borskoe, U.S.S.R. J50+530 61
Borūjerd, Iran J67+339 74
Borzya, U.S.S.R. E21+506 63
Bosco, Switzerland M39+463 45
Boscobel, Wisconsin U04+431 91
Bosiljgrad, Yugoslavia L45+425 58
Boskoop, Netherlands M62+521 44
Bosna-Hercegovina, Yugosl. L72+443 58
Boso Pen, Japan C57+353 68
Bosobolo, Zaire L60+040 82
Bosoli, Botswana L14-210 84
Bosporus, Turkey L06+413 74
Bossier City, Louisiana U22+325 95
Bosso, Niger M10+136 81
Bostan, Pakistan H48+304 70
Boston, England N00+530 37
Boston, Massachusetts S66+424 91
Boston Mts., Arkansas U24+358 95
Botany B., New S. Wales B84-340 109
Botera, Angola M04-118 82
Bothaville, O.F.S. L20-274 84
Bothnia, G. of, N.-W. Europe — 46-47
Botswana (Bechuanaland) L30-216 84
Bouaké, Ivory Coast N30+078 80
Bour, Cent. Afr. Rep. L86+060 81
Bou Arfa, Morocco N12+326 80
Bouches-du-Rhône, dep., Fr. M59+436 55
Bou Djébéha, Mali N16+184 80
Boudoukou, Ivory Coast N18+082 80
Boudry, Switzerland M49+470 45
Bougainville, I., Solomon Is. B60-060 106
Bougaroun C., Algeria M48+368 80
Bougie (Begaia), Algeria M60+366 80
Bougouni, Mali N46+114 80
Bouillon, Belgium M60+498 44
Boularderie I., Nova Scotia S03+463 90
Boulder, Colorado V02+400 94
Boulder, W. Australia D81-309 110
Boulder Mt., Idaho V56+440 98
Boulia, Queensland C61-227 111
Boulogne, France M80+508 54
Bouna, Ivory Coast N18+092 80
Boundary, Brit. Columbia W71+564 88
Bountiful, Utah V42+408 94
Bounty Is., Pacific Ocean A05-475 106
Bourbonnais, prov., France M71+465 54
Bourem, Mali N02+168 80
Bourg, France M59+462 54
Bourg Argental, France M63+453 55
Bourges, France M76+471 54
Bourget, L. du, France M55+457 54
Bourgogne, prov., France M61+471 54
Bourg St Pierre, Switz. M47+460 45
Bourke, New S. Wales C24-302 109
Bourkes, Ontario T31+483 91
Bournemouth, England N11+507 39
Bouvet I., Atlantic Ocean M70-540 27
Bovigny, Belgium M55+502 44
Bovino, Italy L88+413 57
Bow R., Alberta V44+502 88
Bowbells, N. Dakota U74+488 93
Bowen, Queensland C10-200 111
Bowen, C., N.-W. Terr. S88+720 89
Bowie, Texas U47+336 95
Bowling Green, Kentucky T68+370 97
Bowling Green, Missouri U08+394 95
Bowling Green, Ohio T52+414 91
Bowling Green, Virginia T14+380 97
Bowman, N. Dakota U81+462 93
Bowman B., N.-W. Terr. T00+656 89
Bowman I., Antarctica F20-650 27
Bowmanville, Ontario T22+439 91
Bowral, New South Wales B88-345 109
Bowser, Victoria C22-363 109
Box Elder, Montana V30+483 93
Boxholm, Sweden M00+582 47
Boxmeer, Netherlands M54+516 44
Box Tank, New S. Wales C47-322 109
Boxtel, Netherlands M58+516 44
Boydton, Virginia T20+367 97
Boyle, Ireland, Rep. N50+540 42
Boyne, R., Ireland, Rep. N38+537 42
Boyne City, Michigan T60+453 91
Boyoma Falls, Zaire L26+002 82
Bozeman, Montana V36+457 93
Bozoum, Cent. Afr. Rep. L82+062 81
Bra, Italy M43+447 56
Brabant, prov. Belgium M62+508 44
Brabant, Noord, prov., Neth. M60+516 44
Brac, I., Yugoslavia L80+433 56
Bracadale L., Scotland N39+573 40
Bracebridge, Ontario T26+450 91
Bräcke, Sweden L88+628 46
Bracknell, England N05+514 39
Brad, Romania L43+461 58
Braddock, N. Dakota U60+465 93
Braddock, Pennsylvania T29+404 96
Bradford, England N10+538 37
Bradford, Pennsylvania T22+419 96
Braemar, Scotland N20+570 40
Braeriach, Scotland N22+571 40
Braga, Portugal N51+416 52
Bragado, Argentina S03-352 103
Bragança, Brazil R11-011 105
Bragança, Portugal N41+418 52
Bragança Paulista, Brazil R10-228 105
Brahmanbaria, Bangladesh F83+240 71
Brahmaputra R., India F70+265 71
Braidwood, Illinois T79+413 91
Braidwood, New S. Wales C01-354 109
Brail, Switzerland M30+466 45
Brăila, Romania L12+452 58
Braine l'Alleud, Belgium M64+507 44
Braine le Comte, Belgium M65+506 44
Brainerd, Minnesota U25+463 93
Braintree, England M87+519 39
Brak, Libya M04+276 81
Brampton, Ontario T29+437 91
Branchville, S. Carolina T35+333 97
Brandenburg, E. Germany M15+524 48
Brandon, England M86+524 39
Brandon, Manitoba U59+498 88
Brandon B. and Head, Ireland, Rep. N61+523 43
Brandon Mt., Ireland, Rep. N42+525 43
Brandsen, Argentina R80-352 103
Brandvlei, Cape Province L56-304 84
Branford, Florida T48+300 97
Braniewa, Poland L61+544 49
Bransfield Str., Antarctica R60-620 27
Bransk, Poland L43+527 49
Brantford, Ontario T32+431 91
Brantôme, France M86+453 55
Branxholme, Victoria C49-379 109
Bras d'or L., Nova Scotia S05+459 90
Brasilia, Brazil R23-160 105
Brasov, Romania L27+456 58
Brassus, le, Switzerland M53+466 45
Bratislava, Czechoslovakia L78+482 49
Bratsk, U.S.S.R. F19+561 63
Brattleboro, Vermont S76+428 96
Braunau, Austria M12+482 48
Braunlage, W. Germany M26+517 48
Braunschweig, W. Germany M27+523 48
Braunwald, Switzerland M36+469 45
Brava, Somalia K06+012 83
Brawley, California V63+330 92
Bray & Hd., Ireland, Rep. N36+532 43
Bray Hd., Ireland, Rep. N63+519 43
Brazil, Indiana T73+395 95
Brazil, rep., S. America — 104-105
Brazos R., Texas U34+294 95
Brazos Santiago, Texas U43+260 96
Brazzaville, Congo L88-042 82
Brčko, Yugoslavia L67+449 58
Bream B., New Zealand A33-358 112
Brechin, Scotland N16+567 41
Breckenridge, Minnesota U40+463 93
Brecknock, Pen., Chile S70-546 103
Brecknock, See Powys
Břeclav, Czechoslovakia L79+488 49
Brecon, Wales N20+520 38
Brecon Beacons, Wales N20+519 38
Breda, Netherlands M61+516 44
Bredasdorp, Cape Province L60+346 84
Bredene, Belgium M72+512 44
Bredoo, New South Wales C06-360 109
Bredy, U.S.S.R. H89+525 61
Bree, Belgium M56+511 44
Breidha fjördhur, Iceland P54+652 46
Breil, France M45+439 55
Breithorn, mt., Switzerland M43+465 45
Brejo, Brazil Q77-036 105
Bremangerland, Norway M60+618 46
Bremen, W. Germany M37+531 48
Bremerhaven, W. Germany M39+536 48
Bremerton, Washington W16+475 92
Bremgarten, Switzerland M40+474 45
Brenham, Texas U38+302 95
Brenner Pass, Austria-Italy M21+470 56
Breno, Italy M28+459 56
Brent, Ontario T21+461 91
Brentford, England N02+515 39
Brentwood, England M88+516 39
Brescia, Italy M29+455 56
Breskens, Netherlands M69+514 44
Breslau. See Wroclaw
Bressay I., Scotland N06+601 40
Bressuire, France N03+468 54
Brest, France N27+484 54
Brest, Byelorussia L38+521 60
Brest-Litovsk. See Brest
Bretagne, prov., France N17+480 54
Bretcu, Romania L22+460 58
Breton Sd., Louisiana T74+295 95
Breugel, Netherlands M57+515 44
Brevard, N. Carolina T46+352 97
Breves, Brazil R33-116 105
Brevik, Norway M32+590 47
Brewarrina, New S. Wales C19-300 109
Brewer, Maine S52+448 90
Brewster Mt., Antarctica A75-730 27
Brewton, Alabama T72+311 97
Brežice, Yugoslavia L86+459 56
Březová, Czechoslovakia L75+486 49
Brezova, Czechoslovakia L81+496 49
Bria, Cent. Afr. Rep. L48+066 81
Briançon, France M50+449 55
Briare, France M73+476 54
Bribbaree, New S. Wales C12-341 109
Bridgehampton, New York S74+409 96
Bridgend, Wales N21+515 38
Bridgeport, Connecticut S79+412 91
Bridgeport, Nebraska U79+418 94
Bridgeport L., Texas U48+332 95
Bridgeton, New Jersey T01+395 96
Bridgetown, Nova Scotia S31+449 90
Bridgman C., Arctic Ocean Q00+840 26
Bridgnorth, England N15+525 38
Bridgton, Maine S64+440 90
Bridgwater & B., England N18+511 38
Bridlington & B., England N01+541 37
Bridport, Tasmania C16-410 109
Brielle, Netherlands M65+519 44
Brienz, Switzerland M42+468 45
Brienzer See, Switzerland M42+467 45
Brier I., Nova Scotia S38+443 90
Brig, Switzerland M42+463 45
Brigels, Switzerland M36+468 45
Brigham, Utah V42+415 94
Bright, Victoria C18-367 109
Brightlingsea, England M84+518 39
Brighton, Colorado U89+400 94
Brighton, England N01+508 39
Brighton, S. Australia C69-351 109
Brighton, Tasmania C16-427 109
Brignoles, France M54+434 55
Brindaban, India G74+275 72
Brindisi, Italy L72+406 57
Brinkley, Arkansas U08+349 97
Brinkworth, S. Australia C70-337 109
Brione, Switzerland M37+463 45
Brioude, France M70+453 55
Brisbane, Queensland B71-274 111
Brissago, Switzerland M38+461 45
Bristol, England N15+515 38
Bristol, New Brunswick S45+465 90
Bristol, Pennsylvania T00+401 96
Bristol, Rhode Island S68+417 96
Bristol, Tennessee T43+366 97
Bristol B., Alaska Y60+580 99
Bristol Channel, England N23+513 38
Bristol I., South Sandwich Is. P80-580 27
British Columbia, prov. Canada — 88
British Guiana, See Guyana
British Honduras, See Belize
British Isles, N.-W. Europe — 34
Brito, Nicaragua T65+114 101
Britonto, Italy L79+411 57
Britstown, Cape Province L38-306 84
Brive-la-Gaillarde, France M81+452 55
Briviesca, Spain N20+425 52
Brno, Czechoslovakia L80+492 49
Broach, India H12+216 70
Broad B., Scotland N37+582 40
Broadalbin, New York S85+431 91
Broadford, Pennsylvania T27+401 96
Broadford, Scotland N36+572 40
Broadhaven, Ireland, Rep. N60+543 42
Broadus, Montana V02+455 93
Brock I., N.-W. Territories V50+776 88
Brockton, Massachusetts S66+421 96
Brockville, Ontario T04+446 91
Brod, Yugoslavia L53+415 58
Brodeur Pen., N.-W. Terr. T75+723 89
Brodhead, Wisconsin T86+427 91
Brodick, Scotland N31+556 41
Brodribb, Victoria C08-377 109
Broek-in-Waterland, Netherlands M60+524 44
Broglio, Switzerland M38+464 45
Broken B., New S. Wales B83-336 109
Broken Bow, Nebraska U58+414 95
Broken Hill, Zambia L10-144 83
Broken Hill, New S. Wales C51-319 109
Bromberg. See Bydgoszcz
Bromley, England N00+514 39
Bromptonville, Quebec S72+455 91
Brønnøysund, Norway M16+655 46
Bronte, Sicily M01+378 57
Brookfield, Missouri U18+498 95
Brookhaven, Mississippi U02+316 95
Brookings, Oregon W26+421 92
Brookings, S. Dakota U40+444 93
Brooklyn, Iowa U14+417 95
Brooklyn, New York S84+406 96
Brooklyn, Nova Scotia S28+441 90
Brooks Ra., Alaska Y50+674 99
Brook's Point, Philippines E13+089 65
Brookville, Pennsylvania T25+411 96
Broom L., Scotland N31+579 40
Broome, W. Australia D76-178 110
Brora, Scotland N23+580 40
Brosna R., Ireland, Rep. N48+532 43
Brough Hd., Orkney, Scot. N20+592 40
Broughton, England N19+543 37
Broughty Ferry, Scotland N17+565 41
Broumov, Czechoslovakia L82+506 49
Brouwershaven, Netherlands M67+517 44
Brown, Mt., S. Australia C72-325 109
Brown's Valley, Minnesota U41+456 93
Brownsville, Kentucky T68+372 97
Brownsville, Tennessee T86+356 97
Brownsville, Texas U45+259 94
Brownville, Maine S54+453 90
Brownwood, Texas U54+316 95
Brownwood, L., Texas U55+318 95
Broxburn, Scotland N21+559 41
Brozas, Spain N41+396 52
Bruce Coast, Antarctica P25-730 27
Bruce Mt., W. Australia E08-226 110
Bruce Mines, Ontario T53+463 91
Bruck an der Mur, Austria M13+473 48
Bruff, Ireland, Rep. N51+525 43
Bruges, Belgium M71+512 44
Brugg, Switzerland M41+475 45
Brugge, See Bruges
Bruin Pk., Utah V32+396 94
Bruly, Belgium M63+500 44
Brummen, Netherlands M53+521 44
Brunei & state, Borneo E31+050 65
Brunette Downs, N.T., Aust. C85-184 111
Brunflo, Sweden M01+631 46
Brunn. See Brno
Brunner, New Zealand A52-425 112
Brunssum, Netherlands M54+509 44
Brunswick. See Braunschweig
Brunswick, Georgia T39+312 97
Brunswick, Maine S60+439 90
Brunswick, Maryland T15+393 96
Brunswick B., W. Australia D61-152 110
Brunswick, Pen. de, Chile S70-535 103
Bruny I., Tasmania C16-434 109
Brusa. See Bursa
Brusartsi, Bulgaria L42+437 58
Brush, Colorado U82+402 94
Brusio, Switzerland M29+463 45
Brussel (Brussels). See Bruxelles
Bruthen, Victoria C13-377 109
Bruxelles (Brussels), Belgium M64+508 44
Bruzual, Venezuela S56+079 104
Bryan Coast, Antarctica T30-750 27
Bryansk, U.S.S.R. K64+533 60
Bryce Canyon Nat. Park, Ut. V47+377 92
Brynmawr, Wales N19+518 38
Bryson, Quebec T10+457 91
Bryson City, N. Carolina T51+354 97
Brzeg, Poland L75+509 49
Brzesko, Poland L56+500 49
Bsharri, Lebanon K54+343 76
Bua, Angola M10-072 82
Buayan, Philippines D59+061 65
Bubasa, Ethiopia K16+088 83
Bubiyan I., The Gulf J71+298 74
Bubulu, Uganda K64+008 83
Bucaramanga, Colombia S79+072 104
Buchach, Ukraine L27+491 60
Buchan, Victoria C11-374 109
Buchan Ness, Scotland N11+575 40
Buchanan, L., Queensland C25-216 111
Buchanan L., Texas U51+308 95
Buchardo, Argentina S21-347 103
Bucharest. See Bucuresti
Buchs, Switzerland M33+472 45
Buckhannon, West Virginia T31+389 91
Buckie, Scotland N18+577 40
Buckingham, Quebec T03+456 91
Buckingham & co., England N06+520 39
Buckley, New Zealand A10-384 112
Bucksport, Maine S53+446 90
Buctouche, New Brunswick S28+465 90
Bucuresti, Romania L23+444 58
Bud, Norway M48+630 46
Buda, Texas U47+301 95
Budaia, Saudi Arabia K10+230 74
Budapest, Hungary L66+475 49
Budaun, India G65+282 73
Bud Bud, India G14+233 73
Buddh Gaya, India G30+247 73
Bude, England N27+508 38
Budesti, Romania L21+442 58
Budhana, India G76+293 72
Budleigh Salterton, England N20+506 38
Budva, Yugoslavia L67+423 58
Buea, Cameroon M36+042 81
Buenaventura, Colombia T12+040 104
Buena Vista, Georgia T57+323 97
Buena Vista, Virginia T26+377 97
Buenos Aires, Argentina R81-346 103
Buenos Aires, Colombia S60-032 104
Buenos Aires, L., Chile-Argentina S76-465 103
Bufa, mt., Mexico U89+207 100
Buffalo, Minnesota U23+452 93
Buffalo, Missouri U19+377 97
Buffalo, New York T23+429 91
Buffalo L., N.-W. Terr. V63+602 88
Buffalo, S. Dakota U82+456 93
Buffalo, Wyoming V10+444 93
Buff City, Tennessee T44+365 97
Bufumine, Chad L84+150 81
Bug. R., Poland, etc. L51+525 49
Buga, Colombia T08+038 104
Bugulma, U.S.S.R. J43+545 61
Buguruslan, U.S.S.R. J46+536 61
Builth Wells, Wales N20+521 38
Buinsk, U.S.S.R. J70+550 61
Buique, Brazil Q43-086 105
Buitenpost, Netherlands M53+532 44
Bujumbura, Burundi L04-034 83
Buka, I., Solomon Is. B60-050 106
Bukama, Zaire L24-092 82
Bukavu, Zaire L06-026 83
Bukene, Tanzania K74-042 83
Bukhara, Uzbek H64+398 62
Bukoba, Tanzania K78-014 83
Bukwimba, Tanzania K70-028 83
Bülach, Switzerland M39+475 45
Bulagan, Mongolia F09+488 64
Bulan, Philippines D67+125 65
Bulandshahr, India G73+284 72
Bulawayo, Zimbabwe L08-202 84
Bulgaria, Europe L30+425 51
Bulinski, U.S.S.R. D70+680 63
Bullange, Belgium M52+504 44
Buller, Mt., Victoria C21-371 109
Buller R., New Zealand A48-418 112
Bulli, New S. Wales B84-343 109
Bulloo Cr., Queensland C40-280 111
Bull Shoals Res., Arkansas U17+365 95
Bulnes, Chile S74-366 103
Bulo Burti, Somalia J86+038 83
Bulsar, India H12+206 70
Bulu, mt., Borneo E25+028 65
Bulun, U.S.S.R. D46+709 63
Bulun Tokhor, China G15+470 64
Bumba, Zaire L44+020 82
Buna, Kenya K30-012 83
Buna, Papua New Guinea C10-087 111
Bunbury, W. Australia E26-332 110
Bunclody, Ireland, Rep. N40+526 43
Buncrana, Ireland, Rep. N45+551 42
Bundaberg, Queensland B76-248 111
Bundarra, New S. Wales B84-302 109
Bundi, India G86+254 70
Bundoran, Ireland, Rep. N50+545 42
Bungay, England M81+525 39
Bungo, Angola L86-074 82
Bungo Str., Japan D16+330 68
Buninyong, Victoria C37-377 109
Bunker, Missouri U08+374 97
Bunkie, Louisiana U13+309 95
Bunschoten, Netherlands M58+522 44
Buochs, Switzerland M39+470 45
Buolkalakh, U.S.S.R. E02+731 63

Buorkhaya, Guba, U.S.S.R. D20+720 **63**
Buq, Iran H81+286 **75**
Buraida, Saudi Arabia K05+265 **74**
Bur Akaba, Somalia K06+026 **83**
Buram, Sudan L30+108 **81**
Burao, Somalia J86+094 **83**
Buraq, Syria K51+332 **76**
Burazjun, Iran J35+299 **75**
Burchun, China G19+477 **64**
Burd, Jebel, Saudi Arabia K35+272 **74**
Burdekin, R., Queensland C20-200 **111**
Burdur, Turkey K88+377 **74**
Burdwan, India G12+232 **73**
Bureå, Sweden L53+646 **46**
Bureinskiy Khrebet, U.S.S.R. D10+500 **63**
Bureir, Israel K62+316 **76**
Büren, Switzerland M46+471 **45**
Bureya, U.S.S.R. D31+496 **63**
Burg, Den, Netherlands M68+517 **44**
Burgas, Bulgaria L15+425 **58**
Burgaw, N. Carolina T18+346 **97**
Burgdorf, Switzerland M44+471 **45**
Burgenland, prov., Austria L82+473 **49**
Burgess Hill, England N01+509 **39**
Burghersdorp, Cape Province L22-310 **84**
Burgos, Spain N22+423 **52**
Burhanpur, India G82+213 **70**
Buria, India G76+302 **72**
Burity, Brazil Q78-039 **105**
Burkesville, Kentucky T62+368 **97**
Burketown, Queensland C63-176 **111**
Burkeville, Virginia T19+372 **97**
Burks Falls, Ontario T26+457 **91**
Burley, Idaho V54+426 **94**
Burlington, Colorado U74+392 **94**
Burlington, Iowa U07+408 **95**
Burlington, New Jersey S89+402 **96**
Burlington, Ontario T29+434 **91**
Burlington, Vermont S79+445 **91**
Burlington, Wisconsin T80+427 **95**
Burlyuk, U.S.S.R. K68+448 **80**
Burma, S. Asia F50+210 **31**
Burnak, U.S.S.R. K21+518 **61**
Burnham, England N18+512 **38**
Burnham-on-Crouch, Eng. M85+516 **39**
Burnie, Tasmania C25-411 **109**
Burnley, England N14+538 **37**
Burns, New South Wales C54-321 **109**
Burns, Oregon V85+436 **92**
Burnside R., N.-W. Terr. V25+661 **88**
Burntisland, Scotland N19+561 **41**
Burra, S. Australia C66-336 **109**
Burren Junction, N.S.W. C06-301 **109**
Burriana, Spain N01+399 **53**
Burrinjuck & Res., N.S.W. C09-350 **109**
Burrow Hd., Scotland N26+547 **41**
Burrundie, N. Terr., Aust. D19-134 **110**
Burry Port & Inlet, Wales N26+517 **38**
Bursa, Turkey L06+402 **74**
Burt L., Michigan T58+455 **91**
Burton-in-Kendal, England N16+542 **37**
Burtonport, Ireland, Rep. N50+549 **42**
Burton-upon-Trent, England N10+528 **37**
Burträsk, Sweden L56+645 **46**
Burtundy, New S. Wales C47-337 **109**
Buru I., Indonesia D50-034 **65**
Burullus L., Egypt K86+314 **81**
Burum, Yemen, South J66+143 **74**
Burundi, Cent. Africa L00-035 **83**
Burunurt, Mongolia E39+467 **64**
Bury, England N14+536 **37**
Buryatskaya A.S.S.R., U.S.S.R. E60+527 **63**
Bury St Edmunds, England M86+522 **39**
Busembatia, Uganda K68+006 **83**
Bushehr (Bushire), Iran J54+289 **75**
Bushmills, N. Ireland N39+552 **42**
Bushnell, Florida T43+286 **97**
Busra, Syria K51+325 **76**
Bussa, Nigeria M62+102 **80**
Bussaco, Portugal N50+404 **52**
Busselton, W. Australia E28-338 **110**
Bussum, Netherlands M59+523 **44**
Bustam, Iran J30+365 **75**
Buta, Zaire L30+028 **82**
Butana, India G80+292 **72**
Buta Ranquil, Argentina S59-370 **103**
Butaritari, I., Kiribati A40+040 **106**
Bute, S. Australia C72-339 **109**
Bute I., Scotland N31+558 **41**
Bütgenbach, Belgium M53+504 **44**
Buthidaung, Burma F74+210 **71**
Butler, Missouri U26+382 **95**
Butler, Pennsylvania T29+409 **91**
Butschwil, Switzerland M35+474 **45**
Butte, Montana V45+460 **92**
Buttes, Switzerland M51+469 **45**
Buttevant, Ireland, Rep. N52+522 **43**
Button Is., Quebec S27+606 **89**
Butuan, Philippines D57+090 **65**
Butung I., Indonesia D73-050 **65**
Buturlinovka, U.S.S.R. K26+508 **61**
Buxar, India G36+255 **73**
Buxton, England N11+533 **37**
Buy, U.S.S.R. K21+586 **60**
Buyaga, U.S.S.R. D47+597 **63**
Buyr Nuur, lake, Mongolia E15+475 **63**
Buzancais, France M82+469 **54**
Buzău, Romania L19+451 **58**
Buzuluk, U.S.S.R. J46+528 **61**
Buzzards B., Massachusetts S65+416 **96**
Bwahit, mt., Ethiopia K40+132 **83**
Byam Martin Channel North-West Territories V00+762 **88**
Bydgoszcz, Poland L72+531 **49**
Byelaya, R., U.S.S.R. J36+558 **61**
Byelokatay, U.S.S.R. J06+557 **61**
Byelorussia (White Russia) U.S.S.R. L12+540 **60**
Byelyy, Os., U.S.S.R. H30+730 **62**
Bygland, Norway M43+588 **47**
Byglandsfjord, Norway M43+586 **47**
Bylot, I., N.-W. Territories T20+728 **89**
Byng Inlet, Ontario T34+457 **91**
Byrock, New S. Wales C22-306 **109**
Byron, C., New S. Wales B68-286 **111**
Byske, Sweden L53+649 **46**
Bytom, Poland L66+504 **49**
Bytow, Poland L75+542 **49**
Caaguazu, Paraguay R66-254 **103**
Caballo Res., New Mexico V14+330 **94**
Caballo Cocha, Peru S63-038 **104**
Caballos, Sierra de los, New Mexico V13+329 **94**
Cabañas, Cuba T47+229 **101**
Cabanatuan, Philippines D84+155 **65**
Cabar, Yugoslavia M02+456 **56**
Cabedello, Brazil Q28-070 **105**
Cabellos, Uruguay R74-307 **103**
Cabezas, Bolivia S20-188 **104**
Cabezo del Buey, Spain N31+387 **52**
Cabinda, Angola M16-050 **82**
Cabonga Res., Quebec T10+473 **91**
Cabot Hd., Ontario T38+453 **91**
Cabot Str., Nfd., etc. S00+475 **90**
Cabo Blanco, Argentina S35-472 **103**
Cabo Frio, Brazil Q75-226 **105**
Cabosa I., Burma F43+128 **71**
Cabo Verde, Arquipelago de, See Cape Verde Is.
Cabra, Spain N27+375 **52**
Cabrera I., Balearic Is., Spain M72+391 **53**
Cabrobo, Brazil Q56-086 **105**
Cabuérniga, Spain N26+432 **52**
Cabure, Venezuela S58+112 **104**
Caćak, Yugoslavia L58+439 **58**
Cacapon R., W. Virginia T21+394 **96**
Cacequy, Brazil R58-299 **103**
Cáceres, Spain N38+394 **52**
Cachinal, Chile S57-250 **103**
Cachipoque, Angola L64-120 **82**
Cachoeira, Brazil Q54-127 **105**
Cachoeira do Iguacu, Arg. R58-257 **103**
Cachoeira do Sul, Brazil R47-300 **103**
Caconda, Angola M00-138 **82**
Cacouna, Quebec S57+479 **90**
Cadaqués, Spain M71+423 **53**
Caddo L., Louisiana U24+328 **95**
Cadereyta, Mexico U60+256 **100**
Cader Idris, Wales N24+527 **38**
Cadillac, Michigan T63+443 **91**
Cadiz, Spain N38+365 **52**
Cadiz, Gulf of, Spain N43+368 **52**
Caen, France N02+492 **54**
Caerleon, Wales N18+516 **38**
Caernarvon B., Wales N27+525 **38**
Caernarvon, Wales N26+531 **38**
Caerphilly, Wales N19+516 **38**
Cagayan de Oro, Philippines D62+084 **65**
Cagayan Sulu, I., Phil. E09+071 **65**
Cagliari & G. di, Sardinia M35+392 **56**
Caguas, Puerto Rico S36+183 **101**
Caha Mts., Ireland, Rep. N59+517 **43**
Cahir, Ireland, Rep. N48+524 **43**
Cahirsiveen, Ireland, Rep. N61+519 **43**
Cahore Pt., Ireland, Rep. N37+526 **43**
Cahors, France M81+444 **55**
Caibarien, Cuba T27+226 **101**
Caicara, Bolivar, Venezuela S37+074 **104**
Caicara, Brazil S31-032 **104**
Caicara, Monagas, Venezuela S22+098 **104**
Caicos Is., Bahama Is. S70+216 **101**
Caihaique, Chile S70-454 **103**
Cailloma, Peru S70-152 **104**
Caillou B., Louisiana U06+291 **95**
Caimanera, Cuba T02+200 **101**
Caird Coast, Antarctica P40-750 **27**
Cairn Gorm, Scotland N22+571 **40**
Cairns, Queensland C25-168 **111**
Cairn Toul, Scotland N22+570 **40**
Cairo, Egypt K82+300 **81**
Cairo, Georgia T55+308 **97**
Cairo, Illinois T85+370 **95**
Caister, England M80+527 **39**
Caistor, England N02+535 **37**
Caiza, Bolivia S21-217 **104**
Cajamarca, Peru T21-072 **104**
Čakovec, Yugoslavia L82+464 **56**
Cala, Spain N38+380 **52**
Calabar, Nigeria M40+050 **80**
Calabozo, Venezuela S44+089 **104**
Calabria, dep., Italy L80+391 **57**
Calacoto, Bolivia S53-172 **104**
Calafat, Romania L42+440 **58**
Calafate, Argentina S70-503 **103**
Calais, France M79+510 **54**
Calais, Maine S44+452 **90**
Calama, Brazil S17-079 **104**
Calama, Chile S53-224 **103**
Calamar, Colombia S89+102 **104**
Calamar, Colombia S71+019 **104**
Calamian Group, Phil. E00+120 **65**
Calamocha, Spain N08+409 **53**
Calang, Sumatra F57+047 **65**
Calaoria. See Reggio
Calatayud, Spain N10+414 **53**
Calava C., Sicily M00+382 **57**
Calbuco, Chile S79-417 **103**
Calcasieu L., Louisiana U20+296 **95**
Calceta, Ecuador T31-008 **104**
Calchaqui, Argentina S02-299 **103**
Calcutta, India G09+226 **73**
Caldas da Rainha, Portugal N55+394 **52**
Calder R., England N10+537 **37**
Caldera, Chile S65-271 **103**
Caldwell, Idaho V70+437 **92**
Caldwell, Texas U40+305 **95**
Caledonia, Minnesota U09+436 **93**
Calella, Spain M73+416 **53**
Calenzana, Corsica M38+369 **55**
Caleta Buena, Chile S61-199 **103**
Caleta Olivia, Argentina S45-464 **103**
Calgary, Alberta V54+510 **88**
Cali, Colombia T09+036 **104**
Calicut, India G86+114 **70**
California, G. of, Mexico V40+280 **100**
California, state, U.S.A. V17+404 **98**
Calimali, Mexico V50+282 **100**
Calingasta, Argentina S57-313 **103**
Calla, Spain N08+405 **53**
Callabonna & L., S. Aust. C59-298 **109**
Callan, Ireland, Rep. N44+525 **43**
Callander, Ontario T26+462 **91**
Callander, Scotland N25+562 **41**
Callanna, S. Australia C73-296 **109**
Callao, Peru T13-120 **104**
Calmon, Brazil R36-267 **103**
Calmpthout, Belgium M63+514 **44**
Calpulalpam, Mexico U74+221 **100**
Caltagirone, Sicily M03+372 **57**
Caltanissetta, Sicily M06+375 **57**
Calulo, Angola M00-100 **82**
Calumet I., Quebec T10+458 **91**
Calunda, Angola L40-122 **82**
Calvados, dep., France N03+490 **54**
Calverton, Virginia T16+386 **97**
Calvillo, Mexico U77+218 **100**
Calvinia, Cape Province L60-316 **84**
Camabatela, Angola L88-084 **82**
Camaguey, Cuba T18+212 **101**
Camaguey, Is. de, Cuba T18+223 **101**
Camana, Peru S77-166 **104**
Camara, Brazil S16-038 **104**
Camarat C., France M50+432 **55**
Camargo, Bolivia S31-206 **104**
Camargo, Mexico U52+262 **100**
Camargo, Mexico V01+277 **100**
Camarones & B., Argentina S35-448 **103**
Camataqui, Bolivia S32-210 **104**
Ca-Mau, Vietnam E89+092 **69**
Ca-Mau, Vietnam F01+086 **69**
Camaxilo, Angola L66-084 **82**
Cambados, Spain N53+425 **52**
Cambay, India H14+223 **70**
Cambay, G. of, See Khambat
Cambell River, B.C. W32+500 **88**
Cambodia, S. E. Asia F00+120 **69**
Cambodia, C. See Ca-mau, Pt.
Cambrai, France M71+502 **54**
Cambrian Mts., Wales N22+525 **38**
Cambridge, Massachusetts S67+424 **96**
Cambridge, New Zealand A27-379 **112**
Cambridge and Isle of Ely, co. England N00+524 **37**
Camden, Arkansas U17+336 **95**
Camden, Maine S54+443 **90**
Camden, New Jersey T01+399 **96**
Camden, New South Wales B86-340 **109**
Camden, New York T04+433 **91**
Camden, S. Carolina T34+343 **97**
Camden Haven, N.S.W. B74-317 **109**
Camedo, Switzerland M38+462 **45**
Cameron, Missouri U26+398 **95**
Cameron, Texas U42+308 **95**
Cameron Mts., New Zealand A78-460 **112**
Camerota, Italy L88+400 **57**
Cameroon, W. Africa M16+050 **82**
Cameta, Brazil R27-022 **105**
Camilla, Georgia T55+312 **97**
Camina, Chile S57-194 **103**
Caminha, Portugal N53+418 **52**
Caminreal, Spain N08+408 **53**
Camoa, Mexico V25+276 **100**
Camocim, Brazil Q65-030 **105**
Camooweal, Queensland C71-200 **111**
Camorta I., Nicobar Is. F69+081 **71**
Campana, Argentina R84-341 **103**
Campana, I., Chile T02-482 **103**
Campania, dep., Italy M01+411 **57**
Campas, Mexico V28+300 **100**
Campbell, Missouri U00+365 **97**
Campbell B., N.-W. Terr. U85+676 **88**
Campbell I., Pacific Ocean A62-528 **106**
Campbell Mt., Yukon X21+646 **88**
Campbellford, Ontario T17+443 **91**
Campbellpore, Pakistan H16+338 **72**
Campbellton, N.B. S40+480 **90**
Campbelltown, N.S.W. B85-341 **109**
Campbell Town, Tasmania C15-419 **109**
Campbeltown, Scotland N33+554 **41**
Campeche & state, Mexico U03+198 **100**
Campeche, G. of, Mexico U24+190 **100**
Camperdown, Victoria C41-383 **109**
Campiglia Marittima, Italy M27+431 **56**
Campillos, Spain N28+370 **52**
Campina Grande, Brazil Q35-074 **105**
Campinas, Brazil R12-228 **105**
Campobasso, Italy M02+416 **57**
Campo Belo, Brazil T02-210 **105**
Campobello I., N.B S42+449 **90**
Campo Formosa, Brazil Q62-104 **105**
Campo Formoso, Brazil R20-170 **105**
Campo Gallo, Argentina S18-266 **103**
Campo Grande, Brazil R59-206 **105**
Campo Largo, Brazil Q87-116 **105**
Campo Maior, Brazil Q73-048 **105**
Campo Maior, Portugal N42+390 **52**
Campos, Brazil Q67-217 **105**
Campo Sales, Brazil Q63-070 **105**
Campos Novos, Brazil R38-274 **103**
Campsie Fells, Scotland N25+560 **41**
Campulung, Romania L30+453 **58**
Camrose, Alberta V46+532 **88**
Camsell Mt., N.-W. Terr. W21+617 **88**
Canaan, New Brunswick S30+463 **90**
Canaan, New Hampshire S72+436 **91**
Canada, North America **88-89**
Cañada de Gomez, Argent. S09-327 **103**
Canadian, Texas U62+359 **94**
Canadian Channel, Quebec S18+499 **90**
Canadian R., Oklahoma, etc U67+359 **98**
Cañadon de las Vacas Arg. S56-506 **103**
Canakkale, Turkey L22+401 **74**
Canama, Brazil S72-056 **104**
Canandaigua, New York T14+429 **96**
Canandaigua L., New York T14+428 **96**
Cananea, Mexico V33+310 **100**
Cananeia, Brazil R18-250 **103**
Canarias, Islas, Atlantic Oc. P00+280 **80**
Canarreos, Arch. de los, Cuba T44+220 **101**
Canary Is. See Canarias, Islas
Canas, Portugal N47+405 **52**
Canaseraga, New York T17+425 **96**
Canatlan, Mexico U89+244 **100**
Cañaveral, Spain N38+398 **52**
Canaveral, C., Florida T34+284 **99**
Cañaveras, Spain N15+404 **53**
Canavieiras, Brazil Q54-156 **105**
Canbelego, N. South Wales C22-316 **109**
Canberra, Cap. Terr., Aust. C06-353 **109**
Canby, Minnesota U38+447 **93**
Candasnos, Spain N00+415 **53**
Candelo, New South Wales C02-368 **109**
Candia. See Iráklion
Canea. See Khania
Canella, Brazil R35-294 **103**
Canelones, Uruguay R67-345 **103**
Canete, Chile S80-378 **103**
Canete, Peru T09-131 **104**
Cañete, Spain N10+400 **53**
Cangamba, Angola L60-136 **82**
Cangandala, Angola L81-098 **82**
Cangas, Spain N39+431 **52**
Canguaretama, Brazil Q31-064 **105**
Canha, Portugal N52+388 **52**
Canicatti, Sicily M07+373 **57**
Çankiri, Turkey K68+406 **74**
Canna, I., Scotland N40+571 **40**
Cannanore, India G88+120 **70**
Cannelton, Indiana T71+379 **97**
Cannes, France M48+435 **55**
Cannock, England N12+527 **38**
Cannon Ball, N. Dakota U64+464 **93**
Canonba, New South Wales C16-313 **109**
Canon City, Colorado V02+384 **94**
Canora, Saskatchewan U74+514 **88**
Canosa, Italy L84+412 **57**
Canowindra, New S. Wales C08-336 **109**
Canso & C., Nova Scotia S06+454 **90**
Canso, Str. of, Nova Scotia S07+455 **90**
Cantabrica, Cord., Spain N24+429 **52**
Cantal, dep., France M73+452 **55**
Cantanhede, Portugal N52+403 **52**
Canterbury, England M84+513 **39**
Canterbury, New Brunswick S45+459 **90**
Canterbury Bight, N.Z. A46-440 **112**
Canterbury Plains, N.Z. A50-440 **112**
Can Tho, Vietnam E85+100 **69**
Canton (Kwangchow), China E40+232 **67**
Canton, Mississippi U00+326 **95**
Canton, New York T01+446 **91**
Canton, Ohio T38+408 **91**
Canton, S. Dakota U40+432 **93**
Canton I., Phoenix Is. Z42-030 **106**
Canton Res., Oklahoma U52+362 **95**
Canuelas, Argentina R83-351 **103**
Canutama, Brazil S27-066 **104**
Canyon de Chelly Nat. Mon., Arizona V26+362 **94**
Capabarida, Venezuela S63+112 **104**
Capakcur. See Bingol.
Capana, Brazil S10-058 **104**
Capao Bonito, Brazil R21-240 **103**
Cap Chat, Quebec S40+491 **90**
Cap de la Madeleine, Quebec S75+464 **91**
Cape Barren I., Tasmania C12-404 **109**
Cape Breton I., Nova Scotia S06+460 **90**
Cape Breton Highlands Nat. Park, Nova Scotia S04+470 **90**
Cape Charles, Virginia T06+372 **97**
Cape Clear, Ireland, Rep. N57+514 **43**
Cape Coast, Ghana N08+052 **80**
Cape Cod B., Massachusetts S61+419 **96**
Cape Fear R., N. Carolina T22+346 **97**
Cape Girardeau, Missouri T88+373 **95**
Cape Haitien, Haiti S73+198 **101**
Cape May, New Jersey T00+389 **96**
Cape May Court House, New Jersey S89+391 **96**
Cape Province, South Africa L40-300 **84**
Cape Tormentine, N.B. S23+461 **90**
Cape Town, Cape Province L70-340 **84**
Cape Verde Is., Atlantic Ocean P60+160 **80**
Cape York Pen., Queensland C45-132 **111**
Capelle, la, France M67+500 **54**
Capilla, Argentina R85-343 **103**
Capilla del Monte, Argentina S28-309 **103**
Capitan Mts., New Mexico V02+336 **94**
Caplan, Quebec S34+481 **90**
Capoompeta, mt., N.S.W. B78-294 **109**
Capote Mt., Texas U86+300 **94**
Cappoquin, Ireland, Rep. N47+521 **43**
Capraia, I., Italy M31+430 **56**
Capreol, Ontario T35+467 **91**
Caprera, I., Sardinia M33+413 **57**
Capri, I., Italy M04+404 **57**
Capricorn Chan., Queensland B75-226 **111**
Caprivi Strip, Namibia L40-180 **84**
Carabaya, Cord. de, Peru S62-140 **104**
Caracarai, Brazil S05+023 **104**
Caracas, Venezuela S42+105 **104**
Caracol, Brazil Q79-093 **105**
Caragh L., Ireland, Rep. N59+521 **43**
Caraguatay, Paraguay R71-250 **103**
Caransebes, Romania L47+454 **58**
Caraomer, Romania L11+438 **58**
Carapegua, Paraguay R73-257 **103**
Caraquet, New Brunswick S30+478 **90**
Caras, Peru T17-092 **104**
Caratasca Lag., Honduras T54+154 **101**
Caratiá, Brazil S26-060 **104**
Carauari, Brazil S42-048 **104**
Caravaca, Spain N13+381 **53**
Caravelas, Brazil Q56-178 **105**
Caraveli, Peru S81-158 **104**
Carballino, Spain N48+424 **52**
Carballo, Spain N52+432 **52**
Carbonara C., Sardinia M33+391 **57**
Carbondale, Illinois T86+377 **95**
Carbondale, Pennsylvania T03+415 **96**
Carbon Hill, Alabama T75+339 **97**
Carcajou, Alberta V72+580 **88**
Carcassone, France M76+432 **55**
Carcoar, New South Wales C05-337 **109**
Carcross, Yukon W89+601 **88**
Carcura, Libya L60+312 **81**
Cardamom Hills, India G77+100 **70**
Cardenas, Cuba T37+230 **101**
Cardiel, L., Argentina S68-490 **103**
Cardiff, Wales N19+515 **38**
Cardigan, Wales N28+521 **38**
Cardigan B., Wales N27+525 **38**
Cardona, Spain M76+419 **53**
Cardston, Alberta V50+492 **88**
Cardwell, Queensland C24-180 **111**
Carey, L., W. Australia D76-288 **110**
Carhaix, France N21+483 **54**
Carhue. See Adolfo Alsina
Caribbean Sea, S. & Cent. America **101**
Caribou, Maine S48+469 **90**
Caribou, Newfoundland R69+490 **90**
Caribou Mts., Alberta V65+591 **88**
Caribrod. See Dimitrovgrad
Carichic, Mexico V11+278 **100**
Carinda, New South Wales C14-305 **109**
Cariñena, Spain N07+413 **53**
Carinhanha, Brazil Q83-142 **105**
Caripito, Venezuela S19+100 **104**
Carius, Brazil Q57-062 **105**
Carl, L., Oklahoma U44+362 **95**

Carlet, *Spain* N03+392 **53**
Carleton, *Quebec* S36+481 **90**
Carleton, Mt., *N.B.* S42+473 **90**
Carleton Place, *Ontario* T07+451 **91**
Carlingford & L.
Ireland, Rep. N37+540 **42**
Carlinville, *Illinois* U00+392 **95**
Carlisle, *England* N18+549 **37**
Carlisle, *Kentucky* T54+383 **97**
Carlisle, *Pennsylvania* T14+402 **96**
Carlisle, *S. Carolina* T39+346 **97**
Carlos Casares, *Argentina* S08-356 **103**
Carlow & co., *Ireland, Rep.* N42+528 **43**
Carlsbad, *New Mexico* U86+324 **94**
Carlsbad Caverns Nat. Park,
New Mexico U87+320 **98**
Carlton, *Minnesota* U15+467 **93**
Carmacks, *Yukon* X10+617 **88**
Carman, *Manitoba* U46+496 **88**
Carmarthen, *Wales* N26+518 **38**
Carmarthen B., *Wales* N27+516 **38**
Carmaux, *France* M77+440 **55**
Carmel, *New York* S82+414 **96**
Carmel, Mt., *Israel* K60+327 **76**
Carmelo, *Uruguay* R80-340 **99**
Carmen, *Bolivia* S47-115 **104**
Carmen, *Colombia* T01+097 **104**
Carmen, *Mexico* U11+186 **100**
Carmen I., *Mexico* V36+259 **100**
Carmen de Patagones,
Argentina S17-407 **103**
Carmensa, *Argentina* S46-352 **103**
Carmi, *Illinois* T79+382 **97**
Carmona, *Spain* N34+375 **52**
Carnarvon, *Cape Province* L48-312 **84**
Carnarvon, *W. Australia* E37-249 **110**
Carndonagh, *Ireland, Rep.* N44+552 **42**
Carnegie, L., *W. Australia* D74-260 **110**
Carnot, *Cent. Afr. Rep.* L84+050 **81**
Carnoustie, *Scotland* N16+565 **41**
Carnsore Pt., *Ireland, Rep.* N38+522 **43**
Caro, *Michigan* T50+435 **91**
Carolina, *Brazil* R15-072 **105**
Carolina, *Transvaal* K88-262 **84**
Caroline I., *Pacific Ocean* Y00-100 **107**
Caroline Is., *Pacific Ocean* C00+050 **106**
Carora, *Venezuela* S60+102 **104**
Carpathian Mts., *Cent. Europe* L42+490 **49**
Carpatii Meridionali, *Rom.* L42+450 **58**
Carpentaria, G. of, *Aust.* C66-140 **111**
Carrantuohill, *Ireland, Rep.* N59+520 **43**
Carrara, *Italy* M29+441 **56**
Carrathool, *New S. Wales* C28-344 **109**
Carrbridge, *Scotland* N23+573 **40**
Carreño, *Spain* N35+434 **52**
Carrickfergus, *N. Ireland* N35+547 **42**
Carrickmacross, *Ireland, Rep.* N40+540 **42**
Carrick-on-Shannon,
Ireland, Rep. N49+539 **42**
Carrick-on-Suir, *Ireland, Rep.* N45+523 **43**
Carrieton, *S. Australia* C69-324 **109**
Carrington, *N. Dakota* U55+474 **93**
Carrión-de-los-Condes, *Sp.* N28+424 **52**
Carrizo Mts., *Arizona* V26+368 **94**
Carrizo Springs, *Texas* U59+286 **94**
Carrizozo, *New Mexico* V05+336 **94**
Carroll, *Iowa* U30+422 **95**
Carrollton, *Alabama* T79+332 **97**
Carrollton, *Kentucky* T61+387 **91**
Carrollton, *Missouri* U22+394 **95**
Carrowmore L., *Ireland, Rep.* N59+542 **42**
Carroz, le, *Switzerland* M53+466 **45**
Carsamba, *Turkey* K50+411 **74**
Carse of Gowrie, *Scotland* N19+564 **41**
Carson City, *Nevada* V89+392 **92**
Carson Sink, *Nevada* V82+397 **92**
Carstairs, *Scotland* N22+557 **41**
Carstensz G., mt., (Pk. Sukarno)
Irian Jaya, Indon. C76-040 **65**
Cartagena, *Colombia* T03+105 **104**
Cartagena, *Spain* N06+377 **53**
Cartago, *Colombia* T05+047 **104**
Cartago, *Costa Rica* T53+099 **101**
Cartaxo, *Portugal* N53+391 **52**
Cartaya, *Spain* N43+373 **52**
Carter, *Wyoming* V32+414 **93**
Carter Bar, *Scot.-Eng.* N15+553 **41**
Carteret, *France* N11+494 **54**
Cartersville, *Georgia* T59+342 **97**
Carterton, *New Zealand* A27-410 **112**
Carthage, *Illinois* U07+404 **95**
Carthage, *Missouri* U26+372 **95**
Carthage, *New York* T03+440 **91**
Carthage, *N. Carolin* T27+354 **97**
Carthage, *Tennessee* T66+363 **97**
Cartier, *Ontario* T39+467 **91**
Cartwright, *Labrador* R72+530 **89**
Carumbay, *Bolivia* S13-190 **104**
Carupano, *Venezuela* S19+106 **104**
Carutaperá, *Brazil* R06-012 **105**
Caruthersville, *Missouri* T88+362 **95**
Carvoeiro, *Brazil* S12-014 **104**
Casablanca, *Chile* S69-333 **103**
Casablanca, *Morocco* N46+336 **80**
Casaccia, *Switzerland* M32+464 **45**
Casa Grande, *Arizona* V40+328 **99**
Casas Ibañez, *Spain* N09+393 **53**
Cascade, *Montana* V40+473 **93**
Cascade Ra., *Oregon, etc.* W14+426 **98**
Cascais, *Portugal* N56+387 **52**
Casco B., *Maine* S60+437 **90**
Caserta, *Italy* M04+411 **57**
Caseville, *Michigan* T49+439 **91**
Cashel, *Ireland, Rep.* N47+525 **43**
Casilda, *Argentina* S07-331 **103**
Casilda, *Cuba* T30+217 **101**
Casino, *New South Wales* B72-288 **109**
Casma, *Peru* T20-096 **104**
Casmalia, *California* W04+347 **92**
Caspe, *Spain* N00+413 **53**
Casper, *Wyoming* V08+428 **93**
Caspian Sea, *Europe-Asia* J60+400 **30**
Cassai, *Angola* L48-108 **82**
Cassamba, *Angola* L58-132 **82**
Cassel, *France* M75+508 **54**
Casselton, *N. Dakota* U42+470 **93**
Cassiar Mts., *Brit. Columbia* W55+592 **88**
Cassilis, *New South Wales* C00-320 **109**
Cassinga, *Angola* L84-152 **84**
Cassino, *Brazil* R44-323 **99**
Cassino, *Italy* M07+415 **57**
Cassipore, *Brazil* R37+034 **104**
Cassis, *France* M57+432 **55**
Cassopolis, *Michigan* T66+419 **91**
Cassou, *Upper Volta* N12+116 **80**
Cassville, *Missouri* U23+368 **95**
Castanhal, *Brazil* S14-064 **104**
Castanheiro, *Brazil* S34-002 **104**
Castaño, *Argentina* S58-310 **103**
Castasegna, *Switzerland* M33+463 **45**
Casteljaloux, *France* N00+443 **55**
Castellammare & G. di, *Sic.* M13+380 **57**
Castellammare di Stabia,
Italy M03+407 **57**
Castellane, *France* M51+439 **55**
Castellar de Santiago, *Spain* N19+386 **52**
Castelli, *Argentina* R77-360 **103**
Castello, *Brazil* Q69-053 **105**
Castellón de la Plana, *Spain* N00+400 **53**
Castellote, *Spain* N01+408 **53**
Castelnaudary, *France* M78+433 **55**
Castelo Branco, *Portugal* N45+398 **52**
Castelo de Vide, *Portugal* N44+394 **52**
Castelsarrasin, *France* M83+440 **55**
Castelvetrano, *Sicily* M13+377 **57**
Casterton, *Victoria* C52-376 **109**
Castets, *France* N07+439 **55**
Castillo, mt., *Chile* S74-460 **103**
Castine, *Maine* S53+444 **90**
Castlebar, *Ireland, Rep.* N56+539 **42**
Castlebellingham, *Ireland, Rep.* N38+539 **42**
Castleblayney, *Ireland, Rep.* N40+541 **42**
Castlecomer, *Ireland, Rep.* N43+528 **43**
Castlederg, *N. Ireland* N46+547 **42**
Castledermot, *Ireland, Rep.* N41+529 **43**
Castle Douglas, *Scotland* N24+549 **41**
Castleisland, *Ireland, Rep.* N57+522 **43**
Castlemaine, *Ireland, Rep.* N58+522 **43**
Castlemaine, *Victoria* C35-371 **109**
Castlemartyr, *Ireland, Rep.* N48+519 **43**
Castlepollard, *Ireland, Rep.* N44+537 **42**
Castlerea, *Ireland, Rep.* N51+538 **42**
Castlereagh, R., *N.S.W.* C10-308 **109**
Castle Rock, *Utah* V37+412 **94**
Castle Rock, mt., *Oregon* V79+440 **92**
Castle Rock Buttes, *S. Dak.* U81+450 **93**
Castletown, *Scotland* N20+586 **40**
Castletown Bere, *Ireland, Rep.* N60+517 **43**
Castlewellan, *N. Ireland* N35+542 **42**
Castres, *France* M77+436 **55**
Castro, *Brazil* R30-248 **103**
Castro, *Chile* S83-424 **103**
Castro Marin, *Portugal* N44+372 **52**
Castropol, *Spain* N42+435 **52**
Castrovillari, *Italy* L83+398 **57**
Castuera, *Spain* N33+388 **52**
Cat I., *Bahamas, The* T04+243 **101**
Catabola, *Angola* L76-122 **82**
Catak, *Turkey* K14+382 **74**
Catamarca, *Argentina* S35-285 **103**
Catanduanes, I., *Philippines* D64+137 **65**
Catania & G. di, *Sicily* M00+375 **57**
Catanzaro, *Italy* L80+389 **57**
Catarina la Grande, *Mexico* U19+163 **100**
Catarman, *Philippines* D62+124 **65**
Catastrophe, C., *S. Australia* C84-350 **111**
Catabalogan, *Philippines* D60+116 **65**
Catahoula L., *Louisiana* U13+315 **95**
Cateau, le, *France* M69+501 **54**
Cathcart, *New S. Wales* C04-368 **109**
Cathedral Mt., *Texas* U82+302 **94**
Catingueiro, *Brazil* R20-113 **105**
Catlettsburg, *Kentucky* T46+384 **97**
Catonsville, *Maryland* T10+393 **96**
Catorce, *Mexico* U66+237 **100**
Catrilo, *Argentina* S21-363 **103**
Catskill, *New York* S83+422 **96**
Catskill Mts., *New York* S86+422 **96**
Cattaraugus, *New York* T23+424 **96**
Cauquenes, *Chile* S74-359 **103**
Causapscal, *Quebec* S43+484 **90**
Cauto, R., *Cuba* T13+206 **101**
Cauvery R., *India* G72+113 **70**
Caux, *French Guiana* R42+043 **105**
Cavalcante, *Brazil* R15-139 **105**
Cavallo Pass, *Texas* U38+283 **94**
Cavan & co., *Ireland, Rep.* N44+540 **42**
Cave, *New Zealand* A54-443 **112**
Cavendish, *Victoria* C48-375 **109**
Cavergno, *Switzerland* M38+463 **45**
Caviana, I., *Brazil* R31+002 **105**
Cawnpore. *See* Kanpur
Caxias, *Brazil* S72-046 **104**
Caxias, *Brazil* Q80-048 **105**
Caxias do Sul, *Brazil* R37-293 **103**
Cayambe, *Ecuador* T19+011 **104**
Cayenne, *French Guiana* R44+048 **105**
Cayes, Les, *Haiti* S83+182 **101**
Cayo, *Belize* T80+172 **101**
Cayuga, *Ontario* T29+430 **91**
Cayuga, L., *New York* T10+427 **96**
Cazage, *Angola* L56-112 **82**
Cazalla de la Sierra, *Spain* N35+379 **52**
Cazenovia, *New York* T05+429 **96**
Cazin, *Yugoslavia* L85+450 **56**
Cazorla, *Spain* N18+379 **52**
Ceará. *See* Fortaleza
Ceanannus Mór, *see* Kells
Ceara Mirim, *Brazil* Q32-056 **105**
Cebaco, I., *Panama* T37+075 **101**
Cebollar, *Argentina* S39-291 **103**
Cebollera, *Spain* N16+420 **53**
Cebu, *Philippines* D66+104 **65**
Cecil, *Georgia* T50+310 **97**
Ceclavin, *Spain* N41+398 **52**
Cedar, *Utah* V34+394 **94**
Cedar L., *Texas* U74+328 **94**
Cedar Mts., *Oregon* V77+432 **92**
Cedar Ra., *Utah* V47+404 **92**
Cedarburg, *Wisconsin* T78+433 **91**
Cedar City, *Utah* V48+376 **94**
Cedar Falls, *Iowa* U14+426 **95**
Cedar Key, *Florida* T49+293 **99**
Cedar Rapids, *Iowa* U10+420 **95**
Cedar Springs, *Michigan* T63+433 **91**
Cedral, *Mexico* U64+238 **100**
Cedros, I., *Mexico* V62+281 **100**
Ceduna, *S. Australia* D08-320 **111**
Cefalu, *Sicily* M06+380 **57**
Cegled, *Hungary* L61+472 **49**
Cehegin, *Spain* N11+381 **53**
Ceiba, la, *Honduras* T72+157 **101**
Cejita Blanca, *New Mexico* V12+363 **94**
Celanova, *Spain* N48+422 **52**
Celaya, *Mexico* U65+206 **100**
Celebes (Sulawesi), *Indonesia* E00-023 **65**
Celebes Sea, *Indonesia* E00+038 **65**
Celje, *Yugoslavia* L88+462 **56**
Celle, *W. Germany* M30+526 **48**
Celles, *Belgium* M69+507 **44**
Cemisgezek, *Turkey* K36+391 **74**
Cenis, Mte., *France* M49+452 **56**
Center, *Texas* U25+318 **95**
Centerville, *Alabama* T73+329 **97**
Centerville, *Iowa* U17+407 **95**
Centerville, *Missouri* U06+373 **97**
Centerville, *Tennessee* T75+357 **97**
Central, reg., *Scotland* N26+562 **41**
Central, Cord., *Peru* T14-078 **104**
Central African Rep., *Afr.* L60+070 **81**
Central America T66+140 **101**
Central City, *Nebraska* U48+410 **95**
Centralia, *Illinois* T85+386 **95**
Centralia, *Washington* W18+467 **92**
Central Lake, *Michigan* T62+452 **91**
Centreville, *New Brunswick* S46+465 **90**
Cephalonia. *See* Kefallinia
Ceram Sea, *Indonesia* D40-030 **65**
Cerignola, *Italy* L85+413 **57**
Cerigo. *See* Kithira I.
Cerigotto. *See* Andikithira I.
Cerknica, *Yugoslavia* M04+458 **56**
Cermik, *Turkey* K33+382 **74**
Cernauti. *See* Chernovtsy
Cerralvo, *Mexico* U59+261 **100**
Cerralvo, I., *Mexico* V29+243 **100**
Cerreto Sannita, *Italy* M03+413 **57**
Cerro de Pasco, *Peru* T08-107 **104**
Cervera de Pisuerga, *Spain* N27+429 **52**
Cesena, *Italy* M17+441 **56**
Cesis, *Latvia* L29+573 **47**
Ceská Lipa, *Czechoslovakia* M03+507 **48**
Ceské Budějovice, *Czech.* M03+489 **48**
Cessnock, *New S. Wales* B82-329 **109**
Cetinje, *Yugoslavia* L66+424 **58**
Cetraro, *Italy* L84+395 **57**
Cette. *See* Sete
Ceuta, *N. Africa* N32+358 **80**
Ceuta, B. de, *Mexico* V13+241 **100**
Cevennes, France M68+445 **55**
Ceyhan, *Turkey* K58+370 **74**
Ceylon I., & rep. *See* Sri Lanka
Chabatok, *Quebec* S83+504 **90**
Chablis, *France* M67+478 **54**
Chacabuco, *Argentina* S03-346 **103**
Chacance, *Chile* S58-223 **103**
Chachapoyas, *Peru* T17-064 **104**
Chachoengsao, *Thailand* F24+136 **69**
Chaco, R., *New Mexico* V18+360 **94**
Chad, rep., *Cent. Africa* L70+150 **81**
Chad (Tchad), L., *Chad* M04+134 **81**
Chadron, *Nebraska* U78+428 **94**
Chadwick, *Missouri* U18+369 **97**
Chagai, *Pakistan* H62+293 **70**
Chagda, *U.S.S.R.* D26+586 **63**
Chagny, *France* M61+469 **54**
Chagos Arch., *Indian Ocean* H13-057 **77**
Chah Bahār, *Iran* H86+253 **75**
Chaibassa, *India* G25+225 **73**
Chaise Dieu, *France* M68+453 **55**
Chakansur, *Afghanistan* H77+311 **75**
Chakia, *India* G40+251 **73**
Chaksam, *Tibet* F85+293 **71**
Chakwal, *Pakistan* H13+329 **72**
Chala, *Peru* S86-158 **104**
Chalchihuites, *Mexico* U84+236 **100**
Chalcis. *See* Khalkis
Chaleur B., *Quebec-N.B.* S34+479 **90**
Chalham, I., *Chile* S86-507 **103**
Chalhuanca, *Peru* S81-143 **104**
Chaling, *China* E38+269 **67**
Chalisgaon, *India* H00+205 **70**
Chalk River, *Ontario* T14+460 **91**
Challapata, *Bolivia* S41-189 **104**
Chalons-sur-Marne, *France* M64+489 **54**
Chalon-sur-Saône, *France* M61+468 **54**
Chalus, *France* M84+456 **54**
Cham, *W. Germany* M14+492 **48**
Chama, *New Mexico* V08+368 **94**
Chaman, *Pakistan* H51+309 **70**
Chamba, *India* G83+326 **72**
Chambal R., *India* G84+257 **70**
Chamberlain L., *Maine* S56+462 **90**
Chamberlain, *S. Dakota* U56+438 **93**
Chambersburg, *Pennsylvania* T17+399 **96**
Chambéry, *France* M54+456 **54**
Chambivas, *Brazil* R22-066 **105**
Chambord, *Quebec* S72+484 **90**
Chamdo, *China* F46+312 **64**
Chamical, *Argentina* S37-304 **103**
Chamo, L., *Ethiopia* K44+058 **83**
Chamonix, *France* M49+459 **54**
Champa, *India* G44+220 **73**
Champagne, prov., *France* M65+489 **54**
Champaign, *Illinois* T80+402 **95**
Champerico, *Guatemala* U11+142 **100**
Champlain L., *N.Y.-Vermont* S80+442 **91**
Champlitte, *France* M57+476 **54**
Champlon, *Belgium* M57+501 **44**
Chamusca, *Portugal* N51+393 **52**
Chanco, *Chile* S75-356 **103**
Chancy, *Switzerland* M54+462 **45**
Chanda, *India* G60+200 **70**
Chandausi, *India* G68+284 **73**
Chandeleur Is & Sd., *La.* T84+298 **95**
Chanderi, *India* G71+247 **73**
Chandernagore, *India* G10+228 **73**
Chandigarh, *India* G79+307 **72**
Chandod, *India* H08+220 **70**
Chandpur, *Bangladesh* F86+233 **71**
Chandpur, *India* G70+292 **73**
Chanduria, *Bangladesh* G06+229 **73**
Changchih, *China* E42+361 **66**
Changchow, *China* E14+244 **67**
Changchow, *China* E01+318 **66**
Changchun, *China* D57+438 **64**
Ch'angkang, *China* E68+192 **64**
Changkiakow, *China* E31+408 **66**
Changlo, *China* E07+367 **66**
Changpeh, *China* E31+411 **66**
Changping, *China* E22+403 **66**
Changpu, *China* E13+242 **67**
Changsha, *China* E42+282 **67**
Changshan, *China* E09+289 **67**
Changte. *See* Anyang
Changteh, *China* E51+290 **67**
Changting, *China* E22+257 **67**
Changyeh, *China* F26+389 **64**
Changkiang, *China* E58+212 **69**
Channel Is., *English Chan.* N15+494 **54**
Chantada, *Spain* N47+426 **52**
Chanthaburi, *Thailand* F17+126 **69**
Chantilly, *France* M75+492 **54**
Chanute, *Kansas* U33+376 **95**
Chany, Oz., *U.S.S.R.* G75+550 **62**
Chao, R., *Thailand* F27+150 **65**
Chaoan, *China* E20+237 **67**
Chaochow, *China* E20+237 **67**
Chao Hu, *China* F08+273 **66**
Chapala, L., *Mexico* U78+202 **100**
Chapayevsk, *U.S.S.R.* J62+530 **61**
Chapleau, *Ontario* T50+478 **91**
Chapell Is., *Tasmania* C14-403 **109**
Chapra, *India* G31+258 **73**
Char, *Mauritania* N78+216 **80**
Chara, *U.S.S.R.* E10+570 **63**
Charagua, *Bolivia* S19-197 **104**
Charana, *Bolivia* S57-175 **104**
Charcot, I., *Antarctica* S85-700 **27**
Chard, *England* N18+509 **38**
Chardzhou, *Turkmen* H70+390 **62**
Charente, dep., *France* M89+458 **54**
Charente, R., *France* N04+457 **54**
Charente-Maritime, dep.,
France N06+458 **54**
Chari R., *Chad* L80+108 **81**
Charikar, *Afghanistan* H35+350 **75**
Charité, la, *France* M72+472 **54**
Chariton, *Iowa* U20+410 **95**
Charkhari, *India* G62+254 **73**
Charleroi, *Belgium* M63+504 **44**
Charles R., *Massachusetts* S68+424 **96**
Charles City, *Iowa* U16+430 **95**
Charleston, *Illinois* T80+394 **95**
Charleston, *Mississippi* U00+340 **97**
Charleston, *Missouri* T86+370 **95**
Charleston, *Queensland* C38-186 **111**
Charleston, S., *Carolina* T30+328 **97**
Charleston, *W. Virginia* T40+384 **97**
Charleston Pk., *Nevada* V64+362 **92**
Charlestown, *Ireland, Rep.* N52+539 **42**
Charles Town, *W. Virginia* T17+393 **96**
Charleville (Rath Luire),
Ireland, Rep. N52+523 **43**
Charleville, *France* M62+498 **54**
Charleville, *Queensland* C23-264 **111**
Charlevoix, *Michigan* T62+453 **91**
Charlotte, *Michigan* T59+426 **91**
Charlotte, *N. Carolina* T35+352 **97**
Charlotte, *New York* T16+433 **91**
Charlotte Amalie, *Virgin Is.* S29+184 **101**
Charlotte Harbor, *Florida* T43+270 **97**
Charlottenburg, *Germany* M10+525 **48**
Charlottesville, *Virginia* T21+381 **97**
Charlottetown, *P.E.I.* S19+463 **90**
Charlton, *Victoria* C40-363 **109**
Charlton I., *N.-W. Terr.* T26+517 **89**
Charmey, *Switzerland* M47+466 **45**
Charnwood Forest, *England* N08+527 **37**
Charolles, *France* M64+464 **54**
Charrote, Sierra, *Texas* U72+308 **94**
Charsadda, *Pakistan* H19+342 **72**
Charters Towers, *Queensland* C23-200 **111**
Chartres, *France* M81+485 **54**
Charvonnex, *France* M53+460 **45**
Chascomus, *Argentina* R78-356 **103**
Chaska, *Minnesota* U22+448 **93**
Chasseneuil, *France* M87+458 **54**
Châteaubriant, *France* N08+477 **54**
Château Chinon, *France* M67+471 **54**
Château-du-Loir, *France* M87+477 **54**
Châteaudun, *France* M82+481 **54**
Château Gontier, *France* N04+478 **54**
Château-la-Vallière, *France* M88+475 **54**
Chateaulin, *France* N25+482 **54**
Châteauneuf-en-Thymerais,
France M82+486 **54**
Châteaurenault, *France* M85+476 **54**
Châteauroux, *France* M81+468 **54**
Château Salins, *France* M51+488 **54**
Château Thierry, *France* M70+491 **54**
Châteauvillain, *France* M60+480 **54**
Châtelet, *Belgium* M63+504 **44**
Châtellerault, *France* M87+468 **54**
Châtel-St Denis, *Switzerland* M49+465 **45**
Chatfield, *Minnesota* U13+438 **93**
Chatham, *England* M87+514 **39**
Chatham, *New Brunswick* S33+471 **90**
Chatham, *New York* S82+424 **91**
Chatham, *Ontario* T43+424 **91**
Chatham, *Virginia* T27+368 **97**
Chatham Is., *Pacific Ocean* Z70-442 **106**
Chatillon-sur-Seine, *France* M63+478 **54**
Chatra, *India* G31+242 **73**
Chatrapur, *India* G30+194 **71**
Châtre, la, *France* M78+466 **54**
Chattahoochee R., *Georgia* T59+309 **99**
Chattanooga, *Tennessee* T62+350 **97**
Chaudiere R., *Quebec* S67+467 **91**
Chau-doc, *Vietnam* E89+108 **69**
Chauka R., *India* G52+274 **73**
Chaumont-en-Bassigny, *Fr.* M59+481 **54**
Chaunskaya Guba, *U.S.S.R.* A60+695 **63**
Chausa, *India* G36+255 **73**
Chautauqua L., *New York* T26+422 **96**
Chaux de Fonds, la, *Switz.* M49+471 **45**
Chaves, *Brazil* R29-003 **105**
Chaves, *Portugal* N45+418 **52**
Chayu, *Tibet* F47+284 **64**
Chazon, *Argentina* S20-332 **103**
Cheadle, *England* N12+530 **37**
Cheb, *Czechoslovakia* M16+501 **48**
Cheboksary, *U.S.S.R.* J76+562 **61**
Cheboygan, *Michigan* T57+456 **91**
Checmu, *Mexico* T70+213 **100**
Cheduba & I., *Burma* F68+189 **71**
Che foo. *See* Yentai
Chehalis, *Washington* W18+466 **92**
Chekiang, prov. *China* E00+292 **67**
Chekunda, *U.S.S.R.* D16+508 **63**
Chelforó, *Argentina* S39-391 **103**
Chelkar, *Kazakh* J04+479 **62**
Chelm, *Poland* L39+511 **49**
Chelmsford, *England* M87+517 **39**
Chelsea, *Vermont* S75+440 **91**

Chelsea, *Wisconsin* U02+453 **91**
Cheltenham, *England* N12+519 **39**
Chelva, *Spain* N06+397 **53**
Chelyabinsk, *U.S.S.R.* H81+551 **61**
Chemba, *Mozambique* K62-172 **84**
Chembar, *U.S.S.R.* K10+529 **61**
Chemnitz. *See* Karl Marx Stadt
Chenab R., *Pakistan* H22+303 **72**
Chenchow. *See* Hwaiyang
Chengchow, *China* E37+346 **66**
Chengho, *China* E07+274 **67**
Chênghsien, *China* E37+348 **66**
Chengshan Tow, *China* D74+373 **64**
Chêng-têhshih, *China* E12+410 **66**
Chengtu, *China* F06+306 **66**
Chenhsien, *China* E42+258 **67**
Chennan. *See* Tehpao
Chenoa, *Illinois* T83+408 **91**
Chenting, *China* E32+381 **66**
Chenyüan, *China* E69+271 **67**
Chepen, *Peru* T27-072 **104**
Chepes, *Argentina* S40-313 **103**
Cher, R. & dep., *France* M85+473 **54**
Cherbourg, *France* N10+497 **54**
Cherchell, *Algeria* M76+364 **80**
Cheremkhovo, *U.S.S.R.* F11+532 **63**
Cherepovets, *U.S.S.R.* K39+592 **60**
Cherkassy, *Ukraine* K78+494 **60**
Chermoz, *U.S.S.R.* J24+587 **62**
Chernigov, *Ukraine* K82+515 **60**
Chernikovsk, *U.S.S.R.* J25+548 **61**
Chernovsk, *U.S.S.R.* J71+580 **61**
Chernovtsy, *Ukraine* L24+483 **60**
Chernyakhovsk, *U.S.S.R.* L49+546 **47**
Cherokee, *Iowa* U34+427 **95**
Cherokees, L. o' the, *Okla.* U29+367 **95**
Cherra Pungi, *India* F79+252 **71**
Cherryfield, *Maine* S47+446 **90**
Cherskogo, Khrebet, *U.S.S.R.* C20+640 **63**
Chertkovo, *Ukraine* K29+494 **60**
Chervenbyreg, *Bulgaria* L35+433 **58**
Cherwell R., *England* N08+517 **39**
Chesapeake B., *Maryland* T08+388 **99**
Cheshire, co., *England* N15+532 **37**
Cheshskaya Guba, *U.S.S.R.* J80+675 **62**
Chesley, *Ontario* T36+443 **91**
Chester, *England* N17+532 **37**
Chester, *Illinois* T89+379 **97**
Chester, *Pennsylvania* T03+398 **96**
Chester, *S. Carolina* T38+347 **97**
Chesterfield, *England* N09+532 **37**
Chesterfield, *S. Carolina* T31+348 **97**
Chesterfield Inlet, *North-West Territories* U10+639 **89**
Chesterfield Is., *Pacific Oc.* B40+190 **106**
Chester-le-Street, *England* N09+549 **37**
Chestertown, *Maryland* T07+392 **96**
Chesuncook L., *Maine* S56+460 **90**
Chethang, *Tibet* F79+293 **71**
Chetumal & B., *Mexico* T77+184 **100**
Cheviot, *New Zealand* A40-429 **112**
Cheviot, The, *England* N13+555 **37**
Cheviot Hills, *Eng.-Scot.* N14+553 **37**
Cheyenne, *Wyoming* U88+412 **93**
Cheyenne R., *S. Dakota* U70+445 **93**
Chhachrauli, *India* G75+303 **72**
Chhata, *India* G75+277 **72**
Chhatarpur, *India* G62+249 **73**
Chhibramau, *India* G63+271 **73**
Chhindwara, *India* G66+221 **73**
Chiai, *Taiwan* D87+235 **67**
Chiang Mai, *Thailand* F36+188 **69**
Chiang Rai, *Thailand* F31+199 **69**
Chiapa, *Mexico* U18+167 **100**
Chiapas R. & state, *Mexico* U16+170 **100**
Chiasso, *Switzerland* M36+458 **45**
Chiavari, *Italy* M34+443 **56**
Chiba, *Japan* C59+356 **68**
Chibia, *Angola* M08-154 **84**
Chibougamau L., *Quebec* S86+498 **90**
Chicago, *Illinois* T76+418 **95**
Chichagof I., *Alaska* X05+578 **99**
Chichester, *England* N03+508 **39**
Chickasha, *Oklahoma* U48+350 **95**
Chiclayo, *Peru* T29-068 **104**
Chico, *California* W11+397 **92**
Chicoana, *Argentina* S33-252 **103**
Chicopee & R., *Massachusetts* S76+422 **96**
Chicoutimi, *Quebec* S66+484 **90**
Chicundo, *Transvaal* K86-228 **84**
Chidambaram, *India* G62+115 **70**
Chidley, C., *Quebec* S27+603 **89**
Chiang-kan, *Thailand* F20+179 **69**
Chiengue, *Angola* L82-116 **82**
Chienou, *China* E19+268 **67**
Chieti, *Italy* M05+424 **56**
Chièvres, *Belgium* M67+506 **44**
Chigha Khur, *Iran* J54+320 **75**
Chignecto B., *New Brunswick-Nova Scotia* S31+454 **90**
Chignik, *Alaska* Y42+555 **26**
Chichow. *See* Kweichih
Chih-fêng, *China* E06+423 **66**
Chihi, *Tanzania* K50-094 **83**
Chikiang, *China* E62+274 **67**
Chihsien, *China* E34+354 **66**
Chihuahua & state, *Mexico* V06+286 **100**
Chik-Ballapur, *India* G74+135 **70**
Chikien, *China* D85+522 **63**
Chikmagalur, *India* G84+133 **70**
Chikwawa, *Malawi* K60-160 **83**
Chilas, *Kashmir* H05+354 **72**
Childress, *Texas* U62+346 **94**
Chile, rep., *S. America* **103**
Chilecito, *Argentina* S45-292 **103**
Chilete, *Peru* T23-073 **104**
Chilia Veche, *Romania* L04+454 **58**
Chilka L., *India* G27+196 **71**
Chilko L., *Brit. Columbia* W25+512 **88**
Chilko R., *Brit. Columbia* W20+518 **88**
Chillan, *Chile* S73-364 **103**
Chillicothe, *Missouri* U22+398 **95**
Chillicothe, *Ohio* T48+394 **91**
Chillingollah, *Victoria* C42-353 **109**
Chilliwack, *Brit. Columbia* W10+493 **88**
Chiloe, I. de, *Chile* S84-426 **103**
Chilonga, *Zambia* K82-122 **83**
Chilpancingo, *Mexico* U56+174 **100**
Chiltern, *Victoria* C20-362 **109**
Chiltern Hills, *England* N04+518 **39**
Chilton, *Wisconsin* T79+441 **91**
Chiluane, *Mozambique* K60-206 **84**
Chilubula, *Zambia* K86-102 **83**
Chilung, *Taiwan* D80+251 **67**
Chilwa L., *Malawi* K56-154 **83**
Chimay, *Belgium* M64+501 **44**
Chimbai, *Uzbek* J01+430 **62**
Chimbote, *Peru* T21-091 **104**
Chimkent, *Kazakh* H33+423 **62**
Chimpek, *Kazakh* H06+450 **62**
China, rep., *Asia* E60+330 **31**
Chinandega, *Nicaragua* T73+126 **101**
Chincha, *Peru* T07-135 **104**
Chinchaga R., *Alberta* V85+580 **88**
Chinchon, *Spain* N21+402 **52**
Chinchow, *China* D82+412 **64**
Chindwin R., Burma F60+225 **71**
Ching Hai, *China* F28+64
Chingleput, *India* G59+128 **70**
Ching Shan, *China* E54+314 **66**
Chingtao, *China* D88+361 **66**
Chinguetta, *Mauritania* N74+204 **80**
Chinhai, *China* D79+300 **67**
Chin Hill, *Burma* F68+227 **71**
Chini, *India* G70+315 **72**
Chiniot, *Pakistan* H12+316 **72**
Chinishk, *Iran* J06+322 **75**
Chinju, *Korea* D42+353 **64**
Chinkiang, *China* E03+322 **66**
Chin Ling Shan, *China* E80+345 **64**
Chinook, *Montana* V25+486 **93**
Chinsura, *India* G10+229 **73**
Chinwangtao, *China* E02+399 **66**
Chioggia, *Italy* M16+452 **56**
Chios, I. *See* Khios, I.
Chipchiahue, *Argentina* S51-421 **103**
Chipili, *Zambia* L06-110 **83**
Chipman, *New Brunswick* S35+462 **90**
Chippewa Falls, *Wisconsin* U09+449 **93**
Chippewa, R., *Wisconsin* U06+456 **99**
Chipping Norton, *England* N09+519 **39**
Chipping Sodbury, *England* N14+515 **38**
Chiputneticook Ls., *Maine-New Brunswick* S47+457 **90**
Chiquian, *Peru* T12-102 **104**
Chiquimula, *Guatemala* T87+147 **100**
Chiquinquira, *Colombia* S83+056 **104**
Chiras, *Afghanistan* H55+353 **75**
Chirawa, *India* G86+282 **72**
Chi-ri-cahua Mts., *Arizona* V27+320 **93**
Chiriqui, Lag. de, *Panama* T42+093 **101**
Chiriqui Grande, *Panama* T43+090 **101**
Chirpan, *Bulgaria* L28+422 **58**
Chirripo Grande, mt., *Costa Rica* T52+097 **101**
Chisamba Falls, *Zambia* K86-101 **83**
Chishmy, *U.S.S.R.* J28+545 **61**
Chisimaio, *Somalia* K14-002 **83**
Chisinau. *See* Kishinev
Chistopol, *U.S.S.R.* J56+554 **61**
Chita, *U.S.S.R.* E39+520 **63**
Chitipa, *Malawi* K70+098 **83**
Chitorgarh, *India* H01+248 **70**
Chitradurga, *India* G81+142 **70**
Chitral & R., *Pakistan* H19+358 **72**
Chitre, *Panama* T33+080 **101**
Chittagong, *Bangladesh* F79+223 **71**
Chittoor, *India* G65+133 **70**
Chiusi, *Italy* M18+430 **56**
Chiuta, L., *Malawi* K56-146 **83**
Chiva, *Spain* N04+395 **53**
Chivasso, *Italy* M43+452 **56**
Chivay, *Peru* S69-156 **104**
Chivilcoy, *Argentina* S00-349 **103**
Chivota, Sierra, *New Mexico* V14+354 **93**
Chivyu, *U.S.S.R.* J36+635 **62**
Chiwanda, *Tanzania* K60-114 **83**
Chmielnik, *Poland* L55+506 **49**
Choapam, *Mexico* U35+174 **100**
Choban Bey, *Syria* K45+366 **76**
Chocaya, *Bolivia* S38-209 **104**
Chocen, *Czechoslovakia* L83+500 **49**
Cho-chow, *China* E24+395 **66**
Choco, Cord. de, *Colombia* T13+070 **104**
Choconta, *Colombia* S82+052 **104**
Choele Choel, *Argentina* S34-393 **103**
Choiseul, I., *Solomon Is.* B48-070 **106**
Choix, *Mexico* V17+272 **100**
Chojna, *Poland* M03+529 **48**
Choke Mts., *Ethiopia* K44+106 **83**
Cholet, *France* N05+471 **54**
Cholon, *Vietnam* E80+108 **69**
Choluteca, *Honduras* T74+133 **101**
Choma, *Zambia* L18-168 **84**
Chomutov, *Czechoslavakia* M10+505 **48**
Chone, *Ecuador* T31-006 **104**
Chongjin, *Korea* D32+418 **64**
Chong Kal, *Cambodia* F09+139 **69**
Chonos, Arch. de los, *Chile* T00-450 **103**
Chorillos, *Peru* T12-124 **104**
Chorley, *England* N16+537 **37**
Chorrera, *Panama* T28+089 **101**
Chorzele, *Poland* L54+533 **49**
Chorzow, *Poland* L66+503 **49**
Chosi, *Japan* C55+357 **68**
Chos Malal, *Argentina* S62-373 **103**
Chota, *Peru* T22-066 **104**
Choushan I., *China* D77+300 **67**
Christchurch, *England* N11+508 **39**
Christchurch, *New Zealand* A44-435 **112**
Christiansburg, *Virginia* T32+371 **97**
Christianshaab, *Greenland* R40+690 **89**
Christie, Mt., *Yukon* W58+634 **88**
Christmas I., *Indian Ocean* E86-104 **65**
Christmas, I., *Pacific Ocean* Y45+020 **107**
Chrudim, *Czechoslovakia* L85+499 **49**
Chrzanów, *Poland* L64+502 **49**
Chuale L., *Mozambique* K72-250 **84**
Chuambara, *Mozambique* K68-154 **84**
Chuanchow, *China* E09+249 **67**
Chuanhsien, *China* E54+260 **67**
Chubut & R., *Argentina* S40-435 **103**
Chuchow, *China* E40+278 **67**
Chuchow. *See* Lishui
Chucul, *Argentina* S25-330 **103**
Chudovo, *U.S.S.R.* K81+591 **60**
Chudskoye, Oz., *Eston.-U.S.S.R.* L16+58 **47**
Chuho, *China* D42+451 **64**
Chühsien, *China* E07+355 **66**
Chuhsien, *China* E07+289 **67**
Chukai, *Malaysia* F09+042 **65**
Chukhloma, *U.S.S.R.* K14+588 **61**
Chukotskiy Khrebet, *U.S.S.R.* A30+682 **63**
Chulman, *U.S.S.R.* D61+567 **63**
Chulym, *U.S.S.R.* G55+551 **62**
Chumbi, *Tibet* G06+274 **71**
Chumikan, *U.S.S.R.* C88+547 **63**
Chuna, R., *U.S.S.R.* F40+572 **63**
Chunar, *India* G43+250 **73**
Chunchön, *Korea* D43+380 **64**
Chungan, *China* E12+277 **67**
Chunghsien, *China* E72+303 **67**
Chungking, *China* E81+295 **67**
Chungshan, *China* E53+246 **67**
Chungsiang, *China* E44+312 **66**
Chungtien, *China* F32+277 **64**
Chunian, *Pakistan* H06+309 **72**
Chunya, *Tanzania* K70-086 **83**
Chuquibambilla, *Peru* S77-140 **104**
Chuquicamata, *Chile* S53-222 **103**
Chur, *Switzerland* M33+469 **45**
Churapcha, *U.S.S.R.* D16+621 **63**
Churchill, *Manitoba* U25+588 **88**
Churchill C., *Manitoba* U21+590 **89**
Churchill L., *Saskatchewan* V20+560 **88**
Churchill, R. & Falls, *Lab.* S10+530 **89**
Churchill R., *Manitoba* U35+570 **88**
Church's Ferry, *N. Dakota* U55+483 **93**
Churia Ghati Hills, *Nepal* G24+269 **73**
Churu, *India* H00+283 **72**
Chusca, Sierra, *New Mexico* V20+362 **94**
Chusovoi, *U.S.S.R.* J12+582 **62**
Chuvashskaya, aut. rep., *U.S.S.R.* J80+560 **62**
Chwan Ho. *See* Yangtze Kiang
Cibao, Cord. de, *Dom. Rep.* S62+190 **101**
Cicero, *Illinois* T77+418 **95**
Cidones, *Spain* N16+418 **53**
Ciechanow, *Poland* L56+529 **49**
Ciego de Avila, *Cuba* T22+218 **101**
Cienaga, *Colombia* S85+110 **104**
Cienfuegos, *Cuba* T33+222 **101**
Cierfs, *Switzerland* M28+466 **45**
Cieszyn, *Poland* L67+498 **49**
Cieza, *Spain* N08+383 **53**
Cifuentes, *Spain* N16+408 **53**
Cilacap, *Java* E67+077 **65**
Cimaltepec, *Mexico* U39+163 **100**
Cimarron R., *Oklahoma, etc.* U60+370 **98**
Cincinnati, *Ohio* T57+391 **91**
Cioara, *Romania* L15+448 **58**
Ciotat, *France* M57+432 **55**
Circeo C., *Italy* M12+412 **57**
Circle, *Alaska* X56+668 **99**
Circle, *Montana* V04+474 **93**
Circleville, *Ohio* T48+396 **91**
Cirebon, *Java* E69+066 **65**
Cirencester, *England* N12+517 **39**
Ciro, *Italy* L78+394 **57**
Cirque Mt., *Labrador* S22+591 **89**
Citlaltepetl, mt., *Mexico* U44+190 **100**
Citrusdal, *Cape Province* L66-326 **84**
Cittanova, *Italy* L83+384 **57**
Ciudad Bolivar, *Venezuela* S21+082 **104**
Ciudad Chetumal, *Mexico* T79+183 **100**
Ciudad Juarez, *Mexico* V09+316 **100**
Ciudad Madero, *Mexico* U48+223 **100**
Ciudad Real, *Spain* N23+390 **52**
Ciudad Rodrigo, *Spain* N39+406 **52**
Ciudad Victoria, *Mexico* U54+238 **100**
Civray, *France* M88+461 **54**
Civril, *Turkey* L02+383 **74**
Cizre, *Turkey* K17+374 **74**
Clackmannan, *Scotland* N22+561 **41**
Clacton-on-Sea, *England* M83+518 **39**
Claire, L., *Alberta* V42+587 **88**
Clamecy, *France* M69+474 **54**
Clara, *Ireland, Rep.* N46+533 **43**
Clara I., *Burma* F43+108 **71**
Clare, *Michigan* T59+438 **91**
Clare, *S. Australia* C69-338 **109**
Clare, co., *Ireland, Rep.* N53+528 **43**
Clare I., *Ireland, Rep.* N60+538 **42**
Clarecastle, *Ireland, Rep.* N54+528 **43**
Claremont, *New Hampshire* S74+434 **96**
Claremore, *Oklahoma* U34+364 **95**
Claremorris, *Ireland, Rep.* N54+537 **42**
Clarence, *Yukon* X36+658 **88**
Clarence Hd., *N.-W. Terr.* T27+766 **89**
Clarence I., *Antarctica* R54-610 **27**
Clarence, I., *Chile* S72-541 **103**
Clarence, R., *New S. Wales* B74-294 **109**
Clarence, R., *New Zealand* A40-423 **112**
Clarence Str., *N. Terr., Aust.* D24-120 **110**
Clarendon, *Arkansas* U08+347 **97**
Clarinda, *Iowa* U30+406 **95**
Clarion, *Iowa* U22+428 **95**
Clarion, *Pennsylvania* T26+412 **96**
Clarion R., *Pennsylvania* T24+413 **96**
Clark, *S. Dakota* U44+449 **93**
Clarke I., *Tasmania* C12-405 **109**
Clarkesville, *Texas* U30+336 **95**
Clarksburg, *West Virginia* T32+393 **91**
Clarksdale, *Mississippi* U04+342 **97**
Clarksville, *Tennessee* T74+365 **95**
Claro, *Switzerland* M36+463 **45**
Clausthal, *W. Germany* M28+517 **48**
Clay Center, *Kansas* U43+394 **95**
Claydon, *England* M83+521 **39**
Clayton, *Alabama* T63+319 **97**
Clayton, *New Jersey* T01+397 **91**
Clayton, *New Mexico* U80+365 **94**
Clear I., *Ireland, Rep.* N57+514 **43**
Clear L., *California* W17+390 **92**
Clearfield, *Pennsylvania* T21+410 **96**
Clear Lake, *Iowa* U18+432 **95**
Clearmont, *Wyoming* V08+446 **93**
Clearwater L., *Quebec* T00+558 **89**
Clearwater R., *Idaho* V63+461 **92**
Cleburne, *Texas* U44+324 **95**
Clent Hills, *England* N12+524 **37**
Clermont, *Queensland* C15-226 **111**
Clermont, *Transvaal* L12-236 **84**
Clermont-Ferrand, *France* M71+458 **54**
Cleveland, *Ohio* T40+415 **91**
Cleveland, *Tennessee* T59+351 **97**
Cleveland, *Texas* U30+302 **95**
Cleveland Hills, *England* N07+544 **37**
Clew Bay, *Ireland, Rep.* N59+538 **42**
Clifden, *Ireland, Rep.* N60+535 **43**
Clifton, *Arizona* V26+330 **94**
Clifton, *Tennessee* T78+354 **97**
Clifton Forge, *Virginia* T29+378 **97**
Clifton Ville, *Wisconsin* T83+447 **91**
Clinch Mts., *Tenn.-Va.* T48+364 **97**
Clinton, *Arkansas* U16+356 **97**
Clinton, *Illinois* T84+402 **95**
Clinton, *Iowa* U02+418 **95**
Clinton, *Massachusetts* S70+424 **96**
Clinton, *Missouri* U22+384 **95**
Clinton, *Oklahoma* U54+354 **95**
Clinton, *Ontario* T39+436 **91**
Clinton Colden L., *N.W.T.* V18+632 **88**
Clinton Dam, *Tennessee* T55+362 **97**
Clipperton I., *Pacific Ocean* V25+100 **107**
Clisson, *France* N08+471 **54**
Clitheroe, *England* N13+539 **37**
Clogham, *Ireland, Rep.* N47+532 **43**
Clogher, *N. Ireland* N43+544 **42**
Clonakilty & B., *Ireland, Rep.* N53+516 **43**
Cloncurry, *Queensland* C57-207 **111**
Clones, *Ireland, Rep.* N43+542 **42**
Clonmel, *Ireland, Rep.* N46+524 **43**
Clonegal, *Ireland, Rep.* N40+527 **43**
Cloquet, *Minnesota* U15+467 **93**
Clorinda, *Argentina* R77-252 **103**
Cloud Pk., *Wyoming* V12+446 **98**
Clover, *Virginia* T22+369 **97**
Clovis, *New Mexico* U80+344 **94**
Cloyne, *Ireland, Rep.* N49+519 **43**
Cluj, *Romania* L38+468 **58**
Clun Forest, *Wales* N20+524 **38**
Clunes, *Victoria* C37-373 **109**
Clusone, *Italy* M30+458 **56**
Clyde, *New Zealand* A64-451 **112**
Clyde, Firth of, *Scotland* N30+555 **41**
Clyde, Inlet, *N.-W. Terr.* S50+704 **89**
Clyde R., *Scotland* N26+559 **41**
Clydebank, *Scotland* N26+559 **41**
Coahuila, state, *Mexico* U74+270 **100**
Coalcoman, *Mexico* U78+188 **100**
Coamo, *Puerto Rico* S38+180 **101**
Coari, *Brazil* S19-040 **104**
Coast Mts., *Brit. Columbia* W30+510 **88**
Coast Ra., *Oregon, etc.* W23+418 **92**
Coatbridge, *Scotland* N24+558 **41**
Coatepeque, *Guatemala* U11+147 **100**
Coatesville, *Pennsylvania* T05+399 **96**
Coaticook, *Quebec* S71+451 **91**
Coats I., *N.-W. Terr.* T45+620 **89**
Coats Ld., *Antarctica* N75-750 **27**
Cobalt, *Ontario* T28+474 **91**
Coban, *Guatemala* U02+155 **100**
Cobar, *New S. Wales* C25-316 **109**
Cobargo, *New S. Wales* C01-364 **109**
Cobb, Mt., *New Zealand* A45-410 **112**
Cobden, *Victoria* C42-384 **109**
Cobequid Mts., *Nova Scotia* S26+455 **90**
Cobh, *Ireland, Rep.* N50+518 **43**
Cobija, *Bolivia* S53-110 **104**
Cobleskill, *New York* S87+427 **91**
Coboconk, *Ontario* T23+447 **91**
Cobourg, *Ontario* T19+440 **91**
Cobourg Pen., *N. Terr., Aust.* D15-114 **110**
Cobram, *Victoria* C26-359 **109**
Cobre, El, *Cuba* T06+201 **101**
Coburg, *W. Germany* M24+502 **48**
Coburg I., *N.-W. Terr.* T20+760 **89**
Cocahacra, *Peru* S71-170 **104**
Cocamá, *Peru* S68-105 **104**
Cochabamba, *Bolivia* S36-174 **104**
Cochin, *India* G82+100 **70**
Cochin China, *Vietnam* F00+102 **69**
Cochinoca, *Argentina* S35-227 **103**
Cochran, *Georgia* T50+324 **97**
Cochrane, *Ontario* T36+492 **89**
Cochrane, L., *Chile-Argent.* S72-472 **103**
Cockburn, *S. Australia* C54-321 **109**
Cockburn I., *Ontario* T50+459 **91**
Cockburn, Mt., *W. Australia* D45-157 **110**
Cockburnspath, *Scotland* N14+559 **41**
Cockermouth, *England* N20+547 **37**
Cockscomb Mts., *Belize* T84+166 **101**
Coco, I. del, *Pacific Ocean* T70+045 **107**
Cocos Is. (Keeling), *Indian Oc.* F45-120 **77**
Cocula, *Mexico* U83+203 **100**
Cocuy, *Columbia* S75+064 **104**
Cod C., *Massachusetts* S60+421 **96**
Codajas, *Brazil* S12-036 **104**
Codfish I., *New Zealand* A74-467 **112**
Codó *Brazil* Q83-044 **105**
Cod's Hd., *Ireland, Rep.* N61+517 **43**
Cody, *Wyoming* V24+445 **93**
Coe Hill, *Ontario* T17+448 **91**
Coeur d'Alene, *Idaho* V71+477 **92**
Coevorden, *Netherlands* M49+527 **44**
Coeymans, *New York* S83+425 **96**
Coffeyville, *Kansas* U34+370 **95**
Coff's Harbour, *N.S.W.* B71-303 **109**
Cognac, *France* N02+457 **54**
Cogolludo, *Spain* N19+410 **52**
Cohoes, *New York* S82+428 **96**
Cohuna, *Victoria* C35-358 **109**
Coiba, I., *Panama* T40+075 **101**
Coimbatore, *India* G78+110 **70**
Coimbra, *Portugal* N50+402 **52**
Coin, *Spain* N28+366 **52**
Coire. *See* Chur
Cojimies, *Ecuador* T30+003 **104**
Coko Ra., *New S. Wales* C51-305 **109**
Colac, *Victoria* C39-384 **109**
Colair L., *India* G52+166 **70**
Colbeck Arch, *Antarctica* H85-680 **27**
Colby, *Kansas* U66+394 **94**
Colcha, *Bolivia* S47-208 **104**
Colchester, *England* M85+519 **39**
Coldingham, *Scotland* N13+559 **41**
Coldstream, *Scotland* N13+557 **41**
Coldwater, *Mississippi* U00+347 **97**
Colebrook, *New Hampshire* S69+449 **91**
Coleman, *Alberta* V57+496 **88**
Coleman, *Texas* U56+318 **95**
Colemerik. *See* Hakkâri
Coleraine, *N. Ireland* N40+551 **42**
Coleraine, *Victoria* C50-375 **109**
Coleridge, L., *New Zealand* A51-433 **112**
Colgong, *India* G16+252 **73**
Colhué Huapi, L., *Argentina* S53-455 **103**
Colima & state, *Mexico* U82+192 **100**
Colinas, *Honduras* T80+150 **101**
Coll, I., *Scotland* N39+566 **41**
Collahuasi, *Chile* S52-210 **103**
Collarenebri, *New S. Wales* C09-296 **109**
Collie, *New South Wales* C10-317 **109**

Collie, *W. Australia* E21-333 **110**
Collier B., *W. Australia* D65-160 **110**
Collines-de-Normandie, *France* N06+490 **54**
Collingwood, *Ontario* T31+445 **91**
Collingwood, *Queensland* C45-222 **111**
Collo, *Algeria* M50+368 **80**
Collooney, *Ireland, Rep.* N51+542 **42**
Colmar, *France* M46+481 **54**
Colmars, *France* M50+442 **55**
Colmena, *Argentina* S01-286 **103**
Colmenar de Oreja, *Spain* N21+401 **52**
Colmenar Viejo, *Spain* N23+406 **52**
Colmi, *Honduras* T64+150 **101**
Colmonell, *Scotland* N29+551 **41**
Colne, *England* N13+539 **37**
Colne R., *England* M85+519 **39**
Cologne. *See* Köln
Colomb-Bechar (Bechar), *Algeria* N12+314 **80**
Colombia, *Brazil* R23-202 **105**
Colombia, rep., *S. America* **104**
Colombier, *Switzerland* M49+470 **45**
Colombo, *Sri Lanka* G62+070 **70**
Colon, *Argentina* R79-321 **103**
Colon, *Argentina* S07-338 **103**
Colon, *Cuba* T34+227 **111**
Colon, *Panama* T28+093 **111**
Colon, *Venezuela* S74+080 **104**
Colonel Fer. Gomez, *Brazil* R36+008 **105**
Colonelganj, *India* G49+271 **73**
Colonia, *Uruguay* R77-344 **103**
Colonia Alvear, *Argentina* S46-350 **103**
Colonia Sarmiento, *Argent.* S55-457 **103**
Colonsay, I., *Scotland* N37+561 **41**
Colorado, *Texas* U65+323 **94**
Colorado, state, *U.S.A.* V17+391 **98**
Colorado Des., California V66+349 **92**
Colorado Des., *Wyoming* V28+424 **93**
Colorado Plat., *Arizona* V30+360 **94**
Colorado, R., *Argentina* S22-393 **103**
Colorado R., *Texas* U36+292 **95**
Colorado R., *U.S.A.* V57+333 **98**
Colorado R., *Utah, etc.* V30+380 **94**
Colorado R., Little, *Arizona* V38+358 **94**
Colorados, Arch. de los, *Cuba* T56+224 **101**
Colorado Springs, *Colorado* U89+388 **94**
Colotlan, *Mexico* U80+223 **100**
Colpoy B., *Ontario* T36+449 **91**
Colquechaca, *Bolivia* S37-190 **104**
Colton, *California* V74+341 **92**
Columbia, *Alabama* T61+313 **97**
Columbia, *Indiana* T63+412 **91**
Columbia, *Kentucky* T62+371 **97**
Columbia, *Louisiana* U13+321 **97**
Columbia, *Mississippi* T89+312 **99**
Columbia, *Missouri* U14+390 **95**
Columbia, *Pennsylvania* T09+400 **96**
Columbia, *S. Carolina* T36+340 **97**
Columbia, *Tennessee* T72+356 **97**
Columbia C., *Canada* S60+830 **26**
Columbia, Dist. of, *U.S.A.* T12+386 **91**
Columbia, Mt., *Alberta* V75+524 **88**
Colombia Plat., *Wash., etc.* V80+469 **98**
Colombia R., *Canada-U.S.A.* W06+457 **92**
Columbiana, *Alabama* T70+332 **97**
Columbus, *Georgia* T60+325 **97**
Columbus, *Indiana* T65+392 **91**
Columbus, *Kansas* U30+372 **95**
Columbus, *Mississippi* T80+336 **95**
Columbus, *Montana* V26+456 **93**
Columbus, *Nebraska* U42+414 **95**
Columbus, *Ohio* T48+400 **91**
Columbus, *Texas* U39+297 **95**
Colville L., *N.-W. Terr.* W25+678 **88**
Colville Ra., *New Zealand* A26-370 **112**
Colwyn Bay, *Wales* N22+533 **38**
Comacchio, Valli di, *Italy* M18+447 **56**
Comana, *Romania* L23+442 **58**
Comayagua, *Honduras* T76+144 **101**
Combarbala, *Chile* S66-311 **103**
Comber, *N. Ireland* N34+545 **42**
Comblain, *Belgium* M57+505 **44**
Comeragh Mts., *Ireland, Rep.* N45+522 **43**
Comino C., *Sardinia* M31+405 **57**
Comiso, *Sicily* M02+369 **57**
Comitan, *Mexico* U12+162 **100**
Commissioners L., *Quebec* S73+482 **90**
Commonwealth Ra., *Antarc.* Z80-850 **27**
Como, *Italy* M36+458 **56**
Como, L. di, *Italy* M35+460 **56**
Comores, Arch. des, *See* Comoro Is.
Comorin C., *India* G74+081 **70**
Comoro Is., *Ind. Oc.* K06-122 **83**
Compiègne, *France* M73+494 **54**
Comporta, *Portugal* N53+384 **52**
Compostela, *Mexico* U89+213 **100**
Comrie, *Scotland* N24+564 **41**
Conakry, *Guinea* N82+096 **80**
Conceicao do Araguaya, *Brazil* R27-086 **105**
Conceicao do Arroio, *Brazil* R33-299 **103**
Concepcion, *Argentina* S17-312 **103**
Concepcion, *Argentina* R78-284 **103**
Concepcion, *Bolivia* S40-114 **104**
Concepcion, *Chile* S78-368 **103**
Concepcion, *Paraguay* R75-234 **103**
Concepcion del Oro, *Mexico* U68+245 **100**
Concepcion del Uruguay, *Argentina* R80-325 **103**
Conception B., *Nfd.* R48+478 **90**
Conception I., *Bahamas, The* T01+239 **101**
Conception, Pt., *California* W03+346 **98**
Conchas Res., *New Mexico* U86+354 **94**
Conchi, *Chile* S52-219 **103**
Concord, *Massachusetts* S68+425 **96**
Concord, *New Hampshire* S69+432 **91**
Concord, *N. Carolina* T34+354 **97**
Concordia, *Argentina* R79-313 **103**
Concordia, *Kansas,* U46+395 **95**
Concordia, *Mexico* V06+232 **100**
Concordia, *Peru* S63-185 **104**
Condobolin, *New S. Wales* C18-331 **109**
Condom, *France* M88+440 **55**
Condor, Cord. del, *Peru* T20-040 **104**
Conemaugh, *Pennsylvania* T24+404 **96**
Conesa, *Argentina* S28-401 **103**
Confolens, *France* M86+460 **54**
Congo, rep., Cent. Africa. *See* Zaire.
Congo, rep., *Cent Africa* M00+002 **82**
Congo R. (Zaire) *Cent. Afr.* L76-016 **82**
Coniston Water, *England* N19+543 **37**
Coney I., *New York* S83+405 **96**
Conlin, *Montana* V00+469 **93**
Conn L., *Ireland, Rep.* N56+540 **42**
Connacht, prov., *Ireland, Rep.* N51+538 **42**
Connecticut R., *Conn., etc.* S74+413 **96**
Connecticut R., *Vermont* S75+428 **91**
Connecticut, state, *U.S.A.* S80+415 **99**
Connellsville, *Pennsylvania* T28+400 **96**
Connemara, *Ireland, Rep.* N58+535 **43**
Connors, *New Brunswick* S53+472 **90**
Conrad, *Montana* V42+482 **93**
Conroe, *Texas* U33+302 **95**
Conshohocken, *New Jersey* T02+401 **96**
Conselheiro Lafaiete, *Brazil* Q80-204 **105**
Constance. *See Konstanz*
Constance, L. *See* Boden See
Constanta, *Romania* L08+442 **58**
Constantine, *Algeria* M50+362 **80**
Constitucion, *Chile* S75-354 **103**
Consuegra, *Spain* N22+394 **52**
Contamana, *Peru* T00-073 **104**
Conthey, *Switzerland* M46+462 **45**
Contreras, I., *Chile* T00-519 **103**
Contwoyto L., *N.-W. Terr.* V42+657 **88**
Conway, *Arkansas* U14+351 **95**
Conway, *Missouri* U18+376 **95**
Conway, *New Hampshire* S67+440 **91**
Conway, *S. Carolina* T 24+339 **97**
Conwy, *Wales* N23+533 **38**
Coober Pedy, *S. Australia* D03-287 **111**
Cooch Behar, *India* G03+263 **73**
Cook, B. de, *Chile* S60-552 **103**
Cook Inl., *Alaska* Y15+590 **99**
Cook Is., *Pacific Ocean* Y60-200 **106**
Cook, Mt., *New Zealand* A59-436 **112**
Cook Str., *New Zealand* A32-414 **112**
Cook's Passage, *Queensland* C29-147 **111**
Cookshire, *Quebec* S70+454 **91**
Cookstown, *N. Ireland* N40+546 **42**
Cooktown, *Queensland* C28-154 **111**
Coolabah, *New S. Wales* C20-311 **109**
Coolah, *New S. Wales* C02-318 **109**
Coolamon, *New S. Wales* C17-348 **109**
Coolgardie, *W. Australia* D83-309 **110**
Cooma, *New South Wales* C06-362 **109**
Coomacarrea, *Ireland, Rep.* N60+520 **43**
Coonabarabran, *N.S.W.* C04-313 **109**
Coonalpym, *S. Australia* C61-357 **109**
Coonamble, *New S. Wales* C09-309 **109**
Coondiwindi, *Queensland* B88-283 **111**
Cooper Cr., *S. Australia* C66-278 **111**
Cooperstown, *New York* T00+427 **96**
Coorg, *India* G83+122 **70**
Coorong, The, *S. Australia* C62-360 **109**
Cootamundra, *New S. Wales* C12-347 **109**
Cootehill, *Ireland, Rep.* N42+541 **42**
Copenhagen *See* København.
Copetonas, *Argentina* S03-386 **103**
Copiapo, *Chile* S62-273 **103**
Copley, *S. Australia* C69-306 **109**
Coporaque, *Peru* S70-148 **104**
Copper Cliff, *Ontario* T37+465 **91**
Coppermine, *North-West Territories* V65+672 **88**
Coppermine R., *N.-W. Terr.* V60+664 **88**
Coppet, *Switzerland* M53+463 **45**
Coquar, *Quebec* T02+481 **91**
Coquilhatville (Mbandaka), *Zaire* L70+001 **82**
Coquimbo & B. de, *Chile* S68-299 **103**
Corabia, *Romania* L33+438 **58**
Coracoes, *Brazil* R02-217 **105**
Coraki, *New S. Wales* B71-288 **109**
Corangamite, L., *Victoria* C40-382 **109**
Corato, *Italy* L82+411 **57**
Corazon, Sierra, *Texas* U82+295 **94**
Corcaigh. *See Cork*
Corcovado, G. del, *Chile* S80-434 **103**
Corcovado, mt. *Chile* S76-432 **103**
Corcubion, *Spain* N55+429 **52**
Cordell, *Oklahoma* U54+352 **95**
Cordoba, *Mexico* U42+190 **100**
Cordoba, *Peru* T00-139 **104**
Córdoba, *Spain* N29+379 **52**
Cordoba and Sa. de, *Argentina* S26-314 **103**
Cordova, *Alaska* X70+605 **99**
Corfu. *See* Kérkira, I.
Corfu, Str. of *Greece* L60+395 **59**
Coria, *Spain* N39+400 **52**
Corigliano Calabro, *Italy* L81+396 **57**
Corindi, *New S. Wales* B71-300 **109**
Coringa, *India* G47+168 **71**
Corinth. *See* Korinthos
Corinth, *Mississippi* T81+349 **95**
Corinto, *Brazil* Q87-184 **105**
Corinto, *Nicaragua* T73+126 **101**
Coristine, *Ontario* T24+461 **91**
Cork & co., *Ireland, Rep.* N51+519 **43**
Cork Harb., *Ireland, Rep.* N49+518 **43**
Corleone, *Sicily* M10+378 **57**
Corner Inl., *Victoria* C22-387 **109**
Corner Brook, *Nfd.* R78+490 **90**
Corning, *Iowa* U28+410 **95**
Corning, *New York* T13+421 **96**
Cornwall, *New York* S84+414 **96**
Cornwall, *Ontario* S88+450 **91**
Cornwall, co., *England* N28+504 **38**
Coro, *Venezuela* S58+114 **104**
Coroata, *Brazil* Q85-040 **105**
Corocoro, *Bolivia* S52-171 **104**
Coroico, *Bolivia* S47-161 **104**
Corrofin, *Ireland, Rep.* N54+529 **43**
Corona, *New S. Wales* C52-312 **109**
Coronada, B., *Costa Rica* T52+090 **101**
Coronation G., *N. W. Terr.* V40+678 **88**
Coronation I., *Antarctica* R05-610 **27**
Coronel, *Chile* S79-370 **103**
Coronel Pringles, *Argentina* S09-380 **103**
Coronel Suarez, *Argentina* S11-376 **103**
Coronie, *Surinam* R69+058 **105**
Coropuna, mt., *Peru* S76-156 **104**
Corowa, *New South Wales* C22-360 **109**
Corozal, *Belize* T81+184 **101**
Corpen Aike, *Argentina* S56-496 **103**
Corpus Christi & B., *Texas* U44+278 **94**
Corpus Christi L., *Texas* V29+282 **94**
Corpus Christi Pass, *Texas* U43+276 **94**
Corque, *Bolivia* S46-183 **104**
Corrales, *Uruguay* R64-314 **103**
Corralitos, *Mexico* V17+306 **100**
Corregidor, I., *Philippines* D87+144 **65**
Correze, dep., *France* M78+453 **54**
Corrib L. *Ireland, Rep.* N55+534 **43**
Corrientes, *Argentina* R83-276 **103**
Corrientes, C., *Argentina* R76-381 **103**
Corrientes, C., *Mexico* V04+204 **100**
Corrigin, *W. Australia* E12-322 **110**
Corrimal, *New S. Wales* B85-344 **109**
Corry, *Pennsylvania* T28+419 **96**
Corryvreckan, G. of, *Scot.* N35+561 **41**
Corse, I., *France* M36+420 **56**
Corsewall Pt., *Scotland* N31+550 **41**
Corsica. *See* Corse, I.
Corsicana, *Texas* U39+322 **95**
Cortes, G. de, *Cuba* T54+220 **101**
Cortland, *New York* T07+426 **96**
Cortona, *Italy* M18+433 **56**
Coruche, *Portugal* N51+390 **52**
Coruh, R., *Turkey* K24+407 **74**
Corum, *Turkey* K61+405 **74**
Corumba, *Brazil* R75-190 **105**
Corunna. *See* La Coruña.
Corvallis, *Oregon* W20+446 **92**
Corwen, *Wales* N20+530 **38**
Corwin, *Alaska* Y85+685 **99**
Corydon, *Iowa* U20+408 **95**
Cosalo, *Mexico* V09+244 **100**
Coscurita, *Spain* N15+414 **53**
Coseguina, Vol., *Nicaragua* T75+130 **101**
Cosenza, *Italy* L82+393 **57**
Cosquin, *Argentina* S27-312 **103**
Cossonay, *Switzerland* M51+466 **45**
Costa Rica, rep., *Central America* T54+100 **101**
Costermansville. *See* Bukavu
Costillo Pk., *New Mexico* U92+368 **94**
Cotabato, *Philippines* D65+072 **65**
Cotagaita, *Bolivia* S34-208 **104**
Cotahuasi, *Peru* S78-152 **104**
Cote Blanche B., *Louisiana* U10+296 **95**
Cote D'Ivoire. *See* Ivory Coast
Côte-d'Or, dep., *France* M60+474 **54**
Côtes-du-Nord, dep., *France* N18+484 **54**
Cöthen, *E. Germany* M18+517 **48**
Cotonou, *Benin* M76+064 **80**
Cotswold, Hills, *England* N12+519 **39**
Cottbus, *E. Germany* M04+518 **48**
Cottica, *Surinam* R56+038 **105**
Cotulla, *Texas* U55+284 **94**
Coudersport, *Pennsylvania* T18+417 **96**
Coudres, I. aux, *Quebec* S62+474 **91**
Coulagh B., *Ireland, Rep.* N60+517 **43**
Coulman, I., *Antarctica* A62-730 **27**
Council Bluffs, *Iowa* U35+412 **95**
Council Grove, *Kansas* U39+386 **95**
Coupar-Angus, *Scotland* N20+565 **41**
Courantyne, R., *Guyana, etc.* R77+042 **104**
Couronne C., *France* M60+433 **55**
Courtenay, *N. Dakota* U51+472 **93**
Courtmacsherry, *Ireland, Rep.* N52+516 **43**
Courtrai, *Belgium* M70+508 **44**
Court St Etienne, *Belgium* M62+506 **44**
Couterne, *France* N02+485 **54**
Couthuin, *Belgium* M59+505 **44**
Couvin, *Belgium* M63+501 **44**
Covenas, *Colombia* T04+094 **104**
Coventry, *England* N09+524 **37**
Covilhã, *Portugal* N45+403 **52**
Covington, *Kentucky* T57+391 **91**
Covington, *Tennessee* T88+356 **97**
Covington, *Virginia* T30+378 **97**
Cowal, L., *New S. Wales* C15-336 **109**
Cowan, L., *W. Australia* D79-318 **110**
Cowangie, *Victoria* C51-352 **109**
Cowbridge, *Wales* N20+514 **38**
Cowdenbeath, *Scotland* N20+561 **41**
Cowell, *S. Australia* C79-334 **111**
Cowes, *I. of W., England* N08+508 **39**
Cowra, *New South Wales* C07-339 **109**
Coxsackie, *New York* S83+424 **96**
Cox's Bazar, *Bangladesh* F78+214 **71**
Coyame, *Mexico* V01+294 **100**
Coyuca, *Mexico* U64+183 **100**
Cozumel, I., *Mexico* T70+204 **100**
Crabbs, *Newfoundland* R83+482 **90**
Craboon, *N.S.W.* C03-321 **109**
Cracow. *See Krakow*
Cradle Mt., *Tasmania* C24-417 **109**
Craig, *Colorado* V16+404 **94**
Craigavon, *N. Ireland* N38+544 **42**
Craig Harbour, *N.-W. Terr.* T35+760 **89**
Craigue, *Ireland, Rep.* N42+528 **43**
Craigville, *Minnesota* U22+479 **93**
Crail, *Scotland* N16+563 **41**
Craiova, *Romania* L37+443 **58**
Cranborne, *England* N11+509 **39**
Cranbrook, *Brit. Columbia* V65+496 **88**
Crandon, *Wisconsin* T83+455 **91**
Crane I., *Quebec* S63+471 **91**
Cranleigh, *England* N03+511 **39**
Crans, *Switzerland* M45+463 **45**
Crater Lake National Park, *Oregon* W14+430 **92**
Crateus, *Brazil* Q64-052 **105**
Crato, *Brazil* S18-073 **104**
Crato, *Brazil* Q56-072 **105**
Cravo, *Colombia* S62+056 **104**
Crawford, *Nebraska* U80+427 **94**
Crawford, *Scotland* N22+555 **41**
Crazy Mts., *Montana* V32+461 **93**
Creag Meagaidh, *Scotland* N28+569 **40**
Crediton, *England* N22+508 **38**
Cree L., *Saskatchewan* V10+578 **88**
Cree R., *Saskatchewan* V07+584 **88**
Cree R., *Scotland* N27+550 **41**
Cremona, *Italy* M30+452 **56**
Cres, I., *Yugoslavia* M04+448 **56**
Cresco, *Iowa* U14+434 **95**
Cressy, *Victoria* C38-381 **109**
Crest, *Quebec* T24+465 **91**
Cresta, *Switzerland* M33+465 **45**
Creston, *Iowa* U26+410 **95**
Creswell B., *N.-W. Terr.* U20+722 **89**
Creswick, *Victoria* C37-374 **109**
Crete (Kriti), *Greece* L30+350 **59**
Crete, *Nebraska* U42+406 **95**
Crete, Sea of, *Greece* L30+359 **59**
Creuse, dep., *France* M78+460 **54**
Creusot, le, *France* M64+468 **54**
Crewe, *England* N15+531 **37**
Crewkerne, *England* N17+509 **38**
Criccieth, *Wales* N25+529 **38**
Crickhowell, *Wales* N19+519 **38**
Cricklade, *England* N11+516 **39**
Crieff, *Scotland* N23+564 **41**
Crimea (Krym), *U.S.S.R.* K66+450 **60**
Crimmitschau, *E. Germany* M16+508 **48**
Cripple Creek, *Colorado* V02+387 **94**
Crisana, *Romania* L48+468 **58**
Cristobal, *Panama* T29+093 **101**
Crnagora, *Yugoslavia* L64+430 **58**
Croagh Patrick, *Ireland, Rep.* N58+538 **42**
Crockett, *Texas* U33+313 **95**
Croisic le, *France* N15+472 **54**
Croker I., *N. Terr., Aust.* D14-111 **110**
Cromarty, & Firth, *Scotland* N24+577 **40**
Cromer, *England* M82+529 **39**
Cromwell, *New Zealand* A64-449 **112**
Crooked I., *Bahamas, The* S86+228 **101**
Crookston, *Minnesota* U40+478 **93**
Crookwell, *New S. Wales* C03-345 **109**
Croom, *Ireland, Rep.* N52+525 **43**
Croppa Creek, *New S. Wales* B88-291 **109**
Cross Fell, *England* N15+547 **37**
Crosshaven, *Ireland, Rep.* N50+518 **43**
Crossmolina, *Ireland, Rep.* N56+541 **42**
Cross Point, *Quebec* S40+481 **90**
Crotone, *Italy* L77+391 **57**
Crow Agency, *Montana* V15+455 **93**
Crowes, *Victoria* C40-387 **109**
Crowley, *Louisiana* U13+302 **95**
Crown Prince Olav Ld., *Antarctica* K25-690 **27**
Crown Princess Martha Ld., *Antarctica* N30-720 **27**
Crows Nest Pass, *Alberta* V58+498 **88**
Croydon, *England* N01+514 **39**
Croydon, *Queensland* C47-181 **111**
Crozet Is., *Indian Ocean* J60-463 **77**
Crozier, C., *Antarctica* A65-770 **27**
Cruden B., *Scotland* N11+574 **40**
Crumlin, *N. Ireland* N37+546 **42**
Cruz, *Utah* V47+388 **92**
Cruz Alta, *Argentina* S11-330 **103**
Cruz Alta, *Brazil* R52-286 **103**
Cruz del Eje, *Argentina* S29-308 **103**
Cruzeiro do Sul, *Brazil* S76-078 **104**
Cruz Grande, *Chile* S68-294 **103**
Cruz Grande, *Mexico* U55+167 **100**
Crystal Brook, *S. Australia* C71-333 **109**
Crystal Falls, *Michigan* T80+461 **91**
Crystal Springs, *Mississippi* U01+320 **97**
Cuamba, *Mozambique* K50-148 **83**
Cuango, *Angola* L72-092 **82**
Cuanza, R., *Angola* M10-092 **82**
Cuareim, *Brazil* R76-302 **103**
Cuatro Cienegas, *Mexico* U73+269 **100**
Cuba, *New Mexico* V12+360 **94**
Cuba, *New York* T20+423 **91**
Cuba, *Portugal* N47+382 **52**
Cuba, I., *West Indies* T30+220 **101**
Cuchi, *Angola* L78-146 **82**
Cuchillo-Co, *Argentina* S28-384 **103**
Cuchillo Parado, *Mexico* U89+294 **100**
Cucumbi, *Angola* L66-104 **82**
Cucuta, *Colombia* S75+079 **104**
Cudahy, *Wisconsin* T77+430 **91**
Cuddalore, *India* G62+117 **70**
Cuddapah, *India* G66+144 **70**
Cudgewa, *Victoria* C13-362 **109**
Cue, *W. Australia* E12-274 **110**
Cuellar, *Spain* N26+414 **52**
Cuenca, *Ecuador* T24-028 **104**
Cuenca, *Spain* N13+401 **53**
Cuencame, *Mexico* U83+248 **100**
Cuernavaca, *Mexico* U55+188 **100**
Cuero, *Texas* U44+290 **95**
Cuevo, *Bolivia* S21-204 **104**
Cuglieri, *Sardinia* M39+402 **57**
Cuiabá, *Brazil* R80-072 **104**
Cuiaba, *Brazil* R66-156 **105**
Cuicuina, *Nicaragua* T57+136 **101**
Cuilcagh, *Ireland, Rep.* N47+542 **42**
Cuillin Hills, *Scotland* N38+572 **40**
Cuillin Sd., *Scotland* N38+571 **40**
Cuiña, P. de, *Spain* N41+429 **52**
Cuito Cuanavale, *Angola* L64-152 **84**
Culcairn, *New South Wales* C18-357 **109**
Culebra, G. de la, *Costa Rica* T64+108 **101**
Culebra, I., *West Indies* S32+184 **101**
Culgoa, R., *New S. Wales* C20-296 **109**
Culgoa, R., *Queensland* C15-286 **111**
Culiacan, *Mexico* V15+249 **100**
Cullarin Ra., *New S. Wales* C03-346 **109**
Cullera, *Spain* N01+392 **53**
Cullompton, *England* N21+509 **38**
Cully, *Switzerland* M50+465 **45**
Culpeper, *Virginia* T18+384 **97**
Culverden, *New Zealand* A43-427 **112**
Cumana, *Venezuela* S24+104 **104**
Cumaria, *Peru* S84-099 **104**
Cumberland, *Brit. Columbia* W31+496 **88**
Cumberland, *Maryland* T22+397 **96**
Cumberland, *Virginia* T20+375 **97**
Cumberland, *Wisconsin* U12+456 **93**
Cumberland I., *Georgia* T39+308 **97**
Cumberland Mts., *Tenn., etc.* T52+365 **97**
Cumberland Pen., *N.-W. Terr.* T30+664 **89**
Cumberland Plat., *Tenn.* T66+351 **97**
Cumberland R., *Kentucky, etc.* T78+368 **97**
Cumberland Sd., *N.-W. Terr.* S30+650 **89**
Cumbrae, Great, I., *Scotland* N30+558 **41**
Cumbria, co., *England* N18+547 **37**
Cumbrian Mts., *England* N18+545 **37**
Cumbum, *India* G65+156 **70**
Cumnock, *New S. Wales* C07-330 **109**
Cumnock, *Scotland* N26+554 **41**
Cunene R., *Angola* M16-172 **84**
Cuneo, *Italy* M45+444 **56**
Cunnamulla, *Queensland* C26-280 **111**
Cupar, *Scotland* N18+563 **41**
Cuprija, *Yugoslavia* L56+440 **58**
Cura, *Venezuela* S45+100 **104**
Curaca, *Brazil* Q59-090 **105**
Curaçoa, I., *Caribbean Sea* S53+122 **104**
Curaglia, *Switzerland* M37+467 **45**
Curiapo, *Venezuela* S07+086 **104**

Curico, *Chile* S67–350 **103**
Curiplaya, *Colombia* S89+003 **104**
Curitiba, *Brazil* R25–256 **103**
Curitibanos, *Brazil* R34–273 **103**
Curlewis, *New South Wales* B88–311 **109**
Curnamona, *S. Australia* C63–316 **109**
Curora, *Mozambique* K42–116 **83**
Currabubula, *New S. Wales* B86–312 **109**
Curraes Novos, *Brazil* Q39–062 **105**
Curralinho, *Brazil* R28–017 **105**
Currane L., *Ireland, Rep.* N61+518 **43**
Curraun Pen., (Corraun),
Ireland, Rep. N59+539 **42**
Currituck Sd., *N. Carolina* T04+364 **97**
Curtis, I., *Pacific Ocean* Z80–305 **106**
Curua, *Brazil* R52+010 **105**
Curuay, Gde. do, L., *Brazil* R62–022 **105**
Curuca, *Brazil* R17–006 **105**
Curupachi, *Brazil* R76–076 **105**
Curuzú Cuatia, *Argentina* R78–298 **103**
Curwensville, *Pennsylvania* T21+410 **96**
Cury, *Brazil* R63–039 **105**
Cushendall, *N. Ireland* N36+551 **42**
Cushendun, *N. Ireland* N36+551 **42**
Cushing, *Oklahoma* U40+359 **95**
Custer, *S. Dakota* U82+437 **93**
Cut Bank, *Montana* V44+486 **93**
Cuthbert, *Georgia* T59+318 **97**
Cutra L., *Ireland, Rep.* N53+530 **43**
Cuttack, *India* G24+204 **71**
Cuxhaven, *W. Germany* M38+539 **48**
Cuzco, *Peru* S72–135 **104**
Cyclâdes, *See* Kikladhes, Is.
Cygnet, *Tasmania* C18–432 **109**
Cynthiana, *Kentucky* T56+385 **97**
Cyprus, I. and rep., *Mediterranean Sea* K72+350 **76**
Cyrenaica, *Libya* L50+292 **81**
Cyrene. *See Shahhat*
Czechoslovakia, rep., Central Europe **50-51**
Czersk, *Poland* L72+538 **49**
Czestochowa, *Poland* L65+508 **49**
Dabakala, *Ivory Coast* N26+084 **80**
Dabaro, *Somalia* J68+064 **83**
Dabeiba, *Colombia* T07+070 **104**
Dabhoi, *India* H09+220 **70**
Dabie, *Poland* M02+534 **48**
Dabola, *Guinea* N66+108 **80**
Dabrowa Górnicza, *Poland* L65+504 **49**
Dacca, *Bangladesh* F87+237 **71**
Dadanawa, *Guyana* R88+028 **104**
Dade City, *Florida* T43+284 **97**
Dadri, *India* G82+286 **72**
Dagana, *Senegal* P04+164 **80**
Dagarita, *Somalia* K06+106 **83**
Dagash, *Sudan* K70+190 **81**
Dagda, *Latvia* L15+561 **47**
Dagenham, *England* M89+515 **39**
Dagupan, *Philippines* D88+160 **65**
Dahlak Arch, *Ethiopia* K28+156 **83**
Dahomey, rep., *See* Benin
Daimiel, *Spain* N22+391 **52**
Daireaux, *Argentina* S11–365 **103**
Dairen, *See* Luta
Dairut, *Egypt* K86+276 **81**
Daisetsuzan Nat. Park, *Japan* C44+435 **68**
Daishoji, *Japan* C82+363 **68**
Dajarra, *Queensland* C63–218 **111**
Dakar, *Senegal* P14+146 **80**
Dakhla, *Mauritania* P06 + 236 **80**
Dakovica, *Yugoslavia* L58+424 **58**
Dal, *Norway* M22+603 **47**
Dal Alv, *Sweden* L80+602 **47**
Dala, *Angola* L58–112 **82**
Dalan Dszadagad, *Mongolia* F02+437 **64**
Dalat, *Vietnam* E70 + 120 **69**
Dalbandin, *Pakistan* H63+290 **70**
Dalbeattie, *Scotland* N23+549 **41**
Dalbo Sjön, *Sweden* M12+589 **47**
Dalby, *Queensland* B83–270 **111**
Dalby, *Sweden* M12+606 **47**
Dalen, *Netherlands* M49+527 **44**
Dalen, *Norway* M42+595 **47**
Dalgety, *New S. Wales* C07–364 **109**
Dalhart, *Texas* U75+360 **98**
Dalhousie, *India* G84+325 **72**
Dalhousie, *New Brunswick* S38+481 **90**
Dalkeith, *Scotland* N18+559 **41**
Dalkey, *Ireland, Rep.* N36+533 **43**
Dallas, *Oregon* W20+449 **92**
Dallas, *Texas* U41+328 **95**
Dallas, L., *Texas* U42+332 **95**
Dalles, The, *Oregon* W07+456 **92**
Dalmacio Velez, *Argentina* S22–327 **103**
Dalmally, *Scotland* N30+564 **41**
Dalmatia, *Yugoslavia* L82+437 **56**
Dalmatovo, *U.S.S.R.* H73+562 **61**
Dalmau, *India* G54+261 **73**
Dalmellington, *Scotland* N26+553 **41**
Daloa, *Ivory Coast* N38+070 **80**
Dalry, *Scotland* N28+557 **41**
Dalrymple, Mt., *Queensland* C15–206 **111**
Dalton, *England* N19+542 **37**
Dalton, *Ontario* T54+481 **91**
Daltonganj, *India* G35+240 **73**
Dalwhinnie, *Scotland* N25+569 **40**
Daly, *N. Terr., Australia* D22–126 **110**
Daly, R., *N. Terr., Australia* D23–142 **110**
Daly Waters, *N. Terr.*, Aust. D10–162 **111**
Dam, *Surinam* R60+046 **105**
Daman, *India* H12+204 **70**
Damanhur, *Egypt* K88+310 **81**
Damar, I., *Indonesia* D38–072 **65**
Damascus (Damas), *Syria* K52+335 **75**
Damâvand, mt., *Iran* J48+360 **75**
Dambe, *Angola* L88–068 **82**
Damghan, *Iran* J34+362 **75**
Damietta, *Egypt* K80+314 **81**
Damiya, *Jordan* K57+321 **76**
Dammam Ad, *Saudi Arabia* J57+265 **75**
Damoh, *India* G63+238 **73**
Dampier Arch., *W. Aust.* E22–204 **110**
Dampier Land, *W. Australia* D73–174 **110**
Dampier Str., *Indonesia* D26–007 **65**
Damqawt, *Yemen, South* J43 + 166 **75**
Dana, Mt., *California* V85+379 **92**
Danbury, *Connecticut* S81+414 **96**
Danby, *California* V62+347 **92**
Dandenong, *Victoria* C29–380 **109**
Danforth, *Maine* S47+457 **90**
Danger Pt., *Cape Province* L64–348 **84**
Dangra Yum L., *Tibet* G20+310 **71**
Danilov, *U.S.S.R.* K29+582 **60**
Dankaz, *Ethiopia* K44+124 **83**
Danmark Fd., *Greenland* P85+810 **26**
Dannemora, *Sweden* L74+603 **34**
Dannevirke, *New Zealand* A23–400 **112**
Dansville, *New York* T16+426 **96**
Danube (Dunarea, Donau), R.,
Cent. Europe L70+450 **51**
Danville, *Illinois* T76+401 **95**
Danville, *Kentucky* T59+376 **97**
Danville, *Pennsylvania* T10+410 **96**
Danville, *Virginia* T26+366 **97**
Danzig. *See* Gdansk
Danzig, G. of, *Poland* L66+546 **49**
Daolatabad, *Afghanistan* H60+364 **75**
Daqq-e-Patargân,
Iran-Afghanistan H88+341 **75**
Daraban Kalan, *Pakistan* H28+317 **72**
Daraw, *Egypt* K72+240 **81**
Darb, *Saudi Arabia* K16+175 **74**
Darbhanga, *India* G24+262 **73**
Dardanelles, *Turkey* L23+400 **74**
Darende, *Turkey* K45+386 **74**
Dar-es-Salaam, *Tanzania* K34–070 **83**
Dargai, *Pakistan* H19+345 **72**
Dargaon, *India* G33+217 **71**
Dargaville, *New Zealand* A37–359 **112**
Dargo, *Victoria* C16–375 **109**
Darien, *Georgia* T39+314 **97**
Darien, G. of, *Colombia* T10+082 **104**
Dariyah, *Saudi Arabia* J81+247 **74**
Darjeeling, *India* G10+270 **73**
Darling Ra., *W. Australia* E22–314 **110**
Darling, R., *New S. Wales* C44–336 **109**
Darling Downs, *Queensland* C00–276 **111**
Darlington, *England* N09+545 **37**
Darlington, *S. Carolina* T29+343 **97**
Darlington, *Wisconsin* U01+426 **95**
Darlington Point, *N.S.W.* C24–346 **109**
Darłowo, *Poland* L82+544 **49**
Darmstadt, *W. Germany* M38+499 **48**
Daroca, *Spain* N08+411 **53**
Dart, C., *Antarctica* W10–720 **27**
Dart R., *England* N22+505 **38**
Dartmoor, *England* N23+506 **38**
Dartmoor, *Victoria* C53–380 **109**
Dartmouth, *England* N21+503 **38**
Dartmouth, *Nova Scotia* S21+447 **90**
Daru, I., *Papua New Guinea* C41–091 **111**
Darun, *Iran* J58+330 **75**
Daruvar, *Yugoslavia* L77+456 **56**
Darwen, *England* N15+537 **37**
Darwin, *N. Terr., Australia* D24–124 **110**
Darwin, mt., *Chile* S56–548 **103**
Darwin Mt., *Zimbabwe* K80–168 **84**
Daryabad, *India* G51+269 **73**
Daryâcheh e Baktegân L.,
Iran J36+295 **75**
Daryâcheh-ye-Namak, *Iran* J50+348 **75**
Daryâcheh-ye-Rezâ'iyeh, *Iran* J88+378 **74**
Dasara, *Bangladesh* G00+239 **73**
Dashibalbar, *Mongolia* E34+495 **64**
Dasht R., *Pakistan* H78+256 **70**
Dasht Ab, *Iran* J21+289 **75**
Dashtiari, *Iran* H82+255 **75**
Daska, *Pakistan* H04+323 **72**
Daspalla, *India* G31+203 **71**
Daspur, *India* G23+220 **73**
Dasuya, *India* G86+318 **72**
Dataganj, *India* G63+280 **73**
Datia, *India* G69+256 **73**
Daudnagar, *India* G33+250 **73**
Daugavgriva, *Latvia* L36+570 **47**
Daugavpils, *Latvia* L21+559 **47**
Daulatabad, *India* G88+200 **70**
Daulat Yar, *Afghanistan* H55+345 **75**
Daule, *Ecuador* T30–018 **104**
Dauletabad, *Iran* J35+361 **75**
Dauphin, *Manitoba* U60+509 **88**
Dauphine, prov., *France* M56+449 **55**
Davao & G., *Philippines* D57+070 **65**
Davenport, *Iowa* U04+415 **95**
Davenport Ra., *N.T., Aust.* D00–209 **111**
Daventry, *England* N07+523 **37**
David, *Panama* T44+085 **101**
David City, *Nebraska* U43+412 **95**
Davignab, *Namibia* L62–276 **84**
Davis Mts., *Texas* U84+308 **94**
Davis Sea, *Antarctica* F60–650 **27**
Davis Str., *Greenland* R80+660 **26**
Davos Dorf, *Switzerland* M31+468 **45**
Davos Platz, *Switzerland* M31+468 **45**
Davy Sd., *Greenland* P40+720 **26**
Dawna Ra., *Burma* F41+170 **71**
Dawson, *Georgia* T57+318 **97**
Dawson, *Minnesota* U36+449 **93**
Dawson, *New Mexico* V00+366 **94**
Dawson, *N. Dakota* U59+469 **93**
Dawson, *Yukon* X25+643 **88**
Dawson Ra., *Yukon* X22+629 **88**
Dawson, R., *Queensland* C02–255 **111**
Dawson Creek, *B.C.* W02+558 **88**
Dawsonville, *Georgia* T55+344 **97**
Dax, *France* N06+437 **55**
Daylesford, *Victoria* C35–374 **109**
Dayton, *Tennessee* T60+355 **97**
Dayton, *Ohio* T55+398 **91**
Daytona Beach, *Florida* T36+292 **97**
De Aar, *Cape Province* L36–308 **84**
Dead Sea, *Jordan-Israel* K56+314 **76**
Deadwood, *S. Dakota* U82+446 **98**
Deal, *England* M82+512 **39**
Dean, Forest of, *England* N15+518 **38**
Dean Funes, *Argentina* S27–304 **103**
Dease Arm, *N.-W. Terr.* W00+664 **88**
Dease Lake, *Brit. Columbia* W60+580 **88**
Dease R., *Brit. Columbia* W55+592 **88**
Dease Str., *N.-W. Terr.* V20+682 **88**
Death Valley, *California* V72+366 **92**
Deauville, *France* N00+494 **54**
Debar, *Yugoslavia* L57+416 **58**
Debec, *New Brunswick* S46+461 **90**
Debess, *U.S.S.R.* J36+576 **61**
Deblin, *Poland* L49+506 **49**
Debno, *Poland* L92+527 **48**
Debra Markos, *Ethiopia* K42+104 **83**
Debrecen, *Hungary* L51+475 **49**
Decatur, *Alabama* T72+346 **97**
Decatur, *Georgia* T56+338 **97**
Decatur, *Illinois* T84+398 **95**
Decaturville, *Tennessee* T79+355 **97**
Deccan, *India* G80+130 **70**
Deception, I., *South Shetlands* S04–630 **27**
Děčin, *Czechoslovakia* M05+508 **48**
Decize, *France* M69+468 **54**
Decorah, *Iowa* U11+412 **95**
Dedeagach. *See* Alexandroupolis
Dedham, *Massachusetts* S67+423 **96**
Dédougou, *Upper Volta* N20+122 **80**
Dedza, *Malawi* K64–142 **83**
Dee R., *Scotland* N12+571 **40**
Dee R., *Wales* N18+530 **38**
Deel R., *Ireland, Rep.* N54+526 **43**
Deep Creek L., Maryland T26+395 **96**
Deepwater, *New S. Wales* B79–294 **109**
Deer I., *Maine* S52+442 **90**
Deer Lake, *Newfoundland* R74+492 **90**
Deerlijk, *Belgium* M70+508 **44**
Deer Lodge, *Montana* V46+464 **92**
Deer River, *Minnesota* U23+473 **93**
Defferrari, *Argentina* R87–384 **103**
De Funiak Springs, *Florida* T67+307 **97**
Degana, *India* H02+270 **70**
Degerfors, *Sweden* L62+642 **46**
De Gerlache Str., *Antarctica* S20–650 **27**
Degrad, *Brazil* R39+021 **105**
De Grey, R., *W. Australia* E02–204 **110**
Deh Bid, *Iran* J41+306 **75**
Dehdez, *Iran* J58+318 **75**
Dehra, (Dehra Dun), *India* G71+303 **72**
Dehrud, *Iran* J50+290 **75**
Deim Zubeir, *Sudan* L22+078 **81**
Deinze, *Belgium* M69+510 **44**
Deir Abu Said, *Jordan* K56+325 **76**
Deir 'Ali, *Syria* K52+332 **76**
Deir Atiye, *Syria* K49+341 **76**
Deir ez Zor, *Syria* K29+354 **74**
Deir Hafir, *Syria* K44+361 **76**
Deir Shemil, *Syria* K52+352 **76**
Dej, *Romania* L37+471 **49**
Dekalb, *Illinois* T82+419 **95**
De Kalb, *Mississippi* T82+328 **97**
De Kastri, *U.S.S.R.* C55+515 **63**
Dekoven, *Kentucky* T79+376 **97**
Delano Mt., *Utah* V45+385 **98**
Delano Pk., *Utah* V44+384 **94**
Delavan, *Wisconsin* T82+427 **91**
Delaware *N.J., etc.* T02+418 **91**
Delaware, *Ohio* T49+403 **91**
Delaware, state, *U.S.A.* T03+391 **99**
Delaware B., *Del.-New Jersey* T01+391 **96**
Delaware City, *Delaware* T03+396 **96**
Delaware R., *New York, etc.* T01+405 **96**
Delden, *Netherlands* M50+523 **44**
Delegate, *New S. Wales* C06–370 **109**
Deleitosa, *Spain* N33+396 **52**
De Lemmer, *Netherlands* M56+528 **44**
Delémont, *Switzerland* M46+474 **45**
Delfshaven, *Netherlands* M63+519 **44**
Delft, *Netherlands* M64+520 **44**
Delfzijl, *Netherlands* M48+533 **44**
Delgado C., *Mozambique* K26–108 **83**
Delger, *Mongolia* E56+457 **64**
Delgo, *Sudan* K86+200 **81**
Delhi, *India* G77+286 **72**
Delhi, *New York* T00+423 **96**
Dellenbaugh, Mt., *Arizona* V51+363 **92**
Dellys, *Algeria* M66+366 **80**
Delmenhorst, *W. Germany* M39+530 **48**
Del Norte, *Colorado* V08+376 **94**
Deloraine, *Tasmania* C20–415 **109**
Del Rio, *Texas* U66+294 **94**
Delta, *Colorado* V18+387 **94**
Delta, *Louisiana* U06+324 **97**
Delta, *Missouri* T89+372 **97**
Delta, *Pennsylvania* T08+397 **96**
Delta, *Utah* V46+396 **94**
Delungra, *New S. Wales* B85–296 **109**
Demanda, Sa. de la, *Spain* N18+422 **52**
Demchok, *Tibet* G63+326 **70**
Deming, *New Mexico* V18+323 **94**
Demirji Dagh, *Turkey* L10+391 **74**
Demmin, *E. Germany* M12+539 **48**
Demopolis, *Alabama* T77+325 **97**
Denbigh, *Wales* N20+532 **38**
Denderleeuw, *Belgium* M66+509 **44**
Dendermonde, *Belgium* M65+511 **44**
Dendi, mt., *Ethiopia* K42+086 **83**
Denekamp, *Netherlands* M48+524 **44**
Den Haag. *See* s' Gravenhage
Denham Ra., *Queensland* C08–260 **111**
Denia, *Spain* M89+388 **53**
Deniliquin, *New S. Wales* C30–356 **109**
Denison, *Iowa* U32+420 **95**
Denison, *Texas* U39+338 **95**
Denizli, *Turkey* L05+377 **74**
Denman, *New S. Wales* B86–324 **109**
Denmark, *S. Carolina* T37+333 **97**
Denmark, kingdom, *W. Eur.* **47**
Denmark Str., *Greenland, etc.* Q00+670 **25**
Den Oever, *Netherlands* M60+529 **44**
Dent Blanche, mt., *Switz.* M44+460 **45**
Denton, *Maryland* T05+389 **91**
Denton, *Texas* U42+332 **95**
D'Entrecasteaux, Is.,
Papua New Guinea B80–100 **111**
D'Entrecasteaux Pt.,
W. Australia E24–348 **110**
Denver, *Colorado* V00+397 **94**
Deoband, *India* G74+297 **72**
Deobhog, *India* G44+200 **71**
Deogarh, *India* G32+214 **71**
Deoghar, *India* G12+245 **73**
Deoli, *India* G88+257 **70**
Deoria, *India* G37+265 **73**
De Panne, *Belgium* M74+511 **44**
De Pere, *Wisconsin* T78+445 **91**
Deposit, *New York* T03+421 **91**
Depot Harbor, *Ontario* T31+453 **91**
Dera, *Syria* K53+326 **76**
Dera Bugti, *Pakistan* H35+291 **70**
Dera Ghazi Khan, *Pakistan* H26+301 **72**
Dera Ismail Khan, *Pakistan* H25+318 **72**
Dera Nanak, *India* G89+320 **72**
Derbent, *U.S.S.R.* J71+422 **62**
Derby, *W. Australia* D68–172 **110**
Derby & co., *England* N09+529 **37**
Derecske, *Hungary* L51+474 **49**
Derg L., *Ireland, Rep.* N47+546 **42**
Derg L., *Ireland, Rep.* N50+530 **43**
Derg R., *N. Ireland* N46+547 **42**
De Ridder, *Louisiana* U20+308 **95**
De Rijp, *Netherlands* M61+525 **44**
Dermott, *Arkansas* U07+336 **95**
Derna, (Dernah), *Libya* L44+326 **81**
Dernberg C., *Namibia* L86-278 **84**
Derravaragh L., *Ireland, Rep.* N44+537 **42**
Derryveagh Mts.,
Ireland, Rep. N49+550 **42**
Derudeb, *Sudan* K54+174 **81**
De Ruyter, *New York* T05+428 **96**
Derventa, *Yugoslavia* L73+450 **56**
Derwent, R., *England* N12+548 **37**
Derwent R., *England* N05+538 **37**
Derwent R., *Tasmania* C22–424 **109**
Derwent Water, *England* N19+546 **37**
Des Arc, *Arkansas* U09+350 **97**
Descalvados, *Brazil* R76–167 **104**
Deschaillons, *Quebec* S72+466 **91**
Deseado, R., *Argentina* S50–468 **103**
Deshambault L., *Sask.* V00+546 **88**
Des Moines & R., *Iowa* U22+416 **95**
Desna, R., *Ukraine* K84+512 **60**
Desolacion, I., *Chile* S84–532 **103**
Desolation C., *Greenland* R25+610 **26**
De Soto, *Missouri* U04+382 **95**
Dessau, *E. Germany* M16+518 **48**
Deta, *Romania* L53+454 **58**
Detroit, *Michigan* T48+424 **91**
Detroit Lakes, *Minnesota* U35+468 **93**
Dett, *Zimbabwe* L18–186 **84**
Deurne, *Netherlands* M55+515 **44**
Deux Rivières, *Ontario* T20+463 **91**
Deux-Sèvres, dep., *France* N03+466 **54**
Déva, *Romania* L43+459 **58**
Dévávanya, *Hungary* L54+471 **49**
Deventer, *Netherlands* M53+523 **44**
Deveron R., *Scotland* N15+577 **40**
Devil's Elbow, *Scotland* N21+569 **41**
Devils Lake, *N. Dakota* U53+481 **93**
Devin, *Bulgaria* L34+417 **58**
Devizes, *England* N12+513 **39**
Devon, co., *England* N22+508 **38**
Devon I., *N.-W. Territories* T60+750 **89**
Devonport; England N25+504 **38**
Devonport, *New Zealand* A31–368 **112**
Devonport, *Tasmania* C22–412 **109**
De Witt, *Arkansas* U08+343 **97**
Dewsbury, *England* N10+537 **37**
Dexter, *Maine* S56+450 **90**
Dexter, *Missouri* U00+368 **95**
Dezful, *Iran* J70+324 **74**
Dhaba, *Saudi Arabia* K56+274 **74**
Dhahran, *Saudi Arabia* J58+263 **75**
Dhak, *Pakistan* H15+325 **72**
Dhamâr, *Yemen* K04+147 **74**
Dhampur, *India* G69+293 **73**
Dhamra, *India* G18+208 **71**
Dhamtari, *India* G50+208 **70**
Dhang Ra., *Nepal* G48+282 **73**
Dhangain, *India* G34+252 **73**
Dhank, *Oman* J23+236 **75**
Dhankuta, *Nepal* G16+270 **73**
Dhariya, *Saudi Arabia* K13+247 **74**
Dharmjaygarh, *India* G41+224 **73**
Dharmkot, *India* G88+309 **72**
Dharmsala, *India* G82+322 **72**
Dharwar, *India* H00+156 **70**
Dhaulagiri, mt., *Nepal* G40+287 **73**
Dhiban, *Jordan* K55+315 **76**
Dhidhimótikhon, *Greece* L21+413 **58**
Dhionisiadhes. *See* Yianisahes Is.
Dholera, *India* H27+222 **70**
Dholpur, *India* G73+267 **73**
Dhond, *India* H01+184 **70**
Dhubri, *India* G00+260 **73**
Dhula, *Yemen, South* J71+150 **74**
Dhulia, *India* H01+209 **70**
Dhurma, *Saudi Arabia* J84+246 **74**
Dhurwai, *India* G66+255 **73**
Dia I., *Crete* L29+354 **59**
Diamante, *Argentina* S04–320 **103**
Diamantina, *Brazil* R69–144 **105**
Diamantina, *Brazil* Q81–182 **105**
Diamantina, R., *Queensland* C53–242 **111**
Diamond, I., *Burma* F64+159 **71**
Diamond Harbour, *India* G10+222 **73**
Dibah, *U.A.E.* J22+257 **75**
Dibai, *U.A.E.* J28+253 **75**
Dibbah, Jebel, *Saudi Arabia* K56+278 **74**
Dibbéla, *Niger* M14+176 **81**
Dibit, *Somalia* J72+060 **83**
Dibrugarh, *India* F60+274 **71**
Dickinson, *N. Dakota* U77+469 **93**
Dickson, *Tennessee* T75+362 **95**
Die, *France* M60+448 **55**
Diefenbaker L., *Saskatchewan* V10+510 **88**
Diego Garcia, I., *Indian Oc.* H35–100 **25**
Diego Suarez, *Madagascar* J64–124 **83**
Dien Bien Phu, *Vietnam* F12 + 212 **69**
Dieppe, *France* M84+499 **54**
Diest, *Belgium* M60+510 **44**
Dieverbrug, *Netherlands* M52+529 **44**
Dig, *India* G76+274 **72**
Digby, *Nova Scotia* S35+446 **90**
Digby Neck, *Nova Scotia* S37+444 **90**
Dighal, *Yemen, South* J70+146 **74**
Digne, *France* M53+441 **55**
Digoin, *France* M66+465 **54**
Diguel, R., *Irian Jaya, Indon.* C60–072 **65**
Dijon, *France* M60+473 **54**
Diksmuide, *Belgium* M73+510 **44**
Dikwa, *Nigeria* M06+120 **81**
Dilam, *Saudi Arabia* J76+240 **74**
Dili, *Timor I., Indonesia* D56–086 **65**
Dillon, *Montana* V46+452 **92**
Dilolo, *Angola* L48–118 **82**
Dilolo, *Zaire* L46–106 **82**
Dimbokro, *Ivory Coast* N28+068 **80**
Dimitrovo (Pernik), *Bulgaria* L42+426 **58**
Dimitrovgrad, *Yugoslavia* L43+431 **58**
Dimla, *Bangladesh* G06+261 **73**
Dimotika. *See* Dhidhimotikhon.
Dinagat, I., *Philippines* D56+100 **65**
Dinajpur, *Bangladesh* G08+256 **73**
Dinan, *France* N12+485 **54**
Dinanagar, *India* G87+322 **72**
Dinant, *Belgium* M60+503 **44**
Dinapur, *India* G29+256 **73**
Dinar, *Turkey* K89+381 **74**
Dinard, *France* N13+486 **54**

Dinarske Planina, Yugoslavia L82+440 56
Dinas Mawddwy, Wales N22+527 38
Dindigul, India G72+104 70
Dingle & B., Ireland, Rep. N62+521 43
Dingwall, Scotland N27+576 40
Dinosaur Nat. Mon., Colo. V23+406 94
Dinteloord, Netherlands M64+516 44
Diourbel, Senegal P08+146 80
Dipalpur, Pakistan H08+306 72
Dipton, New Zealand A69-459 112
Dir, Pakistan H18+352 72
Direction, C., Queensland C39-129 111
Diredawe, Ethiopia K20+094 83
Diriamba, Nicaragua T66+117 101
Dirk Hartogs I., W. Aust. E42-258 110
Dirksland, Netherlands M65+518 44
Dirranbandi, Queensland C11-284 111
Disappointment, C., Wash. W24+463 92
Disappointment Is.,
Tuamotu Arch. X38-145 107
Disappointment, L., W. Aust. D73-234 110
Disaster B., New S. Wales C00-373 109
Discovery B., Victoria C54-382 109
Disentis, Switzerland M37+467 45
Disko B., Greenland R35+690 26
Disko, I., Greenland R35+700 26
Disna, Byelorussia L11+552 60
Dison, Belgium M55+506 44
District of Columbia, U.S.A. T12+386 91
Diu, India H23+208 70
Diver, Ontario T28+468 91
Dividing Range, mts., Aust. C10-260 111
Diviso, Colombia T20+014 104
Divrigi, Turkey K41+394 74
Diwan Chah, Iran H85+299 75
Diwangiri, India F81+268 71
Diwaniyah, Iraq K01+320 74
Dix, Quebec T07+482 91
Dixmude, Belgium M73+510 44
Dixon, Illinois T87+418 95
Dixon, Kentucky T76+375 97
Dixon Entrance, B.C. W75+545 88
Diyarbakir, Turkey K28+380 74
Dizah, Iran H76+272 75
Djaid, U.A.E. J24+254 75
Djajapura, See Jayapura
Djakarta, See Jakarta
Djambi, See Jambi
Djawa. See Java
Djelfa, Algeria M70+346 80
Djeneien, Tunisia M30+318 81
Djerba, I., Tunisia M26+338 81
Djibouti, E. Africa K12+114 83
Djidjelh, Algeria M54+366 80
Djolu, Zaire L46+08 82
Djougou, Benin M80+098 80
Djursholm, Sweden L72+594 47
Dmitriya Lapteva Proliv,
U.S.S.R. C40+730 63
Dnepr R., Ukraine K68+470 60
Dneprodzerzhinsk, Ukraine K62+486 60
Dnepropetrovsk, Ukraine K60+485 60
Dnester (Dniester), R., Ukr. L28+489 60
Doaktown, New Brunswick S37+466 90
Dobbyn, Queensland C60-198 111
Dobele, Latvia L40+566 47
Doberan, E. Germany M19+541 48
Dobra, Czechoslovakia L50+491 49
Dobřany, Czechoslovakia M11+497 48
Dobrich. See Tolbukhin.
Dobruja, Romania L10+455 58
Dobryanka, U.S.S.R. J22+584 61
Dobrzyn, Poland L66+531 49
Doce Leguas, Cayos de las,
Cuba T25+210 101
Doctor Arroyo, Mexico U61+238 100
Dodecanese, Greece L18+360 59
Dodge City, Kansas U60+378 95
Dodgeville, Wisconsin U01+430 95
Dodman Pt., England N29+502 38
Dodoma, Tanzania K56-062 83
Dodson, Montana V20+484 93
Doel, Belgium M64+513 44
Doesburg, Netherlands M53+520 44
Doetinchem, Netherlands M52+520 44
Dogger Bank, North Sea M78+545 34
Doha, Qatar, Arabia J51+253 75
Dohad, India H04+228 70
Doka, Saudi Arabia K23+199 74
Dokka, Yemen K05+131 74
Dokkum, Netherlands M54+533 44
Dol, France N10+485 54
Dolbeau, Quebec S73+488 90
Dolcigno. See Ulcinj.
Dôle, France M57+471 54
Dolent, Mt., Switzerland M48+459 45
Dolgellau, Wales N23+527 38
Dollar, Scotland N22+562 41
Dolo, Ethiopia K18+040 83
Dolomitiche, Alpi, Italy M18+464 56
Dolores, Argentina R76-364 103
Dolores, Mexico V35+251 100
Dolores, Spain N05+381 53
Dolphin, C., Falkland Is. R84-512 103
Dolunnor. See Tolun.
Dom, mt., Irian Jaya,
Indon. C78-027 65
Domariaganj, India G44+272 73
Dombås, Norway M35+621 46
Domburg, Netherlands M69+516 44
Domel, I., Burma F41+115 71
Dome Rock Mts., Arizona V54+336 92
Domfront, France N04+486 54
Dominica, I., West Indies S07+154 101
Dominican Rep., West Indies S60+190 101
Dömitz, E. Germany M23+531 48
Dom Pedrito, Brazil R58-310 103
Domuyo, mt., Argentina S63-366 103
Domvraina, Greece L42+383 59
Don R., England N07+535 37
Don, R., U.S.S.R. K20+481 62
Don R., Scotland N13+572 40
Donaghadee, N. Ireland N33+546 42
Donald, Victoria C42-364 109
Donaldson, Louisiana U06+301 95
Donau, R., Central Europe M14+489 48
Donaueschingen, W. Germany M39+479 48
Don Benito, Spain N35+388 52
Doncaster, England N07+535 37
Dondo, Angola M04-096 82
Donegal & co., Ireland, Rep. N49+546 42
Donegal B., Ireland, Rep. N52+545 42
Donegal Pt., Ireland, Rep. N58+527 43
Donets, R., U.S.S.R. K25+480 61
Donetsk, Ukraine K43+479 60
Donga, Nigeria M30+076 81
Dongara, W. Australia E30-290 110
Donggala, Celebes, Indon. E02-008 65
Dong-hoi, Vietnam E80+174 69
Dongo, Angola L86-146 82
Dongola, Sudan K88+190 81
Doniphan, Missouri U05+366 97
Donji Miholjac, Yugoslavia L72+457 56
Dønna, Norway M15+661 46
Don Pia-fai, mt., Thailand F22+144 69
Doon R. & L., Scotland N26+553 41
Doorn, Netherlands M58+520 44
Dora, L., W. Australia D72-221 110
Doranda, India G28+233 73
Dorat, le, France M83+462 54
Dorchester, England N15+507 38
Dorchester, New Brunswick S27+459 90
Dorchester, C., N.-W. Terr. T20+654 89
Dordogne, dep., France M85+451 54
Dordogne R., France N03+450 55
Dordrecht, Netherlands M62+518 44
Dore L., Saskatchewan V14+548 88
Dore, Mt., France M72+454 54
Dores, Brazil R39-306 103
Dori, Upper Volta N00+140 80
Dorking, England N02+512 39
Dornie, Scotland N33+573 40
Dornoch & Firth, Scotland N24+579 40
Dorotea, Sweden L81+643 46
Dorrego, Argentina S08-387 103
Dorrigo, New S. Wales B75-304 109
Dorset, co., England N14+508 38
Dorsey, Montana V34+464 93
Dortmund, W. Germany M45+515 48
Dos Bahias, C., Argentina S33-450 103
Doshi, Afghanistan H37+356 75
Dospat, Bulgaria L36+416 58
Dosso, Cameroon M70+130 80
Dossor, Kazakh J43+475 62
Dothan, Alabama T62+312 97
Douai, France M71+504 54
Douala, Cameroon M32+040 81
Douarnenez, France N25+481 54
Doubs, dep., France M51+471 54
Doubtless B., New Zealand A39-349 112
Doucet, Quebec T10+482 91
Douglas, Arizona V27+313 94
Douglas, Cape Province L32-290 84
Douglas, Georgia T47+315 97
Douglas, I. of Man N27+542 37
Douglas, Mt., Montana V32+454 98
Douglas, Wyoming V02+428 93
Douglastown, Quebec S26+488 90
Douglasville, Georgia T58+337 97
Doullens, France M76+502 54
Doulus Hd., Ireland, Rep. N62+520 43
Doume, Cameroon M08+044 81
Doune, Scotland N24+562 41
Dounreay, Scotland N22+586 40
Douro, & R., Spain-Portugal N49+411 52
Dover, Delaware T03+392 96
Dover, England M82+511 39
Dover, New Hampshire S65+434 96
Dover, New Jersey S87+409 96
Dover, Ohio T39+406 91
Dover, Tasmania C18-433 109
Dover, Tennessee T77+365 97
Dover, Str., of,
England-France M81+505 54
Dover Foxcroft, Maine S55+452 90
Dovrefjell, Norway M36+622 46
Dow L., Botswana L32-214 84
Dowa, Malawi K66-136 83
Down, co., N. Ireland N36+543 42
Downham Market, England M88+526 39
Downpatrick, N. Ireland N34+543 42
Downpatrick Hd.,
Ireland, Rep. N56+543 42
Doyles, Newfoundland R85+479 90
Doylestown, Pennsylvania T01+403 96
Drăgăşani, Romania L34+446 58
Draguignan, France M51+436 55
Drake, New S. Wales B76-289 109
Drake Str., Antarctica S00-580 27
Drakensberg, mts., S. Africa L04-270 84
Dráma, Greece L35+411 58
Drammen, Norway M28+598 47
Dranov I., Romania L04+449 58
Dras, Kashmir G85+344 72
Drawsko, Poland L85+535 49
Drayton, N. Dakota U43+486 93
Drazinda, Pakistan H30+318 72
Drem, Scotland N16+560 41
Drenthe, prov., Netherlands M50+528 44
Dresden, E. Germany M07+511 48
Dresden, Ontario T44+426 91
Dreux, France M82+487 54
Drimoleague, Ireland, Rep. N56+516 43
Drin G., Albania L63+417 58
Drina, R., Yugoslavia L66+436 58
Drøbak, Norway M26+597 47
Drogheda & B., Ireland, Rep. N38+537 42
Droitwich, England N13+523 39
Drome, dep. & R., France M65+447 55
Dromod, Ireland, Rep. N47+539 42
Dromore West, Ireland, Rep. N53+542 42
Dromore, N. Ireland N37+544 42
Dromore, N. Ireland N45+545 42
Drongen, Belgium M68+511 44
Drum Hills, Ireland, Rep. N46+520 43
Drumheller, Alberta V45+513 88
Drummond I., Michigan T52+460 91
Drummondville, Quebec S75+459 91
Drumnadrochit, Scotland N27+573 40
Drumshanbo, Ireland, Rep. N48+540 42
Drunen, Netherlands M59+517 44
Druten, Netherlands M56+519 44
Druz, Jeb. ed, Syria K49+326 76
Dryden, Ontario U15+498 89
Drygalski I., Antarctica F78-660 27
Drymen, Scotland N27+561 41
Drysdale River, W. Australia D49-141 110
Dschang, Cameroon M30+056 82
Dubawnt L., N.-W. Terr. U70+636 88
Dubbo, New S. Wales C08-323 109
Dublin, Georgia T47+324 99
Dublin & co., Ireland, Rep. N38+533 43
Dublin, Texas U50+322 95
Dubno, Ukraine L26+504 60
Du Bois, Pennsylvania T23+411 96
Dubrovnik, Yugoslavia L71+427 58
Dubuque, Iowa U04+425 95
Duchcov, Czechoslovakia M08+506 48
Duchesne, Utah V32+402 94
Ducie I., Pacific Ocean W26-254 107
Duck Is., Ontario T48+457 91
Dudinka, U.S.S.R. G26+693 62
Dudley, England N13+525 37
Duero R., Spain N27+416 52
Duffel, Belgium M61+511 44
Dufftown, Scotland N19+574 40
Dugi Otok, I., Yugoslavia M00+440 56
Duifken Pt., Queensland C50-124 111
Duisburg, W. Germany M50+515 48
Dujana, India G80+287 72
Duke of Gloucester Grp.,
Tuamotu Archipelago W80-208 107
Duke of York Arch.,
N.-W. Territories V50+678 88
Duk Faiwil, Sudan K82+076 81
Dulce, G., Costa Rica T49+086 101
Duluth, Minnesota U13+468 93
Dulverton, England N21+510 38
Duma, Syria K52+335 76
Dumas, Arkansas U09+338 97
Dumas, Texas U71+358 94
Dumbarton, Scotland N27+559 41
Dum-Dum, India G09+226 73
Dumeir, Syria K50+336 76
Dumfries, Scotland N22+551 41
Dumfries & Galloway, reg., Scot.
N26+550 41
Dumka, India G16+243 73
Dumraon, India G35+255 73
Dunarea (Danube), R., Cent.
Europe L24+441 51
Dunbar, Scotland N15+560 41
Dunblane, Scotland N24+562 41
Dunboyne, Ireland, Rep. N39+534 43
Duncan, Arkansas U08+346 97
Duncan, Oklahoma U48+345 95
Duncan Pass., Andaman Is. F75+112 71
Duncannon, Ireland, Rep. N41+522 43
Duncansby Hd., Scotland N18+586 40
Dundalk & B., Ireland, Rep. N38+540 42
Dundas, Ontario T30+433 91
Dundas, Tasmania C27-419 109
Dundas Str., N. Terr., Aust. D20-110 110
Dun Dealgan. See Dundalk
Dundee, Natal K88-282 84
Dundee, Scotland N18+565 41
Dundee I., Antarctica R62-630 27
Dundrum & B., N. Ireland N35+543 42
Dundwa Ra., Nepal G46+278 73
Dunedin, New Zealand A 57-459 112
Dunedoo, New S. Wales C04-320 109
Dunfanaghy, Ireland, Rep., N48+552 42
Dunfermline, Scotland N21+561 41
Dungannon, N. Ireland N41+545 42
Dungarpur, India H08+238 70
Dungarven & Harb.,
Ireland, Rep. N46+521 43
Dungbure Ra., Tibet G30+350 71
Dungeness, England M84+509 39
Dungiven, N. Ireland N41+549 42
Dungloe, Ireland, Rep. N50+549 42
Dungog, New S. Wales B80-324 109
Dungu, Zaire L08+034 83
Dunkeld, Scotland N22+566 41
Dunkerque (Dunkirk), France M76+511 54
Dunkirk, New York T26+425 96
Dunkur, Ethiopia K54+118 83
Dunkwa, Ghana N12+060 80
Dún Laoghaire, Ireland, Rep. N38+532 43
Dunlap, Iowa U36+420 95
Dunlavin, Ireland, Rep. N40+530 43
Dunleer, Ireland, Rep. N38+538 42
Dunlop, Scotland N27+557 41
Dunmanus B., Ireland, Rep. N59+516 43
Dunmanway, Ireland, Rep. N55+517 43
Dunmore, Ireland, Rep. N52+536 42
Dunn, N. Carolina T22+353 97
Dunnet Hd & B., Scotland N20+586 40
Dunolly, Victoria C38-369 109
Dunoon, Scotland N30+559 41
Duns, Scotland N14+558 41
Dunstable, England N03+519 39
Dunvegan & L., Scotland N39+574 40
Dupulan, Iran J56+320 75
Du Quain, Illinois T86+380 97
Duque de York, I., Chile T01-506 103
Dura, Jordan K60+315 76
Durango, Colorado V17+372 94
Durango & state, Mexico U88+240 100
Durant, Mississippi T89+330 97
Durant, Oklahoma U38+340 95
Durazno, Uruguay R69-334 103
Durazzo. See Durrës
Durban, Natal K84-298 84
Durbe, Latvia L52+566 47
Durbuy, Belgium M57+503 44
Durdevac, Yugoslavia L78+460 56
Durdurch, Somalia J68+112 83
Dureikish, Syria K53+349 76
Duren, W. Germany M51+508 48
Durga Str., New Guinea C70-073 111
Durham, N. Carolina T23+360 97
Durham, Ontario T35+442 91
Durham & co., England N09+548 37
Durness & Kyle of, Scotland N28+586 40
Durrës, Albania L63+413 58
Durrow, Ireland, Rep. N44+528 43
Dursey I. & Hd., Ireland, Rep. N61+516 43
Dursley, England N14+517 38
Duruh, Iran H86+322 75
Durukhsh, Iran J01+331 75
D'Urville I., New Zealand A37-408 112
Dushanbe, Tadzhik H37+386 62
Dushore, Pennsylvania T09+415 96
Dusky Sound, New Zealand A81-457 112
Düsseldorf, W. Germany M49+513 48
Dussen, Netherlands M60+517 44
Duszniki Zdrój, Poland L82+504 49
Dutch Harb., Aleutian Is. Z10+540 99
Dutch Guiana. See Surinam
Dutton, Mt., Utah V44+380 94
Duvan, U.S.S.R. J12+557 61
Duwadami, Saudi Arabia K04+248 74
Duwwah, Oman J07+205 75
Dvina, R., Latvia L32+568 47
Dyatkovo, U.S.S.R. K64+535 60
Dyce, Scotland N13+572 40
Dyer, C., N.-W. Territories S07+665 89
Dyersburg, Tennessee T87+360 97
Dyfed, co., Wales N26+520 38
Dyfi R., Wales N23+526 38
Dyle R., Belgium M63+510 44
Dyurtyuli, U.S.S.R. J31+554 61
Dzamyn Ude, Mongolia E55+446 64
Dzep, Yugoslavia L47+427 58
Dzerzhinsk, U.S.S.R. K09+563 61
Dzerzhinsh, Byelorussia L17+536 60
Dzhagdy Khrebet, U.S.S.R. D30+538 63
Dzhalal Abad, Kirgiz. H12+407 62
Dzhalinda, U.S.S.R. D67+536 63
Dzhambul, Kazakh. H21+428 62
Dzhetygara, Kazakh. H82+524 62
Dzhezkazgan, Kazakh. H44+480 62
Dzhugdzhur Khrebet,
U.S.S.R. C70+580 63
Dzhungarskiy Ala-Tau,
Kazakh. G60+450 62
Dzierzoniow, Poland L80+508 49
Dzogchen, China F36+322 64
Eagle, Alaska X37+645 99
Eagle I., Ireland, Rep. N60+543 42
Eagle L., Maine S56+463 90
Eagle Ls., Maine S50+471 90
Eagle Grove, Iowa U24+427 95
Eagle Mountain L., Texas U45+328 95
Eagle Pass, Texas U62+287 94
Eaglehawk, Victoria C35-367 109
Eagle River, Wisconsin T86+459 91
Eagles Nest, Ireland, Rep. N58+518 43
Ealing, England N02+515 39
Eardisley, England N18+521 38
Earith, England M89+523 39
Earlston, Scotland N16+556 41
Earlville, New York T04+427 96
Earn L., Scotland N25+564 41
Earn, R., Scotland N20+564 41
Easington, England N08+548 37
East Anglia, S.E. England 39
East Arlington, Vermont S79+431 91
East Aurora, New York T22+428 96
Eastbourne, England M88+508 39
Eastbourne, New Zealand A30-413 112
East Dereham, England M84+527 39
Easter I., Pacific Ocean V25-265 107
Eastern B., Maryland T08+388 96
Eastern States, India G50+230 70
East Grand Forks, Minnesota U42+479 93
East Kilbride, Scotland N25+558 41
Eastland, Texas U53+324 95
East Liverpool, Ohio T34+406 91
East London, Cape Province L12-330 84
East Lothian, co., See Lothian
Eastmain R., Quebec T05+526 89
Eastman, Georgia T49+322 97
Easton, Maryland T06+388 96
Easton, Pennsylvania T02+407 96
Eastport, Maine S42+449 90
East Retford, England N06+533 37
East Riding, Yorks., See Humberside
East St Louis, Illinois U01+386 95
East Sioux Falls, S. Dakota U40+435 93
Eastville, Virginia T06+373 97
Eaton Rapids, Michigan T58+425 91
Eau Claire, Wisconsin U10+448 93
Ebbw Vale, Wales N19+518 38
Eberswalde, E. Germany M07+528 48
Eboli, Italy M00+406 57
Ebolowa, Cameroon M24+028 82
Ebro, R., Spain N09+421 53
Ecaussines, Belgium M65+506 44
Ecclefechan, Scotland N19+550 41
Echallens, Switzerland M50+466 45
Echo L., Tasmania C20-422 109
Echo Cliffs, Arizona V40+364 94
Echt, Netherlands M55+511 44
Echten, Netherlands M52+527 44
Echternach, Luxembourg M51+498 48
Echuca, Victoria C31-362 109
Eck L., Scotland N30+561 41
Ecuador, rep., S. America 104
Edam, Netherlands M60+525 44
Eday, I., Orkney Is., Scot. N16+592 40
Ed Damer, Sudan K66+176 81
Ed Damur, Lebanon K57+337 76
Ed Debba, Sudan K86+180 81
Eddrachillis B., Scotland N31+583 40
Ed Dueim, Sudan K76+140 81
Ede, Netherlands M56+521 44
Edebäck, Sweden M08+601 47
Eden, Maine S50+444 90
Eden, New South Wales C01-371 109
Eden, New York T23+426 96
Eden R., England N17+548 37
Edenburg, Orange Free State L24-296 84
Edendale, New Zealand A67-463 112
Edenderry, Ireland, Rep. N42+533 43
Edenhope, Victoria C52-370 109
Edensburg, Pennsylvania T23+405 96
Edenton, N. Carolina T10+361 97
Edeowie, S. Australia C69-314 109
Ederengin Nuru, Mongolia F40+434 64
Edge Hill, England N09+521 39
Edgeley, N. Dakota U52+464 93
Edgemont, S. Dakota U83+432 93
Edgeøya, I., Arctic Ocean L45+780 62
Edgerton, Wisconsin T84+429 91
Edgeworthstown, Ireland, Rep. N45+537 42
Edhessa, Greece L48+408 59
Edievale, New Zealand A64-458 112
Edina, Missouri U13+402 95
Edinburg, Texas U49+264 94
Edinburgh, Scotland N19+559 41
Edirne, Turkey L21+417 74
Edithburgh, S. Australia C74-351 109
Edith Cavell, Mt., Alberta V78+530 88
Edmonton, Alberta V52+538 88
Edmundston, New Brunswick S50+474 90
Edremit, Turkey L18+397 74
Edsele, Sweden L81+634 46
Edson, Alberta V68+538 88
Eduni, Mt., North-West
Territories W48+644 88
Edward (Amin) L.,
Zaire-Uganda L02-004 83

Edward, R., *New S. Wales* C34–352 **109**
Edwardesabad. *See* Bannu.
Edwards, *New York* T01+443 **91**
Edwards Plat., *Texas* U66+308 **94**
Edwardsville, *Illinois* U00+388 **95**
Eekloo, *Belgium* M69+512 **44**
Efate, I., *Vanuatu* A68–185 **106**
Eferding, *Austria* M06+483 **48**
Effingham, *Illinois* T82+391 **95**
Egadi Is., *Sicily* M17+379 **57**
Egan, *S. Dakota* U40+440 **93**
Egana, *Argentina* R85–369 **103**
Eganville, *Ontario* T13+455 **91**
Eger, *Czechoslovakia. See* Cheb.
Eger, *Hungary* L58+479 **49**
Egersund, *Norway* M54+584 **47**
Egg L., *Quebec* S78+544 **89**
Eggenfelden, *W. Germany* M13+484 **48**
Eghezee, *Belgium* M60+506 **44**
Egin, *Turkey* K39+392 **74**
Eglinton, C., *N.-W. Terr.* S55+707 **89**
Egmont B., *Prince Edward I.* S25+466 **90**
Egmont, Mt., *New Zealand* A35–393 **112**
Egremont, *England* N21+545 **37**
Egridir, *Turkey* K85+378 **74**
Egypt, *N. Africa* L00+250 **81**
Eibergen, *Netherlands* M50+521 **44**
Eichstätt, *Germany* M23+489 **48**
Eidsvoll, *Norway* M22+603 **47**
Eifel, mts., *W. Germany* M50+501 **48**
Eigg I., *Scotland* N37+569 **41**
Eights Coast, *Antarctica* T80–750 **27**
Eighty Mile Beach, *W. Aust.* D95–196 **110**
Eil, *Somalia* J60+078 **83**
Eil L., *Scotland* N31+568 **41**
Eilat, *Israel* K60+296 **76**
Eindhoven, *Netherlands* M57+514 **44**
Eire, *See* Ireland, Rep. of.
Eisden, *Netherlands* M56+508 **44**
Eisenach, *E. Germany* M28+509 **48**
Eisenerz, *Austria* M01+475 **48**
Eisleben, *E. Germany* M21+515 **48**
Ejutla, *Mexico* U40+166 **100**
Ekaterinoslav. *See* Dnepropetrovsk.
Eke, *Belgium* M68+510 **44**
Ekeren, *Belgium* M64+513 **44**
Eketahana, *New Zealand* A26–406 **112**
Ekhinádbes Is., *Greece* L54+384 **59**
Ekimchan, *U.S.S.R.* D12+530 **63**
Eksjö, *Sweden* M00+577 **47**
Ekträsk, *Sweden* L61+644 **46**
Ekwan R., *Ontario* T52+537 **89**
El Aaiun, *Morocco* N80+268 **80**
El Abde, *Lebanon* K54+346 **76**
Elafónisi Chan., *Greece* L42+364 **59**
Élafos I., *Greece* L42+365 **59**
El Agheila (Al'Uqaylah)
Libya L64+302 **81**
El Aguila, *Argentina* S43–363 **103**
El Aina, *Jordan* K55+310 **76**
El Alamein, *Egypt* L07+308 **81**
Elasson, *Greece* L47+399 **59**
Elâzig, *Turkey* K34+386 **74**
Elba, I., *Italy* M28+428 **56**
El Bab, *Syria* K45+364 **76**
El Bahluliye, *Syria* K54+356 **76**
El Banco, *Colombia* S84+090 **104**
El Barco de Valdeorras, *Sp.* N42+424 **52**
Elbasan, *Albania* L60+412 **58**
El Baul, *Venezuela* S50+090 **104**
Elbe R., *Germany* M25+532 **48**
Elbert, Mt., *Colorado* V08+391 **98**
Elbeuf, *France* M83+493 **54**
Elbing. *See* Elblag.
El-Birka, *Saudi Arabia* K27+223 **74**
Elbistan, *Turkey* K47+383 **74**
Elblag, *Poland* L64+542 **49**
El Br'aij, *Syria* K49+343 **76**
Elbrus, mt., *U.S.S.R.* K17+432 **62**
Elburg, *Netherlands* M55+524 **44**
Elburz Mts., *Iran* J56+363 **75**
El Carmen, *Bolivia* S22–145 **104**
El Carmen, *See* Carmen
El Centro, *California* V63+329 **92**
Elche, *Spain* N04+383 **53**
El Chorro, *Argentina* S14–232 **103**
El Cuy, *Argentina* S50–399 **103**
El Dab, *Somalia* J82+088 **83**
El Diwân, *Egypt* K78+224 **81**
El Donfar, *Somalia* J66+104 **83**
Eldora, *Iowa* U18+424 **95**
El Dorado, *Arkansas* U16+332 **95**
El Dorado, *Kansas* U42+378 **95**
El Dorado, *Mexico* V14+242 **100**
El Dorado, *Venezuela* S10+066 **104**
Eldoret, *Kenya* K58+006 **83**
El Djezair (Algiers), *Algeria* M72+366 **55**
El Encanto, *Colombia* S82–012 **104**
Elephant Butte Res., *New Mexico* V13+334 **94**
Elephant I., *Antarctica* R60–610 **27**
El Ergh, *Libya* L50+290 **81**
Eleşkirt, *Turkey* K13+399 **74**
Eleuthera I., *Bahamas, The* T10+250 **101**
Elewijt, *Belgium* M63+510 **44**
El Faiyum, *Egypt* K84+294 **81**
El Fasher, *Sudan* L28+136 **81**
El Fuwara, *Saudi Arabia* K15+262 **74**
Elgena, *Ethiopia* K38+170 **83**
El Geneina, *Sudan* L46+134 **81**
El Geteina, *Sudan* K76+146 **81**
Elgg, *Switzerland* M37+475 **45**
El Ghobbe, *Saudi Arabia* K31+239 **74**
Elgin, *Illinois* T80+420 **95**
Elgin, *New Brunswick* S31+458 **90**
Elgin, *Scotland* N20+576 **40**
El Giof. *See* El Jauf.
El Giza, *Egypt* K82+300 **81**
El Golea, *Algeria* M74+306 **80**
Elgon, Mt., *Uganda* K62+012 **83**
El Hamidiya, *Syria* K49+354 **76**
El Hamra, *Syria* K48+353 **76**
El Hamrat, *Syria* K48+345 **76**
El Hasa, *Saudi Arabia* J67+272 **74**
El-Hayath, *Saudi Arabia* K25+261 **74**
El Hijane, *Syria* K51+333 **76**
El Hilla, *Sudan* L16+134 **81**
El Husn, *Jordan* K55+325 **76**
Elie, *Scotland* N17+562 **41**
Elisabethville. *See* Lubumbashi.
Elisavetgrad. *See* Kirovograd.
Elizabeth, *New Jersey* T86+406 **96**
Elizabeth I., *Massachusetts* S65+414 **96**
Elizabeth, *West Virginia* T38+390 **91**
Elizabeth, mt., *Argentina* S59–483 **103**
Elizabeth City, *N. Carolina* T08+363 **97**
Elizabethtown, *Kentucky* T65+377 **97**
Elizondo, *Spain* N09+433 **53**
El Jafr, *Jordan* K53+303 **76**
El Jauf, *Libya* L40+238 **81**
El Judeide, *Syria* K53+336 **76**
Elk Mts., *New Mexico* V18+337 **94**
Elk, *Poland* L46+538 **49**
Elk City, *Oklahoma* U57+354 **95**
El Kerak, *Jordan* K56+312 **76**
El Kharga, *Egypt* K86+254 **81**
Elkhart, *Indiana* T66+417 **91**
Elkhead Mts., *Colorado* V14+408 **94**
Elkhorn, Mt., *Idaho* V45+424 **92**
El Khushniye, *Syria* K55+330 **76**
Elkins, *West Virginia* T29+389 **91**
Elko, *Nevada* V65+408 **92**
Elk Point, *S. Dakota* U40+427 **93**
Elk River, *Minnesota* U22+453 **93**
Elkton, *Maryland* T05+396 **96**
El Lâdhiqîya. *See* Latakia.
El Laghodeh, *Somalia* J66+094 **83**
Ellas, *Greece* L42+385 **59**
Ellef Ringnes I., *N.-W. Terr.* U65+784 **88**
Ellen, Mt., *Utah* V35+382 **94**
Ellenabad, *India* H02+294 **72**
Ellendale, *N. Dakota* U51+460 **93**
Ellensburg, *Washington* W04+470 **92**
Ellerslie, *Prince Edward I.* S23+466 **90**
Ellesmere I., *N.-W. Terr.* T30+780 **89**
Ellesmere, L., *New Zealand* A44–439 **112**
Ellesmere Port, *England* N17+533 **37**
Ellezelles, *Belgium* M68+507 **44**
Ellice Is., *See* Tuvalu
Ellice R., *N.-W. Territories* V05+666 **88**
Ellichpur, *India* G75+212 **70**
Ellicott City, *Maryland* T11+393 **96**
Elliot, *Cape Province* L12–314 **84**
Elliot B., *N.-W. Territories* U35+676 **88**
Elliot Group, *China* D74+393 **66**
Ellon, *Scotland* N12+574 **40**
Ellora, *India* G88+201 **70**
Ellsworth, *Maine* S50+445 **90**
Ellsworth Mts., *Antarctica* U00–770 **27**
Elm, *Switzerland* M35+469 **45**
El Ma'arra, *Syria* K49+360 **76**
Elma Dagh, *Turkey* K72+398 **74**
El Madhiq, *Saudi Arabia* K32+233 **74**
El Mansura, *Egypt* K82+310 **81**
El Mazar, *Jordan* K56+311 **76**
El Mazra'a, *Jordan* K57+313 **76**
El Meget, *Somalia* J80+032 **83**
El Menzil, *Jordan* K54+311 **76**
Elmira, *New York* T11+421 **96**
El Minya, *Egypt* K86+280 **81**
El Molar, *Spain* N22+408 **52**
Elmore, *Victoria* C32–365 **109**
El Muwaqqar, *Jordan* K53+318 **76**
El Obeid, *Sudan* K88+132 **81**
El Odaiya, *Sudan* L10+120 **81**
Elora, *Tennesse* T68+350 **97**
El Oro, *Mexico* V02+259 **100**
El Pardo, *Spain* N24+405 **52**
El Paso, *Illinois* T84+408 **95**
El Paso, *Texas* V09+316 **98**
Elphin, *Ireland, Rep.* N49+538 **42**
Elphinstone I., *Burma* F42+123 **71**
El Pico, *Bolivia* S28–158 **104**
El Pilar, *Venezuela* S18+104 **104**
El Pintado, *Argentina* S08–246 **103**
El Puente del Arzobispo, *Sp.* N31+398 **52**
El Qadmus, *Syria* K53+351 **76**
El Qanawat, *Syria* K50+327 **76**
El Qaryatein, *Syria* K46+342 **76**
El Qathma, *Saudi Arabia* K17+238 **74**
El Qatrana, *Jordan* K54+312 **76**
El Qatrun, *Libya* M02+250 **81**
El Quds esh Sherif. *See* Jerusalem
El Quneitra, *Syria* K55+331 **76**
El Quseir, *Syria* K50+345 **76**
El Quweira, *Jordan* K58+298 **76**
El Reno, *Oklahoma* U48+353 **95**
Elroy, *Wisconsin* U01+437 **91**
El Sadi. *See* Wajir
El Salvador, *Cent. America* T80+135 **101**
Elsenborn, *Belgium* M53+505 **44**
Elsloo, *Netherlands* M55+509 **44**
Elspeet, *Netherlands* M55+523 **44**
Elst, *Netherlands* M55+519 **44**
Elsterwerda, *E. Germany* M09+515 **48**
Eltham, *New Zealand* A34–394 **112**
El Tigre, *Venezuela* S25+089 **104**
El Toro, *Spain* N04+400 **53**
El Transito, *Chile* S61–288 **103**
Eluru, *India* G53+168 **70**
El Valle, *Colombia* T14+062 **104**
Elvas, *Portugal* N43+389 **52**
El Vigia, *Venezuela* S69+086 **104**
Elvira, C., *N.-W. Territories* V12+728 **88**
Ely, *England* M89+524 **37**
Ely, *Minnesota* U12+478 **93**
Ely, *Nevada* V60+393 **92**
Ely, Isle of, *England* M89+525 **37**
Emangulova, *U.S.S.R.* J28+522 **61**
Emba R., *Kazakh* J28+470 **62**
Embarcacion, *Argentina* S25–232 **103**
Embóna, *Greece* L13+362 **59**
Embrun, *France* M51+445 **55**
Emden, *W. Germany* M47+534 **48**
Emerald, *Queensland* C11–232 **111**
Emerald I., *N.-W. Terr.* V58+756 **88**
Emerson, *Manitoba* U42+492 **88**
Emilia-Romagna, reg., *Italy* M26+445 **56**
Eminabad, *Pakistan* H04+321 **72**
Eminence, *Missouri* U08+372 **97**
Emmaste, *Estonia* L44+587 **47**
Emmaville, *New S. Wales* B81–294 **109**
Emmen, *Netherlands* M49+528 **44**
Emmetsburg, *Iowa* U28+431 **95**
Emmons, Mt., *Utah* V32+406 **94**
Emory Pk., *Texas* U80+292 **94**
Empalme, *Mexico* V34+281 **100**
Empedrado, *Argentina* R83–279 **103**
Empire, *Michigan* T66+448 **91**
Emporia, *Kansas* U37+384 **95**
Emporia, *Virginia* T15+367 **97**
Emporium, *Pennsylvania* T20+415 **96**
Emptinne, *Belgium* M59+503 **44**
Ems, *W. Germany* M44+503 **48**
Enard B., *Scotland* N32+581 **40**
Encarnacion, *Paraguay* R65–273 **103**
Encontrados, *Venezuela* S73+091 **104**
Encounter B., *S. Australia* C68–357 **109**
Encruzilhada, *Brazil* R45–305 **103**
Ende, *Flores I., Indonesia* D80–088 **65**
Enderbury I., *Phoenix Is.* Z36–032 **106**
Enderby Ld., *Antarctica* J60–680 **27**
Enderlin, *N. Dakota* U46+466 **93**
Endicott, *New York* T07+421 **96**
Endicott Mts., *Alaska* Y10+674 **99**
Enez, *Turkey* L23+407 **74**
Enez, G. of, *Greece* L25+407 **59**
Enfe, *Lebanon* K55+343 **76**
Enfield, *England* N00+516 **39**
Engano, C., *Philippines* D76+186 **65**
Engelberg, *Switzerland* M40+468 **45**
Engels, *U.S.S.R.* J83+514 **61**
Enggano, I., *Indonesia* F16–054 **65**
Enghien, *Belgium* M66+507 **44**
England, *Great Britain* N12+520 **34**
Englehart, *Ontario* T29+478 **91**
Englewood, *New Jersey* S84+408 **96**
English Chan., *France-Eng.* N12+500 **54**
English R., *Ontario* U25+502 **88**
English Bazar, *India* G11+250 **73**
English Coast, *Antarctica* T00–740 **27**
Enid, *Oklahoma* U48+364 **95**
Enkhuizen, *Netherlands* M58+527 **44**
Enköping, *Sweden* L78+597 **47**
Enna, *Sicily* M04+375 **57**
En Nahud, *Sudan* L10+126 **81**
En Naqura, *Lebanon* K59+331 **76**
En Nebk, *Syria* K50+340 **76**
Ennell L., *Ireland, Rep.* N44+535 **43**
En Nemara, *Syria* K46+329 **76**
Enngonia, *New S. Wales* C25–294 **109**
Ennis, *Ireland, Rep.* N54+528 **43**
Enniscorthy, *Ireland, Rep.* N39+525 **43**
Enniskillen, *N. Ireland* N46+543 **42**
Ennistimon, *Ireland, Rep.* N56+529 **43**
Enns, *Austria* M03+482 **48**
Enns, R., *Austria* M04+475 **48**
Enontekiö, *Finland* L39+684 **46**
Enriquillo, L.,
Dominican Rep. S70+186 **101**
Ensanche Colonia Sarmiento,
Argentina S60–453 **103**
Ensay, *Victoria* C13–374 **109**
Enschede, *Netherlands* M48+522 **44**
Ensenada, *Argentina* R78–348 **103**
Ensenada, *Mexico* V70+317 **100**
Enshih, *China* E63+302 **67**
Entebbe, *Uganda* K76+001 **83**
Enterprise, *Mississippi* T83+322 **95**
Entraygues, *France* M75+446 **55**
Entre Rios, *Brazil* Q48–120 **105**
Entre Rios, *Brazil* Q79–220 **105**
Eolie, Isole, *Italy* M02+387 **57**
Epe, *Netherlands* M54+523 **44**
Epernay, *France* M66+490 **54**
Ephraim, *Utah* V40+394 **94**
Episkopi & B., *Cyprus* K73+346 **76**
Epping & Forest, *England* M89+517 **39**
Epsom, *England* N02+513 **39**
Equatorial Guinea, *W. Afr.* M30+016 **82**
Ercis, *Turkey* K11+390 **74**
Erd, *Hungary* L66+474 **49**
Erebus Gulf, *Antarctica* R75–640 **27**
Erebus Mt., *Antarctica* B30–780 **27**
Eregli, *Turkey* K81+414 **74**
Ereğli, *Turkey* K67+375 **74**
Erepecú, L., *Brazil* R69–013 **105**
Eressós, *Greece* L25+391 **59**
Erexim, *Brazil* R43–279 **103**
Erfurt, *E. Germany* M24+510 **48**
Erh Hai, *China* F29+256 **64**
Erhlien, *China* E42+422 **63**
Ericht L., *Scotland* N27+568 **41**
Erie, *Pennsylvania* T31+421 **91**
Erie, L., *U.S.A.-Canada* T40+420 **99**
Ericau, *Ontario* T42+423 **91**
Eriha, *Syria* K50+358 **76**
Erisort L., *Scotland* N38+581 **40**
Eritrea, *Ethiopia* K30+150 **83**
Erlach, *Switzerland* M47+470 **45**
Erlangen, *W. Germany* M24+496 **48**
Erlenbach, *Switzerland* M45+467 **45**
Ermelo, *Netherlands* M56+523 **44**
Ermenek, *Turkey* K73+366 **74**
Ernakulam, *India* G82+100 **70**
Erne L., *N. Ireland* N47+545 **42**
Erne L., Up., *N. Ireland* N45+542 **42**
Ernee, *France* N06+483 **54**
Eromanga, I., *Vanuatu* A65–192 **106**
Erquelinnes, *Belgium* M65+503 **44**
Er Rabba, *Jordan* K56+312 **76**
Er Rahad, *Sudan* K86+128 **81**
Er Ramle, *Syria* K46+357 **76**
Er Rastan, *Syria* K50+349 **76**
Errigal, *Ireland, Rep.* N49+550 **42**
Erris Hd., *Ireland, Rep.* N60+543 **42**
Er Rumman, *Jordan* K55+322 **76**
Erudina, *S. Australia* C64–315 **109**
Erval, *Brazil* R49–319 **103**
Erz Geb., *E. Germany* M12+506 **48**
Erzincan, *Turkey* K34+398 **74**
Erzurum, *Turkey* K22+399 **74**
Erzvilkas, *Lithuania* L44+553 **47**
Esashi, *Japan* C45+450 **68**
Esbjerg, *Denmark* M39+555 **47**
Escada, *Brazil* Q31–082 **105**
Escala, la, *Spain* M71+421 **53**
Escalante, *Utah* V40+378 **94**
Escalon, *Mexico* U85+266 **100**
Escanaba & R., *Michigan* T73+458 **91**
Escaut, R., *Belgium* M65+511 **44**
Esch, *Luxembourg* M54+495 **48**
Escholzmatt, *Switzerland* M42+469 **45**
Escudo de Veragua, *Panama* T39+091 **101**
Escuinapa, *Mexico* V04+228 **100**
Escuintla, *Guatemala* U04+142 **100**
Escuminac Pt., *N.B.* S29+471 **90**
Esfahan, *Iran* J50+327 **75**
Eshowe, *Natal* K80–288 **84**
Esk R., *Scotland* N18+559 **41**
Eskdale, *New Zealand* A19–393 **112**
Eske, L., *Ireland, Rep.* N48+547 **42**
Eskilstuna, *Sweden* L81+594 **47**
Eskimo, C., *N.-W. Terr.* U25+610 **89**
Eskisehir, *Turkey* K87+398 **74**
Esla R., *Spain* N35+418 **52**
Eslöv, *Sweden* M10+559 **47**
Esmeralda, I., *Chile* T02–489 **103**
Esmeraldas, *Ecuador* T28+010 **104**
Espalion, *France* M73+445 **55**
Espanola, *Ontario* T40+463 **91**
Esperance, *W. Australia* D79–337 **110**
Esperanza, *Argentina* S06–314 **103**
Espiel, *Spain* N30+382 **52**
Espinho, *Portugal* N52+410 **52**
Espinosa de los Monteros, *Sp.* N21+431 **52**
Espirito Santo, *Brazil* S02–061 **104**
Espirito Santo, *Brazil* Q61–204 **105**
Espiritu Santo, B. del, *Mex.* T74+193 **100**
Espiritu Santo, C., *Argentina* S51–526 **103**
Espiritu Santo, I., *Mexico* V32+244 **100**
Espiritu Santo, I.,
Vanuatu A76–158 **106**
Esquel, *Argentina* S68–428 **103**
Esquimalt, *Brit. Columbia* W21+484 **88**
Esquina, *Argentina* R87–300 **103**
Es Sa'an, *Syria* K46+353 **76**
Es Safi, *Jordan* K57+310 **76**
Es Salt, *Jordan* K56+320 **76**
Es Samra, *Jordan* K53+322 **76**
Es Sanamein, *Syria* K53+331 **76**
Esse & Alv, *Finland* L41+636 **46**
Essen, *Belgium* M63+515 **44**
Essen, *W. Germany* M48+516 **48**
Essequibo, R., *Guyana* R81+068 **104**
Essex, *Ontario* T47+422 **91**
Essex, co., *England* M87+518 **39**
Essex Mt., *Wyoming* V25+419 **98**
Esslingen, *W. Germany* M34+487 **48**
Es Sukhne, *Syria* K37+348 **74**
Es Suweidîya, *Syria* K51+327 **76**
Estabutchie, *Mississippi* T86+314 **97**
Estados, I., de los, *Argentina* S26–548 **103**
Estavayer, *Switzerland* M49+469 **45**
Estcourt, *Natal* L00–290 **84**
Esteli, *Nicaragua* T69+130 **101**
Esternay, *France* M69+487 **54**
Estevan, *Saskatchewan* U79+493 **88**
Estherville, *Iowa* U29+434 **95**
Estin Gol, *China* F26+410 **64**
Estonia, rep., *U.S.S.R.* **47**
Estoril, *Portugal* N56+387 **52**
Estreito, *Brazil* R40–318 **103**
Estremoz, *Portugal* N45+388 **52**
Estrondo, Sa. des, *Brazil* R20–076 **105**
E'Sufeina, *Saudi Arabia* K27+233 **74**
Etah, *India* G68+275 **73**
Etalle, *Belgium* M56+497 **44**
Étampes, *France* M77+484 **54**
Étaples, *France* M80+505 **54**
Etawah, *India* G66+268 **73**
Etawney L., *Manitoba* U47+584 **88**
Eternity Ra., *Antarctica* S20–720 **27**
Ethe, *Belgium* M56+496 **44**
Ethiopia, *E. Africa* **83**
Etivaz, l', *Switzerland* M47+464 **45**
Etive L., *Scotland* N31+565 **41**
Etna, Mt., *Sicily* M00+378 **57**
Eton, *England* N04+515 **39**
Ettelbrück, *Luxembourg* M53+499 **48**
Etten, *Netherlands* M62+516 **44**
Ettrick, *New Zealand* A63–457 **112**
Ettrick R., *Scotland* N18+555 **41**
Euabalong, *New S. Wales* C21–331 **109**
Euboea. *See* Evvoia, I.
Eucla, *W. Australia* D37–316 **110**
Eudunda, *S. Australia* C66–341 **109**
Eufaula, *Alabama* T61+318 **99**
Eufaula & Res., *Oklahoma* U34+353 **95**
Eugene, *Oregon* W19+441 **96**
Eugmö, *Finland* L43+638 **46**
Eugowra, *New S. Wales* C09–334 **109**
Eumungerie, *New S. Wales* C08–320 **109**
Eunice, *Louisiana* U14+304 **95**
Eupen, *Belgium* M54+506 **44**
Euphrates, R., *Iraq, etc.* J89+315 **74**
Eure, dep., *France* M85+491 **54**
Eureka, *California* W25+408 **92**
Eureka, *Kansas* U38+378 **95**
Eureka, *Nevada* V66+396 **92**
Eureka, *Utah* V41+400 **94**
Eure-et-Loir, dep., *France* M28+484 **54**
Euriowie, *New S. Wales* C50–314 **109**
Euroa, *Victoria* C27–367 **109**
Eursinge, *Netherlands* M51+528 **44**
Euston, *New S. Wales* C44–346 **109**
Eutaw, *Alabama* T77+329 **97**
Eutin, *W. Germany* M26+541 **48**
Eutsuk L., *Brit. Columbia* W40+536 **88**
Evale, *Angola* L86–166 **84**
Evandale, *Tasmania* C17–416 **109**
Evans, L., *Quebec* T12+508 **89**
Evanston, *Illinois* T76+421 **95**
Evanston, *Wyoming* V36+412 **93**
Evansville, *Indiana* T76+380 **97**
Evansville, *Minnesota* U34+461 **93**
Eva Peron, La Plata, *Argent* R78–349 **103**
Evaux, *France* M75+462 **54**
Eveleth, *Minnesota* U16+472 **93**
Everard, L., *S. Australia* D00–312 **111**
Everest, Mt., *Nepal-Tibet* G18+280 **71**
Everett, *Washington* W12+478 **98**
Evergem, *Belgium* M68+511 **44**
Everglades, The, *Florida* T35+256 **99**
Everglades Nat. Park, *Florida* T36+255 **97**
Evergreen, *Alabama* T72+315 **97**
Evesham & Vale of, *England* N12+521 **39**
Evijärvi, *Finland* L39+634 **46**
Evje, *Norway* M43+586 **47**
Evolène, *Switzerland* M45+461 **45**
Evora, *Portugal* N47+386 **52**
Evreux, *France* M83+490 **54**
Evros, *Greece* L23+413 **58**
Evrykhou, *Cyprus* K73+350 **76**
Évvoia, G. of, *Greece* L40+387 **59**
Evvoia, I., *Greece* L36+386 **59**
Ewarton, *Jamaica* T13+182 **101**
Ewe, L., *Scotland* N34+578 **40**
Exaltacion, *Bolivia* S33–134 **104**
Exe R., *England* N21+507 **38**
Exeter, *England* N21+507 **38**
Exeter, *New Hampshire* S66+430 **96**
Exloo, *Netherlands* M49+529 **44**
Exminster, *England* N21+507 **38**

Exmoor, *England* N21+512 **38**
Exmouth, *England* N20+506 **38**
Exmouth G., *W. Australia* E33–218 **110**
Expedition Ra., *Queensland* C06–242 **111**
Exuma Is., *Bahamas, The* T10+244 **101**
Exuma Sd., *Bahamas, The* T08+244 **101**
Eyasi L., *Tanzania* K60–036 **83**
Eye L., *Quebec* T10+532 **89**
Eyemouth, *Scotland* N12+559 **41**
Eymoutiers, *France* M79+457 **54**
Eyre, *W. Australia* D52–321 **110**
Eyre Cr., *S. Australia* C67–266 **111**
Eyre, L., *S. Australia* C76–282 **111**
Eyre Pen., *S. Australia* C85–334 **111**
Eyrecourt, *Ireland, Rep.* N49+532 **43**
Eyzies, les, *France* M84+449 **55**
Ezcaray, *Spain* N18+423 **52**
Fab, *Somalia* J72+048 **83**
Fåborg, *Denmark* M28+551 **47**
Facatativa, *Columbia* S86+047 **104**
Fada, *Chad* L50+172 **81**
Fadan' Gourma, *Upper Volta* M88+120 **80**
Faddeyevskiy, Ostrov, *Russia* C35+750 **63**
Faenza, *Italy* M19+443 **56**
Faeröerne, *N. Atlantic Ocean* N40+620 **34**
Faeroes. *See* Faeroerne.
Fafa, *Mali* M86+152 **80**
Făgăras, *Romania* L30+458 **58**
Fagarg, *Sudan* L20+118 **81**
Fagerli, *Norway* L83+671 **46**
Fagernes, *Norway* M34+610 **47**
Fagnano, L., *Argentina* S46–546 **103**
Faid, *Saudi Arabia* K14+271 **74**
Faido, *Switzerland* M37+465 **45**
Fai-fo, (Hoi An), *Vietnam* E70+158 **69**
Fair I., *Scotland* N10+595 **40**
Fairbanks, *Alaska* X75+643 **99**
Fairbury, *Illinios* T81+408 **91**
Fairbury, *Nebraska* U43+402 **95**
Fairfield, *Illinois* T80+384 **95**
Fairfield, *Iowa* U12+410 **95**
Fairfield, *Maine* S58+446 **90**
Fairhaven, *Massachusetts* S65+416 **96**
Fair Head, *N. Ireland* N37+552 **42**
Fairlie, *New Zealand* A55–441 **112**
Fairmont, *Minnesota* U27+437 **93**
Fairmont, *West Virginia* T31+395 **91**
Fairview, *Alberta* V82+559 **88**
Fairville, *New Brunswick* S37+453 **90**
Fairweather, Mt., *Alaska* X15+590 **99**
Faith, *S. Dakota* U73+450 **93**
Faizabad, *Afghanistan* H26+371 **75**
Faizabad, *India* G47+267 **73**
Fajr, *Saudi Arabia* K44+289 **74**
Fakfak, *Irian Jaya, Indon.* D17–029 **65**
Fakiya, *Bulgaria* L18+422 **58**
Falam, *Burma* F68+230 **71**
Falama, *Guinea* N52+106 **80**
Fălciu, *Romania* L11+463 **58**
Falcon, Res., *Texas* U56+269 **94**
Falcone, C. of, *Sardinia* M41+410 **57**
Falkenberg, *Sweden* M15+569 **47**
Falkirk, *Scotland* N23+560 **41**
Falkland, *Scotland* N19+562 **41**
Falkland Is., *S. Atlantic Oc.* S00–517 **103**
Falkland Is. Dependencies,
Antarctica R00–550 **27**
Falknov, *Czechoslovakia* M14+502 **48**
Fallöping, *Sweden* M09+581 **47**
Fall River, *Massachusetts* S67+417 **96**
Falls City, *Nebraska* U34+402 **95**
Falmagne, *Belgium* M61+502 **44**
Falmouth, *Jamaica* T16+185 **101**
Falmouth, *Kentucky* T56+387 **91**
Falmouth & B., *England* N30+501 **38**
False B., *Cape Province* L68–344 **84**
False Point, *India* G19+204 **71**
Falset, *Spain* M85+411 **53**
Falso, C., *Mexico* V30+229 **100**
Falster, I., *Denmark* M18+548 **47**
Faluja, *Israel* K61+316 **76**
Falun, *Sweden* L86+606 **47**
Famagusta & B., *Cyprus* K66+351 **76**
Famatina, *Argentina* S45–290 **103**
Fanad Hd., *Ireland, Rep.* N46+553 **42**
Fannich L., *Scotland* N30+576 **40**
Fanning, I., *Pacific Ocean* Y58+040 **107**
Fanö, I., *Denmark* M39+554 **47**
Fanö Bugt, *Denmark* M41+553 **47**
Fanshawe, C., *N.-W. Terr.* T10+730 **89**
Fanuch, *Iran* J02+266 **75**
Fao, *Iraq* J69+300 **74**
Faradje, *Congo* L02+036 **83**
Farafangana, *Madagascar* J74–230 **83**
Farah, *Afghanistan* H77+324 **75**
Farajja, *Saudi Arabia* J56+218 **75**
Faranah, *Guinea* N64+100 **80**
Faranlep, I., *Caroline Is.* C40+082 **106**
Farasan Is., *Red Sea* K18+168 **74**
Farewell C., *Greenland* Q70+590 **26**
Fargo, *N. Dakota* U41+469 **93**
Faribault, *Minnesota* U20+443 **93**
Faridabad, *India* G76+284 **72**
Faridkot, *India* H02+307 **72**
Faridpur, *India* G63+282 **73**
Faridpur, *Bangladesh* G01+236 **73**
Fariman, *Iran* J02+360 **75**
Farina, *S. Australia* C70–301 **109**
Farmington, *Maine* S61+447 **90**
Farmington, *Missouri* U03+378 **97**
Farmington, *New Mexico* V20+367 **94**
Farmington, *Utah* V42+409 **94**
Farmville, *Virginia* T20+373 **97**
Farnborough, *England* N00+514 **39**
Farne Is., *England* N10+556 **37**
Farnes, *Norway* M43+613 **47**
Farnham, *Quebec* S78+453 **91**
Farnworth, *England* N14+535 **37**
Faro, *Brazil* R71–020 **105**
Faro, *Portugal* N47+370 **52**
Fårön, I., *Sweden* L65+579 **47**
Farrukhabad, *India* G63+274 **73**
Farrukhnagar, *India* G79+284 **72**
Farsala, *Greece* L46+393 **59**
Farsi, *Afghanistan* H71+338 **75**
Farsund, *Norway* M49+581 **47**
Farwell, *Michigan* T59+438 **91**
Farwell, *Texas* U78+340 **98**
Fasa, *Iran* J38+289 **75**
Fatahabad, *India* G87+295 **72**
Fatait ibn Kanat,
Saudi Arabia K10+293 **74**
Fatehabad, *India* G70+271 **73**
Fatehgarh, *India* G62+273 **73**
Fatehpur, *India* H00+280 **72**
Fatehpur, *India* G55+259 **73**
Father L., *Quebec* T02+495 **89**
Fatmomakke, *Sweden* L89+650 **46**
Fatshan, *China* E41+231 **67**
Fatu Hiva, I., *Marquesas Is.* X20–108 **107**
Fawley, *England* N08+508 **39**
Faxaflói, *Iceland* P50+645 **46**
Faxina, *Brazil* R24–238 **105**
Faya. *See* Largeau.
Fayette, *Alabama* T77+337 **95**
Fayette, *Missouri* U16+391 **95**
Fayetteville, *Arkansas* U25+361 **93**
Fayetteville, *N. Carolina* T23+350 **97**
Fayetteville, *Pennsylvania* T14+399 **96**
Fayetteville, *W. Virginia* T37+380 **97**
Fazilka, *India* H06+304 **72**
Fdérik, *Mauritania* N76+226 **80**
Feale R., *Ireland Rep.* N58+525 **43**
Fear, C., *N. Carolina* T16+336 **99**
Featherton, Mt., *Victoria* C17–369 **109**
Fécamp, *France* M87+498 **54**
Fedaracion, *Argentina* R78–309 **103**
Feeagh L., *Ireland, Rep.* N57+539 **42**
Fehmarn, I., *W. Germany* M23+544 **48**
Feifu. *See Faifo.*
Feilding, *New Zealand* A26–400 **112**
Feira de Santana, *Brazil* Q53–124 **105**
Feldbach, *Austria* L85+470 **49**
Feldkirch, *Austria* M33+472 **48**
Felipe Carrillo Puerto, *Mex.* T73+196 **100**
Femund, L., *Norway* M19+623 **46**
Feng chên, *China* E41+405 **66**
Fengshien, *China* E20+346 **66**
Fenghwang, *China* E63+279 **67**
Fengkieh, *China* E63+311 **66**
Fengsiang, *China* E77+343 **66**
Fengyang, *China* E12+328 **66**
Fenit, *Ireland, Rep.* N59+523 **43**
Fenny Stratford, *England* N04+520 **39**
Fens, The, *England* N00+526 **37**
Fenton, *Michigan* T52+428 **91**
Fenyang, *China* E50+373 **66**
Feodosiya & B., *U.S.S.R.* K58+450 **60**
Fergus, *Ontario* T32+437 **91**
Fergus Falls, *Minnesota* U36+463 **93**
Ferguson, *Missouri* U02+387 **97**
Ferguson, *Quebec* S81+478 **91**
Fergusson I., *Papua New Guinea*
B86–095 **111**
Fermanagh, co., *N. Ireland* N46+543 **42**
Fermoy, *Ireland, Rep.* N50+521 **43**
Fernando Poo, I., *See* Macias Nguema
Fernie, *Brit. Columbia* V59+496 **88**
Ferns, *Ireland, Rep.* N39+526 **43**
Ferozepore, *India* H02+309 **72**
Ferrar Gl., *Antarctica* B70–790 **27**
Ferrara, *Italy* M20+448 **56**
Ferrato C., *Sardinia* M32+393 **57**
Ferreira do Zezere, *Portugal* N50+397 **52**
Ferrol del Caudillo, *Spain* N49+434 **52**
Fertile, *Minnesota* U38+476 **93**
Fertö tó, *See* Neusiedler See
Fes, *Morocco* N30+340 **80**
Festus, *Missouri* U02+382 **97**
Fethard, *Ireland, Rep.* N46+524 **43**
Fetlar I., *Scotland* N05+606 **40**
Fez. *See* Fes
Ffestiniog, *Wales* N24+529 **38**
Fiambala, *Argentina* S46–277 **103**
Ficalho, *Portugal* N44+380 **52**
Fichtel Geb., *W. Germany* M18+501 **48**
Fideris, *Switzerland* M31+469 **45**
Fier, *Albania* L63+407 **59**
Fiesch, *Switzerland* M41+464 **45**
Fife, reg., *Scotland* N18+563 **41**
Fife Ness, *Scotland* N15+563 **41**
Figeac, *France* M78+466 **55**
Figline Vald., *Italy* M21+436 **56**
Figueira de Castelo Rodrigo,
Portugal N42+409 **52**
Figueras, *Spain* M72+423 **53**
Figuig, *Morocco* N08+320 **80**
Fiji Is., *Pacific Ocean* A00–175 **106**
Filakovo, *Czechoslovakia* L61+483 **49**
Filchner Ice Shelf,
Antarctica R30–790 **27**
Filey, *England* N02+542 **37**
Filiátes, *Greece* L58+396 **59**
Filicudi, I., *Italy* M03+386 **57**
Filipow, *Poland* L44+542 **49**
Filisur, *Switzerland* M32+467 **45**
Fincastle, *Virginia* T29+374 **97**
Findhorn & R., *Scotland* N22+577 **40**
Findlay, *Ohio* T52+410 **91**
Findlay Grp., *N.-W. Terr.* V00+772 **88**
Fingal, *N. Dakota* U47+468 **93**
Fingal, *Tasmania* C13–417 **109**
Finhaut, *Switzerland* M48+461 **45**
Finistère, dep., *France* N24+483 **54**
Finisterre, C., *Spain* N55+428 **52**
Finke, R., *N. Terr., Aust.* D01–255 **111**
Finland, rep., *N. Europe* **46**
Finland, G. of, *N.-W. Europe* **47**
Finlay R., *Brit. Columbia* W25+564 **88**
Finlay Forks, *Brit. Columbia* W23+559 **88**
Finley, *New S. Wales* C28–357 **109**
Finschhafen,
Papua New Guinea C13–065 **111**
Finspång, *Sweden* L85+587 **47**
Finsteraarhorn, *Switzerland* M41+465 **45**
Fintona, *N. Ireland* N44+545 **42**
Fionn L., *Scotland* N33+577 **40**
Fionnay, *Switzerland* M46+460 **45**
Fiq, *Syria* K56+328 **76**
Firat, R., *Turkey* K36+397 **74**
Firdaus, *Iran* J11+340 **75**
Firenze, *Italy* M23+438 **56**
Firmat, *Argentina* S09–334 **103**
Firnis, *Turkey* K49+379 **74**
Firozabad, *India* G70+272 **73**
Firozpur Jhirka, *India* G78+277 **72**
Firuzabad, *Iran* J45+288 **75**
Firuze, *Iran* J12+378 **75**
Fish Camp, *Kenya* K56+036 **83**
Fisher Str., *N.-W. Terr.* T50+635 **89**
Fishers I., *New York* S72+412 **96**
Fishbuard & B., *Wales* N30+520 **38**
Fitchburg, *Massachusetts* S71+426 **96**
Fitful Hd., *Scotland* N08+599 **40**
Fitzcarrald, *Peru* S70–117 **104**
Fitzgerald, *Alberta* V40+599 **88**
Fitzgerald, *Tasmania* C21–428 **109**
Fitzpatrick, *Alabama* T65+322 **97**
Fitzroy, *W. Australia* D56–181 **110**
Fitz Roy, C., *N.-W. Terr.* T30+755 **89**
Fitzroy, R., *Queensland* C02–230 **111**
Fitzroy, R., *W. Australia* D63–179 **110**
Fitzwilliam I., *Ontario* T41+455 **91**
Fiume. *See* Rijeka
Fivemiletown, *N. Ireland* N44+544 **42**
Fjälläsen, *Sweden* L59+675 **46**
Flagstaff, *Arizona* V40+35 **94**
Flamborough Hd., *England* N00+542 **37**
Flamingo Tk.,
Irian Jaya, Indon. C76–057 **65**
Flat, *Alaska* Y48+624 **99**
Flathead, L., *Montana* V55+478 **92**
Flattery, C., *Queensland* C28–150 **111**
Flattery, C., *Washington* W28+479 **98**
Flèche, la, *France* N00+477 **54**
Fleetwood, *England* N18+539 **37**
Flekkefjord, *Norway* M50+583 **47**
Flemington, *New Jersey* S89+405 **96**
Flensburg, *W. Germany* M34+547 **48**
Flers, *France* N03+488 **54**
Fleurance, *France* M86+439 **55**
Fleurier, *Switzerland* M50+469 **45**
Fleuru, *Belgium* M63+505 **44**
Flims, *Switzerland* M34+468 **45**
Flinders I., *S. Australia* D03–335 **111**
Flinders I., *Tasmania* C12–400 **109**
Flinders Ra., *S. Australia* C70–320 **109**
Flinders, R., *Queensland* C52–194 **111**
Flin Flon, *Manitoba* U71+548 **88**
Flint, *Michigan* T52+431 **91**
Flint, *Wales* N19+532 **38**
Flint I., *Pacific Ocean* Y15–105 **107**
Flint R., *Georgia* T57+310 **99**
Flisa, *Norway* M18+606 **47**
Flora, *Illinois* T81+386 **95**
Florac, *France* M69+443 **55**
Floreffe, *Belgium* M61+504 **44**
Florence. *See* Firenze
Florence, *Alabama* T76+348 **97**
Florence, *Arizona* V40+330 **94**
Florence, *Colorado* V02+384 **94**
Florence, *S. Carolina* T29+342 **97**
Florence, *Wisconsin* T80+460 **91**
Florencia, *Argentina* R86–280 **103**
Florencia, *Colombia* T04+017 **104**
Florennes, *Belgium* M62+502 **44**
Florenville, *Belgium* M58+497 **44**
Flores, *Guatemala* T89+170 **100**
Flores, I., *Atlantic Ocean* Q08+394 **80**
Flores, I. & Sea, *Indonesia* D80–085 **65**
Floriano, *Brazil* Q78–068 **105**
Floriano Peixoto, *Brazil* S44–092 **104**
Florianopolis, *Brazil* R21–276 **103**
Florida, *Sicily* L89+371 **57**
Florida, state, *U.S.A.* T64+306 **99**
Florida B., *Florida* T41+250 **99**
Florida, C., *Florida* T31+257 **99**
Florida Mts., *New Mexico* V16+322 **94**
Florida Str., *Bahamas, The* T30+250 **101**
Florida Str., *Florida* T39+244 **99**
Florida City, *Florida* T33+254 **99**
Florida Keys, *Florida* T34+250 **97**
Floridia, *Uruguay* R67–340 **103**
Florina, *Greece* L51+408 **59**
Flöro, *Norway* M61+617 **46**
Flotta, I., *Orkney Is., Scot.* N19+588 **40**
Floydada, *Texas* U68+340 **94**
Flüelen, *Switzerland* M38+469 **45**
Flushing. *See* Vlissingen
Flushing, *New York* S83+407 **96**
Fly, R., *Papua New Guinea* C50–078 **111**
Flying Fish C., *Antarctica* U65–730 **27**
Foča, *Yugoslavia* L67+435 **58**
Focsani, *Romania* L17+456 **58**
Fofa Cahuel, *Argentina* S65–423 **103**
Foggia, *Italy* L87+415 **57**
Fogo I., *Newfoundland* R55+497 **90**
Föhr, I., *W. Germany* M39+547 **48**
Foix, *France* M80+430 **55**
Fokis, *Greece* L46+386 **59**
Folda, Fd., *Norway* M04+676 **46**
Folégandros, I., *Greece* L30+366 **59**
Foleyet, *Ontario* T45+483 **91**
Foligno, *Italy* M14+430 **56**
Folkestone, *England* M83+511 **39**
Folkston, *Georgia* T42+309 **97**
Folkstone, *N. Carolina* T15+345 **97**
Follega, *Netherlands* M56+529 **44**
Fonda, *New York* S86+429 **96**
Fond du Lac, *Minnesota-*
Wisconsin U09+469 **91**
Fond du Lac, *Saskatchewan* V13+595 **88**
Fond du Lac, *Wisconsin* T81+438 **91**
Fonsagráda, *Spain* N42+431 **52**
Fonseca, G. of, *Honduras* T76+132 **101**
Fontaine, *Belgium* M64+504 **44**
Fontainebleau, *France* M74+484 **54**
Fontana, L., *Argentina* S69–449 **103**
Fontenay le Comte, *France* N05+465 **54**
Foochow, *China* E04+261 **67**
Forbes, *New South Wales* C12+334 **109**
Forbes, Mt., *Alberta* V70+516 **88**
Forcados, *Nigeria* M58+052 **80**
Forcalquier, *France* M56+440 **55**
Førde, *Norway* M55+615 **47**
Fordlandia, *Brazil* R62–038 **105**
Ford Ranges, *Antarctica* X40–770 **27**
Ford's Bridge, *New S. Wales* C27–298 **109**
Fordyce, *Arkansas* U14+338 **95**
Forel, Mt., *Greenland* Q10+670 **26**
Forest, *Ontario* T42+431 **91**
Forestier Pen., *Tasmania* C13–429 **109**
Forfar, *Scotland* N17+566 **41**
Fork, R., N., *Idaho* V42+440 **98**
Forli, *Italy* M18+442 **56**
Forlorn Pt., *Ireland, Rep.* N39+522 **43**
Formentera I., *Balearic Is.* M81+387 **53**
Formia, *Italy* M08+413 **57**
Formosa, *Argentina* R79–261 **103**
Formosa, *Brazil* R13–156 **105**
Formosa. *See* Taiwan, I.
Formosa Str. *See* Taiwan Hai Hsia
Fornos d'Algôdres, *Portugal* N45+407 **52**
Forres, *Scotland* N22+576 **40**
Forrest, *W. Australia* D41–308 **110**
Forrest, *Victoria* C48–386 **109**
Forrest City, *Arkansas* U04+350 **95**
Forsa, *Sweden* L79+617 **47**
Forsayth, *Queensland* C39–185 **111**
Forsnäs, *Sweden* L68+662 **46**
Forssa, *Finland* L38+608 **47**
Forsyth, *Montana* V10+462 **93**
Fort Albany, *Ontario* T40+525 **89**
Fort Alexander, *Manitoba* U37+504 **88**
Fortaleza, *Amazonas, Brazil* S52–064 **104**
Fortaleza, *Ceara, Brazil* Q52–037 **105**
Fortaleza, state of, *Acre,*
Brazil S58–100 **104**
Fort Ann, *New York* S80+435 **96**
Fort Archambault, *See* Sarh
Fort Atkinson, *Wisconsin* T83+429 **95**
Fort Augustus, *Scotland* N28+571 **40**
Fort Beaufort, *Cape Province* L20–328 **84**
Fort Bennett, *S. Dakota* U64+447 **93**
Fort Benton, *Montana* V34+478 **93**
Fort Brabant, *N.-W. Terr.* V42+707 **88**
Fort Bragg, *California* W23+395 **92**
Fort Chipewyan, *Alberta* V36+590 **88**
Fort Collins, *Colorado* V00+406 **94**
Fort Coulonge, *Quebec* T11+459 **91**
Fort Crampel, *Central*
African Republic L64+070 **81**
Ford Dauphin, *Madagascar* J78–250 **83**
Fort Dodge, *Iowa* U25+426 **95**
Fort Edward, *New York* S82+433 **91**
Fortescue, R., *W. Australia* E18–214 **110**
Fort Fairfield, *Maine* S47+467 **90**
Fort Flatters, *Algeria* M50+280 **80**
Fort Fraser, *Brit. Columbia* W28+541 **88**
Fort George, *Scotland* N24+576 **40**
Fort George, R., *Quebec* T20+540 **89**
Fort Gouraud, *See* Fdérik
Fort Grahame, *B.C.* W27+563 **88**
Fort Grey, *New S. Wales* C52–289 **109**
Forth, Firth of, *Scotland* N18+561 **41**
Forth R., *Scotland* N24+561 **41**
Fort Haka, *Burma* F68+226 **71**
Fort Hall, *Kenya* K48–008 **83**
Fort Henrique, *Namibia* M00–174 **84**
Fort Hertz, *Burma* F45+273 **71**
Fort Hill, *See* Chitipa
Fort Howard, *Wisconsin* T78+445 **91**
Fort Hunter, *New York* S85+429 **96**
Fortin Teniente Montania,
Paraguay S00–220 **103**
Fortin Camacho, *Paraguay* S02–221 **103**
Fortin Lopez, *Paraguay* R89–214 **103**
Fortin Munoz, *Paraguay* S04–235 **103**
Fortin Saavedra, *Paraguay* S00–234 **103**
Fort Jameson, *Zambia* K74–138 **83**
Fort Kent, *Maine* S52+472 **90**
Fort Keogh, *Montana* V05+464 **93**
Fort Lallemand, *Algeria* M52+312 **80**
Fort Lamy, *See* N'Djamena
Fort Laperrine. *See* Tamanrasset
Fort Laramie, *Wyoming* U87+422 **93**
Fort Madison, *Iowa* U08+406 **95**
Fort Maginnis, *Montana* V25+472 **93**
Fort Morgan, *Alabama* T78+303 **97**
Fort Morgan, *Colorado* U83+402 **94**
Fort Munro, *Pakistan* H30+229 **72**
Fort Nelson & R., *B.C.* W17+590 **88**
Fort Ogden, *Florida* T41+271 **97**
Fort Peck, *Montana* V08+480 **93**
Fort Peck Res., *Montana* V16+476 **93**
Fort Pierre, *S. Dakota* U62+443 **93**
Fort Plain, *New York* S88+429 **96**
Fort Polignac, *Algeria* M40+262 **80**
Fort Portal, *Uganda* K88+006 **83**
Fort Randall, *Alaska* Y75+547 **26**
Fort Rice, *N. Dakota* U64+465 **93**
Fortrose, *Scotland* N25+576 **40**
Fort Roseberry, *Zambia* L06–112 **83**
Fort St George. *See* Madras
Fort St John, *B.C.* W07+560 **88**
Fort Sandeman, *Pakistan* H31+314 **72**
Fort Saskatchewan, *Alberta* V48+539 **88**
Fort Scott, *Kansas* U28+378 **95**
Fort Sibut, *Cent. Afr. Rep.* L66+058 **81**
Fort Sill, *Oklahoma* U50+346 **95**
Fort Smith, *Arkansas* U26+353 **95**
Fort Smith, N.-W. Terr. V41+600 **88**
Fort Stedman, *Burma* F48+205 **71**
Fort Stockton, *Texas* U76+308 **94**
Fort Sumner, *New Mexico* U85+344 **94**
Fortuna, *California* W25+406 **92**
Fortuna, *Spain* N07+382 **53**
Fortune B., *Newfoundland* R66+471 **90**
Fort Valley, *Georgia* T53+326 **97**
Fort Vermilion, *Alberta* V65+586 **88**
Fort Victoria, *Zimbabwe* K84–202 **84**
Fort Warren, *Wyoming* U89+412 **93**
Fort Wayne, *Indiana* T61+411 **91**
Fort White, *Burma* F67+234 **71**
Fort William, *Scotland* N31+568 **41**
Fort Worth, *Texas* U44+328 **95**
Fort Yates, *N. Dakota* U64+461 **93**
Fort Yukon, *Alaska* X60+663 **99**
Forville, *Belgium* M60+506 **44**
Fosse, *Belgium* M62+504 **44**
Foster, *Victoria* C23–386 **109**
Foster Ls., *Saskatchewan* V03+564 **88**
Fougeres, *France* N07+484 **54**
Foul B., *Egypt* K56+234 **81**
Foul, I., *Burma* F65+182 **71**
Foula, I., *Scotland* N12+602 **34**
Foulness I., *England* M85+516 **39**
Fouly, la, *Switzerland* M47+459 **45**
Foúrnoi, Is., *Greece* L21+376 **59**
Foveaux Strait, *New Zealand* A72–466 **112**
Fowchow. *See* Fowling.
Fowlers B., *S. Australia* D14–320 **110**
Fowling, *China* E76+297 **67**
Fowning, *China* E00+338 **66**
Fowyang, *China* E24+330 **66**
Fox Is., *Aleutian Is.* Z20+530 **99**
Fox R., *Manitoba* U27+556 **88**
Foxe Basin, *N.-W.*
Territories T20+670 **89**
Foxe Chan., *N.-W.*
Territories T30+650 **89**
Foxe Pen., *N.-W. Terr.* T10+647 **89**

Foxford, *Ireland, Rep.* N55+540 **42**
Fox River, *Quebec* S26+490 **90**
Foxton, *New Zealand* A28–404 **112**
Foyle L., *N. Ireland* N43+551 **42**
Foyle R., *N. Ireland* N44+550 **42**
Foynes, *Ireland, Rep.* N55+526 **43**
Foz do Acre, *Brazil* S44–088 **104**
Foz do Cunene, *Angola* M18–172 **84**
Foz Embira, *Brazil* S61–074 **104**
Fraire, *Belgium* M63+503 **44**
Framboise, *Nova Scotia* S02+457 **90**
Frameries, *Belgium* M67+504 **44**
Framingham, *Massachusetts* S69+423 **96**
Franca, *Brazil* R15–206 **105**
Francavilla Fontana, *Italy* L75+405 **57**
France, *W. Europe* M78+470 **50**
Frances, *S. Australia* C54–367 **109**
Frances L., *Yukon* W55+610 **88**
Franceville, *Gabon* M04–018 **82**
Franche-Comte, prov., *France* M50+472 **54**
Francistown, *Botswana* L14–214 **84**
Francois L., *British Columbia* W35+541 **88**
Frankfort, *Kansas* U39+397 **95**
Frankfort, *Kentucky* T59+383 **97**
Frankfort, *Michigan* T67+446 **91**
Frankfurt-am-Main, *W. Germany* M38+501 **48**
Frankfurt-an-der-Oder, *E. Germany* M03+523 **48**
Fränkischer Jura, *W. Germany* M21+492 **48**
Franklin, *Louisiana* U08+298 **95**
Franklin, *New Hampshire* S70+434 **96**
Franklin, *New Jersey* S87+411 **96**
Franklin, *N. Carolina* T50+352 **97**
Franklin, *Pennsylvania* T29+414 **96**
Franklin, *Tasmania* C19–432 **111**
Franklin, *Tennessee* T71+358 **97**
Franklin, *Virginia* T12+367 **97**
Franklin, *W. Virginia* T26+386 **97**
Franklin Dist., *N.-W. Terr.* **88-89**
Franklin, I., *Antarctica* A68–760 **27**
Franklin Mts., *N.-W. Territories* W25+656 **88**
Franklin City, *Virginia* T02+380 **97**
Franklin Falls, *N.H.* S70+434 **91**
Frantsa Iosifa Zemyla, *Arctic Ocean* J30+810 **62**
Franz Josef Fd., *Greenland* P85+740 **26**
Franz Josef Land, *See* Frantsa Iosifa Zemlya.
Fraser R., *British Columbia* W13+514 **88**
Fraserburg, *Cape Province* L50–320 **84**
Fraserburgh, *Scotland* N12+577 **40**
Frasertown, *New Zealand* A15–390 **112**
Frasnes, *Belgium* M68+507 **44**
Frater, *Ontario* T57+473 **91**
Frauenfeld, *Switzerland* M37+476 45
Fray Bentos, *Uruguay* R80–332 **103**
Fredericia, *Denmark* M31+556 **47**
Frederick, *Maryland* T14+394 **96**
Frederick, *Oklahoma* U54+344 **95**
Frederick, *S. Dakota* U51+458 **93**
Fredericksburg, *Virginia* T15+383 **97**
Fredericktown, *Missouri* U02+375 **95**
Fredericton, *New Brunswick* S40+460 **90**
Frederikshåb, *Greenland* R30+620 **26**
Frederikshavn, *Denmark* M27+575 **47**
Fredonia, *Colombia* T04+060 **104**
Fredonia, *Kansas* U35+376 **95**
Fredonia, *New York* T26+425 **96**
Fredrika, *Sweden* L70+641 **46**
Fredrikstad, *Norway* M24+592 **47**
Freehold, *New Jersey* S85+402 **96**
Freeling, *S. Australia* C67–345 **109**
Freeport, *Illinois* T88+423 **95**
Freeport, *Pennsylvania* T29+407 **96**
Freetown, *Sierra Leone* N80+086 **80**
Fregenal de la Sierra, *Spain* N40+382 **52**
Fréhel, C. *France* N14+487 **54**
Freiberg, *E. Germany* M10+510 **48**
Freiburg, *W. Germany* M43+480 **48**
Freirina, *Chile* S67–284 **103**
Freistadt, *Austria* M03+485 **48**
Freital, *E. Germany* M08+511 **48**
Freixiel, *Portugal* N44+413 **52**
Freixo, *Portugal* N41+411 **52**
Fremantle, *W. Australia* E25–320 **110**
Fremont, *Nebraska* U38+414 **95**
Fremont, *Ohio* T49+414 **91**
Fremont Pk., *Wyoming* V28+432 **93**
Fremont R., *Utah* V35+386 **98**
French I., *Victoria* C28–383 **109**
French R., *Ontario* T32+460 **91**
French Guiana, rep., *S. America* R50+036 **105**
Frenchman R., *Saskatchewan* V20+493 **88**
Frenchman Cap, *Tasmania* C24–423 **109**
Frenchpark, *Ireland, Rep.* N50+539 **42**
French River, *Ontario* T36+459 **91**
French Territory of the Afars and the Issas *See* Djibouti
Fresko, *Ivory Coast* N36+050 **80**
Fresnillo, *Mexico* U77+232 **100**
Fria C., *Namibia* M18–184 **84**
Fresno, *California* V89+368 **92**
Frias, *Spain* N20+428 **52**
Fribourg & canton, *Switz.* M47+468 **45**
Fridtjof Nansen Mt., *Antarctica* A10–850 **27**
Friedland, *E. Germany* M09+536 **48**
Friend, *Nebraska* U44+406 **95**
Friesische Is., Nord., *W. Ger.* M39+546 **47**
Friesische Is., Ost., *W. Germany* M52+538 **48**
Friesland, prov., *Netherlands* M54+531 **44**
Friuli-Venezia Giulia, reg., *Italy* M12+462 **56**
Frobisher B., *N.-W. Terr.* S30+618 **89**
Frobisher L., *Saskatchewan* V20+564 **88**
Fro Havet, *Norway* M35+638 **46**
Frome, *England* N14+512 **38**
Frome, L., *S. Australia* C61–308 **109**
Front Ra., *Colorado* V04+400 **94**
Fronteira, *Portugal* N46+390 **52**
Frontera, *Mexico* U16+186 **100**
Fronteras, *Mexico* V27+310 **100**
Front Royal, *Virginia* T18+389 **96**
Frosinone, *Italy* M10+416 **57**
Frostburg, *Maryland* T24+397 **96**
Frøya, *Norway* M38+637 **46**
Frozen Str., *N.-W. Terr.* T55+658 **89**
Frunze, *Kirgiz.* H02+429 **62**
Frutigen, *Switzerland* M44+466 **45**
Frydek, *Czechoslovakia* L70+497 **49**
Fthiótis, *Greece* L45+388 **59**
Fuchin, *China* D20+474 **64**
Fuchow, *China* E22+280 **67**
Fu-chow, *China* D81+397 **66**
Fuente-Alamo de Murcia, *Sp.* N07+378 **53**
Fuente del Arco, *Spain* N35+382 **52**
Fuentes de Onoro, *Spain* N41+406 **52**
Fuertaventura, I., *Canary Islands* N82+284 **80**
Fuerte, El, *Mexico* V20+268 **100**
Fuerte, R., *Mexico* V22+262 **100**
Fuhsin, *China* D80+421 **66**
Fuji yama (Fuji san), *Japan* C66+354 **68**
Fukien, prov., *China* E12+260 **67**
Fukuei Chiao, *Taiwan* D80+255 **64**
Fukui, *Japan* C82+360 **68**
Fukuoka, *Japan* D28+335 **68**
Fukushima, *Japan* C57+377 **68**
Fukuyama, *Japan* C59+415 **68**
Fukuyama, *Japan* D16+345 **68**
Fulda, R., *W. Germany* M33+511 **48**
Fullerton, *Nebraska* U48+414 **95**
Fulton, *Kentucky* T83+365 **97**
Fulton, *Mississippi* T81+343 **97**
Fulton, *Missouri* U12+388 **95**
Fulton, *New York* T07+433 **96**
Fulton Chain Ls., *New York* S89+437 **96**
Funchal, *Madeira I.* P10+326 **80**
Fundão, *Portugal* N45+402 **52**
Fundy, B. of, *N.S., N.B.* S37+448 **90**
Fünen, *See* Fyn.
Fünfkurchen, *See* Pecs.
Funing, *See* Siapu.
Fure, *Japan* C49+446 **68**
Furg, *Iran* J29+283 **75**
Furneaux Grp., *Tasmania* C13–400 **109**
Furnes, *See* Veurne.
Furqlus, *Syria* K47+346 **76**
Fürth, *W. Germany* M24+494 **48**
Furue, *Japan* D25+314 **68**
Fusagasuga, *Colombia* S86+042 **104**
Fushih, *China* E63+365 **66**
Fushimi, *Japan* C85+350 **68**
Fu-shun, *China* D66+419 **66**
Fusio, *Switzerland* M38+464 **45**
Fuyu, *China* D61+452 **64**
Fyn, *Denmark* M28+553 **47**
Fyne, L., *Scotland* N31+561 **41**
Gabaidu, *Kenya* K28–018 **83**
Gabandi, *Iran* J41+272 **75**
Gaberones, *Botswana* L24–246 **84**
Gabès & G. of, *Tunisia* M30+338 **81**
Gabin, *Poland* L62+524 **49**
Gabon, rep., *Cent. Africa* M26–006 **82**
Gabrovo, *Bulgaria* L28+429 **58**
Gach Saran, *Iran* J50+302 **75**
Gadag, *India* G86+155 **70**
Gadsden, *Alabama* T66+340 **97**
Gael Hamkes B., *Greenland* P34+740 **26**
Gaesti, *Romania* L28+447 **58**
Gaeta & G. di, *Italy* M09+412 **57**
Gafsa, *Tunisia* M38+344 **81**
Gagetown, *New Brunswick* S37+457 **90**
Gagnon, *Quebec* S43+516 **89**
Gaibanda, *Bangladesh* G02+253 **73**
Gáidharos, I., *Greece* L18+375 **59**
Gaillac, *France* M78+439 **55**
Gaiman, *Argentina* S34–433 **103**
Gainesboro, *Tennessee* T64+363 **97**
Gainesville, *Alabama* T79+328 **97**
Gainesville, *Florida* T44+296 **97**
Gainesville, *Georgia* T53+342 **97**
Gainesville, *Missouri* U15+366 **97**
Gainsborough, *England* N05+534 **37**
Gainsville, *Texas* U42+336 **95**
Gairdner, L., *S. Australia* C85–316 **111**
Gairloch, *Scotland* N34+577 **40**
Gairlochy, *Scotland* N30+569 **40**
Gala Water, *Scotland* N17+556 **41**
Galag, *Iran* J03+255 **75**
Galangue, *Angola* L82–138 **82**
Galapagos Is., *Pacific Ocean* U00–007 **107**
Galashiels, *Scotland* N17+556 **41**
Galatea, *New Zealand* A20–384 **112**
Galathea B., *Nicobar Is.* F67+066 **71**
Galati, *Romania* L12+454 **58**
Galatz, *See Galati.*
Galax, *Virginia* T36+366 **97**
Galcaio, *Somalia* J76+066 **83**
Galdhøpiggen, mt., *Norway* M40+616 47
Galeana, *Mexico* U60+248 **100**
Galeana, *Mexico* V15+301 **100**
Galena, *Illinois* U03+424 **95**
Galesburg, *Illinois* U02+410 **95**
Galeton, *Pennsylvania* T16+417 **96**
Galich, *U.S.S.R.* K16+584 **61**
Galilee, L., *Queensland* C25–222 **111**
Galilee, Sea of. *See* Tiberias L.
Galiuro Mts., *Arizona* V32+326 **94**
Gallatin, *Tennessee* T69+364 **97**
Galle, *Sri Lanka* G59+060 **70**
Gallego, *Mexico* V08+298 **94**
Gallegos R., *Argentina* S56–516 **103**
Galley Hd., *Ireland, Rep.* N54+515 **43**
Gallipoli (Gelibolu), *Turkey* L20+408 **59**
Gallipoli, *Italy* L72+401 **57**
Gällivare, *Sweden* L56+670 **46**
Gallo Mts., *New Mexico* V20+341 **94**
Galloway, Mull of, *Scotland* N29+546 **41**
Gallup, *New Mexico* V23+356 **94**
Galong, *New South Wales* C09–346 **109**
Galt, *Ontario* T32+434 **91**
Galty Mts., *Ireland, Rep.* N49+523 **43**
Galtymore, Ireland, Rep. N49+524 **43**
Galva, *Illinois* U01+412 **91**
Galveston and B., *Texas* U29+293 **95**
Galvez, *Argentina* S07–320 **103**
Galway (Gaillimh), *Ireland, Rep.* N54+533 **43**
Galway B., *Ireland Rep.* N55+532 **43**
Gambaga, *Ghana* N02+106 **80**
Gambia, The, *W. Africa* P05+130 **80**
Gambia, R., *W. Africa* P00+136 **80**
Gambo, *Newfoundland* R55+488 **90**
Gams, *Switzerland* M33+472 **45**
Gananoque, *Ontario* T07+443 **91**
Gand. *See* Gent
Gandak R., *India* G32+267 **73**
Gandava, *Pakistan* H45+286 **70**
Gander (Airport) & L., *Nfd.* R58+489 **90**
Gandesa, *Spain* M88+411 **53**
Gandia, *Spain* N01+390 **53**
Ganganagar, *India* H07+290 **72**
Gangaw, *Burma* F65+221 **71**
Ganges (Ganga), R., *India* G33+256 **73**
Gangoh, *India* G76+298 **72**
Gangtok, *Sikkim* G08+273 **73**
Ganjam, *India* G29+194 **71**
Ganmam, *New South Wales* C18–348 **109**
Gannat, *France* M71+461 **54**
Gannett Pk., *Wyoming* V28+432 **93**
Gantheame B., *W. Australia* E37–274 **110**
Ganza, *Cent. Afr. Rep.* L44+078 **81**
Gao, *Mali* N00+162 **80**
Gaoual, *Guinea* N80+118 **80**
Gara L., *Ireland, Rep.* N51+539 **42**
Garachine, *Panama* T19+080 **101**
Garah, *New South Wales* C02–290 **109**
Garanhuns, *Brazil* Q38–089 **105**
Garba Tula, *Kenya* K38+004 **83**
Gard, dep., *France* M64+440 **55**
Garda, L. di, *Italy* M26+457 **56**
Gardafui, C., *Somalia* J52+118 **83**
Garden, *Michigan* T69+458 **91**
Garden City, *Kansas* U66+380 **94**
Gardiner, *Maine* S59+442 **90**
Gardiner, *Montana* V35+450 **93**
Gardiner, *Oregon* W24+438 **92**
Gardiners, B. & I., *New York* S73+411 **96**
Gardner I., *Hawaii* Z15+250 **106**
Gardula, *Ethiopia* K44+058 **83**
Garelochhead, *Scotland* N29+561 **41**
Garfield, *Utah* V43+408 **94**
Gar Gunsa, *Tibet* G60+321 **70**
Garha, *India* G72+250 **73**
Garhmuktesar, *India* G73+288 **72**
Garhshankar, *India* G82+312 **72**
Garibaldi, *Brazil* R40–293 **103**
Garibaldi Park, *B.C.* W20+500 **88**
Garies, *Cape Province* L72–306 **84**
Gariganus, *Namibia* L72–262 **84**
Garissa, *Kenya* K30–006 **83**
Garland, *Montana* V06+459 **93**
Garm, *Tadzhik* H27+390 **62**
Garmsar, *Iran* J47+353 **75**
Garo Hills, *India* F87+254 **71**
Garonne, R., *France* M83+438 **55**
Garoua, *Cameroon* M10+092 **81**
Garraway, *Liberia* N48+046 **80**
Garrison & Res., *N. Dakota* U69+477 **93**
Garron Pt., *N. Ireland* N36+550 **42**
Garrovillas, *Spain* N39+397 **52**
Garry, L., *N.-W. Territories* U60+659 **88**
Garsen, *Kenya* K30–024 **83**
Garstang, *England* N17+539 **37**
Gartok, *Tibet* G58+318 **70**
Garvagh, *N. Ireland* N40+550 **42**
Gary, *Indiana* T74+416 **91**
Garza, *Argentina* S22–281 **103**
Garzon, *Colombia* T04+021 **104**
Gascogne, G. de, *Fr.-Sp.* N12+437 **55**
Gascogne, prov., *France* M88+435 **55**
Gasconade R., *Missouri* U11+380 **97**
Gascoyne, R., *W. Australia* E16–252 **110**
Gasharbrum, mt., *Kashmir* G80+358 **72**
Gaspé, *Quebec* S27+488 **90**
Gaspé, B. & C., *Quebec* S25+488 **90**
Gaspé Pen., *Quebec* S33+488 **90**
Gaspésia Park, *Quebec* S38+488 **90**
Gasselte, *Netherlands* M49+530 **44**
Gastonia, *N. Carolina* T37+352 **97**
Gastre, *Argentina* S56–421 **103**
Gat (Ghat), *Libya* M30+246 **81**
Gata, *Spain* N39+402 **52**
Gata, C., *Cyprus* K72+345 **76**
Gate City, *Virginia* T45+366 **97**
Gateshead, *England* N09+550 **37**
Gatineau R., *Quebec* T06+460 **91**
Gatooma, *Zimbabwe* L00–184 **84**
Gatun L., *Panama* T29+092 **101**
Gaud-i-Zirreh, *Afghanistan* H80+297 **75**
Gauhati, *India* F79+262 **71**
Gaurihar, *India* G58+253 **73**
Gavdhos, I., *Crete* L36+348 **59**
Gaviao, *Portugal* N48+394 **52**
Gävle, *Sweden* L78+607 **47**
Gävle Bukten, *Sweden* L75+608 **47**
Gawler, *S. Australia* C68–346 **109**
Gawler Ra., *S. Australia* C85–325 **111**
Gaya, *India* G30+248 **73**
Gaya, *Niger* M70+118 **80**
Gayaza, *Uganda* K86–008 **83**
Gaylord, *Michigan* T58+450 **91**
Gaza, *Cent. Afr. Rep.* L88+046 **81**
Gaza, *Egypt* K63+315 **76**
Gazeh Manzil, *Iran* H85+258 **75**
Gazi Antep, *Turkey* K46+371 **74**
Gazik, *Iran* H89+330 **75**
Gdansk, *Poland* L68+544 **49**
Gdynia, *Poland* L69+545 **49**
Gebeit, *Sudan* K50+190 **81**
Gedaref, *Sudan* K56+140 **81**
Gedinne, *Belgium* M60+500 **44**
Geel, *Belgium* M60+512 **44**
Geelong, *Victoria* C34–382 **109**
Geeraardsbergen, *Belgium* M67+508 **44**
Geeveston, *Tasmania* C19–432 **109**
Geh, *Iran* H89+262 **75**
Geikie R., *Saskatchewan* U88+571 **88**
Gela, *Sicily* M04+371 **57**
Gelderland, *Netherlands* M54+521 **44**
Geldrop, *Netherlands* M57+514 **44**
Gelibolu, *Turkey* L20+405 **74**
Gelinden, *Belgium* M58+508 **44**
Gelsenkirchen, *W. Germany* M47+516 **48**
Gemas, *Malaysia* F14+026 **69**
Gembloux, *Belgium* M62+506 **44**
Gemena, *Zaire* L60+032 **82**
Gemert, *Netherlands* M56+516 **44**
Gemmenich, *Belgium* M54+507 **44**
Gemmi Pass, *Switzerland* M44+464 **45**
Gemville, *New South Wales* C43–309 **109**
Genappe, *Belgium* M63+506 **44**
Gendringen, *Netherlands* M52+519 **44**
Genemuiden, *Netherlands* M54+526 **44**
General Acha, *Argentina* S28–374 **103**
General Alvear, *Argentina* S00–360 **103**
General Capdevila, *Argentina* S09–274 **103**
General Grant Nat. Pk., *Cal.* V84+367 **92**
General Guido, *Argentina* R77–366 **103**
General La Madrid, *Argent.* S08–373 **103**
General Lavalle, *Argentina* R72–364 **103**
General MacArthur, *Phil.* D57+115 **65**
General Pico, *Argentina* S23–356 **103**
General Pinto, *Argentina* S12–348 **103**
General Roca, *Argentina* S46–390 **103**
General Viamonte, *Argentina* S06–350 **103**
General Villegas, *Argentina* S18–350 **103**
Geneseo, *New York* T17+428 **96**
Geneva, *Nebraska* U46+405 **95**
Geneva, *New York* T12+428 **96**
Geneva, L. of. *See* Leman, Lac
Genève (Geneva), *Switz.* M53+462 **45**
Genipapo, *Brazil* R04–044 **105**
Genkai Nada, *Japan* D30+337 **68**
Gennargentu, Mte. del, *Sardinia* M34+400 **57**
Gennep, *Netherlands* M54+517 **44**
Genoa. *See* Genova
Genoa, *Victoria* C03–374 **109**
Genova, *Italy* M37+444 **56**
Genova, G. di, *Italy* M36+440 **56**
Gent, *Belgium* M47+349 **45**
Geographe B., *W. Australia* E28–334 **110**
Geographe Chan., *W. Aust.* E38–250 **110**
Georga Zemlya, *Arctic Oc.* J70+805 **62**
George L., *New S. Wales* C04–352 **109**
George L., *New York* S81+436 **96**
George R., *Quebec* S33+580 **89**
Georgetown, *Guyana* R79+066 **104**
Georgetown, *Delaware* T02+387 **91**
Georgetown, *Georgia* T61+319 **97**
George Town, *Gr. Cayman, W.I.* T38+194 **101**
Georgetown, *Kentucky* T57+382 **97**
George Town, *Pinang I., Malaysia* F28+054 **69**
Georgetown, *Pr. Edward I.* S15+462 **90**
Georgetown, *S. Carolina* T26+333 **97**
George Town, *Tasmania* C19–411 **109**
Georgetown, *Virginia* T13+389 **96**
Georgia, state, *U.S.A.* T50+330 **99**
Georgian B., *Ontario* T36+455 **91**
Georgian B. Is. Nat. Pk., *Ont.* T30+450 **91**
Georgiyevka, *Kazakh.* G51+493 **62**
Georgiyevsk, *U.S.S.R.* K09+442 **62**
Georgina, R., *Queensland* C71–216 **111**
Gera, *E. Germany* M17+509 **48**
Geraldine, *New Zealand* A53–440 **112**
Geraldton, *W. Australia* E32–286 **110**
Geremoabo, *Brazil* Q50–101 **105**
Gérgal, *Spain* N08+371 **53**
Gerlach, *Nevada* V85+408 **92**
Germania, *Argentina* S12–346 **103**
Germania Land, *Greenland* P30+770 **26**
Germany, E. & W., *Central Europe* **48**
Gerona, *Spain* M73+420 **53**
Gers, dep., *France* M87+437 **55**
Gerze, *Turkey* K58+418 **74**
Getafe, *Spain* N22+403 **52**
Gethsemani, *Quebec* S03+503 **90**
Gettysburg, *Pennsylvania* T14+398 **96**
Gettysburg, *S. Dakota* U60+450 **93**
Getz Ice Shelf, *Antarctica* W10–750 **27**
Gevar, *Turkey* K04+376 **74**
Gevgelija, *Yugoslavia* L45+412 **58**
Ghabaghib, *Syria* K53+332 **76**
Ghadames, *Libya* M32+302 **81**
Ghaghra, R., *India* G42+266 **73**
Ghaida, *Yemen, South* J67+142 **74**
Ghail, *Saudi Arabia* J82+226 **74**
Ghana, *W. Afr.* N10+081 **80**
Gharandal, *Jordan* K59+301 **76**
Ghardaia, *Algeria* M68+322 **80**
Gharian, *Libya* M12+322 **50**
Ghat, *Saudi Arabia* K00+260 **74**
Ghatal, *India* G13+227 **73**
Ghatampur, *India* G59+261 **73**
Ghatghat, *Saudi Arabia* J82+245 **74**
Ghats, Eastern, *India* G56+172 **70**
Ghats, Western, *India* H06+177 **70**
Ghauta, *Saudi Arabia* J79+222 **74**
Ghaziabad, *India* G75+286 **72**
Ghazipur, *India* G38+256 **73**
Ghazir, *Lebanon* K56+340 **76**
Ghazni, *Afghanistan* H39+336 **75**
Georgheni, *Romania* L26+467 **58**
Gherabe, *Saudi Arabia* K27+242 **74**
Ghislenghien, *Belgium* M67+507 **44**
Ghizao, *Afghanistan* H53+335 **75**
Ghobreh, *Oman* J08+230 **75**
Ghorak, *Afghanistan* H59+321 **75**
Ghorian, *Afghanistan* H81+344 **75**
Ghotki, *Pakistan* H34+280 **70**
Giant's Causeway, *N. Ireland* N39+552 **42**
Giaour Dagh, *Turkey* K52+366 **74**
Giarabub, *Libya* L34+296 **81**
Giarre, *Sicily* L89+377 **57**
Gibara, *Cuba* T07+211 **101**
Gibeon, *Namibia* L74-252 **84**
Gibraltar, *Spain* N32+361 **52**
Gibraltar, Str. of, *Spain-Morocco* N33+359 **52**
Gibson Desert, *W. Aust.* D60–237 **110**
Giddings, *Texas* U42+302 **95**
Gien, *France* M74+477 **54**
Giessen, *W. Germany* M38+505 **48**
Gifford, *Scotland* N16+559 **41**
Gifhorn, *W. Germany* M27+525 **48**
Gifu, *Japan* C79+353 **68**
Giganta, La, *Mexico* V39+261 **100**
Gijon, *Spain* N34+435 **52**
Gila Desert, *Arizona* V50+323 **98**
Gila R., *Arizona, etc.* V30+330 **94**
Gilau, *Romania* L40+467 **58**
Gilbert Is., *See* Kiribati
Gilbert, R., *Queensland* C47–172 **111**
Gilbués, *Brazil* Q89–096 **105**
Gilehdar, *Iran* J43+276 **75**
Gilgandra, *New S. Wales* C08–317 **109**
Gilgit & R., *Kashmir* H04+359 **72**
Gilgunnia, *New S. Wales* C24–324 **109**
Gill L., *Ireland, Rep.* N50+542 **42**
Gillett, *Arkansas* U09+341 **97**
Gillette, *Wyoming* V03+443 **93**

Gillingham, England M87+514 39
Gimel, Switzerland M52+465 45
Ginir, Ethiopia K26+070 83
Ginzo, Spain N46+420 52
Gioia, G. di, Italy L86+385 57
Giornico, Switzerland M37+464 45
Girardot, Colombia S89+042 104
Girdle Ness, Scotland N12+571 40
Giresun, Turkey K40+409 74
Girga, Egypt K78+264 81
Giridih, India G22+242 73
Girilambone, New S. Wales C19–312 109
Girishk, Afghanistan H62+318 75
Gironde, dep., France N02+448 55
Gironde, R., France N06+453 54
Girvan & R., Scotland N29+553 41
Gisborne, New Zealand A12–387 112
Gisors, France M79+493 54
Giswil, Switzerland M41+468 45
Gitch, mt., Ethiopia K40+132 83
Giurgiu, Romania L24+439 58
Givry, Belgium M66+504 44
Gizhiga, U.S.S.R. B26+621 63
Giżycko, Poland L49+541 49
Gjinokaster, Albania L59+401 59
Gjoa Haven, N.-W. Terr. U43+681 88
Gjøvik, Norway M26+608 47
Glabbeek-Zuurbemde, Belg. M60+509 44
Glace Bay, Nova Scotia S00+462 90
Glacier, British Columbia V75+511 88
Glacier Nat. Park, Montana V50+485 98
Gladstone, Michigan T72+459 91
Gladstone, New S. Wales B73–310 109
Gladstone, Queensland B82–237 111
Gladstone, S. Australia C70–332 109
Gladstone, Tasmania C13–410 109
Gladwin, Michigan T57+440 91
Glamis, Scotland N18+566 41
Glamoc, Yugoslavia L79+441 56
Glamorgan, W. Mid. & S., co., Wales N22+517 38
Glanaruddery Mts., Ireland, Rep. N57+523 43
Glärnisch, mt., Switzerland M36+470 45
Glarus & canton, Switz. M36+471 45
Glasgow, Kentucky T65+370 97
Glasgow, Montana V10+482 93
Glasgow, Scotland N26+558 41
Glass L., Scotland N27+577 40
Glassboro, New Jersey T00+397 96
Glauchau, E. Germany M15+508 48
Glazov, U.S.S.R. J44+582 61
Glen, New Hampshire S67+441 91
Glen Affric, Scotland N30+572 40
Glenarm, N. Ireland N36+550 42
Glenburnie, S. Australia C54–378 109
Glencoe, Minnesota U25+448 93
Glendale, Arizona V44+334 94
Glendale, California V80+342 92
Glencoe, S. Australia C57–377 109
Glen Coe, Scotland N29+567 41
Glendive, Montana U88+471 93
Glendowan Mts., Ireland, Rep. N48+550 42
Gleneagles, Scotland N22+563 41
Glenelg, Scotland N34+572 40
Glenelg, S. Australia C69–350 109
Glenfinnan, Scotland N33+568 41
Glengad Hd., N. Ireland N43+553 42
Glengariff, Ireland, Rep. N57+517 43
Glen Garry, Scotland N30+571 40
Glenhope, New Zealand A44–416 112
Glen Innes, New S. Wales B80–298 109
Glenluce, Scotland N29+549 41
Glen Lyon, Scotland N26+566 41
Glennamaddy, Ireland, Rep. N51+536 42
Glenreagh, New S. Wales B73–300 109
Glenrock, Wyoming V05+428 93
Glenrothes, Scotland N19+562 41
Glens Falls, New York S82+433 91
Glen Shee, Scotland N20+567 41
Glenties, Ireland, Rep. N50+548 42
Glenville, West Virginia T35+389 91
Glenwood, Iowa U34+410 95
Glenwood, Minnesota U33+457 93
Glenwood Springs, Colorado V14+395 94
Gletsch, Switzerland M40+466 45
Glittertind, mt., Norway M38+613 47
Gliwice, Poland L68+503 49
Globe, Arizona V35+333 94
Glogau. See Głogów.
Głogów, Poland L84+517 49
Gloppen, Norway M53+618 46
Glossop, England N12+535 37
Gloucester, Massachusetts S64+426 96
Gloucester, New Jersey T01+399 96
Gloucester, New S. Wales B79–320 109
Gloucester, Virginia T09+374 97
Gloucester & co., England N13+519 39
Gloversville, New York S86+430 96
Glukhov, Ukraine K66+516 60
Glyndebourne, England N00+509 39
Gmünd, Austria M09+469 48
Gmünd, W. Germany M31+488 48
Gmunden, Austria M07+479 48
Gniew, Poland L92+526 48
Gniezno, Poland L75+525 49
Goa, Daman & Diu, India H06+155 70
Goalpara, India F86+261 71
Goalundo, Bangladesh G01+238 73
Gobabis, Namibia L66-224 84
Gobi, des., Mongolia, etc. F00+430 63
Gobindpur, India G20+238 73
Godavari R., India G63+186 70
Godda, India G16+248 73
Godech, Bulgaria L42+430 58
Goderich, Ontario T40+437 91
Godhra, India H07+228 70
Gods L., Manitoba U35+548 88
Gods R., Manitoba U20+552 89
Godthåb, Greenland R32+640 26
Goes, Netherlands M67+515 44
Gogama, Ontario T41+476 91
Gogebic Ra., Michigan T88+467 91
Gog Magog Hills, England M87+522 39
Gogrial, Sudan L10+086 81
Gohana, India G80+291 72
Goiânia, Brazil R26–166 105
Goias, Brazil R31–158 105
Goil L., Scotland N29+561 41
Goirle, Netherlands M60+515 44
Goksun, Turkey K51+381 74
Golaghat, India F66+265 71
Golchikha, U.S.S.R. G37+718 62
Golconda, Illinois T81+374 97
Golconda, India G69+174 70
Gołdap, Poland L46+543 49
Gold Coast. See Ghana
Golden, Colorado V02+398 94
Golden B., New Zealand A42–407 112
Golden Lake, Ontario T14+455 91
Golden Vale, Ireland, Rep. N45+525 43
Goldfield, Nevada V74+379 92
Goldsboro, N. Carolina T18+354 97
Goleniow, Poland M01+535 48
Gol Gol, New South Wales C46–342 109
Golmo, China F60+362 64
Golspie, Scotland N24+580 40
Goltva, Ukraine K67+494 60
Gomal Pass, Pakistan H29+321 72
Gomalcalco, Mexico U20+182 100
Gombe, Nigeria M24+102 81
Gomel, Byelorussia K84+525 60
Gomera, I., Canary Is. P14+280 80
Gómez Farias, Mexico U66+248 100
Gomez Palacio, Mexico U81+256 100
Gonaïves, Haiti S75+194 101
Gonave, I. de la, Haiti S78+189 101
Gonda, India G48+271 73
Gondal, India H25+220 70
Gondo, Switzerland M41+462 45
Gongka Ling, China F26+286 64
Gongolgon, New S. Wales C19–304 109
Gondiądz, Poland L43+535 49
Gonzales, Texas U44+294 95
Goodenough I., Papua New Guinea B89–094 111
Gooderham, Ontario T20+449 91
Good Hope, N.-W. Terr. W52+661 88
Good Hope, C. of, Cape Province L70–344 84
Goodland, Kansas U70+392 94
Goodooga, New S. Wales C16–292 109
Goodrich, Wisconsin U01+452 91
Goodwin Sands, England M79+512 39
Goole, England N05+537 37
Goomalling, W. Australia E19–312 110
Goombalie, New S. Wales C28–300 109
Goor, Netherlands M50+522 44
Goose L., Oregon-California W03+420 92
Goose Bay, Labrador S02+534 89
Gopalpur, India G31+192 71
Göppingen, W. Germany M32+487 48
Gor, Spain N18+374 52
Gora, China F36+292 64
Gorakhpur, India G40+268 73
Gordola, Switzerland M37+462 45
Gordon, S. Australia C71–321 109
Gordon, Nebraska U74+428 94
Gordon R., Tasmania C26–426 109
Gordonsville, Virginia T19+381 97
Gore, Ethiopia K56+080 83
Goré, Chad L80+078 81
Gore, New Zealand A66–461 112
Gore Bay, Ontario T45+459 91
Gorebridge, Scotland N18+558 41
Gorey, Ireland, Rep. N38+527 43
Gorgan, Iran J33+368 75
Gorgona, I., Italy M31+434 56
Gorinchem, Netherlands M60+518 44
Gorizia, Italy M08+460 56
Gor'kiy, U.S.S.R. K06+564 61
Gorlice, Poland L54+496 49
Gorlitz, E. Germany L90+512 48
Gorlovka, Ukraine K42+484 60
Gormanstown, Tasmania C26–421 109
Gorodets, U.S.S.R. K10+567 61
Gorodishche, U.S.S.R. J86+533 61
Gorodnitsa, Ukraine L16+508 60
Goroke, Victoria C51–367 109
Gorontalo, Celebes D72+006 65
Gorrahei, Ethiopia K04+066 83
Gorsel, Netherlands M53+522 44
Gort, Ireland, Rep. N53+531 43
Gorumna I., Ireland, Rep. N58+532 43
Gorzów Wielkopolski, Poland L89+527 48
Gosai Than, mt., Nepal-Tibet G25+283 71
Göschenen, Switzerland M38+467 45
Gosford, New South Wales B83–334 109
Goshanak, Pakistan H60+264 70
Goshen, New York S86+413 96
Gospić, Yugoslavia L88+446 56
Gosport, England N07+508 39
Gossa, Norway M49+629 46
Gossau, Switzerland M34+474 45
Gosselies, Belgium M63+505 44
Gostivar, Yugoslavia L54+418 58
Göta Älv, Sweden M17+581 47
Göteborg, Sweden M18+577 47
Gotha, E. Germany M26+510 48
Gothenburg. See Göteborg.
Gothenburg, Nebraska U61+409 94
Gotland, I., Sweden L68+575 47
Goto Retto, Japan D36+330 68
Gotska Sandon, Sweden L65+583 47
Göttingen, W. Germany M30+515 48
Gottwaldov, Czechoslovakia L74+492 49
Gouda, Netherlands M62+520 44
Goudswaard, Netherlands M65+518 44
Gough I., Atlantic Ocean N30–414 85
Gouin Res., Quebec S88+486 90
Goulburn, New South Wales C02–348 109
Goulburn R., Victoria C29–362 109
Gounarou, Benin M74+108 80
Goundam, Mali N22+164 80
Gouré, Niger M28+140 81
Gournay, France M80+495 54
Gourock, Scotland N29+559 41
Gourock Ra., New S. Wales C04–358 109
Gouverneur, New York T03+443 91
Gowanda, New York T24+424 91
Gower, pen., Wales N25+516 38
Gowna L., Ireland, Rep. N45+539 42
Goya, Argentina R86–292 103
Gozo, I. (Malta), Mediterranean Sea M04+361 57
Graaff Reinet, Cape Province L32–324 84
Grabow, Poland L71+515 49
Gračac, Yugoslavia L85+443 56
Gracefield, Quebec T07+461 91
Gracias, Honduras T82+146 101
Gracias a Dios, Nicaragua T50+149 101
Gradets, Bulgaria L21+428 58
Grado, Spain N37+433 52
Grafton, New South Wales B73–297 109
Grafton, N. Dakota U44+484 93
Grafton, W. Virginia T30+393 91
Grafton, Is., Chile S80–542 101
Grahaju, Brazil Q79–068 105
Graham, Texas U51+331 95
Graham Ld. See Antarctic Pen. S25–660 27
Graham Bell, Os., Arctic Oc. H65+811 62
Grahamstown, Cape Province L20–332 84
Grain, England M86+514 39
Grajewo, Poland L45+537 49
Grammont. See Geeraardsbergen
Grampian Mts., Scotland N26+567 41
Grampian, reg., Scotland N17+573 40
Grampians, mts., Victoria C45–372 109
Gramsbergen, Netherlands M50+526 44
Granada, Nicaragua T66+120 101
Granada, Spain N22+372 52
Granard, Ireland, Rep. N45+538 43
Granby, Quebec S77+454 91
Gran Canaria, I., Canary Is. P04+278 80
Gran Chaco, Argentina S14–270 103
Grand Can., China E24+375 64
Grand I., Michigan T70+465 91
Grand I., New York T24+430 96
Grand L., Louisiana U08+298 95
Grand L., Louisiana U16+298 95
Grand L., Maine-N.B. S45+456 90
Grand L., New Brunswick S36+460 90
Grand L., Newfoundland R74+490 90
Grand R., Colorado V06+400 94
Grand R., Michigan T61+429 91
Grand R., S. Dakota U80+456 98
Grand Bassa, Liberia N60+060 80
Grand Bassam, Ivory Coast N22+052 80
Grand Canyon, Arizona V50+356 98
Grand Canyon Nat. Park, Arizona V45+362 98
Grand Cayman, I., W. I. T38+193 101
Grand Coulee Dam, Wash. V84+479 98
Grande, B., Argentina S50–505 103
Grande, Rio, Brazil R30–198 105
Grande, Sa, Brazil Q66–046 105
Grande Anse, N.B. S31+478 90
Grande Comore, I., Comoro Is., Africa K10-116 83
Grande de Santiago, R., Mexico U84+212 100
Grand Falls, N.B. S47+471 90
Grand Falls, Newfoundland R64+490 90
Grand Forks, B.C. V81+491 88
Grand Forks, N. Dakota U42+479 93
Grand Haven, Michigan T67+431 91
Grandin, L., N.-W. Terr. V88+640 88
Grand Island, Nebraska U50+408 95
Grand Junction, Colorado V22+390 94
Grand Junction, Tennessee T85+350 97
Grand Lahou, Ivory Coast N30+052 80
Grande Ledge, Michigan T58+428 91
Grand Manan I., N.B. S41+448 90
Grand Marais, Minnesota U02+477 91
Grand Mère, Quebec S76+466 91
Grand Mesa, Colorado V18+391 94
Grandola, Portugal N51+381 52
Grand Piles, Quebec S76+467 91
Grand Prarie, Alberta V84+554 88
Grand Rapids, Michigan T64+430 91
Grand Rapids, Minnesota U21+472 93
Grandrieu, Belgium M65+502 44
Grand River, Quebec S27+484 90
Grandson, Switzerland M50+468 45
Grand Teton Mt. & Nat. Park, Wyoming V35+434 98
Grand Tower, Illinois T87+376 97
Grand Victoria L., Quebec T14+476 91
Grane, Norway M10+656 46
Graney L., Ireland, Rep. N52+530 43
Grangemouth, Scotland N22+560 41
Granger, Wyoming V30+416 93
Granite City, Illinois U02+387 95
Granite Falls, Minnesota U33+448 93
Granity, New Zealand A48–416 112
Granja, Brazil Q65–031 105
Grankulla, Finland L32+602 47
Granollers, Spain M76+416 53
Granön, Sweden L64+642 46
Grant, Ontario T69+501 89
Grant Ra., Nevada V63+388 92
Grant City, Missouri U26+404 95
Grantham, England N04+529 37
Granton, Scotland N19+560 41
Grantown-on-Spey, Scotland N21+573 40
Grants, New Mexico V17+351 94
Grants Pass, Oregon W20+425 92
Grantsville, Utah V45+406 94
Granville, New York S79+434 96
Granville, N. Dakota U65+483 93
Granville L., Manitoba U65+562 88
Granvin, Norway M50+605 47
Gras, L., de, N.-W. Terr. V35+646 88
Grasett, Ontario T57+485 91
Graskop, Transvaal K86–250 84
Grasmere, England N18+545 37
Gräsö, Sweden L70+604 47
Grassano, Italy L82+406 57
Grasse, France M49+437 55
Grassier, Switzerland M53+464 45
Graubünden, canton, Switz. M35+467 45
Graus, Spain M88+422 53
Gravarne, Sweden M22+583 47
Grave, Netherlands M56+518 44
Gravelbourg, Saskatchewan V09+499 88
's Gravenhage, Netherlands M64+521 44
Gravenhurst, Ontario T26+449 91
's Gravenzande, Netherlands M65+520 44
Gravesend, England M88+514 39
Gravesend, New S. Wales B88–296 109
Gray, France M57+474 54
Grayling, Michigan T59+447 91
Grayville, Illinois T78+383 97
Graz, Austria L87+471 49
Great L., Tasmania C20–419 109
Great Pt., Massachusetts S60+414 96
Great Australian Bight, Aust. D30–336 110
Great Barrier Reef, Aust. C05–190 111
Great Barrington, Mass. S80+422 96
Great Basin, Nevada V75+402 98
Great Bear L., N.-W. Terr. W00+658 88
Great Bend, Kansas U53+384 95
Great Basket I., Ireland, Rep. N63+521 43
Great Dividing Ra., Aust. C10–260 111
Great Driffield, England N03+540 37
Great Falls, Montana V38+475 93
Great Geysir, Iceland P31+643 46
Great Lake. See Tonle Sap
Great Long L., Quebec S65+562 89
Great Malvern, England N14+521 38
Great North Mts., W. Va., etc. T23+389 96
Great Rapids, Manitoba U57+534 88
Great Salt L., Utah V46+412 92
Great Salt Lake Des., Utah V51+409 92
Great Sand Dunes Nat. Mon., Colorado V04+378 94
Great Sandy Des., W. Aust. D75–202 110
Great Sandy I. (Fraser I.), Queensland B71–252 111
Great Slave L., N.-W. Terr. V60+610 88
Great Smoky Mts., Tennessee T52+356 97
Great Smoky Mts. Nat. Park, Tennessee T52+357 97
Great South B., New York S79+406 96
Great Torrington, England N25+509 38
Great Victoria Des., W. Aust. D40–280 110
Great Wass I., Maine S46+445 90
Great Western Tiers, Tasmania C22–418 109
Great Yarmouth, England M80+526 39
Grebbestad, Sweden M22+587 47
Greco C., Cyprus K65+349 76
Greece, S. Europe L48+380 51
Greeley, Colorado U88+404 94
Green B., Wisconsin T77+448 91
Green Mts., Vermont S77+438 91
Green Mts., Wyoming V14+424 93
Green R., Kentucky T73+375 97
Green R., Utah, etc. V30+386 94
Green Bay, Wisconsin T78+445 91
Greencastle, Indiana T70+396 95
Greenfield, Indiana T65+398 91
Greenfield, Iowa U26+412 95
Greenfield, Massachusetts S75+426 96
Greenland, N. America Q60+700 26
Greenland Sea, Greenland N50+760 26
Greenock, Scotland N29+559 41
Greenore Pt., Ireland, Rep. N38+522 43
Greenport, New York S74+411 91
Green River, Utah V31+390 94
Green River, Wyoming V27+415 93
Greensboro, Georgia T49+335 97
Greensboro, N. Carolina T29+361 97
Greensburg, Kansas U56+376 95
Greensburg, Kentucky T63+373 97
Greensburg, Pennsylvania T28+404 96
Greenville, Alabama T70+318 97
Greenville, Illinois T86+389 95
Greenville, Kentucky T73+372 97
Greenville, Liberia N54+050 80
Greenville, Maine S58+455 90
Greenville, Michigan T62+432 91
Greenville, Mississippi U06+334 95
Greenville, Missouri U03+372 95
Greenville, N. Carolina T14+356 97
Greenville, S. Carolina T45+348 97
Greenville, Tennessee T47+362 97
Greenville, Texas U36+332 95
Greenwich, Connecticut S82+410 95
Greenwich, England N00+515 39
Greenwich, Rhode Island S69+417 96
Greenwood, Mississippi U01+335 97
Greenwood, S. Carolina T43+342 97
Greenwood, Wisconsin U04+449 91
Greenwood L., N.Y.-N.J. S86+412 96
Gregory, S. Dakota U56+432 93
Gregory, L., S. Australia C66–290 109
Gregory Ra., Queensland C40–186 111
Greifen See, Switzerland M38+474 45
Greifswald, E. Germany M10+541 48
Grein, Austria M01+483 48
Greiz, E. Germany M17+506 48
Grenå, Denmark M25+564 47
Grenada, Mississippi T89+338 97
Grenada, I., Windward Is. S10+121 101
Grenadines, Is., Windward Is. S08+127 101
Grenchen, Switzerland M46+472 45
Grenfell, New South Wales C11–339 109
Grenoble, France M56+452 55
Grenora, N. Dakota U83+487 93
Grenville, C., Queensland C41–119 111
Gretna, Louisiana U00+298 95
Gretna, Virginia T27+369 97
Gretna Green, Scotland N18+550 41
Grevená, Greece L51+401 59
Grey Ra., Qnsld.-N.S.W. C50–288 111
Greybull, Wyoming V18+444 93
Greycliff, Montana V28+457 93
Greylock Mt., Massachusetts S79+427 96
Greymouth, New Zealand A52–425 112
Greys Butte, mt., Oregon V89+429 92
Greystones, Ireland, Rep. N36+531 43
Greytown, New Zealand A27–411 112
Greytown. See San Juan del Norte
Griesalp, Switzerland M43+466 45
Griffin, Georgia T56+332 97
Griffith, New South Wales C24–343 109
Grim C., Tasmania C31–407 109
Grimsby, England N01+535 37
Grimstad, Norway M38+583 47
Grindelwald, Switzerland M42+466 45
Grindstone, Michigan T47+440 91
Grinnell, Iowa U16+417 95
Grinnell Pen., N.-W. Terr. U25+766 88
Griquatown, Cape Province L40–288 84
Griva Latvia L21+559 47
Grobina, Latvia L53+565 47
Gröbming, Austria M07+474 48
Grodno, Byelorussia L37+537 60
Grodzisk, Poland L82+522 49
Groenlo, Netherlands M50+520 44
Groix, I. de, France N21+476 54
Groningen & prov., Netherlands M50+532 44
Grono, Switzerland M35+463 45
Groote Eylandt, N. Terr., Aust C80–140 111
Grootfontain, Namibia L80-252 84
Grootfontein, Namibia L70-196 84

Groot Natuna, I., *Indonesia* E70+039 **65**
Grossevichi, *U.S.S.R.* C63+479 **63**
Gross Glockner, *Austria* M15+471 **48**
Grosswardein. *See* Oradea
Groton, *New York* T09+426 **96**
Groton, *S. Dakota* U49+455 **93**
Groznyy, *U.S.S.R.* J87+435 **62**
Grudziadz, *Poland* L67+535 **49**
Grues, I. aux, *Quebec* S63+471 **91**
Gruinard B., *Scotland* N33+579 **40**
Grüsch, *Switzerland* M32+470 **45**
Gruyère, Lac de, *Switz.* M47+467 **45**
Gruz, *Yugoslavia* L71+427 **58**
Gruzinskaya (Georgia), rep., *U.S.S.R.* K10+422 **62**
Grybów, *Poland* L55+496 **49**
Gsteig, *Switzerland* M46+464 **45**
Guabito, Panama T46+096 **101**
Guacanayabo, G. de, *Cuba* T14+206 **101**
Guachipas, *Argentina* S33–256 **103**
Guadalaja, *Spain* N19+406 **52**
Guadalajara, *Mexico* U80+206 **100**
Guadalcanal, *Spain* N35+381 **52**
Guadalcanal, I., *Solomon Is.* B30–095 **106**
Guadalcazar, *Mexico* U62+226 **100**
Guadalquivir, R., *Spain* N30+376 **52**
Guadalupe, *Mexico* U75+227 **100**
Guadalupe I., *Mexico* V82+290 **100**
Guadalupe Mts., *New Mexico, Texas* V00+320 **94**
Guadalupe R., *Texas* U47+296 **98**
Guadalupe-y-Calvo, *Mexico* V11+262 **100**
Guadarrama, *Spain* N25+407 **52**
Guadarrama, Sa. de, *Spain* N24+410 **52**
Guadeloupe, I., *Leeward Is.* S10+162 **101**
Guadiana, R., *Spain* N45+383 **52**
Guadix, *Spain* N19+373 **52**
Guafo & G. de, *Chile* S88–436 **103**
Guaitecas, Is., *Chile* S82–439 **103**
Guajar-a-Mirim, *Brazil* S32–108 **104**
Guajaratuba, *Brazil* S17–050 **104**
Gualeguaychu, *Argentina* R81–330 **103**
Guam, I., *Pacific Ocean* C30+140 **106**
Guamini, *Argentina* S15–370 **103**
Guamo, *Colombia* T00+040 **104**
Guanabacoa, *Cuba* T43+232 **101**
Guanabara, *Brazil* Q82–228 **104**
Guanacevi, *Mexico* V06+259 **100**
Guanahani. *See* San Salvador
Guanajuato, *Mexico* U67+212 **100**
Guanare, *Venezuela* S58+090 **104**
Guanarito, *Venezuela* S54+087 **104**
Guandacol, *Argentina* S52–295 **103**
Guane, *Cuba* T54+223 **101**
Guanica, *Puerto Rico* S41+180 **101**
Guanta, *Venezuela* S27+102 **104**
Guantanamo, *Cuba* T02+202 **101**
Guapi, *Colombia* T17+026 **104**
Guapiles, *Costa Rica* T53+102 **101**
Guapore, *Brazil* R41–289 **103**
Guapore (Rondonia), *Brazil* S31–118 **104**
Guapore, R., *Brazil-Bolivia* S16–128 **104**
Guaqui, *Bolivia* S54–166 **104**
Guarapuava, *Brazil* R40–255 **103**
Guarda, *Portugal* N43+406 **52**
Guasabas, *Mexico* V25+298 **100**
Guasdualito, *Venezuela* S64+072 **104**
Guasipati, *Venezuela* S11+074 **104**
Guatemala, *Guatemala* U03+146 **100**
Guatemala, rep. *Cent. America* U00+154 **100**
Guatrache, *Argentina* S22–378 **103**
Guaviare, R., *Colombia* S56+036 **104**
Guaxupe, *Brazil* R10–212 **105**
Guayabal, *Venezuela* S43+080 **104**
Guayama, *Puerto Rico* S36+181 **101**
Guayaquil, *Ecuador* T29–022 **104**
Guaymas, *Mexico* V35+279 **100**
Guazapares, *Mexico* V15+273 **100**
Guben, *E. Germany* M02+520 **48**
Gubin. *See* Guben
Gudiyatam, *India* G67+130 **70**
Guelma, *Algeria* M46+361 **80**
Guelph, *Ontario* T32+436 **91**
Guemes, *Argentina* S30–246 **103**
Guéret, *France* M79+462 **54**
Guernsey, I., *Channel Is.* N15+495 **54**
Guernsey Res., *Wyoming* U89+424 **93**
Guerrero, *Mexico* V13+284 **100**
Guerrero, *Tamaulipas, Mex.* U56+267 **100**
Guerrero, state, *Mexico* U60+176 **100**
Gugera, *Pakistan* H10+309 **72**
Guiana Highlands, *S. Amer.* R80+028 **104**
Guija, *Mozambique* K74-244 **84**
Guildford, *England* N03+512 **39**
Guildford, *Maine* S56+452 **90**
Guillaumes, *France* M49+441 **55**
Guilo, *Angola* L64–076 **82**
Guimaraes, *Brazil* Q88–020 **105**
Guimarães, *Portugal* N50+414 **52**
Guinea-Bissau, *N.-W. Afr.* P00+120 **80**
Guinea, *West Africa* N60+110 **80**
Guinea, G. of, *N.-W. Africa* M70+030 **82**
Guines, *Cuba* T42+231 **101**
Guingamp, *France* N19+485 **54**
Guiria, *Venezuela* S13+106 **104**
Guise, *France* M68+499 **54**
Guisisil, Vol., *Nicaragua* T67+127 **101**
Gujarat, state, *India* H07+218 **70**
Gujar Khan, *Pakistan* H11+333 **72**
Gujranwala, *Pakistan* H05+321 **72**
Gujrat, *Pakistan* H05+326 **72**
Gulargambone, *N.S.W.* C09–314 **109**
Gulbarga, *India* G78+173 **70**
Gulbene, *Latvia* L20+571 **47**
Gulfport, *Mississippi* T84+304 **95**
Gulgong, *New South Wales* C03–326 **109**
Gulistan, *Pakistan* H50+306 **70**
Gul Koh, *Afghanistan* H42+334 **75**
Gull L., *Quebec* T11+498 **89**
Gullane, *Scotland* N17+560 **41**
Gulpaigan, *Iran* J59+334 **75**
Gulpen, *Netherlands* M55+508 **44**
Gulran, *Afghanistan* H80+351 **75**
Gulu, *Uganda* K76+026 **83**
Gum, *Ethiopia* K20+116 **83**
Gummersbach, *W. Germany* M45+510 **48**
Gümüljina, *See* Komotini
Gümüsane, *Turkey* K33+404 **74**
Guna, *India* G76+246 **73**
Gunbad-i-Qabuz, *Iran* J28+373 **75**
Gunbar, *New South Wales* C28–341 **109**
Gunchu, *Japan* D14+338 **68**
Gundagai, *New S. Wales* C12–351 **109**
Gunisao R., *Manitoba* U40+540 **88**
Gunnedah, *New S. Wales* B88–310 **109**
Gunning, *New South Wales* C05–348 **109**
Gunnislake, *England* N25+505 **38**
Gunnison, *Colorado* V12+386 **94**
Gunnison, *Utah* V42+392 **94**
Gunnison R., *Colorado* V14+385 **94**
Guntakal, *India* G75+152 **70**
Guntersville & L., *Alabama* T68+344 **97**
Guntur, *India* G57+164 **70**
Gurais, *Kashmir* H01+346 **72**
Gurdaspur, *India* G87+320 **72**
Gurdon, *Arkansas* U19+338 **95**
Gurgaon, *India* G78+285 **72**
Gurgl, *Austria* M24+469 **48**
Gurha, *India* H20+252 **70**
Gurkha, *Nepal* G32+280 **73**
Gurla Mandhata, mt., *Tibet* G51+304 **70**
Gurnigel, *Switzerland* M45+468 **45**
Gurskëy, *Norway* M56+623 **46**
Gurupa, *Brazil* R39–015 **105**
Gurupa, I., *Brazil* R39–010 **105**
Guru Sikhar, *India* H13+247 **70**
Gur'yev, *Kazakh* J50+470 **62**
Gusev, *U.S.S.R.* L47+546 **47**
Gusht, *Iran* H78+277 **75**
Guspini, *Sardinia* M38+396 **57**
Gustav Holm, Kap, *Greenland* Q05+670 **26**
Güstrow, *E. Germany* M17+538 **48**
Guthrie, *Iowa* U27+416 **95**
Guthrie, *Kentucky* T73+367 **97**
Guthrie, *Oklahoma* U44+358 **95**
Guyana, *S. America* R84+050 **104**
Guyenne, prov., *France* M82+446 **55**
Guymon, *Oklahoma* U68+368 **94**
Guyra, *New South Wales* B80–302 **109**
Guzman, *Mexico* U82+196 **100**
Gwa, *Burma* F62+176 **71**
Gwabegar, *New S. Wales* C06–306 **109**
Gwadar, *Pakistan* H76+251 **70**
Gwalior, *India* G71+262 **73**
Gwanda, *Zimbabwe* L06–210 **84**
Gwatar, *Iran* H81+251 **75**
Gweebarra B., *Ireland, Rep.* N51+549 **42**
Gwelo, *Zimbabwe* L02–194 **84**
Gwent, co., *Wales* N18+517 **38**
Gwydir, R., *New S. Wales* B83-304 **109**
Gwyned, co., *Wales* N24+530 **38**
Gyangtse, *Tibet* G03+289 **71**
Gydanski Pol., *U.S.S.R.* G80+700 **62**
Gympie, *Queensland* B74–261 **111**
Györ, *Hungary* L74+477 **49**
Gypsumville, *Manitoba* U51+516 **88**
Gyula, *Hungary* L52+465 **49**
Gzhatsk, *U.S.S.R.* K60+555 **60**
Haacht, *Belgium* M62+510 **44**
Haag, *Switzerland* M33+472 **45**
Haaksbergen, *Netherlands* M49+522 **44**
Haarlem, *Netherlands* M62+524 **44**
Habana, *Cuba* T44+232 **101**
Habban, *Yemen, South* J77+146 **74**
Habbaniyah, *Iraq* K07+334 **74**
Habigang, *Bangladesh* F81+244 **71**
Hachinohe, *Japan* C51+405 **68**
Hadda, *Saudi Arabia* K32+214 **74**
Haddington, *Scotland* N16+560 **41**
Hadera, *Israel* K60+324 **76**
Haderslev, *Denmark* M33+552 **47**
Hadhramaut, *Yemen, South* J76+155 **74**
Hadjin, *Turkey* K53+380 **74**
Haeju, *Korea* D58+380 **64**
Haerhpin, *China* D45+455 **64**
Hafar, *Saudi Arabia* J84+284 **74**
Hafar al Ats, *Saudi Arabia* J80+260 **74**
Haffe. *See* Babenna
Hafnarfjördhur, *Iceland* P41+641 **46**
Hagen, *W. Germany* M45+514 **48**
Hageri, *Estonia* L32+591 **47**
Hagerstown, *Maryland* T16+397 **96**
Hagi, *Japan* D21+344 **68**
Hague, C. de la, *France* N12+497 **54**
Hahnville, *Louisiana* U03+299 **97**
Haibak, *Afghanistan* H42+362 **75**
Hai cheng, *China* D74+409 **66**
Haichow. *See* Tunghai
Haidar Pasha, *Turkey* L05+410 **74**
Haifa, *Israel* K60+328 **76**
Haig, *W. Australia* D54–309 **110**
Haik'ou, *China* E58+200 **67**
Hail, *Saudi Arabia* K19+275 **74**
Hailar, *China* E02+490 **64**
Haileybury, *Ontario* T28+475 **91**
Hailun, *China* D48+472 **64**
Hailuoto, *Finland* L32+650 **46**
Hainan I., *China* E60+190 **67**
Hainan Str., *China* E60+200 **67**
Hainaut, prov., *Belgium* M66+505 **44**
Haines, *Alaska* X02+594 **88**
Haiphong, *Vietnam* E80+208 **69**
Hair, *Saudi Arabia* J79+244 **74**
Haiten I., *China* E01+256 **67**
Haiti, rep., *West Indies* S74+190 **101**
Hajduböszörmény, *Hungary* L52+477 **49**
Hajima, Jebel, *Saudi Arabia* K44+245 **74**
Hajipur, *India* G28+257 **73**
Hajjar, *China* F72+369 **64**
Hakkâri, *Turkey* K07+376 **74**
Hakodate, *Japan* C55+418 **68**
Hala, *Pakistan* H40+258 **70**
Halacho, *Mexico* U01+204 **100**
Halba, *Lebanon* K54+346 **76**
Halbe, *Saudi Arabia* K11+198 **74**
Halberstadt, *E. Germany* M24+519 **48**
Halden, *Norway* M21+591 **47**
Haleb. *See* Aleppo
Halebiye, *Syria* K31+357 **74**
Halen, *Belgium* M59+509 **44**
Halesworth, *England* M81+524 **39**
Hali, *Saudi Arabia* K20+189 **74**
Halia, *India* G46+248 **73**
Halib, *Saudi Arabia* J31+227 **75**
Haliburton, *Ontario* T21+450 **91**
Halifax, *England* N11+537 **37**
Halifax, *N. Carolina* T16+363 **97**
Halifax & Harb., *N.S.* S22+446 **90**
Halifax B., *Queensland* C18–190 **111**
Halkett C., *Alaska* Y10+708 **99**
Hall, *W. Germany* M32+491 **48**
Hall Is., *Caroline Is.* B76+080 **106**
Hall Ld., *Greenland* R30+810 **26**
Halle, *E. Germany* M18+515 **48**
Halle, *Belgium* M65+507 **44**
Hallein, *Austria* M11+476 **48**
Halley B., *Antarctica* Q15–738 **27**
Halliste, *Estonia* L27+581 **47**
Hällnäss, *Sweden* L62+643 **46**
Hallock, *Minnesota* U42+488 **93**
Hallowell, *Maine* S59+443 **90**
Halls Creek, *W. Australia* D43–181 **110**
Hallstavik, *Sweden* L69+601 **47**
Hallviken, *Sweden* L87+637 **46**
Halmahera, I., *Indonesia* D42+006 **65**
Halmstad, *Sweden* M13+567 **47**
Halsa, *Norway* M41+631 **46**
Hälsingborg, *Sweden* M14+561 **47**
Halstead, *Kansas* U46+360 **95**
Halys, C., *Turkey* K54+417 **74**
Hama, *Syria* K50+351 **76**
Hamada, *Japan* D17+349 **68**
Hamadan, *Iran* J70+348 **74**
Hamaidan, *Saudi Arabia* J37+208 **75**
Hamam, *Saudi Arabia* J86+208 **74**
Hamamatsu, *Japan* C74+347 **68**
Haman, *Iraq* K05+312 **74**
Hamar, *Saudi Arabia* J83+224 **74**
Hamar, *Norway* M23+608 **47**
Hambantota, *Sri Lanka* G53+061 **70**
Hamburg, *W. Germany* M30+536 **48**
Hamburg, *Iowa* U34+406 **95**
Hamburg, *New York* T23+427 **96**
Hamburg, *Pennsylvania* T06+405 **96**
Hamburg, *S. Carolina* T41+335 **97**
Hämeenlinna, *Finland* L33+610 **47**
Hameln, *W. Germany* M34+521 **48**
Hami, *Yemen, South* J61+148 **74**
Hamidiya, *Syria* K54+347 **76**
Hamilton, *Alabama* T78+342 **97**
Hamilton, *New York* T04+428 **96**
Hamilton, *New Zealand* A28–378 **112**
Hamilton, *N. Carolina* T14+359 **97**
Hamilton, *Ohio* T57+394 **91**
Hamilton, *Ontario* T29+433 **91**
Hamilton, *Scotland* N24+558 **41**
Hamilton, *Tasmania* C19–426 **109**
Hamilton, *Victoria* C48–378 **109**
Hamilton, *Washington* W08+480 **88**
Hamilton Inl., *Labrador* R75+543 **89**
Hamilton, L., *Arkansas* U18+344 **95**
Hamilton, L., *Texas* U51+308 **98**
Hamilton R. (Churchill), *Lab.* S10+530 **89**
Hamina, *Finland* L16+605 **47**
Hamirpur, *India* G59+259 **73**
Hamlet, *N. Carolina* T28+349 **97**
Hamley Bridge, *S. Australia* C68–344 **109**
Hamm, *W. Germany* M43+517 **48**
Hamme, *Belgium* M65+511 **44**
Hammerdal, *Sweden* L88+636 **46**
Hammerfest, *Norway* L38+706 **46**
Hammersley Ra., *W. Aust.* E15–220 **110**
Hammond, *Indiana* T75+416 **91**
Hammond, *Louisiana* U02+305 **95**
Hammond, *New Brunswick* S45+474 **90**
Hammond, *S. Australia* C70–325 **109**
Hammonton, *New Jersey* S85+396 **96**
Hamont, *Belgium* M57+512 **44**
Hampden, *New Zealand* A55–453 **112**
Hampden, *N. Dakota* U52+486 **93**
Hampshire, co., *England* N08+510 **39**
Hampton, *Arkansas* U15+335 **97**
Hampton, *Iowa* U18+427 **95**
Hampton, *New Brunswick* S34+455 **90**
Hampton, *New Hampshire* S65+430 **90**
Hampton, *S. Carolina* T37+329 **97**
Hamun-i-Helmand, *Iran-Afghanistan* H82+314 **75**
Hamun-i-Puzak, *Afghanistan* H80+314 **75**
Han, *Belgium* M59+501 **44**
Hanakiya, *Saudi Arabia* K24+253 **74**
Hanau, *W. Germany* M36+501 **48**
Hanchung, *China* E78+331 **66**
Hancock, *Michigan* T81+473 **99**
Hancock, *New York* T02+419 **96**
Handegg, *Switzerland* M40+466 **45**
Handeni, *Tanzania* K42–054 **83**
Hanford, *California* V88+363 **92**
Hanford, *Washington* V87+466 **92**
Hangchow, *China* D89+303 **67**
Hangchow B., *China* D80+306 **66**
Hangu, *Pakistan* H24+335 **72**
Han Kiang, *China* E60+328 **64**
Hankinson, *N. Dakota* U41+461 **93**
Hankö,(Hango), *Finland* L42+599 **47**
Hankong, *China* E04+254 **64**
Hankow (Wuhan), *China* E34+306 **66**
Hanle, *Kashmir* G66+328 **70**
Hanley, *England* N13+530 **37**
Hanmer, *New Zealand* A43–425 **112**
Hanna, *Alberta* V41+514 **88**
Hanna, *Wyoming* V06+414 **93**
Hannibal, *Missouri* U08+396 **95**
Hannover, *W. Germany* M32+524 **48**
Hannut, *Belgium* M60+507 **44**
Hanö-bukten, *Sweden* M02+558 **47**
Hanoi, *Vietnam* E85+210 **69**
Hanover, *Ontario* T36+442 **91**
Hanover, *Pennsylvania* T12+398 **96**
Hanover, *Virginia* T14+377 **97**
Hanover, I., *Chile* S88–510 **103**
Hansi, *India* G84+291 **72**
Hansweert, *Netherlands* M66+515 **44**
Hanumangarh. *See* Bhatnair
Hanyang, *China* E34+305 **67**
Hanyin, *China* E68+329 **66**
Hanza, *Kashmir* H02+364 **72**
Hao, I., *Tuamotu Arch.* X20–190 **107**
Haparanda, *Sweden* L35+658 **46**
Hapora, *Japan* C50+444 **68**
Hapur, *India* G73+287 **72**
Haqal, *Saudi Arabia* K60+292 **74**
Haraiya, *India* G45+268 **73**
Harak, *Saudi Arabia* K48+256 **74**
Harar, *Ethiopia* K18+092 **83**
Harardera, *Somalia* J74+046 **83**
Hara Usu Nur, *Mongolia* F76+480 **64**
Harbin. *See* Haerhpin
Harbor Beach, *Michigan* T46+438 **91**
Harbor Spring, *Michigan* T60+455 **91**
Harburg Wilhelmsburg, *Ger.* M30+534 **48**
Harda, *India* G77+223 **70**
Hardanger Fjell, *Norway* M42+609 **47**
Hardanger Fd., *Norway* M54+601 **47**
Hardenberg, *Netherlands* M50+526 **44**
Harderwijk, *Netherlands* M56+523 **44**
Hardin, *Montana* V16+457 **93**
Harding, *Natal* L00–306 **84**
Hardoi, *India* G59+274 **73**
Hardwar, *India* G71+299 **72**
Hardwicke B., *S. Australia* C76–348 **109**
Hardy, Pen., *Chile* S52–555 **103**
Hare B., *Newfoundland* R64+512 **90**
Hare I., *Quebec* S58+479 **91**
Hareidland, *Norway* M54+624 **46**
Hare Indian R., *N.-W. Terr.* W35+663 **88**
Harelbeke, *Belgium* M70+509 **44**
Hargeisa, *Somalia* K06+094 **83**
Hari, R., *Sumatra, Indon* F10–016 **65**
Harib, *Saudi Arabia* J85+152 **74**
Harihar, *India* G85+146 **70**
Harim, *Syria* K51+362 **76**
Haripur, *Pakistan* H12+340 **72**
Hariq, *Saudi Arabia* J81+237 **74**
Harishpur, *India* G21+201 **71**
Harlan, *Iowa* U32+416 **95**
Harlan, *Kentucky* T47+368 **99**
Harlech, *Wales* N25+529 **38**
Harlem, *Montana* V22+485 **93**
Harlequin Hills, *Nevada* V84+415 **92**
Harlingen, *Netherlands* M57+532 **44**
Harlingen, *Texas* U46+262 **94**
Harlowton, *Montana* V29+464 **93**
Harmanli. *See* Kharmanli
Harnai, *Pakistan* H42+302 **70**
Harney L., *Oregon* V85+432 **92**
Harney Pk., *S. Dakota* U81+438 **93**
Harney Basin, *Oregon* W00+436 **98**
Harnösand, *Sweden* L73+626 **46**
Har Nuur, lake, *Mongolia* F73+480 **63**
Harper, *Liberia* N46+044 **80**
Harran, *Turkey* K35+370 **74**
Harray, L. of, *Orkney, Scot.* N19+590 **40**
Harrington Harbour, *Quebec* R87+505 **90**
Harris, & Sd., of *Scotland* N41+578 **40**
Harrisburg, *Arkansas* U04+355 **95**
Harrisburg, *Illinois* T82+378 **95**
Harrisburg, *Pennsylvania* T12+403 **96**
Harrison, *Arkansas* U18+362 **95**
Harrison, *Michigan* T59+440 **91**
Harrison, C., *Labrador* R67+548 **89**
Harrison L., *Brit. Columbia* W10+498 **88**
Harrisonburg, *Louisiana* U10+318 **97**
Harrisonburg, *Virginia* T23+384 **97**
Harrisonville, *Missouri* U26+386 **95**
Harrisville, *Michigan* T50+447 **91**
Harrodsburg, *Kentucky* T59+378 **97**
Harrogate, *England* N09+540 **37**
Harrow, *England* N02+516 **39**
Hârsova, *Romania* L12+447 **58**
Harspranget, *Sweden* L61+668 **46**
Harstad, *Norway* L81+689 **46**
Hart, *Michigan* T68+437 **91**
Hartford, *Connecticut* S76+418 **96**
Hartland, *New Brunswick* S45+464 **90**
Hartlepool, *England* N07+547 **37**
Hartsville, *Tennessee* T67+364 **97**
Hartville, *Missouri* U18+373 **97**
Harvard, *Illinois* T82+425 **91**
Harvard, Mt., *Colorado* V08+385 **98**
Harvey, *New Brunswick* S42+457 **90**
Harvey, *N. Dakota* U60+478 **93**
Harwell, *England* N08+516 **39**
Harwich, *England* M82+519 **39**
Haryana, state, *India* G84+291 **72**
Harz, mts., *Germany* M27+516 **48**
Hasan Dagh, *Turkey* K66+382 **74**
Hasan Kuli, *Turkmen* J37+378 **62**
Hasanpur, *India* G70+293 **73**
Hasbeya, *Lebanon* K56+334 **76**
Hassan, *India* G83+130 **70**
Hassayampa, *Arizona* V46+334 **98**
Hasselt, *Belgium* M58+509 **44**
Hasselt, *Netherlands* M53+526 **44**
Hastiere, *Belgium* M61+502 **44**
Hastings, *England* M86+509 **39**
Hastings, *Michigan* T62+427 **91**
Hastings, *Minnesota* U16+448 **93**
Hastings, *Nebraska* U50+406 **95**
Hastings, *New Zealand* A19–396 **112**
Hasting's Ra., *New S. Wales* B80–312 **109**
Hateg, *Romania* L42+456 **58**
Hatfield, *England* N06+536 **37**
Hatfield, *New South Wales* C37–339 **109**
Hatha, *Saudi Arabia* K27+228 **74**
Hathras, *India* G71+276 **73**
Ha-tinh, *Vietnam* E85+184 **69**
Hatteras, C., *N. Carolina* T03+352 **97**
Hattiesburg, *Mississippi* T86+312 **95**
Hatton Headline, N.-W. Terr. S30+611 **89**
Hatvan, *Hungary* L62+477 **49**
Hat Yai, *Thailand* F27+071 **65**
Haudères, les, *Switzerland* M45+461 **45**
Haugesund, *Norway* M58+594 **47**
Haukipudas, *Finland* L28+652 **46**
Haukivesi, *Finland* L10+622 **46**
Haura, *Yemen, South* J74+139 **74**
Hauraki Gulf, *New Zealand* A30–367 **112**
Haurangi Mts., *New Zealand* A28–414 **112**
Hauroko, L., *New Zealand* A76–460 **112**
Hausa, *Jordan* K43+299 **76**
Hausstock, mt., *Switzerland* M36+468 **45**
Haut, Isle, *Maine* S52+441 **90**
Hauta, *Yemen, South* J80+135 **74**
Hauta, *Saudi Arabia* J79+236 **74**
Haut Atlas, mts., *Morocco* N50+320 **80**
Haute-Garonne, dep., *France* M81+434 **55**
Haute-Loire, dep., *France* M67+451 **55**
Haute-Marne, dep., *France* M58+482 **54**
Hautes-Alpes, dep., *France* M53+446 **55**
Haute-Saône, dep., *France* M51+477 **54**
Haute Savoie, dep., *France* M49+460 **54**
Hautes-Pyrénées, dep., *Fr.* M88+431 **55**
Haute Vienne, dep., *France* M85+459 **54**
Haute Volta. *See* Upper Volta
Haut Rhin, dep., *France* M45+479 **54**
Havana. *See* Habana.
Havasu L., *Cal.-Ariz.* V56+346 **92**
Havelange, *Belgium* M59+504 **44**
Havelland, *E. Germany* M14+527 **48**
Havelock, *New Brunswick* S32+460 **90**
Havelock I., *Andaman Is.* F72+119 **71**

Havelock North, *N.Z.* A18–397 **112**
Haverfordwest, *Wales* N30+518 **38**
Haverhill, *Massachusetts* S67+428 **96**
Haverstraw, *New York* S84+412 **96**
Havre, *Belgium* M66+505 **44**
Havre, *Montana* V28+485 **93**
Havre de Grace, *Maryland* T07+396 **96**
Hawaii I., *Hawaii* Y30+200 **107**
Hawaii, state, *U.S.A.* Y60+250 **106**
Hawarden, *Iowa* U38+430 **95**
Hawea Flat, *New Zealand* A64–445 **112**
Hawera, *New Zealand* A34–396 **112**
Hawesville, *Kentucky* T71+379 **97**
Hawick, *Scotland* N16+554 **41**
Hawizeh, *Iran* J71+315 **74**
Hawke, C., *New S. Wales* B76–322 **109**
Hawker, *S. Australia* C70–319 **109**
Hawke's B., *New Zealand* A16–393 **112**
Hawkesbury, *Ontario* S88+456 **91**
Hawr al Hammar, *Iraq* J76+308 **74**
Hawr Saniyah, *Iraq* J80+320 **74**
Hay, *New South Wales* C31–346 **109**
Hay R., *Alberta* V72+595 **88**
Hayes Halvø, *Greenland* S50+770 **26**
Hayling I., *England* N06+508 **39**
Hayneville, *Alabama* T70+322 **97**
Hay-on-Wye, *Wales* N19+521 **38**
Hay River, *North-West Territories* V65+606 **88**
Hays, *Kansas* U56+388 **95**
Hayward, *Wisconsin* U08+460 **93**
Hazara Highlands, *Afghan.* H60+339 **75**
Hazard, *Kentucky* T49+373 **97**
Hazaribagh, *India* G28+240 **73**
Hazaribagh Ra., *India* G36+232 **73**
Hazarjuft, *Afghanistan* H65+310 **75**
Hazelton, *British Columbia* W45+553 **88**
Hazil, *Saudi Arabia* K15+299 **74**
Hazlehurst, *Georgia* T45+318 **97**
Hazleton, *Pennsylvania* T06+410 **96**
Hazro, *Pakistan* H15+339 **72**
Headford, *Ireland, Rep.* N55+535 **43**
Healesville, *Victoria* C27–376 **109**
Heard I., *Indian Ocean* H12–520 **77**
Hearst, *Ontario* T52+498 **89**
Heathcote, *Victoria* C32–369 **109**
Hebbronville, *Texas* U52+274 **94**
Heber, *Utah* V38+406 **94**
Heber Springs, *Arkansas* U12+355 **97**
Hebrides, Outer, *Scotland* N42+580 **40**
Hebron, *Jordan* K59+315 **76**
Hebron, *Labrador* S16+585 **89**
Hebron, *Nebraska* U46+401 **95**
Hebron, *N. Dakota* U72+469 **93**
Hecate Str., *Brit. Columbia* W65+534 **88**
Hecelchakan, *Mexico* U01+202 **100**
Hechingen, *W. Germany* M36+483 **48**
Hechtel, *Belgium* M58+512 **44**
Hectanooga, *Nova Scotia* S36+442 **90**
Hector, Mt., *New Zealand* A28–409 **112**
Hede, *Sweden* M09+624 **46**
Hedemora, *Sweden* L84+603 **47**
Heemstede, *Netherlands* M62+523 **44**
Heer, *Netherlands* M56+508 **44**
Heerenveen, *Netherlands* M54+530 **44**
Heerlen, *Netherlands* M54+509 **44**
Heiberg I., *N.-W. Terr.* U00+782 **89**
Heide, *W. Germany* M36+542 **48**
Heidelberg, *W. Germany* M38+494 **48**
Heidelburg, *Transvaal* L10–266 **84**
Heiden, *Switzerland* M33+474 **45**
Heijen, *Netherlands* M54+517 **44**
Heilbronn, *W. Germany* M35+491 **48**
Heinola, *Finland* L23+612 **47**
Heist, *Belgium* M71+513 **44**
Hejaz (Hijaz), *Saudi Arabia* K40+253 **74**
Hekla, Mt., *Iceland* P28+640 **46**
Helchteren, *Belgium* M58+511 **44**
Helder, Den, *Netherlands* M61+530 **44**
Helena, *Arkansas* U04+346 **95**
Helena, *Montana* V42+466 **93**
Helensburgh, *Scotland* N28+560 **41**
Helensville, *New Zealand* A33–367 **112**
Helgoland, I., *W. Germany* M43+542 **48**
Helgoländer, Bucht, *W. Germany* M42+543 **48**
Hell Gate, *British Columbia* W34+593 **88**
Hellin, *Spain* N10+385 **53**
Helmand Des., *Afghanistan* H60+304 **75**
Helmand R., *Afghanistan* H70+305 **75**
Helme, *Estonia* L25+580 **47**
Helmond, *Netherlands* M56+515 **44**
Helmsdale, *Scotland* N22+581 **40**
Helsingfors. *See Helsinki*
Helsingør, *Denmark* M15+560 **47**
Helsinki, *Finland* L30+602 **47**
Helston, *England* N32+501 **38**
Helvellyn, *England* N18+545 **37**
Helvick Hd., *Ireland, Rep.* N45+520 **43**
Hemelum, *Netherlands* M57+529 **44**
Hemnes, *Norway* M08+662 **46**
Hemse, *Sweden* L70+572 **47**
Hendaye, *France* N10+434 **55**
Henderson, *Kentucky* T76+378 **95**
Henderson, *Minnesota* U24+445 **93**
Henderson, *New York* T07+438 **91**
Henderson, *N. Carolina* T20+363 **97**
Henderson, *Tennessee* T82+354 **97**
Henderson I., *Pacific Ocean* W50–246 **107**
Hendersonville, *N. Carolina* T45+353 **97**
Hengchow. *See* Hengyang
Hengelo, *Netherlands* M49+523 **44**
Henghsien, *China* E64+226 **67**
Hengshan, *China* E43+272 **67**
Hengyang, *China* E44+270 **67**
Henjam, I., *Iran* J25+266 **75**
Henjareh, *Iran* J00+282 **75**
Henley-on-Thames, *England* N05+515 **39**
Henlopen, C., *New Jersey* T00+388 **96**
Hennebont, *France* N20+478 **54**
Henrietta, *Texas* U49+338 **95**
Henrietta Maria C., *Ontario* T44+549 **89**
Henrique de Carvalho, *Angola* L58–096 **82**
Henry Mts., *Utah* V36+380 **94**
Henryetta, *Oklahoma* U36+354 **95**
Henty, *New South Wales* C18–355 **109**
Henzada, *Burma* F58+176 **71**
Heran, *Yemen* K13+161 **74**
Herat, *Afghanistan* H77+344 **75**
Herault, dep., *France* M71+435 **55**
Herberton, *Queensland* C28–172 **111**
Herbertville, *New Zealand* A21–405 **112**
Herbertville, *Quebec* S69+484 **90**
Herbesthal, *Belgium* M54+506 **44**
Herceg Novi, *Yugoslavia* L62+420 **58**
Heredia, *Costa Rica* T54+100 **101**
Hereford, *Texas* U74+348 **94**
Heref. & Worcs., co., *England* N15+522 **38**
Hereheretue, I., *Pacific Oc.* X60–200 **107**
Herford, *W. Germany* M38+521 **48**
Heriot, *New Zealand* A64–458 **112**
Herisau, *Switzerland* M34+474 **45**
Herkimer, *New York* T00+430 **96**
Herma Ness, *Shetland, Scot.* N06+608 **40**
Hermann, *Missouri* U09+387 **95**
Hermidale, *New S. Wales* C20–316 **109**
Hermil, *Lebanon* K52+344 **76**
Hermitage B., *Newfoundland* R72+475 **90**
Hermite, Is., *Chile* S46–560 **103**
Hermon, Mt. *See* Sheikh, Jebel esh
Hermosillo, *Mexico* V36+291 **100**
Herne, *Belgium* M66+507 **44**
Herne Bay, *England* M83+514 **39**
Herning, *Denmark* M36+561 **47**
Héron, *Belgium* M59+506 **44**
Herowabad, *Iran* J68+377 **74**
Herräng, *Sweden* L68+601 **47**
Herrera, *Argentina* S19–285 **103**
Herrera di Pisuerga, *Spain* N26+426 **52**
Herrick, *Tasmania* C13–411 **109**
Herrington, *Kansas* U42+386 **95**
Hersey, *Michigan* T63+439 **91**
Herselt, *Belgium* M61+511 **44**
Herstmonceux, *England* M88+509 **39**
Hertford, *N. Carolina* T09+362 **97**
Hertford & co., *England* N00+518 **39**
's Hertogenbosch, *Netherl'ds* M58+517 **44**
Herval, *Brazil* R39–274 **103**
Hervas, *Spain* N35+402 **52**
Hervé, *Belgium* M56+506 **44**
Hervey B., *Queensland* B73–246 **111**
Hervey Is., *Cook Is.* Y50–200 **106**
Herzberg, *E. Germany* M11+517 **48**
Herzliya, *Israel* K61+322 **76**
Herzogenbuchsee, *Switz.* M44+472 **45**
Hesdin, *France* M78+504 **54**
Hessen, *W. Germany* M38+506 **48**
Heught, Mt., *N. Terr., Aust.* D23–228 **110**
Heusden, *Netherlands* M59+517 **44**
Hève, C. de la, *France* M89+495 **54**
Hexham, *England* N13+550 **37**
Heytesbury, *England* N13+512 **39**
Heywood, *Victoria* C50–381 **109**
Hiakiang, *China* E67+258 **67**
Hiawatha, *Kansas* U34+398 **95**
Hibbing, *Minnesota* U18+474 **93**
Hidalgo, *Mexico* U59+277 **100**
Hidalgo, state, *Mexico* U54+204 **100**
Hieflau, *Austria* M02+476 **48**
Hierro, I., *Canary Is.* P30+276 **80**
Highland, reg., *Scotland* N30+576 **40**
Highland Park, *Illinois* T78+422 **95**
Highmore, *S. Dakota* U57+445 **93**
High Point, *N. Carolina* T30+360 **97**
Highwood Mts., *Montana* V32+475 **93**
Hiimeji, *Japan* D02+348 **68**
Hiiumaa, I., *Estonia* L44+589 **47**
Hijar, *Spain* N03+411 **53**
Hikone, *Japan* C82+353 **68**
Hildesheim, *W. Germany* M30+521 **48**
Hili, *Saudi Arabia* J26+244 **75**
Hillah, al, *Iraq* K03+325 **74**
Hill City, *Kansas* U60+394 **95**
Hill City, *Minnesota* U22+470 **93**
Hillman, *Michigan* T54+451 **91**
Hillsboro, *Illinois* T87+392 **95**
Hillsboro, *N. Carolina* T24+362 **97**
Hillsboro, *Texas* U42+320 **95**
Hilsborough, *N.B.* S28+459 **90**
Hillsdale, *Michigan* T58+419 **91**
Hillston, *New South Wales* C27–335 **109**
Hillsville, *Virginia* T35+368 **97**
Hilversum, *Netherlands* M59+522 **44**
Hilwa, *Saudi Arabia* J80+233 **74**
Hilvan, *Saudi Arabia* K23+222 **74**
Himachal Pradesh, *India* G75+320 **72**
Himalaya Mts., *India, etc.* G60+300 **30**
Himanka, *Finland* L38+641 **46**
Himare, *Albania* L62+401 **59**
Hinckley, *Minnesota* U18+461 **93**
Hindeloopen, *Netherlands* M58+529 **44**
Hindman, *Kentucky* T48+373 **97**
Hindmarsh, L., *Victoria* C49–360 **109**
Hindubagh, *Pakistan* H42+309 **70**
Hindu Kush, mts., *Afghanistan-Pakistan* H20+364 **70**
Hindupur, *India* G75+139 **70**
Hingan. *See* Ankang
Hinganghat, *India* G66+205 **70**
Hingham, *Montana* V33+485 **93**
Hingho, *China* E38+410 **66**
Hinghwa, *China* E01+329 **66**
Hinghwa (Putien), *China* E05+255 **67**
Hingi, *China* F00+251 **67**
Hinglaj, *Pakistan* H57+255 **70**
Hingol R., *Pakistan* H56+250 **70**
Hingoli, *India* G76+196 **70**
Hinnøya, *Norway* L84+687 **46**
Hinsdale, *Montana* V12+484 **93**
Hinsdale, *New Hampshire* S75+428 **96**
Hinton, *W. Virginia* T35+377 **97**
Hiro, *Japan* C40+423 **68**
Hirosaki, *Japan* C57+406 **68**
Hiroshima, *Japan* D15+344 **68**
Hisaronu, *Turkey* K77+416 **74**
Hisban, *Jordan* K55+318 **76**
Hispaniola, I., *West Indies* S70+190 **101**
Hissar, *India* G86+291a72
Hissmofors, *Sweden* M03+634 **46**
Hisua, *India* G27+248 **73**
Hisya, *Syria* K49+344 **76**
Hit, *Iraq* K14+336 **74**
Hitra, *Norway* M38+636 **46**
Hivaoa, I., *Marquesas Is.* X24–100 **107**
Hiwasa, *Japan* D03+338 **68**
Hjälmaren, L., *Sweden* L86+593 **47**
Hjørring, *Denmark* M30+575 **47**
Hkamti, *Burma* F56+260 **71**
Hobart, *Oklahoma* U54+350 **95**
Hobart, *Tasmania* C16–430 **109**
Hobbs, *New Mexico* U78+326 **94**
Hoboken, *Belgium* M64+512 **44**
Hobro, *Denmark* M31+566 **47**
Hochwan, *China* E82+300 **67**
Hodal, *India* G76+279 **72**
Hodeida, *Yemen* K12+148 **74**
Hodgson, *Manitoba* U46+512 **88**
Hodmezövasárhely, *Hungary* L58+464 **49**
Hoek van Holland, *Netherlands* M65+520 **44**
Hoyes Bridge, *Kenya* K58+010 **83**
Hof, *W. Germany* M19+503 **48**
Hofei, *China* E16+319 **66**
Hofmeyr, *Namibia* L70–244 **84**
Höfs Jökull, *Iceland* P24+648 **46**
Hofuf, *Saudi Arabia* J62+254 **74**
Höganäs, *Sweden* M15+562 **47**
Hohe Tauern, *Austria* M15+472 **48**
Hohsien, *China* E51+244 **67**
Hoihong, *China* E59+209 **67**
Hokianga Harb, *N.Z.* A39–354 **112**
Ho-kien-fu, *China* E23+385 **66**
Hokitika, *New Zealand* A54–427 **112**
Hokkaidō I., *Japan* C42+430 **68**
Holbaek, *Denmark* M20+557 **47**
Holberg, *British Columbia* W48+506 **88**
Holbrook, *Arizona* V31+348 **94**
Holbrook, *New South Wales* C17–358 **109**
Holdenville, *Oklahoma* U38+351 **95**
Holdredge, *Nebraska* U54+404 **95**
Holguin, *Cuba* T08+208 **101**
Holinkoerh, *China* E50+404 **66**
Holland, *Michigan* T67+428 **91**
Holland, *New York* T21+426 **96**
Holland, Noord, prov., *Neth.* M61+526 **44**
Holland, Zuid, prov., *Neth.* M63+520 **44**
Holland, *Michigan* T75+428 **91**
Hollange, *Belgium* M56+499 **44**
Hollidaysburg, *Pennsylvania* T21+404 **96**
Hollis, *Oklahoma* U59+347 **95**
Hollogne, *Belgium* M59+507 **44**
Holly, *Colorado* U72+381 **94**
Holly, *Michigan* T52+428 **91**
Holly Springs, *Mississippi* T87+348 **95**
Hollywood, *California* V80+341 **92**
Holmestrand, *Norway* M28+595 **47**
Holmsund, *Sweden* L58+637 **46**
Holstebro., *Denmark* M38+563 **47**
Holstein, *Germany* M32+539 **48**
Holsteinsborg, *Greenland* R40+670 **26**
Holsworthy, *England* N26+508 **38**
Holten, *Netherlands* M51+523 **44**
Holton, *Kansas* U36+394 **95**
Holwerd, *Netherlands* M55+534 **44**
Holy I., *England* N11+557 **37**
Holy I., *Wales* N28+533 **38**
Holy Cross, *Alaska* Y60+624 **99**
Holy Cross, Mt. of the, *Colorado* V09+396 **98**
Holyhead, *Wales* N28+533 **38**
Holyoke, *Colorado* U74+406 **94**
Holyoke, *Massachusetts* S76+422 **91**
Holywood, *N. Ireland* N35+546 **42**
Home B., *N.-W. Territories* S30+678 **89**
Homer, *Alaska* Y10+559 **99**
Homer, *Louisiana* U18+328 **95**
Homer, *New York* T08+427 **91**
Homestead, *Pennsylvania* T29+404 **91**
Homfray Str., *Andaman Is.* F72+124 **71**
Hommelvik, *Norway* M26+634 **46**
Homs, *Libya* M04+326 **81**
Homs, *Syria* K50+347 **76**
Honan. *See* Loyang
Honan, prov., *China* E42+340 **66**
Honda, *Columbia* S89+052 **104**
Honda, B., *Cuba* T49+229 **101**
Hondo, *Mexico* U65+277 **100**
Honduras, rep., *C. America* T76+150 **101**
Honduras, C., *Honduras* T66+160 **101**
Honduras, G. of, *Cent. Amer* T70+165 **101**
Hønefoss, *Norway* M28+602 **47**
Honesdale, *Pennsylvania* T02+415 **96**
Honfleur, *France* N00+494 **54**
Honghai B., *China* E28+227 **67**
Hong Kong I., *S.-E. Asia* E34+223 **67**
Honiara, I., *Solomon Is* B30–095 **106**
Honiton, *England* N19+508 **38**
Honolulu, *Hawaii* Y30+208 **107**
Honor, *Michigan* T66+447 **91**
Honshū, I., *Japan* **68**
Hood, Mt., *Oregon* W10+453 **92**
Hoofdplaat, *Netherlands* M68+514 **44**
Hooger Smilde, *Netherlands* M52+529 **44**
Hoogeveen, *Netherlands* M51+527 **44**
Hoogezand, *Netherlands* M49+532 **44**
Hooghalen, *Netherlands* M51+529 **44**
Hooghly, *India* G10+230 **73**
Hooghly R., *India* G12+216 **73**
Hook Hd., *Ireland, Rep.* N42+521 **43**
Hookina, *S. Australia* C71–318 **109**
Hoopeston, *Illinois* T76+405 **91**
Hoorn Den, *Netherlands* M60+526 **44**
Hoosick Falls, *New York* S80+429 **91**
Hoover Dam, *Arizona* V57+359 **92**
Hope, *Aransas* U21+336 **95**
Hope, *British Columbia* W08+494 **88**
Hopedale, *Labrador* S03+554 **89**
Hopeh, prov., *China* E24+386 **66**
Hopen, I., *Barents Sea* L30+766 **62**
Hopes Advance, C., *Quebec* S56+607 **89**
Hopetoun, *Victoria* C46–357 **109**
Hope Town, *Andaman Is.* F74+117 **71**
Hopetown, *Cape Province* L36–296 **84**
Hopewell, *Virginia* T14+372 **97**
Hopkinsville, *Kentucky* T75+368 **95**
Hoppo, *China* E64+216 **67**
Hoquiam, *Washington* W23+470 **92**
Horaždovice, *Czechoslovakia* M08+493 **48**
Horcasitas, *Mexico* V34+294 **100**
Horgen, *Switzerland* M38+473 **45**
Horka, *E. Germany* L90+513 **48**
Hormuz, *Iran* J31+276 **75**
Hormuz I., *Iran* J21+271 **75**
Hormuz. Str. of, *Saudi Arabia-Iran* J24+266 **75**
Horn, *Austria* L86+487 **49**
Horn, *Iceland* P44+665 **46**
Horn, *Netherlands* M54+512 **44**
Horn, C., *Chile* S44–560 **103**
Horn Mts., *N.-W. Terr.* V85+617 **88**
Hornavan, *Sweden* L74+662 **46**
Horncastle, *England* N01+532 **37**
Hornefors, *Sweden* L61+637 **46**
Hornell, *New York* T16+423 **96**
Hornopiren, mt., *Chile* S75–418 **103**
Hornos, C. de *Chile* S44–560 **103**
Hornsby, *New South Wales* B84–337 **109**
Hornsea, *England* N01+539 **37**
Horonobe, *Japan* C49+451 **68**
Horqueta, *Paraguay* R72–232 **103**
Horseheads, *New York* T11+422 **96**
Horsens, *Denmark* M31+559 **47**
Horse Shoe, *W. Australia* E09–255 **110**
Horseshoe Res., *Arizona* V40+340 **94**
Horsham, *England* N02+511 **39**
Horsham, *Victoria* C47–367 **109**
Horšovský Týn, *Czech.* M13+495 **48**
Horst, *Netherlands* M54+515 **44**
Horten, *Norway* M27+594 **47**
Horton, *Kansas* U34+396 **95**
Horton, *Montana* V06+463 **93**
Horton R., *N.-W. Terr.* W12+682 **88**
Hose Ra., *Sarawak* E38+019 **65**
Hoshangabad, *India* G73+227 **73**
Hoshiarpur, *India* G83+315 **72**
Hospel, *India* G81+153 **70**
Hospenthal, *Switzerland* M39+466 **45**
Hossegor, *France* N08+437 **55**
Hoste, I., *Chile* S56–552 **103**
Hosur, *India* G73+128 **70**
Hotagen, *Sweden* M05+640 **46**
Hotseh, *China* E28+353 **66**
Hot Springs, *N. Carolina* T47+359 **97**
Hot Springs, *S. Dakota* U81+434 **93**
Hot Springs Nat. Pk., *Ark.* U18+346 **95**
Hotton, *Belgium* M57+503 **44**
Houdelaincourt, *France* M57+485 **54**
Houffalize, *Belgium* M55+501 **44**
Houghton L., *Michigan* T59+444 **91**
Houlton, *Maine* S47+461 **90**
Houma, *Louisiana* U04+296 **95**
Hourn, L., *Scotland* N34+571 **40**
Housatonic, R., *Conecticut* S79+414 **96**
House Ra., *Utah* V50+395 **94**
Houstan, *Mississippi* T84+339 **97**
Houston, *Missouri* U12+374 **95**
Houston, *Texas* U32+298 **95**
Houten, *Netherlands* M59+520 **44**
Houtman Abrolhos, *W. Aust.* E42–284 **110**
Hovd, *Mongolia* E80+480 **64**
Hove, *England* N01+508 **39**
Hovsgöl Nuur, lake *Mongolia* F25+520 **63**
Howard, *Michigan* T63+434 **91**
Howard, *Pennsylvania* T16+410 **96**
Howard, *S. Dakota* U45+440 **93**
Howell, *Michigan* T54+426 **91**
Howick, *Natal* L00+294 **84**
Howland I., *Pacific Ocean* Z70+005 **106**
Howley, *Newfoundland* R72+492 **90**
Howrah, *India* G10+226 **73**
Howth, *Ireland, Rep.* N36+534 **43**
Hoy, I. *Orkney, Scotland* N20+588 **40**
Hoyes, *Spain* N41+401 **52**
Hoyt, *New Brunswick* S39+456 **90**
Hoyun, *China* E42+237 **64**
Hozat, *Turkey* K34+393 **74**
Hrubieszów, *Poland* L37+508 **49**
Hsenwi, *Burma* F42+234 **71**
Hsiachwan Shan, *China* E44+216 **67**
Hsiamen, *China* E11+244 **67**
Hsinchu, *Taiwan* D84+248 **67**
Hsinking. *See* Changchun
Hsipaw, *Burma* F46+226 **71**
Hsuchang, *China* E36+340 **66**
Hsuchow. *See* Hsuchang
Huachi, *Bolivia* S44–156 **104**
Huacho, *Peru* T16–111 **104**
Huacrachuco, *Peru* T12–088 **104**
Hualgayoo, *Peru* T22–068 **104**
Hualienkang, *Taiwan* D80+240 **67**
Huambo, *Angola* L86-128 **82**
Huanay, *Bolivia* S48–155 **104**
Huancabamba, *Peru* T27–052 **104**
Huancane, *Peru* S58–152 **104**
Huancavelica, *Peru* T01–126 **104**
Huancayo, *Peru* T01–120 **104**
Huanchaca, *Bolivia* S40–203 **104**
Huanchaco, *Peru* T25–081 **104**
Huanta, *Peru* S85–126 **104**
Huanuco, *Peru* T08–098 **104**
Huaras, *Peru* T16–095 **104**
Huards, L. aux, *Quebec* S65+493 **90**
Huari, *Chile* S59–200 **103**
Huariaca, *Peru* T07–105 **104**
Huarmey, *Peru* T19–101 **104**
Huasco, *Chile* S67–284 **103**
Huatusco, *Mexico* U42+192 **100**
Huaylas, *Peru* T17–090 **104**
Hubli, *India* G88+154 **70**
Huchow, *China* D88+308 **66**
Hucknall Torkard, *England* N07+531 **37**
Huddersfield, *England* N11+536 **37**
Hudiksvall, *Sweden* L77+617 **47**
Hudson, *Maine* S53+451 **90**
Hudson, *Wisconsin* U16+450 **93**
Hudson & R., *New York* S83+423 **96**
Hudson B., *Canada* T60+580 **89**
Hudson R., *New York* S83+420 **91**
Hudson Str., *Canada* S80+620 **89**
Hudson Falls, *New York* S81+433 **91**
Hue, *Vietnam* E75+165 **69**
Hueco Mts., *New Mex.-Texas* V06+320 **94**
Huedin, *Romania* L42+469 **58**
Huehuetenango, *Guatemala* U08+154 **100**
Huejutla, *Mexico* U51+212 **100**
Huelva, *Spain* N41+372 *52*
Huereal Overa, *Spain* N12+374 **53**
Huete, *Spain* N16+402 **53**
Hughenden, *Queensland* C35–209 **111**
Hugo, *Oklahoma* U33+340 **95**
Huhehot, *China* E50+408 **66**
Huiarau Ra., *New Zealand* A18–387 **112**
Hŭichŏn, *Korea* D52+402 **64**
Huj, *Israel* K62+315 **76**
Hukawng Valley, *Burma* F50+266 **71**
Hukow, *China* E23+297 **67**
Hukuntsi, *Botswana* L50–240 **84**
Hula L., *Israel* K56+331 **76**
Hulaiba, *Iraq* J77+301 **74**
Hulin, *China* D10+460 **64**
Hull, *England* N02+537 **37**

Hull, Quebec T04+455 91
Hulst, Netherlands M66+513 44
Hulun. See Hailar
Hulun Chih, China E16+448 64
Hulutao, China D84+407 64
Huma, China D50+515 63
Humacao, Puerto Rico S34+183 101
Humaita, Paraguay R81-271 103
Humansdorp, Cape Province L32-340 84
Humayta, Brazil S18-074 104
Humber, R., England N02+537 37
Humbermouth, Nfd. R77+490 90
Humberside, co., England N03+538 37
Humboldt, Iowa U26+428 95
Humboldt, Saskatchewan V01+519 88
Humboldt, Tennessee T84+358 97
Humboldt B., California W30+408 98
Humboldt Glacier, Greenland R30+790 26
Humboldt R., Nevada V80+404 92
Hume Res., New S. Wales C18-360 109
Humenne, Czechoslovakia L49+490 49
Humphreys, Mt., Arizona Y39+354 94
Humphreys, Mt., California V82+373 92
Humphreys, Mt., Wyoming V31+443 93
Hun, Libya L84+292 81
Húnaflói, Iceland P36+659 46
Hunan, prov., China E54+266 67
Hungary, Central Europe L60+470 51
Hungchiang, China E11+273 67
Hungerford, England N09+514 39
Hungnam, Korea D43+400 64
Hungtse, China E08+332 66
Hunsrück, mts., W. Germany M46+499 48
Hunstanton, England M87+529 39
Hunter Is., Tasmania C31-405 109
Hunter Ra., New S. Wales C00-330 109
Hunter R., New S. Wales B82-326 109
Huntersville, W. Virginia T30+382 97
Huntingburg, Indiana T72+384 97
Huntingdon, Pennsylvania T18+405 96
Huntingdon and Peterborough, co.
See Cambridgeshire
Huntington, New York S81+408 96
Huntington, Utah V36+394 94
Huntington, W. Virginia T45+384 97
Huntley, Montana V20+458 93
Huntly, New Zealand A29-376 112
Huntly, Scotland N17+574 40
Huntsville, Alabama T69+347 97
Huntsville, Ontario T25+453 91
Huntsville, Tennessee T57+364 97
Huntsville, Texas U32+307 95
Hunucma, Mexico T89+210 100
Hun-yüan-chow, China E38+397 66
Hunza, Kashmir H02+364 72
Huon Is., Pacific Ocean B10-180 106
Huon Pen.,
Papua New Guinea C20-064 111
Huon, R., Tasmania C20-431 109
Hupeh, prov., China E42+315 66
Hurd, C., Ontario T40+452 91
Hurghada, Egypt K68+270 81
Huron, S. Dakota U50+444 93
Huron, L., U.S.A.-Canada T40+450 99
Hurtsboro, Alabama T63+323 97
Huskvarna, Sweden M04+578 47
Husum, W. Germany M36+545 48
Hutchinson, Kansas U48+381 95
Hutchinson, Minnesota U26+450 93
Hüttenberg, Austria M03+469 48
Huttwil, Switzerland M43+471 45
Huy, Belgium M59+505 44
Hvar, I., Yugoslavia L79+431 56
Hwahsien, China E40+235 67
Hwaian, China E04+335 66
Hwaijen, China E42+399 66
Hwaining, China E17+305 67
Hwaiyang, China E30+337 66
Hwaiyn. See Tsingkiang
Hwangchow. See Hwangkang
Hwang-Hai. See Yellow Sea
Hwang Ho, R., China E24+360 66
Hwanghsien, China D87+377 66
Hwangkang, China E30+307 66
Hweichow. See Sihsien
Hweimin, China E15+375 66
Hweinan, China D53+428 64
Hweitseh, China F11+264 67
Hwohsien, China E50+365 66
Hyde, England N13+535 37
Hyden, Kentucky T51+372 97
Hyden, W. Australia E06-322 110
Hyde Park, Vermont S75+446 91
Hyderabad, India G69+173 70
Hyderabad, Pakistan H40+254 70
Hyères, France M53+431 55
Hyères, Is. d', France M51+430 55
Hyland R., Yukon W50+602 88
Hyndman Pk., Idaho V54+438 98
Hyogo, Japan D00+347 68
Hyrum, Utah V42+416 94
Hyrynsalmi, Finland L08+647 46
Hythe, England M84+511 39
Hythe, England N08+509 39
Iasi, Romania L14+471 60
Ibadan, Nigeria M66+074 80
Ibague, Colombia T02+044 104
Ibarra, Ecuador T18+005 104
Ibb, Yemen K05+140 74
Ibembo, Zaire L38+026 82
Ibicui, Brazil R70-294 103
Ibiza, I., Balearic Is. M80+390 53
Ibresi, U.S.S.R. J77+553 61
Ibri, Oman J22+231 75
Ibwe Munyama, Zambia L08-162 84
Ica, Peru T04-140 104
Ica, R., Brazil S50-028 104
Icel, Turkey K62+369 51
Iceland, I. & rep., N. Atl. Oc. —34
Ichak, India G28+242 73
Ichang, China E52+307 66
Icheng, China E46+317 66
Ichow. See Lini.
Ichun, China E33+277 67
Idabel, Oklahoma U28+338 95
Ida Grove, Iowa U33+424 95
Idah, Nigeria M50+072 80
Idaho, state, U.S.A. V67+444 98
Idaho Falls, Idaho V42+435 92
Ideles, Algeria M54+236 80
Idfu, Egypt K74+250 81
Idhra, I., Greece L39+374 59
Idirtu, China F50+374 64
Idlib, Syria K50+359 76
Idutywa, Cape Province L10-322 84
Ierissós, G. of, Greece L36+405 59
Ifakara, Tanzania K50-082 83
Iférouane, Niger M48+188 80
Ifni, terr., N.-W. Africa N64+288 80
Igan, Sarawak E49+028 65
Igarapé.Mirim, Brazil R23-020 105
Igarka, U.S.S.R. G20+675 62
Iglesias, Sardinia M39+393 56
Igli, Algeria N12+304 80
Igoma, Tanzania K70-078 83
Igra, U.S.S.R. J41+574 61
Iguaçú, & R., Brazil R58-256 103
Iguala, Mexico U56+183 100
Iguapé, Brazil R16-247 103
Iguatu, Brazil Q56-064 105
Igumira, Tanzania K70-068 83
Ihosy, Madagascar J84-224 83
Ihtiman, Bulgaria L37+424 58
Iida, Japan C73+355 68
Iisalmi, Finland L17+635 46
Ijebu-Ode, Nigeria M66+068 80
IJsselmonde, Netherlands M63+519 44
IJsselmuiden, Netherlands M54+526 44
IJsselstein, Netherlands M60+520 44
IJssel Meer, Netherlands M58+527 44
IJssel R., Netherlands M53+523 44
Ijui, Brazil R54-284 103
Ijzendijke, Netherlands M68+513 44
Ikaria, I., Greece L23+376 59
Ikisu, Tanzania K66-020 83
Ikla, Estonia L33+579 47
Ikonde, Tanzania K88-064 83
Ilagan, Philippines D79+171 65
Ilam, Nepal G12+269 73
Ilam, Iran J82+337 74
Ilanz, Switzerland M35+468 45
Iława, Poland L63+536 49
Iławka, Poland L56+544 490
Ile-à-la Crosse, L., Sask. V18+554 88
Ile-de-France, prov., France M75+490 54
Ilford, England M89+516 39
Ilfracombe, England N25+512 38
Ilhavo, Portugal N52+406 52
Ilhéus, Brazil Q54-148 105
Ili, Kazakh. G76+438 62
Ilia, Greece L51+378 59
Ilic, Turkey K39+394 74
Ilich, Kazakh. H40+410 62
Iligan, Philippines D64+080 65
Ilimsk, U.S.S.R. F08+569 63
Iliodhrómia, I., Greece L37+392 59
Ilion, New York T00+430 96
Ilkeston, England N08+530 37
Ilkley, England N11+539 37
Illapel, Chile S67-315 103
Ille-et-Vilaine, dep., France N11+482 54
Illescas, Spain N23+401 52
Illimani, mt., Bolivia S47-166 104
Illinois, state, U.S.A. U03+398 99
Illinois R., Illinois U04+398 95
Illora, Spain N23+373 52
Ilmen Oz., U.S.S.R. K83+583 60
Ilminster, England N17+509 38
Ilo, Peru S68-175 104
Iloilo, Philippines D75+108 65
Ilorin, Nigeria M62+084 80
Ilpi, U.S.S.R. A41+615 63
Imabaru, Japan D12+340 68
Iman, U.S.S.R. D07+459 63
Imandra, Oz., U.S.S.R. K73+675 62
Imerimandroso, Madagascar J68-176 83
Imi, Ethiopia K16+064 83
Immendingen, W. Germany M38+479 48
Immingham, England N01+536 37
Imperatriz, Brazil S44-054 104
Imperatriz, Brazil R14-056 105
Imperia, Italy M42+439 56
Imperial Dam, Arizona V57+331 98
Imphal, India F66+247 71
Imroz, I., Turkey L26+402 74
Imtan, Syria K49+324 76
Inagua, I. Gt., Bahamas, The S80+211 101
Inagua, I. Lit., Bahamas, The S78+215 101
Inarijärvi, Finland L18+688 46
Inari L., Finland L12+690 46
Inch, Ireland, Rep. N37+527 43
Inchkeith, Scotland N19+560 41
Inchŏn, Korea D50+375 64
Incourt, Belgium M61+507 44
Indaal, L., Scotland N38+557 41
Indals Älv, Sweden L80+629 46
Indaw, Burma F53+242 71
Indawgyi L., Burma F52+253 71
Independence, Iowa U12+425 95
Independence, Kansas U34+372 95
Independence, Missouri U26+390 95
Independencia, Argentina S50-317 103
India, rep., S. Asia — 70-71
Indian Des. See Thar Des.
Indian L., New York S86+437 96
Indiana, Pennsylvania T25+407 96
Indiana, state, U.S.A. T72+402 99
Indianapolis, Indiana T67+398 91
Indian Head, Saskatchewan U82+505 88
Indian House L., Quebec S29+562 89
Indianola, Iowa U22+413 95
Indiga, U.S.S.R. J67+676 62
Indigirka, R., U.S.S.R. C30+678 63
Indonesia, rep., S.-E. Asia E30-050 65
Indore, India G84+226 70
Indre, dep., France M80+467 54
Indre-et-Loire, dep., France M86+472 54
Indur. See Nizamabad
Indus, R., Pakistan, etc. H10+354 70
Inebolu, Turkey K66+419 74
Inez, Kentucky T45+378 97
Infantes, Spain N18+387 52
Ingelmunster, Belgium M70+509 44
Ingersoll, Ontario T35+431 91
Ingham, Queensland C23-188 111
Inglefield Inlet, Greenland S58+770 26
Inglefield Ld., Greenland S00+790 26
Inglewood, New Zealand A34-391 112
Inglewood, Victoria C37-366 109
Ing Luiggi, Argentina S27-353 103
Ingolstadt, W. Germany M22+488 48
Ingrid Christensen Coast,
Antarctica G70-700 27
Inhambane, Mozambique K58-240 84
Ining, China G51+440 62
Inishark I., Ireland, Rep N62+536 42
Inishcrone, Ireland, Rep. N54+542 42
Inishbofin, I., Ireland, Rep. N61+536 42
Inisheer, I., Ireland, Rep. N57+531 43
Inishkea I., Ireland, Rep. N61+541 42
Inishmaan, I., Ireland, Rep. N58+531 43
Inishmore, I., Ireland, Rep. N58+531 43
Inishmurray, I., Ireland, Rep., N52+544 42
Inishowen & Hd.,
Ireland, Rep. N42+552 42
Inishtrahull, Ireland, Rep. N43+554 42
Inishtrahull Sd., Ireland, Rep. N44+554 42
Inishturk, I., Ireland, Rep. N61+537 42
Inklin R., British Columbia W75+590 88
Inner Sd., Scotland N36+574 40
Innerleithen, Scotland N18+556 41
Inner Mongolia, China F00+410 64
Innertkirchen, Switzerland M40+467 45
Innisfail, Queensland C24-172 111
Innsbruck, Austria M22+473 48
Inny R., Ireland, Rep. N47+535 43
Inowrocław, Poland L71+528 49
Inquisivi, Bolivia S43-167 104
Ins, Switzerland M47+470 45
In Salah, (Ain Salah) Alg. M76+270 80
Insar, U.S.S.R. K04+538 61
Insein, Burma F53+168 71
In Shan, China E72+417 66
Insterburg. See Chernyakhovsk.
Interlaken, Switzerland M43+467 45
International Falls, Minnesota U20+486 93
Interview I., Andaman Is. F75+130 71
Intragna, Switzerland M38+462 45
Inutil, B., Chile S60-536 103
Inveraray, Scotland N31+562 41
Inverbervie, Scotland N14+568 41
Invercargill, New Zealand A69-464 112
Inverell, New South Wales B84-288 109
Invergordon, Scotland N25+577 40
Inverkeithing, Scotland N20+560 41
Inverness, Nova Scotia S08+463 90
Inverness, Scotland N25+575 40
Invershin, Scotland N26+579 40
Inverurie, Scotland N14+573 40
Investigator Str., S. Aust. C75-356 111
Inyati, Zimbabwe L08-196 84
Inza, U.S.S.R. J82+538 61
Inzer, U.S.S.R. J14+542 61
Ioannina, Greece L55+397 59
Iola, Kansas U34+379 95
Iona, Nova Scotia S05+460 90
Iona I., Scotland N39+563 41
Ionia, Michigan T60+430 91
Ionia, Montana V14+453 93
Ionian Is., Greece L56+387 59
Ionian Sea, Italy, etc L72+380 51
Íos, I., Greece L28+367 59
Iowa state, U.S.A. U27+418 99
Iowa City, Iowa U09+416 95
Iowa Falls, Iowa U20+426 95
Ipala, Mexico V03+202 100
Ipiales, Colombia T15+008 104
Ipin, China F03+287 67
Ipiros, Greece L55+395 59
Ipoh, Malaysia F24+046 69
Ippy, Cent. Afr. Rep. L54+060 81
Ipswich, England M83+520 39
Ipswich, Queensland B73-274 111
Ipswich, S. Dakota U54+454 93
Ipu, Brazil Q63-043 105
Iquique, Chile S61-202 103
Iquitos, Peru S79-038 104
Iracoubo, French Guiana R49+054 105
Iráklia, I., Greece L27+368 59
Iráklion, Crete L29+353 59
Iran (Persia), S.W. Asia J40+330 75
Irapa, Venezuela S15+105 104
Irapuato, Mexico U68+206 100
Iraq, rep., S.-W. Asia L10+330 74
Irazu, Vol., Costa Rica T53+102 101
Irbid, Jordan K55+326 76
Irbit, U.S.S.R. H72+576 61
Ireland, I., British Isles — 42-43
Ireland, Rep. of
British Isles N48+520 34
Irendyk Mts., U.S.S.R. J12+520 61
Irgiz, Kazakh H83+485 62
Irian Jaya, New Guinea C60-054 65
Iringa, Tanzania K56-078 83
Irish Sea, British Isles N30+536 34
Irkutsk, U.S.S.R. F04+524 63
Iron Mt., Missouri U03+375 97
Iron City, Tennessee T76+350 97
Irondale, Ontario T21+448 91
Iron Knob, S. Australia C76-327 111
Iron Mountain, Michigan T78+458 91
Iron River, Michigan T82+461 91
Iron River, Wisconsin U09+465 93
Ironton, Missouri U04+376 95
Ironton, Ohio T46+386 97
Ironwood, Michigan U01+465 91
Iroquois, Ontario T42+499 91
Iroquois Chute, Quebec S78+477 91
Irrawaddy, Burma F60+172 71
Irrawaddy, R., Burma F54+228 71
Irthing R., England N17+549 37
Irtysh, R., U.S.S.R. H35+595 62
Irumu, Zaire L00+014 83
Irvine & R., Scotland N28+556 41
Irvinestown, N. Ireland N46+545 42
Isa, Mt., Queensland C64-208 111
Isabela I., Galapagos Is. U10-007 107
Isaccea, Romania L09+452 58
Isafjördhur, Iceland P48+661 46
Isai Kalat, Pakistan H66+269 70
Isa Khel, Pakistan H22+327 72
Isangi, Zaire L34+006 82
Isari, Greece L48+374 59
Ischia, I., Italy M07+407 57
Ise B., Japan C80+347 68
Iseghem. See Izegem
Iselin, Pennsylvania T26+406 96
Iseltwald, Switzerland M42+467 45
Isère, dep. & R., France M57+452 55
Isernia, Italy M05+416 57
Isha Baidao, Somalia K08+030 83
Ishan, China E68+245 67
Ishikari, R., Japan C40+435 68
Ishim, U.S.S.R. H34+562 62
Ishimbai, U.S.S.R. J23+534 61
Ishinomaki B., Japan C52+383 68
Ishkamish, Afghanistan H35+364 75
Ishkasham, Afghanistan H26+366 75
Ishpeming, Michigan T76+465 91
Ishqanan, Iran J38+272 75
Isil Kul, U.S.S.R. H23+549 62
Isiolo, Kenya K44+004 83
Isisford, Queensland C35-241 111
Iskenderun, Turkey K53+366 74
Iskilip, Turkey K64+407 74
Iskitim, U.S.S.R. G40+547 62
Iskut R., British Columbia W65+568 88
Islamabad, Pakistan H11+338 72
Islampur, India G29+249 73
Island L., Manitoba U25+538 88
Island Pond, Vermont S71+449 91
Islands, B. of, Newfoundland R84+493 90
Islands, B. of, New Zealand A35-353 112
Islay I., Scotland N37+558 41
Isle of Man., British Is. N28+542 37
Isle of Wight, England N08+507 39
Isleta, New Mexico V11+348 94
Isle Verte, Quebec S56+480 90
Ismailia, Egypt K76+306 81
Isna, Egypt K74+252 81
Isoka, Zambia K74-104 83
Isparta, Turkey K87+378 74
Israel, rep., S.-W. Asia K62+320 76
Issoudun, France M78+469 54
Issyk Kul, Oz., Kirgiz G80+424 62
Istanbul, Turkey L07+411 74
Istmina, Colombia T11+053 104
Istra, Yugoslavia M06+452 56
Itabaiana, Brazil Q31-073 105
Itacare, Brazil Q54-144 105
Itacoatiara, Brazil R8J-030 104
Itaete, Brazil Q67-130 105
Itaituba, Brazil R64-043 105
Itajai, Brazil R22-270 103
Italy, Central Europe M18+440 50
Itapecuru-mirim, Brazil Q86-033 105
Itapemirim, Cachoeiro de,
Brazil Q67-208 105
Itapetininga, Brazil R19-235 105
Itapura, Brazil R39-207 105
Itaqui, Brazil R70-292 103
Itarsi, India G72+225 70
Itasca, L., Minnesota U33+472 98
Itauna, Brazil Q88-201 105
Itéa, Greece L46+385 59
Ithaca, Michigan T58+433 91
Ithaca, New York T09+424 96
Itháci, See Ithaka
Ithaka, Greece L56+384 59
Itiés, Greece L50+401 59
Itula, Congo L12-036 83
Iturbe, Argentina S32-231 103
Ivailovgrad, Bulgaria L23+415 58
Ivanhoe, New South Wales C34-329 109
Ivanic Grad, Yugloslavia L82+457 56
Ivano-Frankovsk, Ukraine L34+490 60
Ivanovka, U.S.S.R. J55+525 61
Ivanovo, U.S.S.R. K24+570 60
Ivdel, U.S.S.R. H87+608 62
Iviza, I. See Ibiza, I.
Ivory Coast, W. Africa N40+080 80
Iwakuni, Japan D17+341 68
Iwaniska, Poland L52+507 49
Ixiamas, Bolivia S49-137 104
Ixtla, Mexico U55+186 100
Ixtlan de Juarez, Mexico U39+174 100
Iyang, China E16+284 67
Iyo Nada, Japan D18+336 68
Izabal & L., Guatemala T85+154 100
Izamal, Mexico T83+208 100
Izegem, Belgium M71+509 44
Izhevsk, U.S.S.R. J40+568 61
Izhma R., U.S.S.R. J37+650 62
Izki, Oman J14+229 75
Izmail, Ukraine L07+454 60
Izmir, Turkey L17+384 74
Izmit, Turkey L01+408 74
Izra, Syria K52+329 76
Iztapa, Guatemala U04+139 100
Izu Pen., Japan C66+348 68
Izu Shichito, Japan C62+343 68
Izyum, Ukraine K47+492 60
Jääski, U.S.S.R. L06+610 47
Jabalpur, India G60+232 73
Jabbeke, Belgium M72+512 44
Jabbul, Syria K45+361 76
Jablonec, Czechoslovakia L89+507 48
Jabrin Oasis, Saudi Arabia J66+232 74
Jaburú, Brazil S39-040 104
Jaca, Spain N03+426 53
Jacarezinho, Brazil R30-232 105
Jachal, Argentina S53-303 103
Jacitara, Brazil S32-019 104
Jacksboro, Tennessee T55+363 97
Jackson, Kentucky T50+375 97
Jackson, Louisiana U07+308 95
Jackson, Michigan T56+423 91
Jackson, Minnesota U30+436 93
Jackson, Mississippi U01+323 97
Jackson, Missouri T88+374 97
Jackson, N. Carolina T15+364 97
Jackson, Ohio T46+391 91
Jackson, Tennessee T83+356 97
Jackson, Wyoming V36+434 93
Jackson Mts., Nevada V81+414 92
Jacksonville, Florida T40+303 97
Jacksonville, Illinois U02+398 95
Jacksonville, N. Carolina T15+348 97
Jacksonville, Texas U32+320 95
Jacmel, Haiti S75+183 101
Jacobabad, Pakistan H49+282 80
Jacobina, Brazil Q63-112 105
Jacques Cartier, Mt., Que. S36+490 90
Jacquet River, N.B. S36+479 90
Jade Mines, Burma F53+256 71
Jadib, Yemen, South J42+166 75
Jaén, Spain N22+377 52
Jafarabad, India H22+209 70
Jaffa (Yafo), Israel K62+320 76
Jaffna, Sri Lanka G60+097 70
Jagadhri, India G76+301 72
Jagdispur, India G33+254 73
Jagodina, Yugoslavia L53+440 58
Jagraon, India G87+308 72
Jaguarão, Brazil R51-324 103

Jaguari, Brazil R58-295 103
Jaguariaira, Brazil R28-242 105
Jaguaruna, Brazil R24-286 103
Jahanabad, India G30+252 73
Jahangirabad, India G71+284 72
Jahra, Kuwait J74+294 74
Jahrum, Iran J38+284 75
Jaicos, Brazil Q66-074 105
Jaipur, India G84+268 70
Jaipur, India G21+208 71
Jais, India G51+263 73
Jaisalmer, India H24+268 70
Jajarm, Iran J22+370 75
Jakarta, Java, Indonesia E79+062 65
Jäkkvik, Sweden L78+663 46
Jakobi, Estonia L21+592 47
Jakobstad. See Pietarsaari
Jalalabad, Afghanistan H28+345 72
Jalalpur, India G44+263 73
Jalalpur, Pakistan H22+295 72
Jalalpur, Pakistan H04+327 72
Jalapa, Nicaragua T65+139 101
Jalapa Enriquez, Mexico U42+195 100
Jalasjärvi, Finland L43+625 46
Jalaun, India G64+260 73
Jaldak, Afghanistan H50+319 75
Jalgaon, India G86+210 70
Jalisco, state, Mexico U80+200 100
Jalk, Iran H74+276 75
Jalor, India H14+252 70
Jalpaiguri, India G07+265 73
Jaluit, I., Marshall Is. A64+060 106
Jamaica, I., West Indies T14+181 101
Jamaja, Estonia L48+580 47
Jamalabad, Iran J73+373 74
Jamalpur, Bangladesh G00+249 73
Jamalpur, India G21+253 73
Jamberoo, New S. Wales B86-346 109
Jambi, Sumatra, Indonesia F08-016 65
Jamdena, I., See Yamdena
James B., Canada T30+530 89
James Ras., N. Terr., Aust. D15-241 110
James R., S. Dakota U50+442 98
James R., Virginia T20+377 97
Jamesburg, California W10+364 92
James Ross, I., Antarctica R75-640 27
Jamestown, New York T25+421 91
Jamestown & Res., N. Dakota U52+469 93
Jamestown, S. Australia C68-332 109
James W. Ellsworth Ld,
Antarctica U40-770 27
Jamiltepec, Mexico U47+162 100
Jammer Bugt, Denmark M36+573 47
Jammu & Kashmir H01+327 72
Jammu & Kashmir, India-
Pakistan H00+350 70
Jamnagar, India H30+224 70
Jampur, Pakistan H26+296 72
Jamrad, Afghanistan H42+331 75
Jamrao, Pakistan H35+255 70
Jämsä Finland L29+619 47
Jamshedpur, India G22+228 73
Jamui, India G22+249 73
Jamuna R., Bangladesh G02+250 73
Jandaq, Iran J34+341 75
Jandiala, India G89+315 72
Janesville, Wisconsin T84+427 95
Jangipur, India G11+245 73
Jani Khel, Pakistan H27+328 72
Janjira, India H12+184 70
Jan Mayen, I., Arctic Ocean N55+710 62
Janos, Mexico V18+310 100
Jansath, India G73+293 72
Jansenville, Cape Province L30-330 84
Januaria, Brazil Q86-154 105
Janze, France N09+480 54
Jaoho, China D06+472 64
Jaora, India G89+236 70
Japan & Sea of, E. Asia C60+400 64
Japen, I., See Yapen I.
Japur R., Brazil S45+019 104
Japvo Mt., India F65+256 71
Jaragua, Brazil R25-265 103
Jaragua, Brazil R26-157 105
Jarales, New Mexico V12+346 94
Jaramillo, Argentina S43-472 103
Jarandilla, Spain N34+402 52
Jardim, Brazil Q40-065 105
Jardines de la Reina, Cuba T24+211 101
Jarji, Nigeria M46+108 80
Jarocin, Poland L75+520 49
Jaromer, Czechoslovakia L85+504 49
Jarosław, Poland L44+500 49
Järpen, Sweden M09+634 46
Jarrow, England N09+550 37
Jarvis I., Pacific Ocean Y60-002 106
Järvsö, Sweden L83+617 47
Jashpurnagar, India G35+229 73
Jask, Iran J13+257 75
Jason I., Falkland Is. S07-510 103
Jasper, Florida T48+305 97
Jasper, Georgia T57+345 97
Jasper, Texas U24+310 95
Jasper & Park, Alberta V80+533 88
Jassy. See Iasi.
Jastrowie, Poland L79+534 49
Jaswantnagar, India G66+269 73
Jaszberény, Hungary L60+475 49
Jath, India G88+170 70
Jativa, Spain N03+390 53
Jatoba, Brazil Q50-092 105
Jaú, Brazil R21-222 105
Jauche, Belgium M60+507 44
Jauf, Saudi Arabia K31+299 74
Jauhari, Saudi Arabia J46+165 75
Jauja, Peru T02-117 104
Jaumave, Mexico U57+234 100
Jaunjelgava, Latvia L29+566 47
Jaunpur, India G44+258 73
Java, I., Indonesia E60-073 65
Javari, R., Peru-Brazil S78-065 104
Javier, I., Chile S86-471 103
Jawa, Nigeria M24+128 81
Jawalamukhi, India G82+318 72
Jayapura, Indonesia C57+026 65
Jazir, Oman J20+186 75
Jebba, Nigeria M62+090 80
Jeble, Syria K54+354 76
Jech Doab, Pakistan H14+321 72
Jedabya, Libya L58+306 81
Jedburgh, Scotland N15+555 41
Jedede, Saudi Arabia K29+218 74
Jefferson, Georgia T51+341 97
Jefferson, Wisconsin T82+430 95
Jefferson, Mt., Oregon W11+446 92
Jefferson City, Missouri U13+386 95
Jeffersonville, Indiana T64+383 97
Jehol. See Chêng-têhshih.
Jekabpils, Latvia L25+565 47
Jelgava, Latvia L37+566 47
Jelsava, Czechoslovakia L59+486 49
Jemeppe, Belgium M62+505 44
Jena, E. Germany M21+509 48
Jenin, Jordan K58+325 76
Jenipapo, Brazil R84-064 104
Jennings, Louisiana U16+302 95
Jenolan Caves, New S. Wales C00-339 109
Jeparit, Victoria C48-362 109
Jeppo, Finland L44+634 46
Jerablus, Syria K42+368 76
Jerash, Jordan K55+323 76
Jeremie, Haiti S84+187 101
Jerez, Mexico U78+228 100
Jerez de la Frontera, Spain N37+367 52
Jeriban, Somalia J66+072 83
Jericho, Jordan K57+319 76
Jericho, Queensland C24-234 111
Jerilderie, New S. Wales C26-354 109
Jerome, Arizona V43+348 94
Jerruck, Pakistan H40+250 70
Jersey, I., Channel Is. N13+492 54
Jersey City, New Jersey S84+407 96
Jerseyshore, Pennsylvania T14+412 96
Jerusalem, Israel-Jordan K59+318 76
Jervis B., New South Wales B86-351 109
Jervois Ra., N. Terr., Aust. C83-225 111
Jesenik, Czechoslovakia L77+503 49
Jesselton, Sabah E24+060 65
Jessore, Bangladesh G04+231 73
Jesup, Georgia T41+316 97
Jesus I., Quebec S81+457 91
Jesus Maria, Argentina S25-310 103
Jesus Maria, Mexico V16+282 100
Jetalsar, India H26+217 70
Jeypore, India G44+189 71
Jezzin, Lebanon K57+335 76
Jhal, Pakistan H45+282 70
Jhalrapatan, India G82+246 70
Jhang Maghiana, Pakistan H16+313 72
Jhansi, India G68+254 73
Jhau, Pakistan H56+262 70
Jhelum, Pakistan H08+330 72
Jhelum R., Pakistan H14+325 72
Jhunjhunu, India G87+281 72
Jiachan, Tibet G53+316 70
Jianpur, India G40+262 73
Jibhalanta, Mongolia F49+480 63
Jicaro, Nicaragua T65+138 101
Jičin, Czechoslovakia L88+505 49
Jidd, Iraq K32+328 74
Jidda, Saudi Arabia K35+215 74
Jiggitai L., Tibet G19+350 71
Jihlava, Czechoslovakia L87+494 49
Jildiah, Jebel, Saudi Arabia K15+277 74
Jimena de la Frontera, Spain N32+365 52
Jimenez, Mexico U64+290 100
Jimenez, Mexico V00+270 100
Jimma, Ethiopia K48+076 83
Jim Thorpe, Pennsylvania T05+408 96
Jind, India G82+293 72
Jinotega, Nicaragua T66+131 101
Jipijapa, Ecuador T33-012 104
Jirgalanta, Mongolia F80+480 63
Jirm, Afghanistan H25+368 75
Jisha, Saudi Arabia J61+253 74
Jisresh Shughur, Syria K52+358 76
Jiul R., Romania L37+441 58
Jiza, Jordan K54+317 76
João Pessoa, Brazil Q28-071 105
Jodhpur, India H12+263 70
Joensuu, Finland L01+626 46
Jofane, Mozambique K64-214 84
Jogjakarta, See Yogyakarta
Johannesburg, Transvaal L12-262 84
John o' Groats, Scotland N18+586 40
Johnsonburg, Pennsylvania T22+415 96
Johnson City, Tennessee T44+363 97
Johnston I., Pacific Ocean Z28+170 106
Johnstown, Ireland, Rep. N41+534 43
Johnstown, New York S85+430 96
Johnstown, Pennsylvania T24+403 96
Johore Baharu, Malaysia F08+015 69
Joinville, Brazil R23-263 103
Joinville, France M59+484 54
Joinville I., Antarctica R60-630 27
Jokkmökk, Sweden L61+666 46
Jol Plat., Saudi Arabia J65+154 74
Joliet, Illinois T78+415 95
Joliette, Quebec S81+460 91
Jolo, I., Philippines D82+059 65
Jonava, Lithuania L34+551 47
Jonesboro, Arkansas U04+358 95
Jonesboro, Georgia T56+335 97
Jonesboro, Illinois T86+374 97
Jonesboro, Louisiana U16+322 97
Jonesport, Maine S46+445 90
Joniškis, Lithuania L39+562 47
Jönköping, Sweden M05+578 47
Jonquière, Quebec S67+484 90
Jonuta, Mexico U13+180 100
Joplin, Missouri U27+372 95
Jordan, Minnesota U22+447 93
Jordan, Montana V12+473 93
Jordan, S.-W. Asia K53+310 74
Jordan, R., Israel K57+323 76
Jordan R., Utah V42+407 94
Jorhat, India F65+267 71
Jorje Montt, I., Chile S88-513 103
Jorna da Del Muerto,
New Mexico V11+330 94
Joseph Bonaparte Gulf,
W. Australia D40-130 110
Jostedalsbre Glacier, Norway M47+616 47
Jotunheimen, Norway M42+615 34
Joux, L. de, Switzerland M52+466 45
Jowai, India F76+254 71
Juan de Fuca Str.,
U.S.A.-Canada W20+479 98
Juan Fernandez I.,
Pacific Ocean T25-345 107
Juan Stuven, I., Chile T00-479 103
Juárez, Argentina R89-376 103
Juarez, Mexico U01+188 100
Juba, Sudan K80+050 81
Jubba, Saudi Arabia K23+280 74
Jubbulpore. See Jabalpur
Jubeil, Lebanon K56+341 76
Jubi, C., Morocco N78+280 80
Jucaro, Cuba T23+216 101
Juchitan, Mexico U31+164 100
Judenburg, Austria M02+471 48
Judique, Nova Scotia S09+459 90
Judith, Montana V28+477 93
Judith Pt., Rhode Island S67+414 91
Juian, China D85+278 67
Juichow. See Kaoan
Juist, I., W. Germany M48+537 48
Juiz de Fora, Brazil Q80-217 105
Jujuy, Argentina S32-242 103
Jukao, China D86+324 66
Jukkasjarvi, Sweden L52+679 34
Julaco, Bolivia S46-209 104
Julesburg, Colorado U74+410 94
Juli, Peru S57-162 104
Juliaca, Peru S61-156 104
Julianstown, Ireland, Rep. N38+537 42
Julio de Castilhos, Brazil R52-293 103
Jullundur, India G86+313 72
Jumaima, Iraq K08+298 74
Jumet, Belgium M63+504 44
Jumilla, Spain N08+385 53
Jumin, Iran J08+345 75
Jumla, Nepal G47+293 73
Jumna (Yamuna), R., India G58+260 73
Junagarh, India H27+216 70
Junan, China E33+330 66
Junction City, Kansas U41+390 95
Jundiai, Brazil R11-232 105
Juneau, Alaska W86+585 99
Junee, New South Wales C14-349 109
Jungfrau, mt., Switzerland M42+465 45
Jungfraujoch, Switzerland M42+465 45
Jungkiang, China E68+259 67
Junin, Argentina S67-400 103
Junin, Argentina S06-345 103
Junin, Chile S61-198 103
Junin, Peru T06-112 104
Juning. See Junan
Juniper, New Brunswick S43+466 90
Juniye, (Jounie) Lebanon K56+340 76
Junsele, Sweden L78+637 46
Juojarvi, Finland L08+628 46
Jupia, Brazil R39-208 105
Juquila, Mexico U45+163 100
Jura, dep., France M54+467 54
Jura, mts., France-Switz. M54+463 54
Jura I. & Sd. of, Scotland N35+560 41
Jurado, Colombia T17+072 104
Jurbarkas, Lithuania L43+551 47
Jurf ed Darawish, Jordan K55+307 76
Jüri, Estonia L30+594 47
Juruá, R., Brazil S40-045 104
Juruena & R., Brazil R83-128 104
Juruty, Brazil R67-020 105
Jusiye, Syria K50+344 76
Jussy, Switzerland M52+462 45
Justlahuaco, Mexico U48+174 100
Justo Daract, Argentina S31-338 103
Jutahy, Brazil S42-027 104
Juticalpa, Honduras T64+146 101
Jutland. See Jylland
Juuka, Finland L05+632 46
Juwain, Afghanistan H80+316 75
Juwara, Oman J16+190 75
Jylland, Denmark M36+562 47
Jylland, South, Denmark M36+552 47
Jyväskylä, Finland L26+623 46
K2, Mt, Kashmir G81+359 72
Kabaena, I., Indonesia D79-054 65
Kabala, Sierra Leone N70+096 80
Kabale, Uganda L00-014 83
Kabalega Falls, Uganda K80+020 83
Kabba, Nigeria M54+078 80
Kabia, I., Indonesia D87-061 65
Kabinda, Zaire L32-062 82
Kabongo, Zaire L26-074 82
Kabul & R., Afghanistan H34+346 75
Kabunda, Zaire L04-126 83
Kabwe, Zambia L10-144 83
Kačanik, Yugoslavia L53+424 58
Kachiry, Kazakh G84+530 62
Kachkar, U.S.S.R. H84+544 61
Kachuga, U.S.S.R. E84+540 63
Kadaura, India G61+260 73
Kadina, S. Australia C74-340 109
Kadiri, India G70+141 70
Kadiyevka, Ukraine K39+486 60
Kadoka, S. Dakota U69+438 93
Kadom, U.S.S.R. K15+546 61
Kadugli, Sudan L02+110 81
Kaduna, Nigeria M46+106 80
Kadur, India G84+136 70
Kadyy, U.S.S.R. K11+577 61
Kadzand, Netherlands M70+514 44
Kaesong, Korea D52+380 64
Kaf, Saudi Arabia K46+315 74
Kafakumba, Congo L38-096 82
Kafanchan, Nigeria M40+096 80
Kafia Kingi, Sudan L34+092 81
Kafra, Chad L44+162 81
Kafr Behum, Syria K50+351 76
Kafrun, Syria K52+348 76
Kagan, Uzbek H63+396 62
Kagi. See Chiai
Kagmar, Sudan K88+144 81
Kagoshima, Japan D27+316 68
Kagoshima B., Japan D28+311 68
Kagul, Moldavia L11+459 60
Kahafa, Saudi Arabia K10+270 74
Kahama, Tanzania K74-038 83
Kahoka, Missouri U10+404 95
Kahra, Yemen J89+161 74
Kahror, Pakistan H18+296 72
Kahta, Turkey K38+381 74
Kahuta, Pakistan H09+336 72
Kai-Kep, Indonesia D14-058 65
Kaiama, Nigeria M66+096 80
Kaiapoi, New Zealand A44-434 112
Kai-chow, China E30+357 66
Kaieteur Fall, Guyana R87+052 104
Kai fêng, China E33+348 66
Kaigo, Sudan K80+060 81
Kaihwa. See Wenshan
Kaikoura, New Zealand A38-424 112
Kaikoura Ra., New Zealand A40-421 112
Kailas Ra., India-Tibet G78+352 70
Kaimanawa Mts., N.Z. A24-390 112
Kaimganj, India G64+275 73
Kaimur Ra., India G48+245 73
Kaipara Harb., New Zealand A35-364 112
Kaira, India H13+226 70
Kairana, India G77+294 72
Kairouan, Tunisia M30+358 81
Kairovo, U.S.S.R. J16+558 61
Kaisarie. See Kayseri
Kaišedorys, Lithuania L33+549 47
Kaiserslautern, W. Germany M43+494 48
Kaiser Wilhelm II Ld.,
Antarctica G00-670 27
Kaitangata, New Zealand A61-463 112
Kaithal, India G81+297 72
Kai-yuan, China D66+427 66
Kajaani, Finland L13+642 46
Kajiado, Kenya K50-018 83
Kajiki, Japan D26+317 68
Kajuri Kach, Pakistan H31+321 72
Kakamari, Uganda K64+034 83
Kakamega, Kenya K60+002 83
Kakh, Iran J08+342 75
Kakhovskoye Vdkhr., Ukr. K62+471 60
Kakia, Botswana L40-248 84
Kakisa, L., N.-W. Terr. V76+607 88
Kakori, India G55+269 73
Kakoyarra, New S. Wales C51-317 109
Kaksha, U.S.S.R. J80+582 61
Kalabagh, Pakistan H21+330 72
Kalabaka, Greece L50+397 59
Kalabo, Zambia L44-150 84
Kalabsha, Egypt K74+234 81
Kalach, U.S.S.R. K24+504 61
Kaladan, Burma F72+211 71
Kalahari Des., Botswana L40-238 84
Kalajoki, Finland L36+643 46
Kalakan, U.S.S.R. E19+552 63
Kalakepen, Sumatra F43+028 65
Kalámai, Greece L47+370 59
Kalamáta. See Kalámai.
Kalamazoo, Michigan T63+424 91
Kalamboa, Sudan L30+126 81
Kalamos I., Greece L55+386 59
Kala Nao, Afghanistan H71+350 75
Kalanaur, India G82+289 72
Kalangali, Tanzania K66-062 83
Kalannie, W. Australia E18-302 110
Kala Sarkari, Afghanistan H46+358 75
Kalat, Pakistan H50+270 70
Kalat-i-Ghilzai, Afghanistan H49+320 75
Kalat-i-Nadiri, Iran J01+371 75
Kalaw, Burma F50+207 71
Kale, Burma F65+232 71
Kalediran, Turkey K74+362 74
Kalémié Zaire L04-060 83
Kalewa, Burma F64+232 71
Kalgan. See Changkiakow
Kalgoorlie, W. Australia D82-307 110
Kalikino, U.S.S.R. J35+528 61
Kalimnos, I., Greece L19+370 59
Kalingapatnam, India G35+184 70
Kalinin, U.S.S.R. K56+568 60
Kaliningrad, U.S.S.R. L57+547 47
Kalinino, U.S.S.R. E70+599 63
Kalispell, Montana V56+479 98
Kalisz, Poland L71+518 49
Kaliua, Tanzania K80-050 83
Kalix Älv, Sweden L56+676 46
Kalixfors, Sweden L59+677 46
Kalka, India G78+308 72
Kalkaska, Michigan T61+448 91
Kalkfeld, Namibia L84-208 84
Kalkfontein, Botswana L54-222 84
Kalkwerk, Namibia L76-268 84
Kallavesi, Finland L14+628 46
Kallim, Chad L54+128 81
Kalloni, Greece L23+392 59
Kall Sjön, Sweden M12+637 46
Kalmar, Sweden L82+567 47
Kalmar Sund, Sweden L82+565 47
Kalmykovo, Kazakh J50+490 62
Kalna, India G10+232 73
Kalocsa, Hungary L66+465 49
Kalokhorio, Cyprus K72+351 76
Kalol, India H14+234 70
Kalpi, India G62+261 73
Kaltag, Alaska Y50+640 99
Kaluga, U.S.S.R. K52+545 60
Kalule, Zaire L24-096 82
Kalundborg, Denmark M23+557 47
Kalundu, Zambia L02-104 83
Kalutara, Sri Lanka G61+065 70
Kalvariya, Lithuania L41+544 47
Kalyan, India H11+192 70
Kalyazin, U.S.S.R. K44+572 60
Kama, R., U.S.S.R. J22+608 62
Kamah, Labrador S22+590 89
Kamaishi, Japan C48+393 68
Kamalampaka, Tanzania K86-056 83
Kamalia, Pakistan H08+307 72
Kaman, India G77+276 72
Kamaran, I., Red Sea K14+154 74
Kamasin, India G54+255 73
Kamassa, Cameroon M10+078 81
Kamchatka, U.S.S.R. B40+560 63
Kamen, U.S.S.R. G52+538 62
Kamenets Podolskiy, Ukraine L21+488 60
Kamenskoye, U.S.S.R. B00+625 63
Kamensk Shakhtinski,
U.S.S.R. K28+483 61
Kamensk Ural'skiy, U.S.S.R. H79+564 61
Kamet, Mt., India G64+309 70
Kami Iwani, Japan D10+351 68
Kamina, Zaire L30-088 82
Kamloops, Brit. Columbia W02+507 88
Kamnik, Yugoslavia M02+462 56
Kamouraska, Quebec S59+476 90
Kampa Dzong, Tibet G09+283 71
Kampala, Uganda K74+002 83
Kampen, Netherlands M54+526 44
Kampot, Cambodia F05+106 69
Kamptee, India G64+212 70
Kamsack, Saskatchewan U71+513 88
Kamyshin, U.S.S.R. J88+501 61
Kamyshlov, U.S.S.R. H74+568 61
Kanab, Utah V45+370 94
Kannauj, India G61+270 73

Kanawha, R., W. Virginia T38+382 97
Kanayama, Japan C77+356 68
Kanazawa, Japan C80+366 68
Kanchanaburi, Thailand F33+140 69
Kanchipuram, India G61+126 70
Kanchenjunga, mt., Nepal G11+277 73
Kandahar, Afghanistan H56+316 75
Kandalaksha, U.S.S.R. K73+674 62
Kandaya, Latvia L43+570 47
Kandavu, I., Fiji A10-190 106
Kandhla, India G76+293 72
Kandi, India G11+239 73
Kandole, Zaire L38-034 82
Kandos, New South Wales C00-329 109
Kandy, Sri Lanka G57+073 70
Kane, Pennsylvania T23+416 96
Kane Basin, Greenland S60+790 26
Kanev, Ukraine K81+497 60
Kangan, Iran J47+278 75
Kangar, Malaysia F28+064 69
Kangaroo I., S. Australia C76-358 111
Kangāvar, Iran J72+346 74
Kangmar, Kashmir G70+334 70
Kango, Gabon M30+002 82
Kangpao, China E31+418 66
Kangra, India G82+321 72
Kangsa R., Bangladesh F88+250 71
Kanhsien, China E30+259 67
Kani, Burma F61+224 71
Kaniva, Victoria C53-364 109
Kankakee, Illinois T77+411 95
Kankan, Guinea N56+104 80
Kanker, India G50+202 70
Kankesanturai, Sri Lanka G60+098 70
Kan Kiang, China E28+274 64
Kannus, Finland L37+639 46
Kano, Nigeria M38+118 80
Kanpetlet, Burma F67+214 71
Kanpur, India G58+265 73
Kansas, state, U.S.A. U60+387 98
Kansas R., Kansas U36+390 95
Kansas City, Kansas U28+391 95
Kansas City, Missouri U28+390 95
Kansk, U.S.S.R. F55+563 63
Kansu, prov., China E84+350 66
Kantai, India G28+262 73
Kantchari, Upper Volta M82+124 80
Kanturk, Ireland, Rep. N53+522 43
Kanuma, Japan C61+365 68
Kanus, Namibia L68-278 84
Kanyinchaung, Burma F76+210 71
Kaoan, China E27+284 67
Kao-bang, Indo-China E82+227 69
Kaocheng, China E30+349 66
Kaohsiung, Taiwan D88+226 67
Kaolack, Senegal P06+142 80
Kaolan. See Lanchow
Kao Lu-ang, mt., Thailand F32+086 69
Kaomi, China E01+363 66
Kaoyi, China E31+376 66
Kaoyu, China E03+328 66
Kaoyu Hu, China E04+328 66
Kapal, Kazakh G65+452 62
Kapalu, Kashmir G82+352 72
Kapfenberg, Austria L88+473 48
Kapiri Mposhi, Tanzania L06-140 83
Kapiskau R., Ontario T52+526 89
Kapiti I., New Zealand A31-408 112
Kapoeas, R., Borneo E52+001 65
Kapoeta, Sudan K68+048 81
Kaposvár, Hungary L73+464 58
Kapsabet, Kenya K60+002 83
Kapsukas, Lithuania L40+545 47
Kapunda, S. Australia C66-343 109
Kapurthala, India G88+313 72
Kapuskasing, Ontario T46+496 89
Kara, U.S.S.R. H66+692 62
Kara Sea, U.S.S.R. H00+750 62
Kara Bogaz Gol, Turkmen. J40+413 62
Karabuk, Turkey K74+411 74
Karabuta, Iran J73+370 74
Karacabey, Turkey L10+402 74
Karaca Dagh, Turkey K74+394 74
Karachev, U.S.S.R. K60+531 60
Karachi, Pakistan H47+248 70
Karaga, U.S.S.R. B11+592 63
Karaganda, Kazakh H10+500 62
Karaginskiy Os., U.S.S.R. B05+590 63
Karak, Tibet G67+322 70
Kara Kalpakskaya, Uzbek. J12+430 62
Karakelong, I., Indonesia D49+042 65
Karakoram Ra., Kashmir G84+364 72
Karakose, Turkey K12+398 74
Kara Kum, Turkmen J10+393 62
Kara Kum Can., Turkmen H75+370 75
Karaman, Turkey K71+372 74
Karamea, New Zealand A47-412 112
Karamea Bight, N.Z. A50-413 112
Karamsur Pass, Pakistan H08+368 72
Karand, Iran J82+343 74
Karasa, U.S.S.R. J56+547 61
Karasburg, Namibia L66-282 84
Kara Shahr, Sinkiang, China G22+421 62
Karasjok, Norway L27+694 46
Karatina, Kenya K46-004 83
Karatsu, Japan D30+336 68
Karaul, U.S.S.R. G37+701 62
Karauli, India G78+265 73
Karaurgan, Turkey K17+404 74
Kardam, Tibet G54+304 70
Kardhitsa, Greece L48+394 59
Karelskaya A.S.S.R. (Karelia), rep., U.S.S.R. K80+642 62
Karenni, Burma F45+194 71
Karesuando, Sweden L45+684 46
Karganrud, Iran J66+379 74
Karghalik, Sinkiang, China G75+379 72
Kargil, Kashmir G83+345 72
Kargopol, U.S.S.R. K36+615 60
Karhal, India G66+270 73
Kariba, Dam & L., Zam.- Zimb. L06-164 84
Karibib, Namibia L84-218 84
Karikal, India G61+110 70
Karimata, I., Indonesia E67-015 65
Karin, Somalia J86+108 83
Karis, (Karjaa), Finland L38+601 47
Kariz, Iran H85+349 75
Karkaralinsk, U.S.S.R. G87+495 62
Karkkila, Finland L34+605 47
Karla Marksa, Pik, mt., Tad. H16+372 75
Karl-Marx Stadt, E. Germany M09+508 48
Karlovac, Yugoslavia L87+455 56
Karlovy Vary, Czechoslovakia M13+502 48
Karlsbad. See Karlovy Vary
Karlsborg, Sweden M03+585 47
Karlshamn, Sweden M01+562 47
Karlskrona, Sweden L86+561 47
Karlsruhe, W. Germany M38+490 48
Karlstad, Sweden M09+595 47
Karlukovo, U.S.S.R. B43+688 63
Karmöy, I., Norway M58+593 47
Karnal, India G78+297 72
Karnataka, India G79+123 70
Karnes, Texas U47+289 94
Karnten, prov., Austria M06+467 48
Karona Fall, Guyana R8^+040 104
Karoonda, S. Australia C61-352 109
Karora, Sudan K40+176 83
Karpáthos, I. & Str., Greece L17+356 59
Karperon, Greece L50+400 59
Karroo Great, Cape Province L46-326 84
Kars, Turkey K12+406 74
Karsakpai, Kazakh H50+480 62
Kärsämäki, Finland L25+640 46
Kārsava, Latvia L14+568 47
Karshi, Uzbek H56+388 62
Karstula, Finland L31+629 46
Karsun, U.S.S.R. J78+542 61
Kartaly, U.S.S.R. H86+530 61
Kartarpur, India G87+314 72
Kartse, Kashmir G83+343 72
Karungi, Sweden L37+661 46
Karungu, Kenya K66-010 83
Karunki, Finland L36+661 46
Karur, India G71+112 70
Karvina, Czechoslovakia L69+498 49
Karwar, India H05+149 70
Karymskoye, U.S.S.R. E34+517 63
Kasai R., Zaire L60-034 82
Kasama, Zambia K82-104 83
Kasanga, Tanzania K84-084 83
Kasauli, India G78+309 72
Kasba L., N.-W. Territories U74+604 88
Kasempa, Zambia L26-134 82
Kasenga, Zaire L08-106 83
Kasenga, Zambia L20-158 84
Kasganj, India G68+278 73
Kashan, Iran J53+340 75
Kashgar, China G83+395 62
Kashing, China D85+308 66
Kashira, U.S.S.R. K40+548 60
Kashiwazaki, Japan C68+374 68
Kashmir, see Jammu and Kashmir
Kashmor, Pakistan H32+283 70
Kasimov, U.S.S.R. K22+549 61
Kasinka, Botswana L34-184 84
Kaskinen, (Kasko) Finland L53+624 46
Kasongo, Zaire L20-044 82
Kásos, I., Greece L19+354 59
Kásós Str., Crete L20+352 59
Kaspichan, Bulgaria L17+433 58
Kassala, Sudan K52+154 83
Kassandra, Greece L39+400 59
Kassel, W. Germany M33+515 48
Kastamonu, Turkey K66+414 74
Kastélli, Crete L38+355 59
Kasterlee, Belgium M60+512 44
Kastoria, Greece L53+405 59
Kastrosikiá, Greece L56+391 59
Kasulu, Tanzania L00-046 83
Kasungu, Malawi K70-132 83
Kasur, Pakistan H03+311 72
Katahdin, Mt., Maine S53+459 90
Katahdin Iron Works, Maine S55+455 90
Katákolon, Greece L52+377 59
Katanga, See Shaba
Katanning, W. Australia E14-336 110
Katav Ivanovsk, U.S.S.R. J11+548 61
Katerini, Greece L45+403 59
Katha, Burma F52+242 71
Kathawachaga, L., N.-W.T. V40+661 88
Katherine, N. Terr., Aust. D16-144 110
Kathmandu, Nepal G28+277 73
Kathua, Kashmir G87+324 72
Katihar, India G14+256 73
Katmai Vol., Alaska T32+580 99
Kato Akhaia, Greece L51+381 59
Káto Nevrokópion, Greece L37+413 58
Katoomba, New S. Wales B88-338 109
Katowice, Poland L66+503 49
Katrine, L., Scotland N27+563 41
Katrineholm, Sweden L83+590 47
Katsina, Nigeria M44+128 80
Kattegat, Sweden-Denmark M24+570 47
Kattowitz. See Katowice
Katwa, India G11+236 236 73
Katwewe, Zaire L10-084 83
Katwijk-aan-Zee, Netherlands M64+522 44
Kauai, I., Hawaii Y58+220 107
Kaufbeuren, W. Germany M26+478 48
Kauhava, Finland L42+631 46
Kaukauna, Wisconsin T80+443 91
Kaunus, Lithuania L36+549 47
Kauriya, India G44+212 71
Kautokeino, Norway L42+689 46
Kavak, Turkey K54+411 74
Kavali, India G60+150 70
Kaválla, Greece L33+411 58
Kaválla, Greece L34+409 59
Kavkas, Bolshoi & Maly, mts., U.S.S.R. K80+415 62
Kawakawa, New Zealand A35-354 112
Kawambwa, Zambia L06-098 83
Kawanoe, Japan D08+340 68
Kawardha, India G53+220 73
Kawasaki, Japan C62+355 68
Kawhia, New Zealand A31-381 112
Kawich Ra., Nevada V71+379 92
Kawkareik, Burma F40+165 71
Kaw Peunan, Thailand F30+097 69
Kaw Samui, Thailand F30+094 69
Kayes, Mali N68+142 80
Kayseri, Turkey K58+387 74
Kaysville, Utah V42+410 94
Kazachye, U.S.S.R. C82+707 63
Kazakhskaya, rep., U.S.S.R. H60+470 62
Kazalinsk, Kazakh H78+457 62
Kazan, U.S.S.R. J66+558 61
Kazanlük, Bulgaria L28+426 58
Kazérun, Iran J50+296 75
Kazvin, Iran J60+363 74
Kdyne, Czechoslovakia M12+494 48
Kéa (Tziá), I., Greece L34+374 59
Kearney, Nebraska U54+406 95
Keban Maden, Turkey K38+388 74
Ke-bao I., Vietnam E75+212 69
Kecherma, Niger M12+172 81
Kechika R., Brit. Columbia W40+588 88
Kecskemét, Hungary L62+469 49
Kedainiai, Lithuania L36+553 47
Kedgwick, New Brunswick S44+476 90
Kediri, Java, Indonesia E48-079 65
Keele Pk., N.-W. Terr. W60+637 88
Keele R., N.-W. Territories W38+642 88
Keelung (Chilung), Taiwan D80+251 67
Keene, New Hampshire S74+429 96
Keeper Hill, Ireland, Rep. N50+527 43
Keeseville, New York S81+445 91
Keetmanshoop, Namibia L72-266 84
Keewatin, Dist., N.-W. Terr. — 88-89
Keewong, New S. Wales C30-323 109
Kefallinia, Greece L57+382 59
Kegaska, Quebec S07+502 9
Keighley, England N11+539 37
Keila, Estonia L33+593 47
Keita, Chad L42+174 81
Keitele, Finland L22+631 46
Keith, Scotland N18+575 40
Keith, S. Australia C58-361 109
Keith B., N.-W. Territories W10+654 88
Kelamet, Ethiopia K38+160 83
Kelang, Malaysia F22+031 69
Kelcyre, Albania L59+403 59
Kellet, C., N.-W. Terr. W32+718 88
Kelloselkä, Finland L01+670 34
Kells, Ireland, Rep. N41+537 42
Kelme, Lithuania L42+557 47
Kelowna, British Columbia V86+500 88
Kelso, Scotland N15+556 41
Kem, Karelia, U.S.S.R. K62+651 62
Ké Macina, Mali N32+140 80
Kemal Paşa, Turkey L16+383 74
Kemerovo, U.S.S.R. G24+553 62
Kemi, Finland L33+657 46
Kemijärvi Finland L15+667 46
Kemijoki, Finland L28+662 46
Kemmerer, Wyoming V34+418 93
Kemp, L., Texas U55+336 95
Kemp Ld., Antarctica J05-670 27
Kempele, Finland L27+649 46
Kempsey, New South Wales B74-311 109
Kempt L., Quebec S86+475 91
Kempten, W. Germany M28+477 48
Kenai Pen., Alaska Y00+605 99
Kendal, England N16+543 37
Kendall, New York T18+333 96
Kendall, C., N.-W. Terr. T72+640 89
Kendari, Celebes, D75-038 65
Kendawangan, Borneo E59-024 65
Kenema, Sierra Leone N68+080 80
Ken-tung, Burma F32+212 71
Kenhardt, Cape Province L52-292 84
Kenilworth, England N09+524 37
Kenitra, Morocco N40+344 80
Kenmare, N. Dakota U72+487 93
Kanmare & R., Ireland, Rep. N58+519 43
Kenmore, Scotland N24+566 41
Kennebec, S. Dakota U59+439 93
Kennebec R., Maine S59+443 90
Kennebunk, Maine S63+434 96
Kennet R., England N06+514 39
Kennett, Missouri U01+363 97
Kenogami & L., Quebec S68+483 90
Keno Hill, Yukon X01+643 88
Kenora, Ontario U27+499 88
Kenosha, Wisconsin T77+426 95
Kensington, Prince Ewdard I. S21+464 90
Kent, New Brunswick S32+466 90
Kent, co., England M86+512 39
Kent I., Maryland T08+389 96
Kent Peninsula, N.-W. Territories V15+680 88
Kentford, England M87+523 39
Kentucky, state, U.S.A. T70+374 99
Kentucky L., N. Dakota T78+362 95
Kentville, Nova Scotia S27+450 90
Kenya, E. Africa K40+010 83
Kenya, Mt., Kenya K46-004 83
Keokuk, Iowa U08+404 95
Keonjhar, India G26+215 71
Keos (Tzia). See Kea, I.
Kepler Mts., New Zealand A76-454 112
Keppel, I., Falkland Is. S00-512 103
Kerala, state, India G80+100 70
Kerang, Victoria C37-357 109
Kerava, Finland L29+604 47
Kerch, U.S.S.R. K51+454 60
Kerchoual, Mali M88+170 80
Keren, Ethiopia K40+158 83
Kerena, Papua New Guinea C26-081 111
Kerguelen Is., Indian Ocean H30-495 77
Kericho, Kenya K58-004 83
Kerinci, mt., Sumatra F22-016 65
Kerkenbosch. See Zuidwolde
Kerkenna Is., Tunisia M24+346 81
Kerki, Turkmen. H58+377 62
Kérkira & I., Greece L61+396 59
Kerkrade, Netherlands M54+509 44
Kermadec Is., Pacific Ocean Z80-295 106
Kermān, Iran J17+303 75
Kerman Desert, Iran J04+290 75
Kermanshah, Iran J77+343 74
Kerry, co., Ireland, Rep. N58+520 43
Kerry Hd., Ireland, Rep. N60+524 43
Kerzers, Switzerland M47+470 45
Kesagami L., Ontario T30+502 89
Kesariya, India G30+264 73
Kesteren, Netherlands M57+519 44
Kestilä, Finland L22+644 46
Keswick, England N19+546 37
Keszthely, Hungary L76+468 49
Ketapang, Borneo E60-017 65
Ketchikan, Alaska W65+555 99
Ketrzyn, Poland L52+541 49
Kettering, England N04+524 37
Keuka L., New York T13+425 96
Kewanee, Illinois U00+412 95
Kewaunee, Wisconsin T75+445 91
Keweenaw B., Michigan T80+469 91
Keweenaw Pen., Wisconsin T84+466 99
Key L., Ireland, Rep. N50+540 42
Key Harbour, Ontario T34+459 91
Key Largo, Florida T32+251 97
Keyser, W. Virginia T24+395 96
Keysville, Virginia T21+371 97
Key West, Florida T41+246 97
Kezhma, U.S.S.R. F24+590 63
Khabab, Syria K52+330 76
Khabarovsk, U.S.S.R. D00+483 63
Khaburah, Oman J18+240 75
Khadasan, Mongolia F06+478 64
Khadhra, Saudi Arabia K09+285 74
Khadro, Pakistan H37+261 70
Khafs Maqran, Saudi Arabia J83+214 74
Khagaul, India G29+255 73
Khaibar, Saudi Arabia K33+258 74
Khairabad, India G55+274 73
Khairpur, Pakistan H37+275 70
Khairpur, Pakistan H16+296 72
Khaiwan, Yemen K07+165 74
Khalis-ed-Daff, Saudi Arabia K35+220 74
Khalki, I., Greece L14+362 59
Khalkidhki, Greece L40+404 59
Khalkis, Greece L38+385 59
Khal-Mer-Sede, U.S.S.R. G69+675 62
Khalturin, U.S.S.R. J66+586 61
Khaluf, Saudi Arabia J12+204 75
Kham, Iran J25+290 75
Khambat, G. of, H14+223 70
Khamiab, Afghanistan H55+374 75
Khamis, Mushait, Saudi Arabia K10+183 74
Kham-kheut, Laos F03+182 69
Khamr, Yemen K06+161 74
Khanabad, Afghanistan H35+367 75
Khanaqin, Iraq J88+344 74
Khān Baghdādi, Iraq K14+339 74
Khandela, India G87+275 72
Khandwa, India G81+218 70
Khan-ez-Zebib, Jordan K53+315 76
Khanfar, Yemen, South J89+133 74
Khangai Shan, Mongolia F50+480 31
Khangarh, Pakistan H23+299 72
Khanh-hoa, Vietnam E66+122 69
Khania, Crete L36+355 59
Khaniadhana, India G71+250 73
Khanka Oz., U.S.S.R. D15+449 63
Khanntor, Syria K47+344 76
Khanpur, Pakistan H26+286 72
Khan Sheikhun, Syria K50+354 76
Khan Tengri, Kirgiz. G58+420 62
Khanty Mansiysk, U.S.S.R. H35+610 62
Khanu, Iran J13+280 75
Khan Yunis, Egypt K64+314 76
Kharaghoda, India H19+232 70
Kharan, Pakistan H57+285 70
Kharar, India G13+227 73
Kharkov, Ukraine K53+500 60
Kharmanli, Bulgaria L25+419 58
Kharovsk, U.S.S.R. K29+599 60
Kharsawan, India G25+228 73
Khartaksho, Kashmir G83+349 72
Khartoum, Sudan K74+156 81
Khasab, U.A.E. J23+262 75
Khasfa, Saudi Arabia J35+197 75
Khasi Hills, India F80+254 71
Khaskovo, Bulgaria L27+419 58
Khasmel Girba, Sudan K56+150 81
Khatanga, U.S.S.R. F16+721 63
Khatangsky Guba, U.S.S.R. E50+745 63
Kheralu, India H14+236 70
Kheri, India G55+279 73
Kherlen R., Mongolia E44+480 64
Kherson, Ukraine K74+466 60
Khetri, India G85+280 72
Khilok, U.S.S.R. E56+515 63
Khinis, Turkey K19+394 74
Khinjan, Afghanistan H37+355 75
Khios & I., Greece L24+384 59
Khisfin, Syria K55+329 76
Khiva, Uzbek H86+413 62
Khmel'nitskiy, Ukraine L18+494 60
Khmer, See Cambodia
Kholm. U.S.S.R. K83+572 60
Kholmsk, U.S.S.R. C47+469 63
Khōng, Laos E84+139 69
Khor, U.S.S.R. D00+479 63
Khóra Sfakion, Crete L35+352 59
Khor Dhahiya, Saudi Arabia J50+189 75
Khor Kalba, Saudi Arabia J22+252 75
Khorramabad, Iran J70+336 74
Khormali, China G04+452 64
Khorramshahr, Iran J70+305 74
Khotan, Sinkiang, China G61+369 62
Khrisoúpolis, Greece L32+410 58
Khrojna, Bulgaria L32+418 58
Khudhfiya, Saudi Arabia J53+190 75
Khujur, Iran J69+358 74
Khulna, Bangladesh G02+228 73
Khumain, Iran J59+338 75
Khungcha, Burma F71+218 71
Khunsar, Iran J58+332 75
Khur, Iran J09+329 75
Khur, Iran J30+338 75
Khurai, India G70+241 73
Khurja, India G73+282 72
Khurma, Saudi Arabia K17+218 74
Khusf, Iran J06+328 75
Khushab, Pakistan H16+323 72
Khvalynsk, U.S.S.R. J72+525 61
Khvoy, Iran K00+386 74
Khyber Pass, Pakistan H23+340 72
Kiama, New South Wales B86-347 109
Kiambi, Zaire L20-056 82
Kiambi, Zaire L12-074 83
Kiamichi Mts., Oklahoma U28+346 95
Kiamusze, China D28+468 64
Kian, China E30+271 67
Kiangchow. See Kiangling
Kiangling, China E46+303 67
Kiangpeh, China E80+296 67
Kiangsi, prov., China E24+274 67
Kiangsu, prov., China E00+332 66
Kiangtu. See Yangchow
Kiangyin, China D88+317 66
Kiantajarvi, Finland L05+650 46
Kiao-chow B., China D88+360 66
Kiaohsien, China D89+362 66
Kiating. See Loshan
Kibangula, Zaire L16-048 82
Kibombo, Zaire L24-040 82

Kibondo, Tanzania K86-036 83
Kicevo, Yugoslavia L54+415 58
Kichiga, U.S.S.R. B09+598 63
Kichiginsk, U.S.S.R. H82+545 61
Kicking Horse Pass, Alberta V68+512 88
Kidal, Mali M82+182 80
Kidderminster, England N14+524 37
Kidnappers, C., New Zealand A17-396 112
Kidodi, Tanzania K48-076 83
Kiel, W. Germany M29+543 48
Kiel (Nord-Ostsee) Kanal.
W. Germany M35+540 84
Kielce, Poland L56+510 49
Kieldrecht, Belgium M65+513 44
Kieler Bucht, W. Germany M27+545 48
Kienchang. See Nancheng
Kiencheng, China E62+282 67
Kienko, China E87+321 66
Kienning. See Kienow
Kienow, China E09+271 67
Kienping, China E02+419 66
Kienshui, China F13+237 64
Kienteh, China E03+296 67
Kiev. See Kiyev
Kiffa, Mauritania N68+166 80
Kigali, Rwanda L00-020 83
Kiganga, Tanzania K60-078 83
Kigoma, Tanzania L02-048 83
Kihsien, China E16+401 66
Kii Chan., Japan D00+336 68
Kijabe, Kenya K50-010 83
Kikhchik, U.S.S.R. B53+535 63
Kikinda, Yugoslavia L57+458 58
Kikkertaksoak I., Quebec S27+603 89
Kikládhes, Is., Greece L30+370 59
Kikori & R., Papua New Guinea C35-074 111
Kikwit, Zaire L66-054 82
Kila Drosh, (Drosh), Pak. H19+355 72
Kilbeggan, Ireland, Rep. N45+534 43
Kilbourn, Wisconsin T89+437 91
Kilbrennan Sd., Scotland N33+556 41
Kilchu, Korea D34+410 64
Kilcormac, Ireland, Rep. N46+532 43
Kilcullen, Ireland, Rep. N40+531 43
Kildare & co., Ireland, Rep. N41+532 43
Kilfrinnane, Ireland, Rep. N51+524 43
Kilgarvan, Ireland, Rep. N57+519 43
Kilian, China G73+372 72
Kilifi, Kenya K30-036 83
Kilimanjaro Mt., Tanzania K46-030 83
Kilindini, Kenya K32-040 83
Kilkee, Ireland, Rep. N58+527 43
Kilkeel, N. Ireland N36+540 42
Kilkenny & co., Ireland, Rep. N43+526 43
Kilkieran B., Ireland, Rep. N58+533 43
Kilkis, Greece L44+411 58
Kilkis, Greece L43+409 59
Kilkivan, Queensland B77-260 111
Kill, Ireland, Rep. N39+533 43
Killala B., Ireland, Rep. N55+542 42
Killaloe, Ireland, Rep. N51+528 43
Killarney, Ireland, Rep. N57+520 43
Killarney, Ontario T39+460 91
Killary Harb., Ireland, Rep. N60+536 42
Killashandra, Ireland, Rep. N45+540 42
Killiecrankie, Pass of,
Scotland N22+568 41
Killimor, Ireland, Rep. N50+532 43
Killin, Scotland N26+565 41
Killini, Greece L53+379 59
Killorglin, Ireland, Rep. N59+521 43
Killybegs, Ireland, Rep. N51+546 42
Killyleagh, N. Ireland N34+544 42
Kilmacthomas, Ireland, Rep. N45+522 43
Kilmallock, Ireland, Rep. N51+524 43
Kilmarnock, Scotland N27+556 41
Kilmore, Victoria C30-373 109
Kilosa, Tanzania K48-068 83
Kilrea, N. Ireland N39+549 42
Kilrush, Ireland, Rep. N57+526 43
Kilsyth, Scotland N24+560 41
Kiltamagh, Ireland, Rep. N54+538 42
Kilwa Kivinje, Tanzania K34-088 83
Kilwinning, Scotland N28+557 41
Kima, Zaire L18-016 82
Kimball, S. Dakota U54+437 93
Kimberley, Cape Province L32-288 84
Kimi, Greece L35+386 59
Kimito, (Kemiö), Finland L44+601 47
Kimolos, I., Greece L33+368 59
Kimvula, Zaire L84-058 82
Kinabulu, mt., Sabah E20+062 65
Kinbrace, Scotland N24+583 40
Kincardine, Ontario T40+442 91
Kincardine, Scotland N14+569 40
Kincardine-on-Forth, Scot. N22+561 41
Kinchow Wan, China D80+391 66
Kincraig, Scotland N24+571 40
Kindat, Burma F63+237 71
Kindersley, Saskatchewan V22+512 88
Kindia, Guinea N76+100 80
Kindu-Port Empain, Zaire L24-030 82
Kinel, U.S.S.R. J56+532 61
Kinel Cherkkassy, U.S.S.R. J49+535 61
Kineo, Maine S58+457 90
Kineshma, U.S.S.R. K17+575 61
King I., Burma F40+125 71
King I., Tasmania C36-400 111
King and Queen, Virginia T11+376 97
King Christian IX Ld.,
Greenland Q10+680 26
King Edward VIII Fall,
Guyana R88+056 104
King Edward VII Land,
Antarctica Y40-770 27
Kingfisher, Oklahoma U48+358 95
King Frederick VIII Ld.,
Greenland P40+790 26
King Frederick VI Ld.,
Greenland Q70+630 26
Kingfu, China F04+284 64
King George I,
South Shetlands R75-620 27
King George Is., Pacific Oc. X60-150 107
King George, Mt, B.C. V61+504 88
King George Sd., W. Aust. E10-351 110
King George V Ld., Antarc. C00-790 27
King George VI Sd., Antarc. S50-700 27
King George VI Falls,
Guyana S08+058 104
Kingku, China F25+236 64
King Leopold Ra., W. Aust. D60-170 110
King Leopold & Queen Astrid
Coast, Antarctica G40-670 27
Kingman, Kansas U49+376 95
Kingmen, China E47+310 66
Kings Pk., Utah V32+407 94
Kingsbridge, England N23+503 38
King's Canyon Nat. Park,
California V84+371 92
Kingsclere, England N08+513 39
Kingscote, S. Australia C74-356 109
Kingscourt, Ireland, Rep. N41+539 42
King's Lynn, England M88+528 39
King Sound, W. Australia D70-166 110
Kingsport, Tennessee T46+366 97
Kingston, Jamaica T11+179 101
Kingston, New York S84+419 96
Kingston, New Zealand A68-453 112
Kingston, Ontario T09+443 91
Kingston, S. Australia C61-368 109
Kingston Ra., California V71+366 92
Kingston-on-Thames, Eng. N02+514 39
Kingstree, S. Carolina T29+336 97
Kingswear, England N21+503 38
Kingtung, China F24+243 64
Kingushi, Zaire L80-052 82
Kingussie, Scotland N24+571 40
King William I., N.-W. Terr. U45+684 88
King William Ld., Greenland P40+750 26
Kingwood, W. Virginia T28+395 91
Kingyang, China E74+361 66
Kingyüan, See Ishan
Kinhsien, China D80+391 66
Kinhwa, China E02+291 67
Kinki, China E83+378 66
Kinlochewe, Scotland N32+576 40
Kinlochleven, Scotland N30+567 41
Kinloch Rannoch, Scotland N25+567 41
Kinross, Scotland N21+562 41
Kinsale, Ireland, Rep. N51+517 43
Kinsale, Old Hd. of, Ireland,
Rep. N51+516 43
Kinshasa, Zaire L88-044 82
Kintap, Borneo E29-038 65
Kintyre, Scotland N34+556 41
Kintyre, Mull of, Scotland N35+553 41
Kinvarra, Ireland, Rep. N54+531 43
Kinyangiri, Tanzania K62-044 83
Kiowa, Kansas U51+370 95
Kiparissia, Greece L50+372 59
Kiparissia, G. of, Greece L52+374 59
Kipawa & L., Quebec T24+468 91
Kipini, Kenya K26-026 83
Kirá Panayiá, See Pélagos, I.
Kirchberg, Switzerland M45+471 45
Kirensk, U.S.S.R. E72+580 63
Kirgizskaya, rep., U.S.S.R. H10+420 62
Kiribati, Pac. Oc. A35+007 106
Kirin, China D50+438 64
Kirit, Somalia J84+088 83
Kiriwina, I.,
Papua New Guinea B84-086 111
Kirkagac, Turkey L14+390 74
Kirkby Lonsdale, England N16+542 37
Kirkcaldy, Scotland N19+561 41
Kirkcudbright., Scot., N24+548 41
Kirkee, India H06+186 70
Kirkenes, Norway L00+697 46
Kirkintilloch, Scotland N25+559 41
Kirkland Lake, Ontario T30+482 91
Kirksville, Missouri U16+402 95
Kirkuk, Iraq K04+357 74
Kirkwall, Orkney, Scot. N18+590 40
Kirong Dzong, Nepal G28+284 73
Kirov, U.S.S.R. K64+541 60
Kirov, U.S.S.R. J62+586 61
Kirovgrad, U.S.S.R. J01+574 61
Kirovograd, Ukraine K77+486 60
Kirovsk, U.S.S.R. K67+675 62
Kirriemuir, Scotland N18+567 41
Kirsanov, U.S.S.R. K14+526 61
Kirsehir, Turkey K65+391 74
Kirthar Ra., Pakistan H46+270 70
Kirun. See Chilung
Kiruna, Sweden L58+678 46
Kisamba, Zaire L36-074 82
Kisbér, Hungary L72+475 49
Kisangani, Zaire L28+006 82
Kishanganj, India G12+261 73
Kishangarh, India H01+264 70
Kishangarh, India H27+279 72
Kishi, Nigeria M66+090 80
Kishinev, Moldavia L07+470 60
Kishtwar, Kashmir G85+333 72
Kisii, Kenya K62-008 83
Kisiju, Tanzania K34-074 83
Kiska, I., Aleutian Is. A15+511 99
Kiskisink, Quebec S73+479 90
Kiskunfélegyháza, Hungary L61+467 49
Kismayu See Chisimaio
Kispest, Hungary L65+475 49
Kissaraing I., Burma F39+118 71
Kissidougou, Guinea N60+092 80
Kisujszallás, Hungary L55+472 49
Kisumu, Kenya K60-002 83
Kisvárda, Hungary L48+482 49
Kiswe, Syria K52+333 76
Kita, Mali N56+130 80
Kitab, Uzbek. H48+390 62
Kitakyushu, Japan D25+338 68
Kitchener, Ontario T33+434 91
Kitchioh, China E25+228 67
Kitgum, Uganda K72+030 83
Kithira I., Greece L42+363 59
Kithirai Chan, Greece L42+360 59
Kithnos, I., Greece L33+374 59
Kitima, Cyprus K76+348 76
Kittanning, Pennsylvania T28+408 96
Kittatinny Mts., New Jersey S89+411 96
Kittila, Finland L30+676 46
Kitui, Kenya K42-012 83
Kityang, China E22+235 67
Kitzingen, W. Germany M29+497 48
Kiuchuan, China F38+397 64
Kiungchow. See Kiungshan
Kiungchow Str. See Hai Nan
Kiungchow Hai Hsia,
China E60+202 67
Kiungshan, Hainan I., China E57+200 67
Kiuruvesi, Finland L20+637 46
Kivijarvi, Finland L29+632 46
Kivu L., Zaire-Rwanda L06-020 83
Kiwai I., Papua New Guinea C39-087 111
Kiyev, Ukraine K87+505 60
Kiyma, Kazakh H44+518 62
Kizel, U.S.S.R. J23+592 62
Kizil Irmak, Turkey K68+400 74
Kizil Jilga, Kashmir K65+353 70
Kizyl Arvat, Turkmen J24+390 62
Kjerringøy, Norway M02+675 46
Kladanj, Yugoslavia L68+442 58
Kladno, Czechoslovakia M06+501 48
Klagenfurt, Austria M04+466 48
Klaipeda, Lithuania L53+558 47
Klamath R., California W22+414 92
Klamath Falls, Oregon W11+422 92
Klamath Mts., California W18+414 92
Klang, See Kelang
Klar Älv, Sweden M12+607 47
Klerksdorp, Transvaal L20-268 84
Kleszczele, Poland L40+525 49
Klimpfjall, Sweden M01+650 46
Klisura, Bulgaria L33+427 58
Kliuchi, U.S.S.R. J89+526 61
Ključ, Yugoslavia L79+445 56
Klodawa, Poland L66+523 49
Klofta, Norway M23+601 47
Klomnice, Poland L64+510 49
Klondike R., Yukon X15+642 88
Kloosterzande, Netherlands M66+513 44
Klosters, Switzerland M31+469 45
Kluane, L., Yukon X22+610 88
Klundert, Netherlands M63+517 44
Knighton, Wales N18+523 38
Knin, Yugoslavia L83+440 56
Knob, C., W. Australia E05-345 110
Knobel, Arkansas U04+364 97
Knockboy, Ireland, Rep. N57+518 43
Knockbrack, Ireland, Rep. N57+519 43
Knockmealdown Mts.,
Ireland, Rep. N48+522 43
Knockower, Ireland, Rep. N58+517 43
Knokke, Belgium M70+513 44
Knox, Pennsylvania T28+412 96
Knox Coast, Antarctica F10-660 27
Knoxville, Iowa U18+412 95
Knoxville, Tennessee T54+360 97
Knysna, Cape Province L40-340 84
Knyszyn, Poland L43+534 49
Kobarid, Yugoslavia M09+463 56
Kōbe, Japan C88+348 68
København, Denmark M14+557 47
Koblenz, W. Germany M45+504 48
Kobrin, Byelorussia L34+522 60
Kobroör, I., Indonesia D02-063 65
Kocaeli. See Izmit
Kočane, Yugoslavia L46+419 58
Kočevje, Yugoslavia M01+456 56
Kochi, Japan D09+335 68
Kochiki Retto, Japan D32+317 68
Kochow. See Mowming
Kodavere, Estonia L17+587 47
Kodiak & I., Alaska Y20+578 99
Koeala (Kuala), Sumatra F40+034 65
Koemai, Borneo E50-026 65
Koepang (Kupang), Timor I.,
Indonesia D69-102 65
Koetai, R., Borneo E26+004 65
Koffiefontein, Orange Free
State L30-294 84
Koforidua, Ghana N02+062 80
Kofu, Japan C68+356 68
Kogaluk R., Quebec T05+594 89
Køge B., Greenland Q58+650 26
Kohat, Pakistan H21+336 72
Koh Chang, Thailand F16+120 69
Kohima, India F65+257 71
Koh Kong, Cambodia F12+113 69
Koh Kut, Thailand F15+116 69
Koh Rong, Cambodia F10+107 69
Kojnic, Yugoslavia L72+439 58
Kojonup, W. Australia E17-338 110
Kokand, Uzbek H24+408 75
Kokchetav, Kazakh H33+533 62
Kokhtla Yarva, Estonia L15+594 47
Kokkola, Finland L41+639 46
Koko, Chad L70+096 81
Kokoda,
Papua New Guinea C13-090 111
Kokomo, Indiana T67+405 91
Koko Nor. See Ching Hai
Kokoshili Ra., Tibet G30+357 71
Kokpekty, Kazakh. G46+488 62
Kokstad, Cape Province L04-306 84
Kokura, Japan D25+338 68
Kokyar, Sinkiang, China G77+374 72
Ko-lan-chow, China E50+389 66
Kolar, India G71+132 70
Kolari, Finland L38+673 46
Kolarovgrad, Bulgaria L19+433 58
Kolberg. See Kołobrzeg
Kolda, Senegal P00+130 80
Kolding, Denmark M33+555 47
Kole, Zaire L28+020 82
Kolguyev Ostrov, U.S.S.R. J65+690 62
Kolhapur, India H05+168 70
Kolin, Czechoslovakia L89+500 48
Kolkas Rags, Latvia L44+577 47
Kollick Kenyon Plateau,
Antarctica V00-770 27
Köln, W. Germany M48+509 48
Kolno, Poland L48+534 49
Kolo, Poland L68+522 49
Kolo, Tanzania K56-046 83
Kołobrzeg, Poland L86+542 49
Kologriv, U.S.S.R. K04+588 61
Kolokani, Mali N48+134 80
Kolomna, U.S.S.R. K38+550 60
Kolomyya, Ukraine L30+486 60
Kolossia, Kenya K56+016 83
Kolozsvár, See Cluj
Kolpashevo, U.S.S.R. G42+583 62
Kolwezi, Zaire L26-108 82
Kolyma, R., U.S.S.R. B60+675 63
Kolymskiy, Khrebet, U.S.S.R. B30+634 63
Komandorskiye Ostr., U.S.S.R. A80+550 63
Komariya, Sri Lanka G49+070 70
Komarno, Czechoslovakia L71+478 49
Komatsu, Japan C81+364 68
Komi, aut. rep., U.S.S.R. J40+650 62
Komintern, U.S.S.R. K31+477 61
Kommunarsk, Ukraine U38+485 60
Kommunizma, Pk., Tadzhik. H17+388 62
Komotini, Greece L28+410 58
Kompong Chan, Cambodia E87+120 69
Kompong Chnang, Cambodia F02+123 69
Kompong Som, Cambodia F07+111 69
Kompong-thom, Cambodia F01+127 69
Komsomolets Ostrov, U.S.S.R. F60+808 63
Komsomolsk, U.S.S.R. C77+505 63
Kondinskoe, U.S.S.R. H56+625 62
Kondoa, Tanzania K56-048 83
Kong, Ivory Coast N28+092 80
Kong Karl's Land, Arctic Oc. L05+790 62
Kongmoon, China E41+226 67
Kongor, Sudan K82+072 81
Kongsberg, Norway M32+597 47
Kongsmoen, Norway M16+648 46
Kongsvinger, Norway M18+602 47
Kongwa, Tanzania K52-064 83
Königsberg, See Kaliningrad
Konispol, Albania L59+397 59
Konotop, Ukraine K71+513 60
Konstantinovka, Ukraine K43+485 60
Konstantinovsk, U.S.S.R. K23+476 61
Konstanz, Switz. M35+476 48
Kontiomaki, Finland L11+643 46
Konya, Turkey K76+380 74
Konza, Kenya K48-018 83
Koondrook, Victoria C35-357 109
Koonenberry, New S. Wales C46-305 109
Koorawatha, New S. Wales C08-341 109
Kootenay Park, B.C. V70+506 88
Kootwijk, Netherlands M55+522 44
Koo-wee-rup, Victoria C27-382 109
Kopeisk, U.S.S.R. H80+550 61
Kopervik, Norway M58+593 47
Köping, Sweden L84+595 47
Kopparberg, Sweden M00+599 47
Koppigen, Switzerland M44+471 45
Koprivnica, Yugoslavia L79+462 56
Kora, India G58+261 73
Korce, Albania L56+407 59
Korcheva, U.S.S.R. K50+568 60
Korcula, I., Yugoslavia L78+429 56
Korea, N., Asia D30+412 64
Korea, S., Asia D30+368 64
Korea Strait, Asia D36+393 64
Korinthia, & Argolis, Greece L43+378 59
Kórinthos, Greece L42+379 59
Kórinthos, G. of, Greece L44+382 59
Koritza. See Korce
Kormakiti, Cyprus K72+354 76
Kornat, I., Yugoslavia L88+438 56
Korneuburg, Austria L82+484 49
Korogwe, Tanzania K40-052 83
Koroit, Victoria C46-383 109
Korong Vale, Victoria C38-364 109
Körös R., Hungary L58+468 58
Korosten, Ukraine L08+510 60
Koro Toro, Chad L70+160 81
Korppoo, Finland L50+602 47
Korsakov, U.S.S.R. C44+466 63
Korsnas, Finland L53+628 46
Korsnes, Norway L84+683 46
Kortessem, Belgium M58+509 44
Kortgem, Netherlands M67+516 44
Korti, Sudan K80+180 81
Kortrijk (Courtrai), Belgium M70+508 44
Korumburra, Victoria C25-384 109
Korwai, India G72+241 73
Koryakskiy Khrebet, U.S.S.R. A60+623 63
Korzum, Turkey L03+371 74
Kos, I., Greece L17+368 59
Koscierzyna, Poland L72+541 49
Kosciusko, Mississippi T88+330 95
Kosciusko, Mt., N.S.W. C10-364 109
Kosha, Sudan K86+206 81
Koshchagyl, Kazakh. J37+470 62
Koshki, U.S.S.R. J57+542 61
Kosi, India G75+277 72
Košice, Czechoslovakia L52+497 49
Kosima, Kuwait J73+295 74
Koslan, U.S.S.R. J66+634 62
Köslin, See Koszalin
Koso Gol, Mongolia F28+510 63
Kosovo Metohija, Yugoslavia L54+425 58
Kostainica, Yugoslavia L81+452 56
Kosti, Sudan K74+132 81
Kostroma, U.S.S.R. K24+578 60
Koszalin, Poland L83+542 49
Kota Baharu, Malaysia F17+061 69
Kotah, India G85+252 70
Kota Kinabalu, Sabah E24+060 65
Kotalpur, India G14+230 73
Kota Tinggi, Malaysia F07+018 69
Kotcha L., British Columbia W08+592 88
Kotehandpur,
Bangladesh G06+234 73
Kotel, Bulgaria L21+429 58
Kotelnich, U.S.S.R. J70+584 61
Kotelnyy, Ostrov, U.S.S.R. C65+754 63
Kotido, Uganda K66+030 83
Kotka, Finland L18+605 47
Kot Kapura, India H01+306 72
Kot Kasim, India G79+280 72
Kotkhai, India G74+311 72
Kotlas, U.S.S.R. J80+612 62
Kotli, Kashmir H07+335 72
Kotonkoro, Nigeria M54+110 80
Kotri, Pakistan H41+253 70
Kotturu, India G82+148 70
Kotzebue Sd., Alaska Z00+665 99
Kouango, Cent. Afr. Rep. L60+050 81
Koudougou, Upper Volta N13+120 80
Koulikoro, Mali N46+128 80
Kounde, Cent. Afr. Rep. M02+060 81
Kourou, French Guiana R46+052 105
Koutiala, Mali N32+122 80
Kouvola, Finland L19+608 47
Kovel, Ukraine L34+512 60
Kovno. See Kaunas
Kovrov, U.S.S.R. K22+563 61
Kowloon, China E35+224 67
Koyiu, China E45+231 67
Koyukuk, R., Alaska Y30+655 99
Kozan, Turkey K55+375 74
Kozani, Greece L49+403 59
Kozhikode. See Calicut
Kra & Isthmus of, Thailand F37+104 69
Kracheh, Cambodia E84+125 69
Kragerø, Norway M34+588 47
Kragujevac, Yugoslavia L53+440 58

Krakow, Poland L60+501 49
Kramatorsk, Ukraine K45+487 60
Krammer, Netherlands M65+517 44
Kranj, Yugoslavia M04+463 56
Kranystaw, Poland L41+510 49
Kranz, U.S.S.R L57+549 47
Krapina, Yugoslavia L85+462 56
Krasino, Novaya Zemlya J35+708 62
Krasnobród, Poland L44+505 49
Krasnodar, U.S.S.R. K37+451 62
Krasnograd, Ukraine K58+494 60
Krasnoufimsk, U.S.S.R. J14+566 61
Krasnovisher, U.S.S.R. J17+602 62
Krasnovodsk, Turkmen J44+401 62
Krasnoyarsk, U.S.S.R. F71+562 63
Krasnyi Kholm, U.S.S.R. K48+581 60
Krasny Kut, U.S.S.R. J78+509 61
Krasnyy Yar, U.S.S.R. K02+507 61

Krefeld, W. Germany M51+513 48
Kremenchug, Ukraine K69+491 60
Kremensk, U.S.S.R. K10+497 61
Krems, Austria L87+484 49
Kretinga, Lith. L53+559 47
Kreuzlingen, Switzerland M35+476 45
Kribi, Cameroon M30+030 81
Krimml, Austria M17+472 48
Krishna, R., India G63+166 70
Krishnanagar, India G09+234 73
Krishnaraja Res., India G81+126 70
Kristiansand, Norway M42+581 47
Kristianstad, Sweden M05+561 47
Kristiansund, Norway M43+631 46
Kristiinankaupunki, Finland L52+623 46
Kristinehamn, Sweden M05+594 47
Kriti, I., Greece L30+350 59
Kriva Palanka, Yugoslavia L45+422 58
Krivoy Rog, Ukraine K70+478 60
Krizevci, Yugoslavia L81+460 56
Krk, I., Yugoslavia M02+451 56
Krnov, Czechoslovakia L74+501 49
Kroken, Norway M04+653 46
Kroměříz, Czechoslovakia L76+493 49
Kronoby, Finland L42+637 46
Kronshtadt, U.S.S.R. L02+600 60
Kroonstad, Orange Free State L16-276 84
Kropotkin, U.S.S.R. K28+454 62
Krotoszyn, Poland L76+517 49
Krško, Yugoslavia L87+459 56
Krugersdorp, Transvaal L14-262 84
Kruishoutem, Belgium M69+509 44
Krujë, Albania L62+415 58
Krumbach, W. Germany M28+482 48
Krumlov, Czechoslovakia M04+488 48
Krunga, Kenya K22-018 83
Krung Thep, Thailand F27+138 69
Krupnik, Bulgaria L40+418 58
Krusevac, Yugoslavia L52+436 58
Krustpils, Latvia L24+565 47
Krzyz, Poland L84+529 49
Ksar el Boukhari, Algeria M74+358 80
Kuala, Sumatra F40+034 65
Kuala Kangsar, Malaysia F25+049 69
Kuala Kerai, Malaysia F16+054 65
Kuala Klawang, Malaysia F18+030 69
Kuala Lipis, Malaysia F17+042 69
Kuala Lumpur, Malaysia F20+032 69
Kuandang, Celebes D72+008 65
Kuantan, Malaysia F10+037 65
Kub, Namibia L74-242 84
Kucha, Sinkiang, China G43+418 62
Kuching, Sarawak E58+016 65
Kuchow. See Jungkiang
Kudat, Sabah E20+069 65
Kudymkar, U.S.S.R. J33+593 62
Kuhak, Iran H71+271 75
Kuhak, Iran H79+309 75
Kuh Banan, Iran J22+315 75
Kuh-e-Bul, Iran J55+305 75
Kuh Furgan, Iran J22+279 75
Kuh-i-Bul, Iran J43+308 75
Kuh-i-Dinar, Iran J51+310 75
Kuh-i-Kashigah, Iran J28+284 75
Kuhmo, Finland L03+641 46
Kuhpayeh, Iran J45+327 75
Kuhrud, Iran J53+337 75
Kuhsan, Afghanistan H82+347 75
Kuibis, Namibia L80-268 84
Kuibyshevka, U.S.S.R. D39+509 63
Kuikiang, China E23+297 67
Kuinre, Netherlands M55+528 44
Kukan, Thailand F05+146 69
Kukatush, Ontario T43+481 91
Kukawa, Nigeria M08+128 81
Kukes, Albania L58+421 58
Kukong, China E41+249 64
Kukong (Shiukwan), China E38+248 67
Kulachi, Pakistan H27+320 72
Kulaikh, Saudi Arabia K25+212 74
Kuldiga, Latvia L48+570 47
Kuldja, Sinkiang, China G51+440 62
Kulhakangri Mt., Tibet F87+280 71
Kulin, China E85+281 67
Kulmbach, W. Germany M21+501 48
Kulu, India G78+319 72
Kulunda, U.S.S.R. G67+526 62
Kulwin, Victoria C44-350 109
Kumai, Borneo, Indon. E50-026 65
Kumamoto, Japan D26+328 68
Kumara, New Zealand A52-426 112
Kumara, U.S.S.R. D48+517 63
Kumasi, Ghana N10+068 80
Kumbakonam, India G63+110 70
Kumher, India G76+273 73
Kumora, U.S.S.R. E52+559 63
Kumta, India H04+144 70
Kunda, Estonia L21+595 47
Kunduz, Afghanistan H36+367 75
Kungchang. See Lungsi
Kungnung, India F70+240 71
Kungrad, Uzbek J06+431 62
Kungur, U.S.S.R. J19+574 61
Kunhsien, China E53+327 66
Kunlun Shan, China-Tibet 30-31
Kunming, China F14+250 64
Kunsan, Korea D50+360 64
Kuopio, Finland L14+629 46
Kupa R., Yugoslavia M00+455 56
Kupang, Timor I., Indon. D69-102 65
Kupishkis, Lithuania L30+558 47
Kupyansk, Ukraine K45+497 60
Kure, Japan D15+342 68
Kure, I., Hawaii Z80+288 106
Kureika, U.S.S.R. G05+670 62
Kuressare, Estonia L45+582 47
Kurgan, U.S.S.R. H57+556 62
Kuria Muria Is., Arabian Sea J22+175 75
Kurigram, Bangladesh G02+258 73
Kurilskiye Ostrova, U.S.S.R. C00+458 63
Kurnool, India G72+159 70
Kurow, New Zealand A57-446 112
Kurram, Pakistan H29+339 72
Kurri Kurri, New S. Wales B82-328 109
Kursk, U.S.S.R. K53+517 60
Kurski Zaliv, U.S.S.R. L55+550 47
Kurtalan, Turkey K18+384 74
Kuru, Finland L37+619 47
Kuruman, Cape Province L40-276 84
Kurume, Japan D27+332 68
Kurunegala, Sri Lanka G58+076 70
Kusa, U.S.S.R. J04+553 61
Kusaie, I., Caroline Is. B10+053 106
Kushersk, U.S.S.R. J30+584 61
Kushiro, Japan C33+430 68
Kushk, Afghanistan H75+348 75
Kushka, Turkmen. H77+352 62
Kushtia, Bangladesh G05+239 73
Kushva, U.S.S.R. J02+584 61
Kuskokwim B., Alaska Y80+590 99
Kusma, Nepal G38+282 73
Kustanay, Kazakh H70+531 62
Kütahya, Turkey L01+393 74
Kutai, R., Borneo, Indon. E26+004 65
Kut-al-Hai, Iraq J84+322 74
Kutatjane, Sumatra, Indon. F44+034 65
Kutch, & Gulf of, India H23+232 70
Kutch, Rann of, India H30+240 70
Kutchan, Japan C56+429 68
Kutin, Yugoslavia L80+455 56
Kutno, Poland L64+522 49
Kütsing, China F07+255 67
Kutu, Ethiopia K64+090 83
Kutum, Sudan L32+140 81
Kuusamo, Finland L05+659 46
Kuusjärvi, Finland L07+627 46
Kuwait & state, The Gulf J72+294 74
Kuyang, China E60+414 66
Kuybyshev, U.S.S.R. J58+531 61
Kuybyshev, U.S.S.R. G68+559 62
Kuybyshevskoye Vdkhr., U.S.S.R. J60+548 61
Kuytan, U.S.S.R. F22+544 63
Kuzhbal, U.S.S.R. K05+585 61
Kuzino, U.S.S.R. J04+571 61
Kuzmin, Yugoslavia L64+450 58
Kuznetsk, U.S.S.R. J81+530 61
Kuzovatovo, U.S.S.R. J75+536 61
Kvaløy, N., Norway L65+702 46
Kvaløy, S., Norway L68+697 46
Kvarken, Ostra, Sweden L56+634 46
Kvarner, G. of, Yugoslavia M05+448 56
Kvarneric, G. of, Yugoslavia M01+445 56
Kvesmenes, Norway L60+693 46
Kwajalein, Is., Marshall Is. A80+088 106
Kwakhanai, Botswana L52-218 84
Kwakoegron, Surinam R62+051 105
Kwangchang, China E23+267 67
Kwangchow, China E40+232 67
Kwangchow Wan, China E56+210 67
Kwang-nam, Vietnam E70+159 69
Kwangnan, China F00+241 67
Kwangping. See Yungnien
Kwangshun, China E82+261 67
Kwangsichuang prov., China E72+238 67
Kwangsin. See Shangjao
Kwangtung, prov., China E36+235 67
Kwania L., Uganda K74+016 83
Kwan-tung (Luta) Pen., Ch. D86+388 66
Kweichih, China E15+307 66
Kweichow. See Fengkieh
Kweichow, prov., China E84+268 67
Kweihwa. See Huhehot
Kweihwa. See Tzeyun
Kweilin, China E59+254 67
Kweiping, China E59+233 67
Kweisui. See Huhehot
Kweiteh, China F22+360 64
Kweiteh. See Shangkiu
Kweiyang, China E80+266 67
Kweiyang, China E45+258 67
Kwi-chu, Vietnam E88+194 69
Kwidzyń, Poland L66+538 49
Kwitao, Burma F44+257 71
Kwoka, mt., New Guinea D15-006 65
Kyabram, Victoria C30-363 109
Kyakhta, U.S.S.R. E81+504 63
Kyalite Crossing, N.S.W. C40-349 109
Kyangin, Burma F58+182 71
Kyaring Nor, China F46+348 64
Kyaukiaw, Burma F72+208 71
Kyaukpyu, Burma F69+195 71
Kyaukse, Burma F53+215 71
Kybybolite, S. Australia C54-369 109
Kyelang, India G78+326 72
Kyi R., Tibet F80+298 71
Kymi, Finland L19+605 47
Kyneton, Victoria C33-373 109
Kyoga L., Uganda K74+014 83
Kyoto, Japan C85+350 68
Kyrenia, Cyprus K70+353 76
Kyshtym, U.S.S.R. H86+557 61
Kythrea, Cyprus K69+352 76
Kyûshû, I., Japan D24+330 68
Kyustendil, Bulgaria L44+423 58
Kyusyur, U.S.S.R. D45+708 63
Kywong, New South Wales C20-350 109
Kyzl, U.S.S.R. F63+517 63
Kyzyl Kum, Uzbek, etc. H70+423 62
Kyzylsk, U.S.S.R. J06+526 61
Kzyl Orda, Kazakh H57+450 62
Laanila, Finland L16+684 46
La Argentina, Argentina S70-503 103
La Ascención, Mexico V18+310 100
La Asuncion, Venezuela S23+110 104
Laban, Jordan K56+309 76
La Banda, Argentina S25-277 103
Labang, Sarawak E40+033 65
Labe, Guinea N74+114 80
Labelle, Quebec S89+463 91
Laberge, L., Yukon X00+610 88
Labouheyre, France N06+442 55
Laboulaye, Argentina S20-341 103
Labrador, Canada 89
Labrea, Brazil S28-072 104
La Brea, Honduras T76+134 101
La Brea, Trinidad S08+102 104
Labuan, I., Sabah E29+054 65
Labuk B., Sabah E14+061 65
La Canoa, Venezuela S23+086 104
La Carlota, Argentina S20-334 103
La Carolina, Spain N22+383 52
Laccadive Is., Lakshadweep H13+115 70
La Ceiba, Venezuela S66+094 104
Lacepede B., S. Australia C62-367 109
Lac Frontiere, Quebec S60+467 90
Lachen, Switzerland M37+472 45
Lachine, Quebec S82+455 91
Lachlan R., New S. Wales C30-338 109
Lachmangarh, India G89+278 72
Lachute, Quebec S87+457 91
Lackawanna, New York T23+428 96
Lackawaxen, Pennsylvania T00+415 96
Lacken Res., Ireland, Rep. N39+532 43
La Cocha, Argentina S33-278 103
Lacombe, Alberta V53+522 88
La Concordia, El Salvador T85+134 101
Laconia, New Hampshire S69+435 96
La Copelina, Argentina S46-372 103
La Coruña, Spain N51+433 52
La Crosse, Wisconsin U07+438 93
La Cruz, Columbia T11+015 104
La Cruz, Mexico V01+279 100
Ladakh Ra., Tibet G60+322 70
Ladis, Iran H82+289 75
Ladoga, L. See Ladozhskoye Ozero
La Dorada, Columbia S88+055 104
Ladozhskoye Oz., U.S.S.R. K84+606 60
Ladwa, India G77+300 72
Lady Neunes B., Antarctica A70-730 27
Ladysmith, British Columbia W23+490 88
Ladysmith, Natal L02-288 84
Ladysmith, Wisconsin U07+455 93
Lae, Papua New Guinea C18-068 111
Laeken, Belgium M64+509 44
Laesö, I., Denmark M24+573 47
La Esperanza, Honduras T81+143 101
La Estrada, Spain N51+427 52
Lafayette, Georgia T62+347 97
La Fayette, Indiana T71+404 91
Lafayette, Louisiana U12+302 95
La Florencia, Argentina S13-241 103
Lafontaine, Quebec S59+471 90
Lagakalaka, Somalia J66+060 83
Lagan R., N. Ireland N35+546 42
Lages, Brazil Q37-056 105
Laggan, Scotland N26+570 40
Laggan L., Scotland N27+570 40
Laghouat, Algeria M72+332 80
Lagonegro, Italy L85+401 57
Lagos, Mexico U72+214 100
Lagos, Nigeria M70+064 80
Lagos, Portugal N52+371 52
La Grande, Oregon V79+453 92
Lagrange, Georgia T60+330 97
Lagrange, Indiana T62+416 91
Lagrange, Kentucky T62+384 97
La Grange, W. Australia D79-186 110
La Granja, Spain N24+409 52
La Guaira, Venezuela S41+106 104
La Guardia, Argentina S33-295 103
La Guardia, Spain N53+419 52
Laguna, Brazil R23-284 103
Lagunas, Peru T04-053 104
Lagunillas, Bolivia S22-196 104
Laharpur, India G54+276 73
Lahej, Yemen, South K00+130 74
Lahijan, Iran J60+372 75
Laholm, Sweden M12+565 47
Lahore, Pakistan H04+316 72
Lahti, Finland L26+610 47
Lai, C., Vietnam E77+171 69
Laibach. See Ljubljana
Lai-chau, Vietnam F11+222 69
Laichow. See Yehsien
Laigle, France M86+488 54
Laila, Saudi Arabia J79+223 74
Laingsburg, Cape Province L56-330 84
Lairg, Scotland N26+580 40
Laishev, U.S.S.R. J63+554 61
Laives, Italy M22+465 45
Laja, L., Chile S68-374 103
Lajao, Brazil Q69-192 105
La Japonesa, Argentina S39-386 103
Lajes, Brazil R32-278 103
La Junquera, Spain M73+424 53
La Junta, Colorado U81+380 94
Lakatrask, Sweden L53+663 46
Lake Andes, S. Dakota U52+432 93
Lake Butler, Florida T45+300 97
Lake Charles, Louisiana U19+302 95
Lake City, Florida T46+302 97
Lake City, Michigan T61+444 91
Lake District, England N19+546 37
Lake Edward, Quebec S73+477 91
Lakefield, Ontario T20+444 91
Lake Geneva, Wisconsin T80+426 91
Lake George, New York S82+434 96
Lake Harbour, N.-W. Terr. S59+632 89
Lakeland, Florida T42+280 97
Lake Majella, California W12+365 92
Lake Pleasant, New York S86+434 96
Lake Providence, Louisiana U07+328 95
Lakes Entrance, Victoria C12-378 109
Lakeview, Minnesota U12+469 93
Lakeview, Oregon W02+422 92
Lakewood, New Jersey S85+400 96
Lakewood, New York T26+422 96
Lakewood, Ohio T40+415 91
Lakhimpur, India F65+272 71
Lakhimpur, India G55+280 73
Lakki, Pakistan H24+325 72
Lakkor Tso, Tibet G36+320 71
Lakonia, Greece L45+369 59
Lakonia, G. of, Greece L44+366 59
Lakota, Ivory Coast N34+060 80
Lakota, N. Dakota U50+481 93
Lakse Fd., Norway L20+705 46
Lakshadweep, Indian Ocean H13+115 70
Laktsang, Tibet G42+303 71
Lala Musa, Pakistan H06+327 72
Lalbagh, India G10+242 73
Lalganj, India G29+259 73
La Libertad, Ecuador T35-022 104
La Libertad, Guatemala U01+167 100
La Libertad, Nicaragua T61+123 101
La Ligua, Chile S67-324 103
Lalin, Spain N49+426 52
Lalitpur, India G69+247 73
La Maddalena, I., Sardinia M34+413 57
La Malbaie, Quebec S61+476 91
Lamar, Colorado U76+381 94
Lamar, Missouri U26+374 95
Lamastre, France M63+450 55
Lambach, Austria M07+481 48
Lamballe, France N15+485 54
Lambay I., Ireland, Rep. N36+535 43
Lambayeque, Peru T30-066 104
Lambert's Ld., Greenland P30+790 26
Lambertville, New Jersey T00+403 96
Lámbia, Greece L49+379 59
Lamb's Hd., Ireland, Rep. N61+517 43
Lamé, Chad M02+092 81
Lamego, Portugal N47+411 52
Lameroo, S. Australia C57-354 109
Lamesa, Texas U70+326 94
Lamia, Greece L45+389 59
Lamlash, Scotland N31+555 41
Lammermuir Hills, Scotland N16+559 41
Lamotrek Is., Caroline Is. C30+075 106
La Moure, N. Dakota U50+464 93
Lampa, Peru S80-153 104
Lampazos, Mexico U62+270 100
Lampedusa, I., Medit. Sea M12+355 81
Lampeter, Wales N25+521 38
Lamphun, Thailand F35+186 69
Lampi, I., Burma F41+108 71
Lampton, C., N.-W. Terr. W20+710 88
Lamu, Kenya K24-024 83
Lamud, Peru T17-063 104
Lanark, Scotland N23+557 41
Lancashire, co., England N16+537 37
Lancaster, England N17+540 37
Lancaster, Missouri U16+404 95
Lancaster, New Hampshire S69+445 91
Lancaster, New York T22+429 96
Lancaster, Pennsylvania T08+401 96
Lancaster, S. Carolina T34+347 97
Lancaster, Wisconsin U04+429 91
Lancaster Sd., N.-W. Terr. T60+734 89
Lanchow, China F07+360 66
Landeck, Austria M27+471 48
Landen, Belgium M60+508 44
Lander, Wyoming V22+429 93
Landerneau, France N26+484 54
Landes, dep., France N04+440 55
Landfall, I., Chile S85-534 103
Landi Khana, Pakistan H23+342 72
Landi Kotal, Pakistan H23+342 72
Landon, Sweden M04+636 46
Landovery, Wales N23+520 38
Landsberg, W. Germany M25+481 48
Landsberg. See Gorzow Wielkopolski
Land's End, England N34+500 38
Landshut, W. Germany M17+490 48
Landskrona, Sweden M13+559 47
Langå, Denmark M31+563 47
Langadhas, Greece L41+408 59
Langana L., Ethiopia K38+076 83
Langchung, China E84+315 66
Langeac, France M70+451 55
Langeland, I., Denmark M26+549 47
Längelmavesi, Finland L34+615 47
Langenthal, Switzerland M43+472 45
Langholm, Scotland N18+552 41
Lang Jökull, Iceland P30+646 46
Langkawi, I., Malaysia F31+063 69
Langlade, I., Atlantic Oc. R68+468 90
Langogne, France M67+447 55
Langon, France N02+445 55
Langøya, Norway M00+687 46
Langport, England N17+511 38
Langres, France M58+478 54
Langsa, Sumatra F42+045 65
Långsele, Sweden L78+632 46
Lang-Son, Vietnam E79+218 69
Långträsk, Sweden L58+654 46
Languedoc, prov., France M66+430 55
Lanklaar, Belgium M56+510 44
Lankor Tso, Tibet G42+325 71
Lannion, France N21+488 54
Lansdale, Pennsylvania T02+402 96
Lansing, Michigan T57+428 91
Lansingburg, New York S82+428 91
Lan Tao, China E36+223 67
Lanzarote, I., Canary Is. N82+290 80
Laoag, Philippines D87+182 65
Lao Bao, Vietnam E80+165 69
Lao-chang-Ho R., China E23+378 66
Lao-Cai, Vietnam F07+225 69
Laon, France M69+496 54
La Oroya, Peru T06-115 104
Laos, S.-E. Asia F10+192 69
Lao shan, China D86+363 66
Lapalisse, France M68+462 54
La Palma, I., Canary Is. P30+286 80
La Paragua, Venezuela S21+070 104
La Paz, Argentina R88-307 103
La Paz, Argentina S45-334 103
La Paz, Bolivia S49-165 104
La Paz, Honduras T76+143 101
La Paz, Mexico V32+241 100
Lapchung L., Tibet G27+300 71
Lapeer, Michigan T50+431 91
La Pelada, Argentina S06-309 103
Lapinlahti, Finland L16+634 46
Lapithos, Cyprus K71+353 76
La Plata, Argentina R78+349 103
La Porte, Indiana T70+416 95
Laporte, Pynnsylvania T09+414 96
La Porte City, Iowa U13+424 95
Lapovo, Yugoslavia L54+442 58
Lappa Järvi, Finland L38+631 46
Lappeenranta, Finland L11+610 47
Lappland, N. Europe L57+680 46
Lapptrask, Sweden L39+660 46
Laprida, Argentina S06-378 103
Laptevykh Sea, U.S.S.R. D70+750 63
Lăpusul Românesc Romania L36+475 49
Lapy, Poland L43+530 49
Laqit, Kuwait J71+290 74
La Quiaca, Argentina S34-222 103
Lar, Iran J33+276 75
Larache, Morocco N38+350 80
Laragne, France M55+443 55

Laramate, *Peru* S89–142 **104**
Laramie, *Wyoming* V04+413 **93**
Laramie Mts., *Wyoming* V06+424 **93**
Laramie Pk., *Wyoming* V02+422 **93**
Larangeiras, *Brazil* S11–132 **104**
La Rasse, *Switzerland* M49+471 **45**
Larbert, *Scotland* N23+560 **41**
Larchwood, *Ontario* T38+466 **91**
Laredo, *Texas* V39+275 **94**
Largeau (Faya), *Chad* L66+180 **81**
Largo, *New Mexico* V17+366 **94**
Largs, *Scotland* N29+558 **41**
Larino, *Italy* M01+418 **57**
La Rioja, *Argentina* S41–294 **103**
Larisa, *Greece* L44+396 **59**
Larkana, *Pakistan* H41+275 **70**
Larnaca & B., *Cyprus* K68+349 **76**
Larne & L., *N. Ireland* N35+549 **42**
Larned, *Kansas* U56+382 **95**
La Robla, *Spain* N34+428 **52**
Laroche, *Belgium* M56+502 **44**
La Rochelle, *France* N07+462 **54**
La Roda, *Spain* N13+392 **53**
Lars Christensen Coast,
Antarctic H50–680 **27**
Laruns, *France* N03+430 **55**
Larvik, *Norway* M30+590 **47**
Laryak, *U.S.S.R.* G60+612 **62**
La Salle, *Illinois* T84+413 **95**
Las Animas, *Colorado* U80+380 **94**
Las Anod, *Somalia* J76+082 **83**
Las Cejas, *Argentina* S29–269 **103**
Las Coloradas, *Argentina* S64–396 **103**
Las Cruces, *New Mexico* V11+323 **94**
Las Cruces, *New Mexico* V11+325 **98**
La Serena, *Chile* S67–299 **103**
Last Flores, *Argentina* R86–361 **103**
Lasgird, *Iran* J43+353 **75**
Lash, *Afghanistan* H81+316 **75**
Las Heras, *Argentina* S53–465 **103**
Lashio, *Burma* F43+228 **71**
Lashkar, *India* G71+262 **73**
Lasithi, *Crete* L24+350 **59**
Las Khoreh, *Somalia* J70+110 **83**
Las Lajas, *Argentina* S62–385 **103**
Las Lomitas, *Argentina* S03–247 **103**
Las Palmas, *Canary Is.* P04+280 **80**
Las Plumas, *Argentina* S44–436 **103**
Lassen Pk., *California* W09+405 **92**
Lassen Peak Nat. Park, *Cal.* W08+405 **98**
Las Tablas, *Panama* T31+078 **101**
Last Mountain L., *Sask.* V00+510 **88**
Lastovo, I., *Yugoslavia* L79+427 **56**
Las Vacas, *Mexico* U67+295 **100**
Las Vegas, *Nevada* V60+362 **92**
Las Vegas, *New Mexico* V02+356 **94**
Latacunga, *Ecuador* T22–009 **104**
Latakia, *Syria* K55+355 **76**
La Tamba, *Guinea* N60+108 **80**
Laterrière, *Quebec* S67+483 **90**
Latheron, *Scotland* N20+583 **40**
Latrobe, *Pennsylvania* T27+404 **96**
Latrobe, *Tasmania* C22–412 **109**
Latrun, *Jordan* K60+318 **76**
La Tuque, *Quebec* S77+475 **91**
Latvia, rep., *U.S.S.R.* **47**
Lauder, *Scotland* N16+557 **41**
Laufen, *Switzerland* M45+474 **45**
Launceston, *England* N26+506 **38**
Launceston, *Tasmania* C18–414 **109**
Laune R., *Ireland, Rep.* N59+519 **43**
Launggyang, *Burma* F40+260 **71**
La Union, *Chile* S78–403 **103**
La Union, *Mexico* U70+180 **100**
La Union, *El Salvador* T77+134 **101**
La Union, *Spain* N05+377 **53**
Laura, *Queensland* C33–156 **111**
Laura, *S. Australia* C70–331 **109**
La Urbana, *Venezuela* S41+070 **104**
Laurel, *Maryland* T11+391 **96**
Laurel, *Mississippi* T83+316 **95**
Laurel, *Montana* V22+456 **93**
Laurel Hill, *Pennsylvania* T25+402 **96**
Laurens, *S. Carolina* T42+345 **97**
Laurent, *Quebec* S73+471 **91**
Laurentide Mts., *Quebec* S82+465 **90**
Laurentides Park, *Quebec* S68+477 **91**
Lauria, *Italy* L85+400 **57**
Laurie, I., *South Orkneys* Q87–610 **27**
Laurinburg, *N. Carolina* T27+348 **97**
Lausanne, *Switzerland* M50+465 **45**
Lautaro, *Chile* S75–384 **103**
Lautem, *Timor I., Indonesia* D48–084 **65**
Lauzon, *Quebec* S67+468 **91**
Lavacherie, *Belgium* M57+501 **44**
Laval, *France* N05+481 **54**
Laval B., *Quebec* S54+487 **90**
Lavalle, *Argentina* S52–327 **103**
Lavalleja, *Uruguay* R60–340 **103**
Lavamund, *Austria* L90+466 **48**
Lavardac, *France* M88+442 **55**
La Vega, *Dominican Rep.* S63+193 **101**
La Vela, *Venezuela* S57+114 **104**
Laverton, *W. Australia* D75–284 **110**
Laviana, *Spain* N33+432 **52**
Lavina, *Montana* V24+463 **93**
Lavongai, *Bismarck Arch.* B96–030 **106**
Lavos, *Portugal* N53+401 **52**
Lavras, *Brazil* R00–213 **105**
Lavras, *Brazil* R53–308 **103**
Lavras, *Brazil* Q54–068 **105**
Lavrentiya, *U.S.S.R.* Z36+654 **63**
Lávrion, *Greece* L36+377 **59**
Lawk Sawk, *Burma* F48+212 **71**
Lawra, *Ghana* N16+106 **80**
Lawrence, *Kansas* U32+390 **95**
Lawrence, *Massachusetts* S67+427 **96**
Lawrence, *New Zealand* A61–459 **112**
Lawrenceburg, *Tennessee* T75+352 **97**
Lawrenceville, *Illinois* T76+387 **95**
Lawton, *Oklahoma* U50+345 **95**
Laxford L., *Scotland* N31+584 **40**
Laysan I., *Hawaii* Z42+260 **106**
Lazarevac, *Yugoslavia* L59+444 **58**
Lazio, dep., *Italy* M16+420 **57**
Lead, *S. Dakota* U83+444 **93**
Leadhills, *Scotland* N22+554 **41**
Leadville, *Colorado* V08+392 **94**
Leaf R., *Quebec* S65+587 **89**
Leakesville, *Mississippi* T81+311 **97**
Leaksville, *N. Carolina* T28+365 **97**
Leamington, *England* N09+523 **37**
Leamington, *Ontario* T46+421 **91**
Leane L., *Ireland, Rep.* N57+520 **43**
Leatherhead, *England* N03+513 **39**
Leavenworth, *Indiana* T68+382 **97**
Leavenworth, *Kansas* U30+393 **95**
Łeba, *Poland* L74+547 **49**
Lebanon, *Kentucky* T61+375 **97**
Lebanon, *Missouri* U16+377 **95**
Lebanon, *New Hampshire* S74+437 **96**
Lebanon, *Pennsylvania* T09+403 **96**
Lebanon, rep., *W. Asia* K56+340 **74**
Lebesby, *Norway* L18+705 **46**
Lebombo Mts., *S. Africa* K78–250 **84**
Lebork, *Poland* L74+545 **49**
Lebu, *Chile* S82–375 **103**
Lebye, *Lebanon* K52+342 **76**
Lecce, *Italy* L71+404 **57**
Lecco, *Italy* M34+458 **56**
Lectourre, *France* M86+439 **55**
Ledbury, *England* N15+520 **38**
Ledesma, *Argentina* S29–238 **103**
Ledesma, *Spain* N36+411 **52**
Ledo, *India* F55+272 **71**
Lee R., *Ireland, Rep.* N51+519 **43**
Leech Lake, *Minnesota* U28+472 **93**
Leeds, *England* N09+538 **37**
Leende, *Netherlands* M57+513 **44**
Leerbeek, *Belgium* M65+508 **44**
Leerdam, *Netherlands* M59+519 **44**
Leesburg, *Virginia* T15+391 **96**
Leesville, *Louisiana* U20+311 **95**
Leeton, *New South Wales* C21–346 **109**
Leeuwarden, *Netherlands* M55+532 **44**
Leeuwin, C., *W. Australia* E29–340 **110**
Leeward Is., *West Indies* S10+172 **101**
Lefka, *Cyprus* K73+351 **76**
Lefkara, *Cyprus* K70+348 **76**
Lefkoniko, *Cyprus* K67+353 **76**
Lefroy, L., *W. Australia* D80–312 **110**
Legaspi, *Philippines* D68+130 **65**
Legge Pk., *Tasmania* C14–416 **109**
Leghorn, *See* Livorno
Legnica, *Poland* L83+512 **49**
Leh, *Kashmir* G74+342 **72**
Le Havre, *France* M89+495 **54**
Lehi, *Utah* V41+404 **94**
Lehututu, *Botswana* L48–240 **84**
Leiah, *Pakistan* H24+310 **72**
Leicester & co., *England* N07+526 **37**
Leichhardt, R., *Queensland* C62–186 **111**
Leiden, *Netherlands* M63+522 **44**
Leigh Creek, *S. Australia* C70–305 **109**
Leighlinbridge, *Ireland, Rep.* N42+527 **43**
Leighton Buzzard, *England* N04+519 **39**
Leignon, *Belgium* M59+503 **44**
Leimuiden, *Netherlands* M62+522 **44**
Leinster, prov., *Ireland, Rep.* N42+530 **43**
Leinster, Mt., *Ireland, Rep.* N41+526 **43**
Leipzig, *E. Germany* M16+514 **48**
Leisele, *Belgium* M74+510 **44**
Leitchfield, *Kentucky* T68+375 **97**
Leith, *Scotland* N19+560 **41**
Leitrim, co., *Ireland, Rep.* N49+543 **42**
Leix (Laois), co., *Ireland, Rep.* N44+534 **43**
Leixlip, *Ireland, Rep.* N39+534 **43**
Leiyang, *China* E43+264 **67**
Leka, *Norway* M20+650 **46**
Le Kef, *Tunisia* M38+360 **81**
Leksands Noret, *Sweden* M00+607 **47**
Leksvik, *Norway* M26+637 **46**
Leland, *Michigan* T64+451 **91**
Leland, *Mississippi* U05+334 **95**
Leleque, *Argentina* S66–424 **103**
Le Maire, Estrecho de, *Arg.* S30–550 **103**
Léman, Lac, *Switzerland* M51+464 **45**
Le Mans, *France* M89+480 **54**
Le Mars, *Iowa* U37+428 **95**
Lemberg. *See* Lvov
Lemnos. *See* Limnos, I.
Lemvethna, *Burma* F59+174 **71**
Lena, R., *U.S.S.R.* D65+692 **63**
Lenina Pk., *Kirgiz.* H13+393 **62**
Leninabad, *Uzbek* H33+403 **62**
Leninakan, *Armyanskaya* K04+408 **62**
Leningrad, *U.S.S.R.* K88+599 **60**
Leninka, *U.S.S.R.* A14+647 **63**
Leninogorsk, *Kazakh.* G40+505 **62**
Leninsk, *Turkmen.* H70+390 **62**
Leninsk Kuznetskiy, *U.S.S.R.* G23+545 **62**
Lenk, *Switzerland* M45+465 **45**
Lennox, I., *Chile & Argent.* S42–553 **103**
Lenoir, *N. Carolina* T39+359 **97**
Lens, *France* M73+504 **54**
Lent, *Netherlands* M55+519 **44**
Lentiira, *Finland* L01+644 **46**
Lenvik, *Norway* L71+694 **46**
Lenya, *Burma* F36+115 **71**
Lenz, *Switzerland* M32+467 **45**
Lenzerheide, *Switzerland* M32+467 **45**
Leoben, *Austria* L89+473 **48**
Leola, *S. Dakota* U54+458 **93**
Leominster, *England* N17+522 **38**
Leominster, *Massachusetts* S71+426 **96**
León, *France* N08+439 **55**
Leon, *Mexico* U70+212 **100**
Leon, *Nicaragua* T72+125 **101**
León, *Spain* N33+426 **52**
León, Monts de, *Spain* N37+426 **52**
Leongatha, *Victoria* C25–384 **109**
Leonidhion, *Greece* L43+372 **59**
Leonora, *W. Australia* D83–286 **110**
Leonteva, *U.S.S.R.* K50+590 **60**
Leopoldsburg, *Belgium* M58+511 **44**
Leopold II L., *See* Mai-Ndomba L.
Leopoldville. *See* Kinshasa
Lepepe, *Botswana* L24–234 **84**
Lepontine, Alpi, *Switz.-Italy* M41+463 **45**
Lepreau, *New Brunswick* S39+452 **90**
Lercara Friddi, *Sicily* M08+378 **57**
Lerdo, *Mexico* U82+255 **100**
Lerida, *Spain* M86+416 **53**
Lerma, *Argentina* S34–250 **103**
Lerma, *Spain* N22+420 **51**
Lermoos, *Austria* M25+474 **48**
Léros, I., *Greece* L19+372 **59**
Le Roy, *New York* T18+429 **91**
Lerwick, *Shetland, Scot.* N07+601 **40**
Lesbos. *See* Lesvos I.
Les Escoumains, *Quebec* S56+483 **90**
Leskovac, L48+430 **58**
Lesotho (Basutoland), *Afr.* L10–294 **84**
Lesozavodsk, *U.S.S.R.* D09+454 **63**
Lesparre, *France* N06+453 **55**
Lesser Slave L., *Alberta* V65+554 **88**
Lessines, *Belgium* M67+507 **44**
Lestijärvi, *Finland* L32+635 **46**
Lesvos, I., *Greece* L22+392 **59**
Leszno, *Poland* L81+518 **49**
Letcher, *S. Dakota* U49+439 **93**
Letchworth, *England* N01+520 **39**
Letea I., *Romania* L04+453 **58**
Lethbridge, *Alberta* V46+497 **88**
Leti Kep., *Indonesia* D42–084 **65**
Leticia, *Colombia* S60–043 **104**
Letpadan, *Burma* F56+177 **71**
Lette, *New South Wales* C42–344 **109**
Letterfrack, *Ireland, Rep.* N60+535 **43**
Letterkenny, *Ireland, Rep.* N46+550 **42**
Letty Harbour, *N.-W. Terr.* W28+690 **88**
Letur, *Spain* N13+384 **53**
Leucate, *France* M72+429 **55**
Leuchars, Scotland N17+564 **41**
Leucite Hills, *Wyoming* V24+418 **93**
Leuk, *Switzerland* M44+463 **45**
Leuser, mt., *Sumatra* F47+038 **65**
Leuven (Louvain), *Belgium* M62+509 **44**
Leuze, *Belgium* M68+506 **44**
Levádhia, *Greece* L43+385 **59**
Levanger, *Norway* M22+638 **46**
Leven, *Scotland* N18+562 **41**
Leven L., *Scotland* N20+562 **41**
Levêque, C., *W. Australia* D72–163 **110**
Levice, *Czechoslovakia* L69+483 **49**
Levick, Mt., *Antarctica* B20–740 **27**
Levin, *New Zealand* A28–406 **112**
Levis, *Quebec* S67+468 **91**
Levitha, I., *Greece* L21+370 **59**
Levkás, I., *Greece* L56+387 **59**
Levoča, *Czechoslavakia* L57+490 **49**
Lewes, *England* N00+509 **39**
Lewes R., *Yukon* X05+616 **88**
Lewis, Butt of, *Scotland* N37+585 **40**
Lewis I., *Scotland* N40+581 **40**
Lewis Ra., *Montana* V52+482 **98**
Lewisburg, *Pennsylvania* T11+410 **91**
Lewisburg, *Tennesee* T73+354 **97**
Lewisburg, *W. Virginia* T33+378 **97**
Lewiston, *Idaho* V72+464 **92**
Lewiston, *Maine* S61+441 **90**
Lewiston, *Michigan* T56+449 **91**
Lewiston, *N. Carolina* T13+362 **97**
Lewistown, *Illinois* U01+404 **91**
Lewistown, *Montana* V27+470 **93**
Lewistown, *Pennsylvania* T16+406 **96**
Lexington, *Georgia* T49+338 **97**
Lexington, *Kentucky* T57+380 **97**
Lexington, *Missouri* U23+392 **95**
Lexington, *Nebraska* U58+408 **95**
Lexington, *N. Carolina* T32+358 **97**
Lexington, *Tennessee* T80+356 **97**
Lexington, *Virginia* T27+377 **97**
Leydsdorp, *Transvaal* K86–240 **84**
Leyte, I., *Philippines* D60+108 **65**
Lezajsk, *Poland* L46+503 **49**
Lha-kang Dzong, *Tibet* F83+281 **71**
Lhasa, *Tibet* F83+296 **71**
Lha-tse Dzong, *Tibet* G14+291 **71**
Lhontse Dzong, *Tibet* F76+284 **71**
Lianchow, *See* Wuwei
Liangsiang, *China* E22+396 **66**
Liant, C., *Thailand* F26+127 **69**
Liao R., *China* D70+422 **64**
Liaocheng, *China* E24+365 **66**
Liaohsien, *China* E39+370 **66**
Liao-tung, G. of, *China* D86+398 **66**
Liao yang-chow, *China* D71+412 **66**
Liard, *N.-W. Territories* W23+602 **88**
Liard R., *N.-W. Territories* W23+608 **88**
Liari, *Pakistan* H51+256 **70**
Liberal, *Kansas* U66+370 **94**
Liberdade, *Brazil* S70–072 **104**
Liberec, *Czechoslovakia* L90+508 **48**
Liberia, *Costa Rica* T61+106 **101**
Liberia, rep., *W. Africa* N60+070 **80**
Libertad, *Mexico* V46+298 **100**
Liboi, *Kenya* K24+004 **83**
Libourne, *France* N02+449 **55**
Libreville, *Gabon* M32+004 **82**
Libya, *N. Africa* L60+250 **81**
Licata, *Sicily* M07+371 **57**
Licheng. *See* Tsinan
Lichfield, *England* N11+527 **37**
Licking R., *Kentucky* T56+387 **97**
Lida, *Byelorussia* L29+539 **60**
Lida-di-Roma, *Italy* M16+417 **57**
Liddel R., *Scot.-Eng.* N17+551 **41**
Liddes, *Switzerland* M47+460 **45**
Liddon G., *N.-W. Terr.* V45+750 **88**
Lidjombo, *Cameroon* L84+026 **82**
Lidköping, *Sweden* M11+585 **47**
Lidzbark, *Poland* L57+541 **49**
Liechtenstein, *Europe* M32+472 **45**
Liège & prov., *Belgium* M57+506 **44**
Liegnitz. *See* Legnica
Lieksa, *Finland* L00+633 **46**
Lienkong, *China* E23+263 **67**
Lienyunkang, *China* E03+347 **66**
Lienz, *Austria* M14+468 **48**
Liepāja, *Latvia* L54+565 **47**
Lierneux, *Belgium* M55+503 **44**
Lierre, *Belgium* M63+511 **44**
Liers, *Belgium* M57+507 **44**
Liestal, *Switzerland* M44+475 **45**
Lievre, R. du, *Quebec* T03+467 **91**
Lifford, *Ireland, Rep.* N45+548 **42**
Lifu, I., *Loyalty Is.* A75–212 **106**
Ligure, Appennino, *Italy* M36+446 **56**
Liguria, dep. *Italy* M38+445 **56**
Ligurian Sea, *Italy* M39+433 **56**
Lihsien, *China* E50+296 **67**
Likiang, *China* F28+268 **64**
Likimi, *Zaire* L56+028 **82**
Liling, *China* E38+277 **67**
Lilla Edet, *Sweden* M17+581 **47**
Lille, *Belgium* M61+512 **44**
Lille, *France* M71+507 **54**
Lillehammer, *Norway* M27+611 **47**
Lillesand, *Norway* M39+582 **47**
Lillo, *Belgium* M64+513 **44**
Lillo, *Spain* N20+397 **52**
Lillooet, *British Columbia* W11+506 **88**
Lilongwe, *Malawi* K66–140 **83**
Lim Fd., *Denmark* M40+566 **47**
Lima, *Ohio* T55+408 **91**
Lima, *Peru* T12–120 **104**
Limache, *Chile* S68–330 **103**
Limassol, *Cyprus* K72+347 **76**
Limavady, *N. Ireland* N42+550 **42**
Limay, R., *Argentina* S52–392 **103**
Limay Mahuida, *Argentina* S40–372 **103**
Limbazhi, *Latvia* L32+575 **47**
Limbourg, *Belgium* M54+506 **44**
Limburg, *W. Germany* M42+504 **48**
Limburg, prov. *Belgium* M58+510 **44**
Limchow. *See* Hoppo.
Limeira, *Brazil* R14–225 **105**
Limerick (Luimneach)
Ireland, Rep. N52+527 **43**
Limes, *Belgium* M58+496 **44**
Limestone, *Maine* S47+470 **90**
Limmen, *Netherlands* M62+526 **44**
Limmen Bight,
N. Terr., Australia C86–148 **111**
Limni, *Greece* L40+388 **59**
Limnos, I., *Greece* L29+400 **59**
Limoges, *France* M82+458 **54**
Limon, *Colorado* U83+392 **94**
Limon, *Costa Rica* T48+100 **101**
Limousin, prov., *France* M78+454 **54**
Limoux, *France* M77+431 **55**
Limpopo R.,
Mozambique etc. K68–250 **84**
Lina, mt., *New Guinea* D07–014 **65**
Linares, *Chile* S70–358 **103**
Linares, *Mexico* U57+248 **100**
Linares, *Spain* N22+381 **52**
Lincheng, *China* E16+349 **66**
Linchwan. *See* Fuchow
Lincoln, *Argentina* S09–349 **103**
Lincoln, *England* N03+532 **37**
Lincoln, *Illinois* T86+402 **95**
Lincoln, *Maine* S51+454 **90**
Lincoln, *Michigan* T51+447 **91**
Lincoln, *Nebraska* U40+408 **95**
Lincoln, *New Zealand* A45–436 **112**
Lincoln, co., *England* N01+532 **37**
Lincoln Sea, *Arctic Ocean* R35+840 **26**
Lincoln Wolds, *England* N01+534 **37**
Lincolnton, *N. Carolina* T37+355 **97**
Lindau, *W. Germany* M32+475 **48**
Lindesay, Mt., *Queensland* B68–281 **111**
Lindesnes, *Norway* M47+580 **47**
Lindi, *Tanzania* K32–100 **83**
Lindley, *Orange Free State* L12–278 **84**
Lindos, *Greece* L11+361 **59**
Lindsay, *Ontario* T23+444 **91**
Line Is., *Pacific Ocean* Y30+020 **107**
Linfen, *China* E51+360 **66**
Lingchwan, *China* E58+255 **67**
Lingen, *W. Germany* M46+525 **48**
Lingga, I., *Riau Kep., Indonesia* F02–003 **65**
Lingling, *China* E51+263 **67**
Linguère, *Senegal* P00+154 **80**
Lingyun, *China* E81+244 **67**
Linhai, *China* D83+290 **67**
Linhares, *Brazil* Q61–194 **105**
Linho, *China* E75+408 **66**
Linhsien, *China* E45+248 **67**
Lini, *China* E10+351 **66**
Linkiang, *China* D49+416 **64**
Linkiang (Tsingkiang), *China* E27+280 **67**
Linköping, *Sweden* L86+584 **47**
Linkuva, *Lithuania* L36+561 **47**
Linlithgow, *Scotland* N21+560 **41**
Linn, *Missouri* U11+385 **97**
Linnhe, L., *Scotland* N33+566 **41**
Linosa, I., *Medit. Sea* M13+359 **57**
Linping, *China* E33+244 **67**
Lins, *Brazil* R29–218 **103**
Linsi, *China* E11+434 **64**
Lintan, *China* F10+348 **66**
Linth, *R., Switzerland* M36+472 **45**
Linthal, *Switzerland* M36+469 **45**
Linton, *Quebec* S73+473 **91**
Linyu, *China* E01+400 **66**
Linz, *Austria* M04+483 **48**
Lion, G. du, *France* M66+430 **55**
Lion Pt., *N.-W. Territories* W25+727 **88**
Lio Porgyul, *Tibet* G67+320 **70**
Liouesso, *Congo* L86+010 **82**
Lipa, *Yugoslavia* L84+447 **56**
Lipari. & I., *Italy* M01+385 **57**
Lipetsk, *U.S.S.R.* K33+526 **60**
Liping, *China* E66+263 **67**
Lipovets, *Ukraine* L06+492 **60**
Lippstadt, *W. Germany* M40+517 **48**
Lipsoi, I., *Greece* L19+373 **59**
Lira, *Uganda* K74+022 **83**
Lircay, *Peru* S89–130 **104**
Liria, *Spain* N04+396 **53**
Lisala, *Zaire* L50+022 **82**
Lisboa, *Portugal* N55+387 **52**
Lisbon. *See* Lisboa
Lisburn, *N. Ireland* N36+545 **42**
Lisburne, C. *Alaska* Z00+685 **99**
Liscannor B., *Ireland, Rep.* N57+529 **43**
Lisdoonvarna, *Ireland, Rep.* N56+530 **43**
Lishih, *China* E53+375 **66**
Lishui, *China* E00+285 **67**
Lisianski, I., *Hawaii* Z55+260 **106**
Lisieux, *France* M89+492 **54**
Liskeard, *England* N27+504 **38**
L'Isle, *Switzerland* M52+466 **45**
L'Islet, *Quebec* S62+471 **91**
Lismore, *Ireland, Rep.* N48+521 **43**
Lismore, *New South Wales* B70–286 **111**
Lismore I., *Scotland* N33+565 **41**
Lisnaskea, *N. Ireland* N45+542 **42**
Lissar, *Iran* J66+380 **74**
Listowel, *Ireland, Rep.* N57+524 **43**
Listowel, *Ontario* T36+437 **91**
Lisu, *Ethiopia* K50+100 **83**
Litchfield, *Illinois* T88+392 **95**
Litchfield, *Minnesota* U27+451 **93**
Lith Ai, *Saudi Arabia* K28+202 **74**
Lithgow, *New South Wales* B89–335 **109**
Lithinon, C., *Crete* L32+349 **59**
Lithuania, rep., *U.S.S.R.* **47**

Litoměrice, *Czechoslovakia* M05+505 48
Little R., *Missouri* T88+363 97
Little Belt Mts., *Montana* V34+468 93
Little Current, *Ontario* T42+460 91
Little Falls, *Minnesota* U26+460 93
Little Falls, *New York* S89+430 96
Little Horn Mts., *Arizona* V52+334 92
Little River, *Newfoundland* R85+478 90
Little River, *New Zealand* A43-437 112
Little Rock, *Arkansas* U14+348 95
Little Rocky Mts., *Montana* V22+479 93
Little Smoky R., *Alberta* V74+546 88
Littleton, *Colorado* V00+396 94
Littleton, *New Hampshire* S70+443 91
Little Valley, *New York* T23+423 96
Littoria, *Italy* M13+415 57
Liuan, *China* E22+318 64
Liuchow, *China* E64+243 67
Liupan Shan, *China* E84+356 66
Liusvaara, *Karelia* K77+626 46
Live Oak, *Florida* T48+303 97
Liverpool, *New South Wales* B85-339 109
Liverpool, *Nova Scotia* S28+440 90
Liverpool & B., *England* N18+534 37
Liverpool Coast, *Greenland* P35+710 26
Liverpool Plains, *N.S.W.* C00-312 109
Liverpool Ra., *New S. Wales* B88-318 109
Livingston, *Alabama* T79+326 97
Livingston, *Guatemala* T82+158 100
Livingston, *Montana* V33+457 93
Livingston, *Tennessee* T62+364 97
Livingston, *Texas* U30+307 95
Livingston, I., *S. Shetlands* S04-630 27
Livingstone, *See* Maramba
Livingstonia, *Malawi* K66-108 83
Livno, *Yugoslavia* L78+438 56
Livny, *U.S.S.R.* K45+524 60
Livo Joki, *Finland* L18+655 46
Livorno, *Italy* M28+435 56
Livramento, *Brazil* R63-308 103
Liwa, *Oman* J21+246 75
Liwale, *Tanzania* K42-098 83
Lizard & Pt., *England* N31+500 38
Ljubljana, *Yugoslavia* M03+461 56
Ljubuški, *Yugoslavia* L75+432 56
Ljungdalen, *Sweden* M13+628 46
Ljusdal, *Sweden* L83+618 47
Llandaff, *Wales* N19+515 38
Llandeilo, *Wales* N24+519 38
Llandrindod Wells, *Wales* N20+522 38
Llandudno, *Wales* N23+533 38
Llanelli, *Wales* N25+517 38
Llanerchymedd, *Wales* N26+533 38
Llanes, *Spain* N29+434 52
Llangollen, *Wales* N19+530 38
Llanguihuie, L., *Chile* S76-411 103
Llanllyfni, *Wales* N26+530 38
Llano Estacado, *New Mex.* U78+340 94
Llanrhaiadr, *Wales* N20+528 38
Llanrwst, *Wales* N23+531 38
Llerena, *Spain* N36+383 52
Lleyn Pen., *Wales* N27+529 38
Lliamna, L., *Alaska* Y30+595 99
Llico, *Chile* S72-347 103
Lloydminster, *Saskatchewan* V30+534 88
Lluchmayor, *Balearic Is.* M72+395 53
Loango, *Congo* M20-046 82
Lobbes, *Belgium* M64+504 44
Loberia, *Argentina* R83-382 103
Lobito, *Angola* M08-124 82
Lobos, *Argentina* R86-352 103
Lobstick L., *Labrador* S30+540 89
Locarno, *Switzerland* M37+462 45
Lochalsh, *Ontario* T56+484 91
Lochalsh, Kyle of, *Scotland* N34+573 40
Lochbuie, *Scotland* N35+564 41
Lochcarron, *Scotland* N33+574 40
Lochearnhead, *Scotland* N26+564 41
Lochem, *Netherlands* M51+522 44
Lochgelly, *Scotland* N20+561 41
Lochgilphead, *Scotland* N33+560 41
Lochgoilhead, *Scotland* N29+562 41
Lochinver, *Scotland* N31+582 40
Lochmaben, *Scotland* N21+551 41
Lochmaddy, *Scotland* N43+576 40
Lochnagar, *Scotland* N20+570 40
Lochy, L., *Scotland* N29+570 40
Lockerbie, *Scotland* N20+551 41
Lockhart, *New South Wales* C21-353 109
Lock Haven, *Pennsylvania* T15+411 96
Lockport, *New York* T22+431 96
Locle, le, *Switzerland* M49+471 45
Loc Ninh, *Vietnam* E81+118 65
Lochristi, *Belgium* M67+511 44
Lodeynoye Pole, *U.S.S.R.* K69+608 60
Lodhran, *Pakistan* H20+295 72
Lodi, *Wisconsin* T87+434 91
Lødingen, *Norway* L84+684 46
Lodwar, *Kenya* K56+030 83
Lodz, *Poland* L63+518 49
Loenen, *Netherlands* M54+521 44
Loewoek, *Celebes* D73-010 65
Lofer, *Austria* M14+476 48
Lofoten, Is., *Norway* M16+680 46
Logan, *Montana* V39+459 93
Logan, *Utah* V42+418 94
Logan, Mt., *Quebec* S40+489 90
Logan, Mt., *Yukon* X30+606 88
Logansport, *Indiana* T68+408 95
Logone R., *Cameroon-Chad* M00+104 81
Logrona, *Spain* N15+424 53
Lohardaga, *India* G32+234 73
Loharu, *India* G85+285 72
Loikaw, *Burma* F46+197 71
Loir, R., *France* N02+476 54
Loire, dep., *France* M67+457 54
Loire R., *France* N09+472 54
Loire Atlantique, dep., *Fr.* N11+474 54
Loiret, dep., *France* M77+479 54
Loir-et-Cher, dep., *France* M82+475 54
Loja, *Ecuador* T25-040 104
Loja, *Spain* N25+372 52
Lokerer, *Belgium* M66+511 44
Lokka, *Finland* L14+678 46
Løkken, *Denmark* M32+574 47
Lökken, *Norway* M32+631 46
Loko, *Sudan* K84+044 81
Lokoja, *Nigeria* M50+078 80
Loks I., *N.-W. Territories* S26+620 89
Lola, *Angola* M08-144 82
Lolland, *Denmark* M20+546 47
Lom, *Bulgaria* L41+438 58
Loman, *Minnesota* U23+485 93
Lomas, *Argentina* R80-348 103
Loma Tina, mt., *Dom. Rep.* S64+186 101
Lombard, *Montana* V39+461 93
Lombardia, dep., *Italy* M30+457 56
Lomblen, I., *Indonesia* D70-085 65
Lombok, I. & Str., *Indonesia* E24-088 65
Lome, *Togo* M84+062 80
Lomela, *Zaire* L40-022 82
Lomie, *Cameroon* M08+032 81
Lommel, *Belgium* M58+512 44
Lomond Hills, *Scotland* N20+562 41
Lomond L., *Scotland* N28+562 41
Łomża, *Poland* L48+532 49
Loncoche, *Chile* S77-394 103
Loncopue, *Argentina* S64-381 103
Londiani, *Kenya* K54-002 83
London, *England* N01+515 39
London, *Ontario* T37+430 91
Londonderry, & co.,
Northern Ireland N44+550 42
Londonderry, C., *W. Aust.* D49-138 110
Londonderry, I., *Chile* S64-550 103
Long Beach, *S. Carolina* T23+334 99
Long I., *Bahamas, The* T01+234 101
Long I., *New York* S78+408 96
Long I., *Nova Scoia* S38+443 90
Long L., *Maine* S56+466 90
Long L., *Ontario* T70+496 89
Long L., *Scotland* N29+562 41
Long Ra., *Newfoundland* R74+500 90
Longa, *Brazil* Q73-054 105
Long Beach, *California* V79+338 92
Long Beach, *New Jersey* S85+396 96
Long Branch, *New Jersey* S84+403 96
Longchamps, *Belgium* M56+500 44
Longford, *Tasmania* C18-416 109
Longford & co., *Ireland, Rep.* N47+537 42
Long Island Sd., *N.Y., etc.* S77+411 96
Long Island City, *New York* S84+407 96
Long Melford, *England* M86+521 39
Longmont, *Colorado* V01+402 94
Long Point I., *Ontario* T32+426 91
Long Prairie, *Minnesota* U29+460 93
Longreach, *Queensland* C35-232 111
Longs Pk., *Colorado* V04+402 94
Longtown, *England* N18+550 37
Longué, *France* N01+474 54
Longueuil, *Quebec* S81+456 91
Longuyon, *France* M57+494 54
Longview, *Texas* U28+324 95
Longview, *Washington* W18+461 92
Longwy, *France* M55+495 54
Long-Xuyen, *Vietnam* E87+104 69
Lonneker, *Netherlands* M48+522 44
Lons Saunier, *France* M57+467 54
Looc, *Philippines* D78+123 65
Looe, E. & W., *England* N27+504 38
Lookout, C., *N. Carolina* T07+347 99
Loolmalasin, mt., *Tanzania* K56-030 83
Loop Hd., *Ireland, Rep.* N60+526 43
Lopei, *China* D24+476 64
Lopez C., *Gabon* M38-006 82
Lopik, *Netherlands* M60+520 44
Lop Nor, *Sinkiang, China* F88+404 64
Lopphavet, *Norway* L54+704 46
Lora Hamun, *Pakistan* H61+292 70
Lorain, *Ohio* T43+414 91
Loralai, *Pakistan* H38+304 70
Lorca, *Spain* N10+377 53
Lord Howe I., *Pacific Ocean* B35-314 106
Lordsburg, *New Mexico* V22+324 94
Loreno, *Brazil* R00-226 105
Loreto, *Brazil* R02-073 105
Loreto, *Mexico* V38+260 100
Lorica, *Colombia* T04+092 104
Lorient, *France* N20+478 54
Lorne, *Victoria* C36-386 109
Lorn, Firth of, *Scotland* N34+563 41
Lorrach, *W. Germany* M44+476 48
Lorraine, prov., *France* M53+487 54
Los Andes, *Chile* S64-328 103
Los Angeles, *California* V79+341 92
Los Angeles, *Chile* S74-375 103
Los Blancos, *Argentina* S16-235 103
Loshan, *China* F08+296 67
Lošinj I., *Yugoslavia* M04+445 56
Los Lamentos, *Mexico* V04+305 100
Los Menucos, *Argentina* S49-408 103
Los Pozos, *Chile* S62-265 103
Los Santos, *Panama* T32+080 101
Los Santos de Maimona, *Spain* N38+385 52
Lossie R., *Scotland* N20+577 40
Lossiemouth, *Scotland* N20+577 40
Los Teques, *Venezuela* S42+103 104
Los Tigres, *Argentina* S16-258 103
Lostwithiel, *England* N28+504 38
Los Vilos, *Chile* S69-319 103
Lot, dep., *France* M80+446 55
Lot, R., *France* M85+445 55
Lota, *Chile* S79-371 103
Lotbinière, *Quebec* S72+466 91
Lot-et-Garonne, dep., *France* M87+443 55
Lothian, reg., *Scotland* N18+559 41
Lottigna, *Switzerland* M36+465 45
Loubet Coast, *Antarctica* S25-680 27
Loudeac, *France* N16+482 54
Loudima, *Congo* M12-042 82
Loudon, *Malawi* K69-122 83
Loudon, *Tennessee* T56+357 97
Loudun, *France* N00+470 54
Louga, *Senegal* P08+154 80
Loughborough, *England* N07+528 37
Loughborough's I., *Burma* F43+104 71
Loughor, *Wales* N24+517 38
Loughrea, *Ireland, Rep.* N51+532 43
Louhans, *France* M59+466 54
Louisa, *Kentucky* T46+381 97
Louisburg, *N. Carolina* T20+362 97
Louiseville, *Quebec* S78+463 91
Louisiade Arch.
Papua New Guinea B70-110 111
Louisiana, state, *U.S.A.* U20+306 99
Louis Trichardt, *Transvaal* L00-232 84
Louisville, *Colorado* V02+400 94
Louisville, *Kentucky* T65+383 97
Louisville, *Mississippi* T84+331 97
Loule, *Portugal* N48+371 52
Loup City, *Nebraska* U54+412 95
Lourdes, *France* N01+431 55
Lourenço Marques, *See* Maputo
Lourical, *Portugal* N53+401 52
Lourinha, *Portugal* N56+392 52
Louth, *England* N00+534 37
Louth, *New South Wales* C29-306 109
Louth & co., *Ireland, Rep.* N39+539 42
Louvain, *Belgium* M62+509 44
Louveigne, *Belgium* M56+505 44
Louviers, *France* M83+492 54
Lövanger, *Sweden* L52+643 46
Loveland, *Colorado* V00+404 94
Lovell, *Wyoming* V21+448 93
Loviisa (Lovisa), *Finland* L23+605 47
Lovington, *New Mexico* U80+329 94
Lövlid, *Sweden* L80+647 46
Low, C., *N.-W. Territories* T64+634 89
Lowa, *Zaire* L24-014 82
Lowell, *Massachusetts* S68+427 91
Lowell, *Michigan* T62+429 91
Lower Brule, *S. Dakota* U57+441 93
Lowestoft, *England* M80+525 39
Lowicz, *Poland* L60+521 49
Lowland, *N. Carolina* T09+353 97
Lowriet, *Belize* T81+182 101
Lowville, *New York* T03+438 91
Loxton, *S. Australia* C57-345 109
Loyalty Is., *Pacific Ocean* A80-210 106
Loyang, *China* E45+348 66
Loyung, *China* E63+244 67
Lozère, dep., *France* M68+444 55
Loznica, *Yugoslavia* L65+445 58
Luampa, *Zambia* L34-152 84
Luan. *See* Changchih
Luanda, *Angola* M10-090 82
Luang Prabang, *Laos* F17+198 69
Luarca, *Spain* N40+435 52
Luashi, *Zaire* L38-110 82
Lubaczow, *Poland* L42+501 49
Lubana, *Latvia* L20+569 47
Lubartow, *Poland* L45+515 49
Lubben, *E. Germany* M07+520 48
Lubbock, *Texas* U70+336 94
Lübeck, *W. Germany* M26+539 48
Lubeck, *Victoria* C45-368 109
Lübecker B.,
E. & W. Germany M24+541 48
Lubefu, *Zaire* L34-046 82
Lubin, *Poland* L82+514 49
Lublin, *Poland* L45+512 49
Lubliniec, *Poland* L68+507 49
Lubnaig, L., *Scotland* N26+563 41
Lubumbashi, *Zaire* L14-118 83
Luc, le, *France* M52+434 55
Lucala, *Angola* L88-094 82
Lucan, *Ireland, Rep.* N39+534 43
Lucania. *See* Basilicata.
Lucca, *Italy* M27+439 56
Lucca, *Jamaica* T19+185 101
Luce B., *Scotland* N29+548 41
Lucena, *Spain* N27+374 52
Lučenec, *Czechoslovakia* L62+483 49
Lucera, *Italy* L88+415 57
Lucerne. *See* Luzern.
Luch, *U.S.S.R.* K17+570 61
Luchow, *China* E88+288 67
Luchow (Hofei), *China* E17+319 66
Lucinda, *Pennsylvania* T27+413 96
Lucindale, *S. Australia* C58-370 109
Luckau, *E. Germany* M08+519 48
Luckenwalde, *E. Germany* M11+521 48
Lucknow, *India* G54+268 73
Lucknow, *Ontario* T39+440 91
Luçon, *France* N07+465 54
Luderitz, *Namibia* L88-266 84
Ludhiana, *India* G85+309 72
Ludington, *Michigan* T69+440 91
Ludlow, *England* N16+524 38
Ludvika, *Sweden* L89+601 47
Ludwigshafen, *W. Germany* M40+495 48
Ludwigslust, *E. Germany* M21+533 48
Ludza, *Latvia* L14+565 47
Luebo, *Zaire* L52-054 82
Luga, *U.S.S.R.* L01+587 60
Lugano & L. di, *Switz.* M36+460 45
Lugansk, *Ukraine* K34+486 60
Lugh Ferrandi, *Somalia* K14+036 83
Lugo, *Spain* N45+430 52
Lugoj, *Romania* L49+457 58
Lugovaia, *Kazakh.* H13+430 62
Luhaiya, *Yemen* K14+157 74
Luhit R., *India* F54+276 71
Luhsien. *See* Luchow.
Luhwang Shan I., *China* D77+297 67
Luichow. *See* Hoihong
Luichow Pen., *China* E66+208 64
Luime, *Angola* L84-108 82
Luitpold Cst., *Antarctica* Q20-770 27
Lujan, *Argentina* R85-345 103
Lujan, *Argentina* S53-330 103
Lujan, *Paraguay* R75-252 103
Lukala, *Zaire* M04-056 82
Lukovit, *Bulgaria* L35+432 58
Lukoyanov, *U.S.S.R.* K03+550 61
Lukula, *Zaire* M12-054 82
Lule Älv, *Sweden* L54+663 46
Lulea, *Sweden* L47+656 46
Luluabourg, *Zaire* L46-058 82
Lulung, *China* E07+398 66
Lumberton, *N. Carolina* T24+346 97
Lumbres, *France* M78+507 54
Lummen, *Belgium* M59+510 44
Lumsden, *New Zealand* A69-457 112
Luna, *Arkansas* U06+334 97
Lunan B., *Scotland* N15+566 41
Lund, *Sweden* M11+557 47
Lundy I., *England* N28+512 38
Lune, R., *England* N16+542 37
Lüneburg, *W. Germany* M28+533 48
Lunel, *France* M66+437 55
Luneville, *France* M51+486 54
Lungan. *See* Pingwu.
Lungki, *China* E13+246 67
Lungnan, *China* E32+248 67
Lungsi, *China* F03+349 66
Lungyen, *China* E18+252 67
Luni, *India* H11+260 70
Lunino, *U.S.S.R.* J89+536 61
Lunz, *Austria* L90+478 48
Lupeh, *China* D83+446 64
Lupiro, *Tanzania* K50-084 83
Lupkow, *Poland* L48+493 49
Luputa, *Zaire* L38-072 82
Luray, *Virginia* T21+387 91
Lurgan, *N. Ireland* N38+544 42
Luribay, *Bolivia* S46-170 104
Lurøy, *Norway* M13+664 46
Lusaka, *Zambia* L10-154 84
Lusambo, *Zaire* L40-050 82
Lusambo, *Zaire* L44-084 82
Lushai Hills, *India* F72+233 71
Lushnjë, *Albania* L62+409 59
Lushun, *China* D82+388 66
Lusk, Wyoming U86+427 93
Luss, *Scotland* N28+561 41
Lut Des., *Iran* J10+310 30
Lüta, *China* D80+389 66
Luther, *Michigan* T65+441 91
Luton, *England* N02+519 39
Lutsen, *Minnesota* U04+476 91
Lutsk, *Ukraine* L28+508 60
Luttre, *Belgium* M64+505 44
Luvia, *Finland* L50+613 47
Luxembourg, and Grand-duchy of,
N.-W. Europe M54+497 48
Luxembourg, prov., *Belg.* M57+500 44
Luxeuil, *France* M52+478 54
Luxor, *Egypt* K74+256 81
Luzern & canton, *Switz.* M40+471 45
Luzon, I., *Philippines* D85+150 65
Luzon Str. *Philippines* D75+200 64
Luzy, *France* M66+468 54
Lvov, *Ukraine* L36+498 60
Lwanhsien, *China* E07+397 66
Lwan-ping, *China* E13+409 66
Lyallpur, *Pakistan* H15+314 72
Lybster, *Scotland* N20+583 40
Lycksele, *Sweden* L68+646 46
Lydavėnai, *Lithuania* L41+556 47
Lydda, *Israel* K61+320 76
Lydenburg, *Transvaal* K88-252 84
Lydney, *England* N16+517 38
Lyell, Mt., *Brit. Columbia* V72+17 88
Lyell, Mt., *California* V85+378 92
Lyell Ra., *New Zealand* A46-416 112
Lykens, *Pennsylvania* T11+405 96
Lyme B., *England* N18+506 38
Lyme Regis, *England* N18+507 38
Lymington, *England* N09+508 39
Lynchburg, *Virginia* T25+374 97
Lyndhurst, *S. Australia* C70-303 109
Lynn, *Massachusetts* S65+425 96
Lynton, *England* N23+512 38
Lyon, *France* M61+458 54
Lyon, *Montana* V39+448 93
Lyonnais, prov., *France* M65+458 54
Lyons, *Georgia* T44+322 97
Lyons, *Kansas* U49+384 95
Lyons, *New York* T12+430 96
Lyons, R., *W. Australia* E27-243 110
Lys, R., *Belgium, etc.* M69+509 44
Lysamis, *Kenya* K42+016 83
Łyse, *Poland* L51+534 49
Lysekil, *Sweden* M21+583 47
Lyss, Switz. M46+471 45
Lyster, *Quebec* S69+464 91
Lysva, *U.S.S.R.* J14+581 61
Lytham St Annes, *England* N18+537 37
Lyttelton, *New Zealand* A43-436 112
Lytton, *British Columbia* W09+502 88
Ma'an, *Jordan* K56+302 76
Maarheeze, *Netherlands* M57+513 44
Maarianhamina. *See* Mariehamn.
Ma'arret en Numan, *Syria* K50+357 76
Maas, R., *Netherlands* M55+518 44
Maasbree, *Netherlands* M54+514 44
Maaseik, *Belgium* M55+511 44
Ma'asir, *Saudi Arabia* K41+307 74
Maassluis, *Netherlands* M65+519 44
Maastricht, *Belgium* M56+508 44
Maatsuyker Is., *Tasmania* C22-436 109
Mabote, *Mozambique* K66-222 84
Mabrouk, *Mali* N08+194 80
Mabuki, *Tanzania* K70-030 83
McAdam, *New Brunswick* S44+456 90
Macahe, *Brazil* Q71-225 105
Macahyba, *Brazil* Q32-059 105
McAlester, *Oklahoma* U34+350 95
McAlister, mt., *New S. Wales* C02-345 109
Macaloje, *Mozambique* K52-120 83
Macao (Port.), *China* E38+223 67
Macapa, *Brazil* R36+001 105
Macás, *Ecuador* T19-024 104
Macau, *Brazil* Q40-051 105
McCammon, *Idaho* V43+426 94
Macclesfield, *England* N13+533 37
McClintock Chan., *N.-W. Ter.* U70+714 88
McClure, C., *N.-W. Terr.* W08+746 88
McClure Str., *N.-W. Terr.* V70+738 88
McComb, *Mississippi* U03+312 97
McConnellsburg, *Pa.* T18+399 96
McCook, *Nebraska* U66+402 94
Macdonald, L., *W. Australia* D37-234 110
Macdonnel Ranges, *N. Terr., Aust.* D15-232 110
McDouall Ra., *N. Terr., Aust.* D00-196 111
Macdougall, L., *N.-W. Terr.* U50+660 88
Maceio, *Brazil* Q34-095 105
Macerata, *Italy* M09+433 56
McGill, *Nevada* V59+395 92
Macgillycuddy's Reeks,
Ireland, Rep. N59+520 43
McGregor, *Texas* U44+314 95
McGregor Ra., *Queensland* C43-268 111
Mach, *Pakistan* H48+298 70
Machala, *Ecuador* T29-032 104
Machareti, *Bolivia* S19-208 104
Machias, *Maine* S45+448 90
Machias B., *Maine* S44+446 90
Machiasport, *Maine* S44+447 90
Machicha, *Mozambique* K58-240 84
Machilipatnam (Bandar), *India* G52+162 70
Machiques, *Venezuela* S75+100 104
Machiwara, *India* G83+309 72
Machu Picchu, *Peru* S77-128 104
Machynlleth, *Wales* N23+526 38
Macias Nguema, *Equat - Guinea* M38+036 80
Măcin, *Romania* L11+452 58
McIntosh, *S. Dakota* U68+459 93
Mackay, *Alberta* V40+570 88
Mackay, *Queensland* C00-211 111
Mackay L., *N.-W. Terr.* V32+640 88
Mackay, L., *W. Australia* D37-226 110
McKeesport, *Pennsylvania* T29+404 96

Mackenna, Argentina S27-338 103
McKenzie, Tennessee T81+361 97
Mackenzie B., Antartica H05-680 27
Mackenzie Dist., N.-W. Terr. W00+640 88
Mackenzie B., N.-W. Terr. X15+688 88
Mackenzie Mts., N.-W. Terr. W60+642 88
Mackenzie R., N.-W. Terr. W45+654 88
Mackenzie King I., N.-W. T. V30+776 88
Mackillop, L., Queensland C52-262 111
Mackinac I. & Str. of, Mich. T58+458 91
Mackinaw, Michigan T59+458 91
McKinley, Mt., Alaska Y05+628 99
Macksville, New S. Wales B74-308 109
Maclean, New S. Wales B71-294 109
McLeansboro, Illinois T81+381 97
Macleay, R., New S. Wales B76-308 109
Macleod, Alberta V50-498 88
McLeod R., N.-W. Terr. V35+632 88
Macloutsi, Botswana L10-222 84
MacMahon Fort, Algeria M80+292 80
McMillan, L., New Mexico U86+326 94
Macmillan Ra., Yukon X10+636 94
Macmillan R., Yukon W85+635 88
McMinnville, Tennessee T65+357 97
McMullen Pk., Arizona V24+330 94
McMurdo Sd., Antarctica A90-770 27
McNary, Arizona V29+340 94
Macomb, Illinois U06+404 95
Macomer, Sardinia M37+402 57
Macon, Belgium M65+501 44
Mâcon, France M61+463 54
Macon, Georgia T52+328 97
Macon, Mississippi T82+331 95
Macon, Missouri U15+398 95
McPherson, Kansas U46+384 95
McPherson, N.-W. Terr. W89+672 88
Macpherson Ra., Queensland B75-280 111
Macquarie Harb., Tasmania C28-423 109
Macquarie I., Pacific Ocean B35-510 106
Macquarie, L., New S. Wales B81-331 109
Macquarie Mt., N.S.W. C05-337 109
Macquarie, R., N.S.W. C15-306 109
Macquarie, R., Tasmania C17-417 109
McRae, Georgia T48+320 97
Mac-Robertson Ld., Antarc. H75-690 27
Macroom, Ireland, Rep. N54+519 43
Macuje, Colombia S80+004 104
Macusani, Peru S62-140 104
McVicar Arm, N.-W. Terr. V85+652 88
Madaba, Jordan K55+317 76
Madadi, Chad L56+182 81
Madagascar I., Indian Oc. J76-200 83
Madahy, Brazil Ro6-050 105
Madain Salih, Saudi Arabia K41+269 74
Madan, Iran J10+366 74
Madaripur, Bangladesh F89+232 71
Madawaska, Ontario T18+455 91
Madeira Is., Atlantic Ocean P10+326 80
Madeira, R., Brazil S08-056 104
Madeleine, C. de la, Quebec S32+493 90
Madhepur, India G22+262 73
Madhipura, India G19+259 73
Madhopur, India G81+260 70
Madhopur, India G86+323 72
Madhubani, India G23+264 73
Madhupur, India G20+243 73
Madhya Pradesh, India G75+236 70
Madinat ash Sh'ab, Yemen, South K01+127 74
Madison, Georgia T51+338 97
Madison, Kansas U37+382 95
Madison, Nebraska U45+418 95
Madison, New Jersey S87+407 96
Madison, N. Carolina T30+364 97
Madison, S. Dakota U42+440 93
Madison, Wisconsin T86+430 95
Madisonville, Kentucky T75+372 97
Madoc, Ontario T15+445 91
Madona, Latvia L23+569 47
Madras, India G58+132 70
Madre, Laguna, Texas U44+266 94
Madre, Sa., Mexico V04+250 100
Madre, Sierra, Wyoming V12+412 93
Madre Austral, Lag. de la, Mexico U47+246 100
Madre de Dios, I., Chile T00-502 103
Madre de Dios, R., Peru-Bol. S54-123 104
Madre del Sur, Sa., Mexico U65+174 100
Madrid, New Mexico V08+354 94
Madrid, Spain N22+404 52
Madridejos, Spain N21+395 52
Madura, I., Indonesia G72+100 70
Madurai, I., Indonesia E40+069 65
Maebashi, Japan C65+364 68
Maeseyck, Belgium M55+511 44
Maestra, Sa., Cuba T10+202 101
Mafeking, Cape Province L26-260 84
Mafia I., Tanzania K32-078 83
Mafra, Portugal N56+390 52
Mafraq, Jordan K53+324 76
Magad Plat. See Jol Plat
Magadan, U.S.S.R. B86+595 63
Magadi & L., Kenya K52-020 83
Magadino, Switzerland M37+462 45
Magallanes. See Punta Arenas
Magallanes, Estrecho de, Chile S82-532 103
Magangue, Colombia S89+092 104
Magas, Iran H80+271 75
Magaz, Spain N27+420 52
Magburaka, Sierra Leone N72+088 80
Magdala, Ethiopia K34+112 83
Magdalen Is., Quebec S13+474 90
Magdalena, Bolivia S25-133 104
Magdalena, Mexico V35+306 100
Magdalena, New Mexico V14+342 94
Magdalena, B., Mexico V42+245 100
Magdalena, I., Chile S78-447 103
Magdalena, R., Colombia S88+095 104
Magdalena, R., Mexico V45+308 100
Magdeburg, E. Germany M20+521 48
Magee I., N. Ireland N34+548 42
Magellan, Str. of, Chile S60-528 103
Magerøya, Norway L26+709 46
Maggia, Switzerland M38+462 45
Maggiore, L., Italy M37+460 56
Maghang Tsangpo, R., Tibet G25+292 71
Maghara, Geb., Egypt K70+306 76
Magharee Is., Ireland, Rep. N60+523 43
Maghera, N. Ireland N50+548 42
Magheratelt, N. Ireland N40+548 42
Maglaj, Yugoslavia L71+446 58
Maglie, Italy L70+401 57
Magnetic Pole, N., N.-W. T. U70+760 88
Magnitogorsk, U.S.S.R. J06+533 61
Magnolia, Alabama T76+322 97
Magnolia, Arkansas U19+332 95
Magnolia, Mississippi U02+311 95
Magnolia, N. Carolina T20+350 97
Magog, Quebec S73+453 91
Magpie, Quebec S27+503 90
Magpie L., Quebec S28+510 90
Maguse L., N.-W. Terr. U44+614 88
Magwe, Burma F60+202 71
Mahabad, Iran J86+368 74
Mahabaleshwar, India H07+180 70
Mahaban, India G73+274 72
Mahabharat Ra., Nepal G30+274 73
Mahaddei Uen, Somalia J86+028 83
Mahadeo Hills, India G72+223 73
Mahail, Saudi Arabia K17+190 74
Mahajamba B. de, Madag. J78-154 83
Mahajan, India H07+287 72
Mahalapye, Botswana L20-232 84
Mahallat, Iran J58+339 75
Maham, India G82+290 72
Mahanadi R., India G31+206 71
Mahanoro, Madagascar J68-200 83
Mahanoy City, Pennsylvania T07+408 96
Maharashtra, state, India H00+190 70
Mahbubnagar, India G71+168 70
Mahdia, Tunisia M24+354 81
Mahé, India. G87+117 70
Mahendragiri, mt., India G33+192 71
Mahia Pen., New Zealand A12-392 112
Mahmed-Hussein-magala, Iran J55+368 75
Mahmudabad, India G53+273 73
Mahmudabad, Iran J47+366 75
Mahot I., Saudi Arabia J12+205 75
Mahunda, Mozambique K32-118 83
Mahuva, India H18+211 70
Maibud, Iran J35+322 75
Maida, Yemen K13+163 74
Maidan, Afghanistan H49+324 75
Maidenhead, England N04+515 39
Maidstone, England M87+513 39
Maiduguri, Nigeria M10+118 81
Maienfeld, Switzerland M33+470 45
Maihar, India G55+243 73
Maikal Ra., India G52+224 73
Maikop, U.S.S.R. K29+445 62
Maimana, Afghanistan H60+358 75
Mai-Ndombe, L., Zaire L70-020 82
Main, R., Germany M33+498 48
Main R., N. Ireland N38+547 42
Main Barrier Ra., N.S.W. C52-316 109
Maine, prov., France N01+483 54
Maine, state, U.S.A. S60+450 99
Maine, G. of, Maine, etc. S54+433 90
Maine-et-Loire, dep., France N04+472 54
Maing Kaing, Burma F58+248 71
Maingkwan, Burma F50+263 71
Mainpuri, India G66+272 73
Mainstream, Maine S57+449 90
Mainz, W. Germany M40+500 48
Maipo, mt., Argentina S59-342 103
Maipu, Argentina R77-368 103
Maique R., Ireland, Rep. N53+526 43
Maison Carrée (El Harrach), Algeria M72+366 80
Maissin, Belgium M59+500 44
Mait & I., Somalia J78+108 83
Maitland, New South Wales B81-327 109
Maitland, S. Australia C74-343 109
Maitland, L., W. Australia D83-269 110
Maiz, Mexico U58+224 100
Maizura, Japan C88+354 68
Maja, I., Indonesia E63-011 65
Majagua, Colombia S88+085 104
Majitha, India H00+317 72
Majmaa, Saudi Arabia J88+259 74
Majorca. See Mallorca
Majunga, Madagascar J82-158 83
Majuro, Is., Marshall Is. A50+065 106
Makale, Ethiopia K32+134 83
Makania, Tanzania K44-044 83
Makariev, U.S.S.R. K07+578 61
Makarvey, U.S.S.R. J89+561 61
Makasar, Celebes, see Ujung Pandang
Makassar Str., Indonesia E15-032 65
Makatea, I., Tuamotu Arch. X80-158 107
Makedhonia, Greece L48+407 59
Makemo, I., Tuamotu Arch. X54-162 107
Makhachkala, U.S.S.R. J76+430 62
Makhai, China F66+381 64
Makikihi, New Zealand A53-446 112
Makindu, Kenya K42-024 83
Makkinga, Netherlands M53+530 44
Makla, Jebel el, Saudi Arabia K58+286 74
Mako, Hungary L57+462 58
Makongolosi, Tanzania K70-084 83
Makorako, mt., N.Z. A23-391 112
Makram, Saudi Arabia K32+205 74
Makri, India G48+198 70
Makri, Turkey L05+367 74
Maksamaa, Finland L47+632 46
Maku, Iran K03+393 74
Makum, India F57+274 71
Makurdi, Nigeria M38+078 80
Makwiro, Zimbabwe K88-178 84
Makeyevka, Ukraine K42+481 60
Mal B., Ireland, Rep. N57+528 43
Mal B., Quebec S25+486 90
Mala, Peru T10-127 100
Malå, Sweden L68+652 46
Malabang, Philippines D65+076 65
Malabar Coast, India H00+120 70
Malabo, Macias Nguema M37+038 80
Malacca, Str. of, Sumatra-Pen-Malaysia F26+025 65
Malad City, Idaho V44+422 94
Maladeta, mt., Spain M86+426 53
Malaga, Spain N26+367 52
Malaita, Solomon Is. B25-090 106
Malakal, Sudan K80+094 81
Malakand & Pass, Pakistan H19+345 72
Malang, Java E43-080 65
Malange, Angola L82-096 82
Malaren, L., Sweden L78+595 47
Malargue, Argentina S57-355 103
Malas, Ethiopia K42+164 83
Malawi (Nyasaland), E. Afr. K66-120 83
Malayir, Iran J68+343 74
Malaysia, S. E. Asia 65
Malazgirt, Turkey K13+391 74
Malbork, Poland L66+540 49
Malchow, E. Germany M15+535 48
Malda, India G11+250 73
Maldegem, Belgium M69+512 44
Malden, Massachusetts S66+424 96
Malden, Missouri U00+366 95
Malden, I., Pacific Ocean Y30-045 107
Maldive Is., Indian Ocean H10+050 30
Maldon, England M86+517 39
Maldonado, Uruguay R60-349 103
Maléa, C., Greece L41+365 59
Malé Karpaty, Czech. L77+484 49
Malekula, I., Vanuatu A73-173 106
Máleme, Crete L37+355 59
Maler Kotla, India G85+305 72
Malesherbes, France M75+483 54
Malheur L., Oregon V83+433 92
Mali, rep., W. Africa N00+160 80
Malia, India H25+230 70
Malihabad, India G56+269 73
Malin Hd., Ireland, Rep. N44+554 42
Malinau, Borneo E20+036 65
Malindi, Kenya K30-032 83
Malines, Belgium M61+510 44
Malkangiri, India G48+185 71
Malko Trnovo, Bulgaria L15+420 58
Mallacoota & Inl., Victoria C02-376 109
Mallaig, Scotland N35+570 40
Mállia, G., Crete L27+354 59
Malloggia, Switzerland M32+464 45
Mallorca I., Balearic Is. M72+395 53
Mallow, Ireland, Rep. N52+521 43
Malmberget, Sweden L56+671 46
Malmédy, Belgium M54+504 44
Malmesbury, England N13+516 39
Malmö, Sweden M12+556 47
Malmyzh, U.S.S.R. J56+565 61
Malombe L., Malawi K58-146 83
Malone, New York S86+449 91
Malonga, Zaire L40-106 82
Malpeque B., P.E.I. S23+466 90
Malta, Montana V17+484 93
Malta Chan., Medit. Sea M02+364 57
Malta, I., Mediterranean Sea M03+359 57
Malters, Switzerland M41+470 45
Malton, England N05+541 37
Malung, Sweden M08+607 47
Malvaglia, Switzerland M36+464 45
Malvan, India H09+161 70
Malvern, Arkansas U16+344 95
Malvern Hills, England N14+521 38
Malvina, Quebec S69+452 91
Malvinas, Islas. See Falkland Is.
Mama, U.S.S.R. E42+583 63
Maman, Sudan K50+160 83
Mamantel, Mexico U07+184 100
Mambasa, Zaire L06+012 83
Mammoth Cave, Kentucky T66+372 97
Mammoth Cave Nat. Park, Kentucky T68+372 97
Mamonal, Colombia T03+104 104
Mamou, Guinea N72+104 80
Mampoko, Zaire L68+008 82
Maputo, Mozambique K74-260 84
Mamu, Afghanistan H67+296 75
Mamudju, Celebes, E07-026 65
Man, Ivory Coast N46+076 80
Man, I. of, Irish Sea N27+542 37
Manacapuru, Brazil S03-033 104
Manacor, Balearic Is. M71+395 53
Manado, Celebes, D61+015 65
Managua, Nicaragua T68+122 101
Managua L., Nicaragua T68+124 101
Manakha, Yemen K08+151 74
Manama, Bahrain I. J57+263 75
Mananjary, Madagascar J70-214 83
Manankoro, Mali N44+104 80
Manantenina, Madagascar J76-244 83
Manapouri L., New Zealand A75-455 112
Manasarowar L., Tibet G52+307 70
Manasquan, New Jersey S85+401 91
Manassas, Virginia T15+387 91
Manaus, Brazil S00-030 104
Mancelona, Michigan T61+449 91
Manche, dep., France N09+492 54
Manchester, England N13+535 37
Manchester, Greater, co., Eng. N14+535 37
Manchester, Iowa U09+424 95
Manchester, New Hampshire S69+429 91
Manchester, Tennessee T67+354 97
Manchester, Virginia T15+375 97
Manchouli, China E14+492 64
Manchuria, China D60+460 64
Mancinik, Turkey K48+392 74
Manda, Tanzania K62-106 83
Mandal, Norway M45+580 47
Mandalay, Burma F53+220 71
Mandal Gobi, Mongolia E83+452 64
Mandan, N. Dakota U65+468 93
Mandarin B., China E58+209 67
Mander, Netherlands M49+524 44
Mandera, Kenya K20+038 83
Mandeville, Louisiana U01+304 97
Mandi, India G78+317 72
Mandie, Mozambique K68+164 84
Mandla, India G58+226 73
Mandritsara, Madagascar J68-158 83
Mandvi, India H34+228 70
Manfred, New South Wales C37-334 109
Manfredonia, G., di, Italy L84+416 57
Manfuha, Saudi Arabia J79+246 74
Mangaia, I., Cook Is. Y50-220 107
Mangaldai, India F77+264 71
Mangalme, Chad L62+122 81
Mangalore, India H01+129 70
Mangareva, I., Tuamotu Archipelago W88-235 107
Mangaweka, New Zealand A26-398 112
Mangfall Geb., W. Germany M18+476 48
Manglaralto, Ecuador T34-018 104
Mangoche, Malawi K58-144 84
Mangoni, New Zealand A39-350 112
Mangrol, India H30+210 70
Mangualde, Portugal N47+406 52
Mangueria, L. da, Brazil R48-332 103
Manhatten, Kansas U40+392 95
Manhay, Belgium M56+503 44
Manhuassu, Brazil Q72-204 105
Manicoré, Brazil S07-058 104
Manifold, C., Queensland B85-225 111
Manihiki, I., Pacific Ocean Y66-105 106
Manikarchar, India G01+256 73
Manikganj. See Dasara
Manikpur, Bangladesh F77+218 71
Manikuagan R., Quebec S52+508 90
Manila, Philippines D84+146 65
Manilla, New South Wales B86-307 109
Manipur, India F65+250 71
Manisa, Turkey L15+386 74
Manistee, Michigan T68+443 91
Manistee R., Michigan T64+445 91
Manistique, Michigan T68+460 91
Manitoba, prov., Canada 88
Manitoba, L., Manitoba U52+510 88
Manitou Gorge, Quebec S57+578 89
Manitou Is., Michigan T66+451 91
Manitoulin I., Ontario T42+457 91
Manitowaning, Ontario T41+457 91
Manitowoc, Wisconsin T76+442 9
Maniwaki, Quebec T06+464 91
Maniya, Iraq K12+308 74
Manizales, Colombia T03+051 104
Manja, Madagascar K04-214 83
Manjhi, India G32+258 73
Manjimup, W. Australia E23-340 110
Manka, Taiwan D81+250 67
Mankato, Minnesota U24+442 93
Mankheri, India G33+237 73
Manlleu, Spain M76+420 53
Manly, New South Wales B83-338 109
Manmad, India H03+203 70
Mannahill, S. Australia C60-324 109
Mannar, Sri Lanka G61+090 70
Mannar, G. of, India G67+086 70
Mannargudi, India G64+107 70
Mannheim, W. Germany M39+495 48
Manning, S. Carolina T31+337 97
Mannum, S. Australia C64-349 109
Manoa, Bolivia S33-097 104
Manoel Vieira, Brazil S02-104 104
Manokwari, New Guinea D06-008 65
Manono, Zaire L16-074 82
Manorhamilton, Ireland, Rep. N49+543 42
Manosque, France M55+439 55
Manresa, Spain M79+417 53
Mansehra, Pakistan H10+344 72
Mansel I., North-West Territories T30+616 89
Mansfield, England N07+531 37
Mansfield, Louisiana U22+320 95
Mansfield, Massachusetts S67+421 91
Mansfield, Ohio T45+408 91
Mansfield, Pennsylvania T13+418 96
Mansfield, Victoria C24-370 109
Mansfield, Mt., Vermont S77+446 91
Mansi, Burma F54+248 71
Mansilla de Las Mulas, Spain N33+425 52
Manta, Ecuador T34+009 104
Manti, Utah V40+392 94
Mantilla, Argentina R82-288 103
Mantova, Italy M25+451 56
Mantua. See Mantova
Manu, Peru S65-123 104
Manu'a, I., Samoa Is. Z28-150 106
Manuel Rodrigue, I., Chile S84-528 103
Manujan, Iran J15+274 75
Manus I., Admiralty Is. C20-023 106
Many, Louisiana U21+315 95
Manyoni, Tanzania K62-058 83
Manzala L., Egypt K78+312 81
Manzanares, Spain N20+390 52
Manzanillo, Cuba T13+204 101
Manzanillo, Mexico U86+190 100
Manzanillo, Pta., Panama T27+096 101
Mao, Chad L88+140 81
Mapia Is., Pacific Ocean D00+005 106
Mapimi, Mexico U83+259 100
Maping. See Liuchow
Mapire, Venezuela S28+076 104
Maple Creek, Saskatchewan V26+499 88
Maqainama, Saudi Arabia J67+223 74
Maqatin, Yemen, South J81+135 74
Maqna, Suadi Arabia K62+284 74
Maquela do Zombo, Angola L88-062 82
Maquinchao, Argentina S53-412 103
Maquoketa, Iowa U04+420 95
Mara, Transvaal L04+232 84
Maraã, Brazil S33-019 104
Maraba, Brazil R24-053 105
Maracá, I. de, Brazil R32+020 105
Maracaibo, Venezuela S70+106 104
Maracaibo, L. de, Venezuela S70+100 104
Maracana, Brazil R15-008 105
Maracassume, Brazil R06-020 105
Maracay, Venezuela S45+103 104
Marada, Libya L64+290 81
Maradi, Niger M46+132 80
Maragheh, Iran J82+374 74
Maragogi, Brazil Q32-090 105
Marakei, I., Kiribati A40+025 106
Marakwet, Kenya K56+010 83
Maralinga, S. Aust. D20-302 110
Maramba, Zambia L24-178 84
Marand, Iran J86+384 74
Maranguape, Brazil Q52-038 105
Marañon, R., Peru S74-034 104
Maras, Turkey K48+376 74
Marau, Brazil Q54-141 105
Maravilha, Brazil S48-061 104
Marazion, England N33+501 38
Mabella, Spain N29+365 52
Marble Bar, W. Australia E02-211 110
Marblehead, Massachusetts S65+425 96
Marcellino, Brazil S44+008 104
Marche, Belgium M58+502 44
Marche, dep., Italy M11+433 56
Marche, prov. France M80+462 54
Marchena, Spain N32+373 52
Marchin, Belgium M58+505 44
Mar Chiquita, Argentina S16-306 103
Marcus I., Pacific Ocean B70+250 106
Marcy, Mt., New York S84+441 91

Mardan, *Pakistan* H17+342 **72**
Mar del Plata, *Argentina* R76–379 **103**
Mardin, *Turkey* K26+373 **74**
Mare, I., *Loyalty Is.* A70–220 **106**
Marechal Deodoro, *Brazil* Q34–098 **105**
Maree L., *Scotland* N33+577 **40**
Marengo, *Wisconsin* U05+465 **91**
Margarita, I., *Venezuela* S24+110 **104**
Margarites, *Crete* L32+354 **59**
Margate, *England* M82+514 **39**
Maria I., *Tasmania* C12–427 **109**
Marianao, *Cuba* T45+230 **101**
Marianas, Is., *Pacific Ocean* C25+150 **106**
Marianna, *Arkansas* U05+347 **97**
Marianna, *Florida* T62+308 **97**
Marianske Lázně, *Czech.* M14+499 **48**
Marias, *Montana* V33+479 **93**
Marias R., *Montana* V48+483 **98**
Marib, *Yemen* K00+157 **74**
Maribor, *Yugoslavia* L86+466 **56**
Maridi, *Sudan* L04+050 **81**
Marie Byrd Ld., *Antarctica* W60–780 **27**
Mariefred, *Sweden* L77+592 **47**
Marie Galante, I., *Leeward Is.* S07+159 **101**
Mariehamn, *Finland* L60+601 **47**
Marienbad. *See* Marianske Lázně
Marienberg, *Netherlands* M51+525 **44**
Marienbourg, *Belgium* M63+501 **44**
Marienburg. *See* Malbork
Mariental, *Namibia* L72-244 **84**
Marienville, *Pennsylvania* T25+415 **96**
Mariestad, *Sweden* M07+587 **47**
Marietta, *Georgia* T57+339 **97**
Marietta, *Ohio* T39+394 **91**
Mari Indus, *Pakistan* H20+329 **72**
Mariiskaya, aut. rep., *U.S.S.R.* J70+564 **62**
Marina Fall, *Guyana* R88+055 **104**
Marine City, *Michigan* T45+427 **91**
Marinette, *Wisconsin* T76+451 **91**
Marinha Grande, *Portugal* N54+398 **52**
Marion, *Arkansas* U02+352 **97**
Marion, *Illinois* T84+377 **95**
Marion, *Iowa* U10+420 **95**
Marion, *Indiana* T64+406 **91**
Marion, *Kentucky* T80+372 **97**
Marion, *N. Carolina* T42+357 **97**
Marion, *N. Dakota* U50+466 **93**
Marion, *Ohio* T49+406 **91**
Marion, *Virginia* T39+368 **97**
Marion B., *Tasmania* C12–428 **109**
Maritsa R., *Bulgaria, etc* L24+419 **58**
Mariyampole. *See* Kapsukas
Marj, Al., *Libya* L54+324 **81**
Marjamaa, *Estonia* L33+589 **47**
Markala, *Mali* N34+140 **80**
Markapur, *India* G60+157 **70**
Markelo, *Netherlands* M51+522 **44**
Marken, I., *Netherlands* M59+524 **44**
Market Deeping, *England* N02+527 **37**
Market Drayton, *England* N15+529 **37**
Market Harborough, *Eng.* N05+525 **37**
Markethill, *N. Ireland* N39+543 **42**
Markham, L., *Tibet* G42+350 **71**
Markham, Mt., *Antartica* B50–830 **27**
Markovo, *U.S.S.R.* A57+644 **63**
Marks, *U.S.S.R.* J79+517 **61**
Markstay, *Ontario* T33+465 **91**
Marlboro, *Massachusetts* S69+424 **96**
Marlborough, *Guyana* R82+075 **104**
Marlborough, *England* N10+514 **39**
Marlette, *Michigan* T48+433 **91**
Marlo, *Victoria* C09–378 **109**
Marmande, *France* M89+445 **55**
Marmara, Sea of, *Turkey* L10+407 **74**
Marmaris, *Turkey* L10+369 **74**
Marne, dep., *France* M64+488 **54**
Marnoo, *Victoria* C43–367 **109**
Maroni, R., *Fr. Guiana* R53+029 **105**
Maroua, *Cameroon* M04+106 **81**
Marquesas, Is., *Pacific Oc.* X30–100 **107**
Marquette, *Michigan* T74+465 **91**
Marquina, *Spain* N15+433 **53**
Marra, R., *New S. Wales* C17–306 **109**
Marrakech, *Morocco* N48+316 **80**
Marrawah, *Tasmania* C32–410 **109**
Marree, *S. Australia* C72–296 **109**
Marsabit, *Kenya* K42+022 **83**
Marsa Hali, *Saudi Arabia* K22+187 **74**
Marsala, *Sicily* M15+378 **57**
Marsden, *New South Wales* C14–338 **109**
Marseille, *France* M58+433 **55**
Marsh, I., *Louisiana* U12+295 **95**
Marshall, *Illinois* T76+394 **95**
Marshall, *Michigan* T60+423 **91**
Marshall, *Minnesota* U35+445 **93**
Marshall, *Missouri* U20+391 **95**
Marshall, *Texas* U26+326 **95**
Marshall Is., *Pacific Ocean* A60+075 **106**
Marshall Pass, *Colorado* V08+382 **98**
Marshalltown, *Iowa* U17+421 **95**
Marshfield, *Missouri* U18+374 **95**
Marshfield, *Oregon* W26+434 **92**
Marshfield, *Wisconsin* U01+447 **91**
Mars Hill, *Maine* S48+465 **90**
Marstrand, *Sweden* M20+579 **47**
Marsum, *Netherlands* M56+532 **44**
Martaban, *Burma* F45+166 **71**
Martaban, G. of, *Burma* F50+155 **71**
Martelange, *Belgium* M56+498 **44**
Marthas Vineyard, I., *Mass.* S64+412 **96**
Martigny-Ville, *Switzerland* M48+461 **45**
Martin, *S. Dakota* U71+432 **93**
Martin L., *Alabama* T65+328 **97**
Martina, *Switzerland* M27+469 **45**
Martinho, *Brazil* R71–059 **105**
Martinique, I., *Windward Is.* S06+146 **101**
Martinsburg, *W. Virginia* T18+395 **96**
Martinsville, *Virginia* T29+367 **97**
Marton, *New Zealand* A27–401 **112**
Martos, *Spain* N24+377 **52**
Martre, Lac la, *N.-W. Terr.* V85+634 **88**
Maruf, *Afghanistan* H48+315 **75**
Marugame, *Japan* D07+342 **68**
Marum, *Netherlands* M52+531 **44**
Marutea, I., *Tuamotu Arch.* X45–180 **107**
Marvejols, *France* M71+445 **55**
Mary, *Turkmen.* H79+375 **62**
Maryborough, *Queensland* B74–255 **111**
Maryborough. *See* Portlaoise
Maryborough, *Victoria* C38–371 **109**
Marydale, *Cape Province* L48–294 **84**
Maryland, state, *U.S.A.* T10+392 **99**
Maryport, *England* N21+547 **37**
Marysville, *California* W10+391 **92**
Marysville, *New Brunswick* S39+460 **90**
Maryville, *Kansas* U40+398 **95**
Maryville, *Missouri* U30+404 **95**
Mas-afuera, *Pacific Ocean* T35–345 **107**
Masaka, *Uganda* K80–004 **83**
Masangena, *Mozambique* K72–216 **84**
Masara, *Mozambique* K66–182 **84**
Masasi, *Tanzania* K38–108 **83**
Masaya, *Nicaragua* T67+120 **101**
Masbate, I., *Philippines* D70+121 **65**
Mascara, *Algeria* N00+354 **80**
Maseru, *Lesotho* L14–292 **84**
Mashaki, *Afghanistan* H40+333 **75**
Masharbrum, mt., *Kashmir* G82+356 **72**
Mashhad, *Iran* J02+363 **75**
Mashkol, Hamun-i-, *Pak.* H72+281 **70**
Masi-Manimba, *Zaire* L72–048 **82**
Masindi, *Uganda* K80+016 **83**
Masira Chan., *Saudi Arabia* J08+207 **75**
Masira, G. of, *Saudi Arabia* J10+197 **75**
Masira I., *Oman* J08+204 **75**
Masjed Soleymān, *Iran* J63+314 **74**
Mask L., *Ireland, Rep.* N56+536 **42**
Masoala C., *Madagascar* J58–160 **83**
Mason, *Michigan* T57+426 **91**
Mason City, *Iowa* U19+432 **95**
Masøy, *Norway* L30+709 **46**
Massa, *Italy* M29+440 **56**
Massachusetts, state, *U.S.A.* S80+421 **99**
Massachusetts B., *Mass.* S63+424 **96**
Massafra, *Italy* L77+406 **57**
Massakori, *Chad* L86+130 **81**
Massapê, *Brazil* Q62–034 **105**
Massawa, *Ethiopia* K34+156 **83**
Massena, *New York* S89+449 **91**
Massénya, *Chad* L82+114 **81**
Masseube, *France* M87+434 **55**
Massey, *Ontario* T42+462 **91**
Massillon, *Ohio* T39+409 **91**
Masterton, *New Zealand* A26–409 **112**
Mastuj, *Pakistan* H15+363 **72**
Mastung, *Pakistan* H49+298 **70**
Mastura, *Saudi Arabia* K37+231 **74**
Masulipatnam (Bandar), *India* G52+162 **70**
Masyaf, *Syria* K52+351 **76**
Mat, *India* G73+276 **72**
Mata Amarilla, *Argentina* S68–496 **103**
Matagalpa, *Nicaragua* T65+130 **101**
Matagorda, B. & Pen., *Texas* U36+286 **94**
Matagorda, I., *Texas* U40+282 **94**
Matakana I., *New Zealand* A23–376 **112**
Matale, *Sri Lanka* G57+076 **70**
Matam, *Senegal* N80+156 **80**
Matamoros, *Mexico* U79+256 **100**
Matamoros, *Mexico* U45+258 **100**
Matane, *Quebec* S45+488 **90**
Matang, *Malaysia* F26+048 **69**
Matanuska, *Alaska* Y00+614 **99**
Matanzas, *Cuba* T39+230 **101**
Matapedia, *Quebec* S42+480 **90**
Matapedia, L., *Quebec* S45+486 **90**
Matapozuelos, *Spain* N28+414 **52**
Matara, *Sri Lanka* G57+060 **70**
Mataram, *Lombok I., Indon.* E24–085 **65**
Mataro, *Spain* M75+415 **53**
Matatiele, *Cape Province* L08–304 **84**
Mataule, *Brazil* R47+015 **105**
Mataura, *New Zealand* A66–462 **112**
Matehuala, *Mexico* U63+236 **100**
Matera, *Italy* L80+407 **57**
Mátészalka, *Hungary* L46+479 **49**
Mateur, *Tunisia* M32+370 **81**
Matfors, *Sweden* L78+624 **46**
Mathew Town, *Bahamas, The* S82 + 210 **101**
Mathura, *India* G74+274 **73**
Matiara, *India* G16+263 **71**
Matlock, *England* N09+531 **37**
Matna, *Sudan* K60+138 **81**
Matrah, *Oman* J09+236 **75**
Matruh, *Egypt* L16+312 **81**
Matsue, *Japan* D12+354 **68**
Matsumoto, *Japan* C69+362 **68**
Matsushima, *Japan* C53+384 **68**
Matsuyama, *Japan* D13+338 **68**
Mattawa, *Ontario* T22+463 **91**
Matterhorn, mt., *Switz.-It.* M44+460 **45**
Matto Grosso, *Brazil* S00–150 **104**
Mattoon, *Illinois* T80+394 **95**
Matucana, *Peru* T09–118 **104**
Matun, *Afghanistan* H30+334 **75**
Matura, *Brazil* S49–035 **104**
Maturin, *Venezuela* S19+097 **104**
Matvaieva, *U.S.S.R.* J13+578 **61**
Mau, *India* G59+222 **73**
Mau Aimma, *India* G48+257 **73**
Maubeuge, *France* M66+503 **54**
Maubin, *Burma* F56+166 **71**
Maubourguet, *France* N00+435 **55**
Maudaha, *India* G59+257 **73**
Maude, *New South Wales* C34–345 **109**
Mauele, *Mozambique* K66–244 **84**
Maues, *Brazil* R73–034 **105**
Mauganj, *India* G48+246 **73**
Maugerville, *New Brunswick* S39+459 **90**
Maui, I., *Hawaii* Y30 + 208 **107**
Mauleon Licharre, *France* N04+432 **55**
Maurawan, *India* G55+264 **73**
Maurice, L., *S. Australia* D24–292 **110**
Mauritania, rep., *W. Africa* N60+200 **80**
Mauritius, I., *Indian Ocean* J17–200 **77**
Maurs, *France* M77+448 **55**
Mauston, *Wisconsin* U01+438 **91**
Maumturk Mts., *Ireland, Rep.* N58+535 **43**
Mawk Mai, *Burma* F43+202 **71**
Mawson, *Antarctica* H78–680 **27**
Maxcanu, *Mexico* U00+205 **100**
Maxton, *N. Carolina* T26+348 **97**
Maxwelltown, *Scotland* N22+551 **41**
May, C., *New Jersey* T00+389 **96**
May, I. of, *Scotland* N15+562 **41**
Maya, I., *Indonesia* E63-O11 **65**
Mayaguez, *Puerto Rico* S42+182 **101**
Mayari, *Cuba* T04+207 **101**
Mayavaram, *India* G62+112 **70**
Mayen, *W. Germany* M46+503 **48**
Mayenne, dep., *France* N05+482 **54**
Mayersville, *Mississippi* U06+329 **97**
Mayfield, *Kentucky* T82+367 **97**
Maymyo, *Burma* F51+220 **71**
Maynooth, *Ireland, Rep.* N39+534 **43**
Maynooth, *Ontario* T18+452 **91**
Mayo, co., *Ireland, Rep.* N56+537 **42**
Mayoumba, *Gabon* M26–036 **82**
Mayran, L., *Mexico* U77+258 **100**
Mays Landing, *New Jersey* S88+394 **96**
Maysville, *Kentucky* T52+386 **97**
Mayville, *New York* T22+423 **96**
Maza, *Argentina* S20–367 **103**
Mazabuka, *Zambia* L14–158 **84**
Mazagan (El Jadida), *Morocco* N52+330 **80**
Mazagão, *Brazil* R39–002 **105**
Mazamet, *France* M76+435 **55**
Mazan, *Argentina* S39–288 **103**
Mazan, *Peru* S78–036 **104**
Mazapil, *Mexico* U70+247 **100**
Mazara del Vallo, *Sicily* M14+376 **57**
Mazaredo, *Argentina* S40–470 **103**
Mazar-i-Sharif, *Afghanistan* H47+366 **75**
Mazarron, *Spain* N08+377 **53**
Mazatenango, *Guatemala* U09+144 **100**
Mazatlán, *Mexico* V09+232 **100**
Mazheikyai, *Lithuania* L45+563 **47**
Mbabane, *Swaziland* K82–264 **84**
Mbalama, *Mozambique* K38–134 **83**
Mbale, *Uganda* K66+008 **83**
Mbandaka, *Zaire* L70+001 **82**
Mbarangandu, *Tanzania* K50–104 **83**
Mbarara, *Uganda* K86–006 **83**
Mbeya, *Tanzania* K70–090 **83**
Mbozi, *Tanzania* K72–090 **83**
Mbuji-Mayi, *Zaire* L38–062 **82**
Mcuburi, *Mozambique* K36–146 **83**
Mead L., *Nevada, etc.* V57+361 **92**
Meadville, *Pennsylvania* T31+416 **91**
Meaford, *Ontario* T33+446 **91**
Meath, co., *Ireland, Rep.* N39+537 **42**
Mecatina I. Gt. *Quebec* R83+508 **90**
Mecatina I. Lit., *Quebec* R86+506 **90**
Mecca, *Saudi Arabia* K31+214 **74**
Mechanicville, *New York* S82+429 **96**
Mechelen, *Belgium* M56+509 **44**
Mechelen (Malines), *Belg.* M63+510 **44**
Mecheria, *Algeria* N02+332 **80**
Mecklenburg, *W. Germany* M18+535 **48**
Medak, *India* G70+181 **70**
Medak, *Yugoslavia* L87+444 **56**
Medan, *Sumatra* F38+036 **65**
Medanos, *Argentina* S17–389 **103**
Medellin, *Colombia* T04+061 **104**
Medemblik, *Netherlands* M59+528 **44**
Medenine, *Tunisia* M28+334 **81**
Meder, *Ethiopia* K26+146 **83**
Medford, *Oregon* W17+423 **92**
Medford, *Wisconsin* U02+451 **91**
Medgidia, *Romania* L10+443 **58**
Media, *Pennsylvania* T02+399 **96**
Medias, *Romania* L34+461 **58**
Medicine Bow Ra., *Wyo.-Colo.* V06+408 **93**
Medicine Hat, *Alberta* V34+500 **88**
Medina, *Saudi Arabia* K30+246 **74**
Medina, *New York* T20+432 **96**
Medina, *N. Dakota* U56+469 **93**
Medina, *Ohio* T41+411 **91**
Medinaceli, *Spain* N15+412 **53**
Medina del Campo, *Spain* N29+413 **52**
Medina de Rioseco, *Spain* N30+419 **52**
Medina Sidonia, *Spain* N36+365 **52**
Médine, *Mali* N68+142 **80**
Mediterranean Sea, *S. Europe* **50-51**
Mednogorsk, *U.S.S.R.* J14+518 **61**
Medora, *N. Dakota* U81+469 **93**
Medvezhegorsk, *Karelia* K64+628 **62**
Medvezhi Osa., *U.S.S.R.* B20+710 **63**
Medvezhi Yar, *U.S.S.R.* F80+706 **63**
Medway R., *England* M87+513 **39**
Meekatharra, *W. Australia* E10–266 **110**
Meenin. *See* Menin
Meerle, *Belgium* M61+515 **44**
Meerlo, *Netherlands* M54+515 **44**
Meersburg, *W. Germany* M35+477 **48**
Meersen, *Netherlands* M55+509 **44**
Meerut, *India* G74+290 **72**
Meeuwen, *Belgium* M57+511 **44**
Mega, *Ethiopia* K40+040 **83**
Megalópolis, *Greece* L47+374 **59**
Mégantic, & L., *Quebec* S65+456 **91**
Mégara, *Greece* L40+380 **59**
Meghalaya, state, *India* F82+254 **71**
Megiskan, *Quebec* T13+483 **91**
Mehar, *Pakistan* H43+272 **70**
Meherpur, *Bangladesh* G08+238 **73**
Mehndawal, *India* G41+270 **73**
Meihsien, *China* E23+244 **67**
Meiktila, *Burma* F55+208 **71**
Meiningen, *E. Germany* M28+505 **48**
Meiringen, *Switzerland* M41+467 **45**
Meissen, *E. Germany* M09+512 **48**
Meitene, *Latvia* L38+564 **47**
Mejillones, *Chile* S62–230 **103**
Mekatina, *Ontario* T55+471 **91**
Meknes, *Morocco* N34+340 **80**
Me-kong, R., *S.-E. Asia* E84+125 **69**
Melaka, *Malaysia* F17+022 **69**
Melanesia, *Pacific Oc.* B30–050 **106**
Melbourne, *Victoria* C30–378 **109**
Meleuz, *U.S.S.R.* J24+528 **61**
Melfi, *Italy* L86+410 **57**
Melfort, *Saskatchewan* U87+531 **88**
Meligalá, *Greece* L48+372 **59**
Melilla, *Morocco* N18+352 **80**
Melipilla, *Chile* S67–336 **103**
Melitopol, *Ukraine* K58+469 **60**
Melk, *Austria* L88+483 **48**
Melle, *France* N01+462 **54**
Mellier, *Belgium* M57+498 **44**
Mellingen, *Switzerland* M40+474 **45**
Melo, *Uruguay* R56–322 **103**
Melona, *Israel* K59+330 **76**
Melreux, *Belgium* M57+503 **44**
Melrose, *Minnesota* U29+457 **93**
Melrose, *Scotland* N16+556 **41**
Melton Mowbray, *England* N05+528 **37**
Melun, *France* M74+485 **54**
Melut, *Sudan* K76+104 **81**
Melvich, *Scotland* N24+586 **40**
Melville, *Saskatchewan* U77+508 **88**
Melville B., *Greenland* S00+760 **26**
Melville, C., *Queensland* C32–142 **111**
Melville I., *N. Terr., Aust.* D23–116 **110**
Melville I., *N.-W. Terr.* V30+756 **88**
Melville L., *Labrador* R85+538 **89**
Melville Pen., *N.-W. Terr.* T55+679 **89**
Melvin L., *N. Ireland-Ireland, Rep.* N49+544 **42**
Memba & B., *Mozambique* K26–142 **83**
Membij, *Syria* K42+365 **76**
Memel. *See* Klaipeda
Memphis, *Tennessee* U00+352 **97**
Memphremagog, L., *Quebec* S74+451 **91**
Memramcook, *N.B.* S27+460 **90**
Mena, *Arkansas* U26+346 **95**
Menai Bridge, *Wales* N25+532 **38**
Menai Str., *Wales* N26+531 **38**
Menairi, *Chad* L44+152 **81**
Ménaka, *Mali* M76+158 **80**
Menasha, *Wisconsin* T80+442 **91**
Mendak, *Saudi Arabia* K22+203 **74**
Mendawai, R., *Borneo* E40–017 **65**
Mende, *France* M69+445 **55**
Mendebo Mts., *Ethiopia* K32+068 **83**
Menderez, R., *Turkey* L08+379 **74**
Mendip Hills, *England* N16+513 **38**
Mendocino, C., *California* W27+404 **92**
Mendota, *Illinois* T85+416 **91**
Mendota, L., *Wisconsin* T86+431 **95**
Mendoza, *Argentina* S53–328 **103**
Mendrisio, *Switzerland* M36+459 **45**
Menfi, *Sicily* M12+376 **57**
Menga, *Cameroon* M16+062 **81**
Meng Chai Nat, *Thailand* F29+152 **69**
Meng Chumporn, *Thailand* F35+106 **69**
Meng Fang, *Thailand* F35+198 **69**
Meng Kalamasai, *Thailand* F09+165 **69**
Meng Kemmarat, *Thailand* E98+160 **69**
Meng Krabin, *Thailand* F19+139 **69**
Meng Kuwi, *Thailand* F31+121 **69**
Meng Pran Kao, *Thailand* F31+124 **69**
Meng Pre, *Thailand* F29+182 **69**
Meng Teun, *Thailand* F35+176 **69**
Mengtsz, *China* F10+232 **64**
Meng Uthen, *Thailand* F03+175 **69**
Menin, *Belgium* M71+508 **44**
Menindee, *New S. Wales* C45–324 **109**
Menindee L., *New S. Wales* C46–324 **109**
Meningie, *S. Australia* C64–357 **109**
Menjapa, mt., *Borneo* E24+011 **65**
Menominee & R., *Michigan* T76+451 **91**
Menomonie, *Wisconsin* U12+448 **93**
Menorca I., *Balearic Is.* M65+400 **53**
Mentawai Is., *Indonesia* F40+020 **31**
Mentok, *Bangka I., Indonesia* E89+020 **65**
Menton, *France* M45+438 **55**
Menzelinsk, *U.S.S.R.* J41+557 **61**
Menzies, *W. Australia* D84–296 **110**
Meoqui, *Mexico* V03+282 **100**
Me-ping, R., *Thailand* F30+160 **69**
Meppel, *Netherlands* M53+527 **44**
Merabello G., *Crete* L25+352 **59**
Merano, *Italy* M23+467 **56**
Merasheen I., *Nfd.* R55+475 **90**
Merauke, *New Guinea* C57–085 **65**
Mercara, *India* G85+126 **70**
Merced, *California* W03+373 **92**
Mercedaria, mt., *Argentina* S61–320 **103**
Mercedes, *Argentina* R86–346 **103**
Mercedes, *Argentina* R79–293 **103**
Mercedes, *Bolivia* S41–126 **104**
Mercedes, *Uruguay* R78–333 **103**
Mercer, *New Zealand* A29–373 **112**
Mercer, *Pennsylvania* T32+413 **91**
Merchtem, *Belgium* M65+510 **44**
Mercy, C., *N.-W. Terr.* S20+650 **89**
Meredith, *Michigan* T57+442 **91**
Meredith, C., *Falkland Is.* S04–522 **103**
Mereg, *Somalia* J76+038 **83**
Mergentheim, *W. Germany* M32+494 **48**
Mergui, *Burma* F38+124 **71**
Mergui Arch., *Burma* F48+116 **71**
Meribah, *S. Australia* C55–347 **109**
Merida, *Mexico* T88+209 **100**
Merida, *Spain* N38+390 **52**
Merida & Cord. de, *Venez.* S67+084 **104**
Meriden, *Connecticut* S77+415 **96**
Meridian, *Mississippi* T82+324 **97**
Meringur, *Victoria* C52–344 **109**
Merioneth, co., *see* Gwyned
Merj Uyun, *Lebanon* K57+334 **76**
Merka, *Somalia* K01+018 **83**
Merksplas, *Belgium* M61+514 **44**
Merowe, *Sudan* K80+182 **81**
Merredin, *W. Australia* E09–314 **110**
Merrill, *Wisconsin* T88+452 **91**
Merrimack R., *New Hamp.-Mass.* S68+427 **96**
Merriwa, *New S. Wales* B88–322 **109**
Merrygoen, *New S. Wales* C05–319 **109**
Mersey R., *England* N16+534 **37**
Merseyside, co., *England* N18+534 **37**
Mersin, *Turkey* K62+369 **74**
Mersing, *Malaysia* F07+024 **65**
Mersis, *Somalia* J84+046 **83**
Mersrags, *Latvia* L41+573 **47**
Merta, *India* H06+266 **70**
Merthyr Tydfil, *Wales* N20+518 **38**
Mertola, *Portugal* N46+376 **52**
Meru, *Kenya* K44+002 **83**
Merwe, *Zambia* K82–142 **83**
Merzig, *W. Germany* M50+494 **48**
Mesa, *Arizona* V40+334 **94**
Mesabi Ra., *Minnesota* U20+477 **93**
Mesagne, *Italy* L73+405 **57**
Mesará B., *Crete* L32+350 **59**
Mesa Verde Nat. Park, *Colo.* V22+376 **98**
Mesen, *Belgium* M73+508 **44**
Meshghara, *Lebanon* K56+336 **76**
Meskene, *Syria* K41+360 **76**
Mesmiye, *Syria* K52+331 **76**
Mesocco, *Switzerland* M35+464 **45**
Mesolóngion, *Greece* L51+384 **59**
Messancy, *Belgium* M55+496 **44**
Messina, *Sicily* L89+382 **57**
Messina, Str. di, *Italy* L87+380 **57**
Messinia, *Greece* L49+372 **59**
Messinia, G. of, *Greece* L48+367 **59**
Mesudiye, *Turkey* K43+405 **74**
Metan, *Argentina* S30–255 **103**
Metangula, *Mozambique* K60–128 **83**
Metaripuá, *Brazil* S40–077 **104**
Méthana Pen., *Greece* L40+376 **59**

Methil (Buckhaven & Methil), Scotland N18+562 41
Methven, New Zealand A50-436 112
Metis Ls., Quebec S46+483 90
Metis Beach, Quebec S48+487 90
Metkovic, Yugoslavia L74+430 58
Metlakatla, Alaska W65+551 99
Metlika, Yugoslavia L88+456 56
Metropolis, Illinois T83+372 95
Metropolitan, Michigan T77+460 91
Métsovon, Greece L53+398 59
Mettet, Belgium M62+503 44
Mettlen, Switzerland M42+470 45
Mettur Dam, India G74+119 70
Metulla, Israel K57+333 76
Metz, France M53+491 54
Meulebeke, Belgium M70+510 44
Meurthe-et-Moselle, dep., France M51+485 54
Meuse, dep., France M57+490 54
Meuse, R., Belgium, etc. M56+490 54
Mexcala & R., Mexico U58+177 100
Mexiana, I., Brazil R27+000 105
Mexicali, Mexico V62+326 100
Mexico, Mexico U55+194 100
Mexico, New York T07+434 96
Mexico, rep. Cent. America 100
Mexico B., New York T08+435 96
Mexico, G. of U00+250 100
Meyadin, Syria K27+350 74
Meyersdale, Pennsylvania T24+398 96
Meymac, France M77+455 54
Mèze, France M68+435 55
Mezen, U.S.S.R. J94+658 62
Mezieres, France M62+497 54
Mezöbereny Békés, Hungary L54+468 49
Mezökövesd, Hungary L57+478 49
Mesötúr, Hungary L56+470 49
Mezquitic, Mexico U82+226 100
Mgori, Tanzania K60-050 83
Mhow, India G85+224 70
Miahuatlan, Mexico U39+165 100
Miajadas, Spain N35+391 52
Miami, Arizona V36+333 94
Miami, Florida T31+257 97
Miami, Oklahoma U30+369 95
Miandowab, Iraq K05+326 74
Miandrivazo, Madagascar J88-196 83
Mianeh, Iran J73+374 74
Miani, India G86+317 72
Miani, Pakistan H11+325 72
Mian Kalai, Pakistan H20+348 72
Mianwali, Pakistan H21+325 72
Miao-tao I., China D86+383 66
Miass, U.S.S.R. J00+558 61
Miastko, Poland L78+540 49
Micay, Colombia T15+029 104
Michailovsk, U.S.S.R. H80+536 61
Micheh, China E59+378 66
Michigan, state, U.S.A. T73+462 99
Michigan, L., U.S.A.-Canada T70+434 99
Michigan City, Indiana T71+417 91
Michipicoten, Ontario T60+482 89
Michipicoten I. & B., Ont. T64+477 91
Michoacan, state, Mexico U72+188 100
Michurinsk, U.S.S.R. K27+529 61
Mickelson, Michigan T59+444 91
Micronesia, Pacific Oc. B30+100 106
Mid Canyon, Montana V41+471 93
Middleboro, Massachusetts S65+419 96
Middelburg, Netherlands M68+515 44
Middelburg, Transvaal L04-258 84
Middelharnis, Netherlands M66+518 44
Middelkerke, Belgium M73+512 44
Middleburg, New York S86+426 91
Middleburg, Pennsylvania T13+408 96
Middlebury, Vermont S79+441 91
Middleham, England N11+543 37
Middlemarch, New Zealand A59-455 112
Middleport, New York T21+431 96
Middlesboro, Kentucky T52+366 97
Middlesbrough, England N07+546 37
Middlesex, Belize T80+172 101
Middleton, Nova Scotia S30+449 90
Middleton-in-Teesdale, Eng. N13+546 37
Middletown, Connecticut S76+416 96
Middletown, Delaware T04+394 91
Middletown, New York S87+414 96
Middletown, Ohio T56+395 91
Middletown, Pennsylvania T11+402 96
Midland, Michigan T55+436 91
Midland, Ontario T29+447 91
Midland, Texas U72+320 94
Midlands, West, co., Eng. N11+525 37
Midleton, Ireland, Rep. N49+519 43
Midlothian, co., see Lothian
Midnapur, India G16+224 73
Midway Is., Hawaii Z60+290 106
Midwest, Wyoming V08+435 93
Midye, Turkey L12+416 74
Miécourt, Switzerland M47+474 45
Miedzyrzec, Poland L44+520 49
Mienning, China F30+239 64
Mienyang, China E40+302 67
Mienyang, China F01+313 66
Mier, Mexico U55+264 100
Mieres, Spain N35+432 52
Mifflintown, Pennsylvania T15+405 96
Migdal Gad, Israel K62+317 76
Mikhaylovgrad, Bulgaria L41+434 58
Mikhaylovka, U.S.S.R. K10+500 61
Mikkeli, Finland L16+617 47
Mikonos, I., Greece L28+375 59
Milaca, Minnesota U22+458 93
Milan, Italy. See Milano
Milan, Missouri U19+402 95
Milan, New Hampshire S67+446 91
Milan, Tennessee T82+364 95
Milang, S. Australia C67-354 109
Milano, Italy M35+455 56
Milas, Turkey L14+373 74
Milazzo, Sicily L89+382 57
Milbank, S. Dakota U40+452 93
Mildenhall, England M87+523 39
Mildura, Victoria C47-342 109
Miléai, Greece L41+393 59
Miles, Queensland C00-267 111
Milesburg, Pennsylvania T17+409 96
Miles City, Montana V05+464 93
Milford, Delaware T02+389 96
Milford, Massachusetts S69+422 96
Milford, Nova Scotia S21+451 90
Milford, Pennsylvania S89+413 96
Milford, Utah V48+384 94
Milford Haven, Wales N30+517 38
Milford Sound, N.Z. A72-447 112
Mili Is., Marshall Islands A44+060 106
Miliana, Algeria M76+362 80
Milk R., Montana V16+486 93
Milkovo, U.S.S.R. B37+549 63
Mill, Netherlands M55+517 44
Mill I., Antarctica F26-650 27
Mill Is., N.-W. Territories T15+642 89
Millau, France M72+441 55
Millbridge, Ontario T16+447 91
Mille Lacs, Minnesota U22+462 93
Miller, S. Dakota U54+446 93
Millerovo, U.S.S.R. K28+489 61
Millersburg, Ohio T41+406 91
Miller's Flat, New Zealand A63-457 112
Mille Vaches, Quebec S55+486 90
Millford, Ireland, Rep. N46+551 42
Millicent, S. Australia C58-376 109
Millinocket, Maine S52+457 90
Millport, Scotland N29+558 41
Millridge, Maine S47+445 90
Millstreet, Ireland, Rep. N54+520 43
Milltown Malbay, Ireland, Rep. N56+528 43
Millville, New Jersey T00+394 96
Milne B., Papua New Guinea B86+05 111
Milnor, N. Dakota U45+463 93
Milo, Maine S54+452 90
Milos, I., Greece L33+367 59
Milparinka, New S. Wales C49-294 109
Milton, New Zealand A70-461 112
Milton, Ontario T29+435 91
Milton, Pennsylvania T12+410 96
Milwaukee, Wisconsin T78+430 95
Mimika, New Guinea C82-047 65
Mina al Ahmadi, Kuwait J71+293 74
Minab, Iran J18+271 75
Minaki, Ontario U27+500 88
Minas, Uruguay R62-343 103
Minas de Riotinto, Spain N39+377 52
Minas Novas, Brazil Q76-174 105
Minatitlan, Mexico U27+180 100
Minbu, Burma F60+202 71
Minch Little, Scotland N39+577 40
Minch North, Scotland N36+580 40
Mindanao, I., Philippines D60+074 65
Mindarie, S. Australia C59-349 109
Minden, W. Germany M37+523 48
Minden, Louisiana U20+326 95
Mindoro, I. & Str., Phil. D86+125 65
Mine Hd., Ireland, Rep. N46+520 43
Minehead, England N21+512 38
Mineola, New York S82+407 96
Mineral Ra., Michigan T88+467 91
Mineral Point, Wisconsin U01+429 91
Mineral Wells, Texas U49+328 95
Minga, Zambia K84-144 83
Mingan Is., Quebec S23+502 90
Mingary, S. Australia C55-321 109
Mingin, Burma F63+229 71
Minglanilla, Spain N10+395 53
Mingoyo, Tanzania K32-102 83
Mingshui, China F53+422 64
Minhla, Burma F59+199 71
Minho, Spain-Portugal N49+422 52
Minhow, China E04+261 67
Minicoy, I., Laccadives H11+082 70
Minna, Nigeria M50+096 80
Minneapolis, Minnesota U20+450 93
Minnedosa, Manitoba U60+502 88
Minnesota, state, U.S.A. U36+464 98
Minnesota R., Minn., etc. U36+450 98
Minnik, Syria K48+365 76
Minorca. See Menorca
Minot, N. Dakota U68+483 93
Min Shan, China F12+343 66
Minsk, Byelorussia L15+538 60
Minsk Mazowiecki, Poland L51+522 49
Minto, N. Dakota U44+483 93
Minto Inl., N.-W. Terr. V70+712 88
Minto L., Quebec T02+568 89
Minusinsk, U.S.S.R. F79+537 63
Minya Konka, China F19+295 64
Minyip, Victoria C45-365 109
Mio, Michigan T54+446 91
Miquelon Is., Atlantic Ocean R68+470 90
Mirador, Brazil Q88-063 105
Miraflores, Colombia S78+051 104
Miraj, India H02+169 70
Miramar, Argentina R78-382 103
Mirambeau, France N04+453 55
Miramichie B., N.B. S29+472 90
Miramont, France M87+446 55
Miram Shah, Pakistan H29+330 72
Miranda, Argentina R86-364 103
Miranda, Brazil R69-202 105
Miranda, Nicaragua T57+140 101
Miranda de Ebro, Spain N18+427 52
Miranda do Corvo, Portugal N50+401 52
Miranda do Douro, Portugal N37+415 52
Mirande, France M88+435 55
Mirandela, Portugal N43+415 52
Mirandilla, Spain N37+391 52
Mirdum, Netherlands M57+528 44
Mirebeau, France M89+468 54
Mirim, L., Brazil R48-327 103
Mirjâveh, Iran H81+290 75
Mirnoe, U.S.S.R. G04+623 62
Mirosi, Romania L30+444 58
Mirpur, Kashmir H07+332 72
Mirpur Khas, Pakistan H36+255 70
Mirtoan Sea, Greece L38+368 59
Mirtos, Crete L27+350 59
Mirt Padam, India F58+284 71
Mirzapur, India G44+251 73
Miscou I., New Brunswick S27+480 90
Mishikamau, L., Labrador S25+542 89
Mishrif, Saudi Arabia K01+205 74
Miska, Saudi Arabia K13+249 74
Miskolc, Hungary L55+481 49
Misoöl, I., New Guinea D30-018 65
Misquah Hills, Minnesota U062+478 91
Misque, Bolivia S32-178 104
Missis, Turkey K56+370 74
Mississippi, state, U.S.A. U00+328 99
Mississippi Delta, Louisiana T70+290 95
Mississippi R., U.S.A. U03+380 99
Mississippi Sd., Mississippi T84+303 95
Missolónghi, See Mesolóngion.
Missoula, Montana V54+469 92
Missouri, state, U.S.A. U20+381 99
Missouri R., U.S.A. U33+408 98
Missouri Valley, Iowa U36+416 95
Mistassini L., Quebec S83+508 89
Mistretta, Sicily M04+379 57
Misurata, (Misrâtah), Libya M00+322 81
Mitala Maria, Uganda K76+001 83
Mitchell, Ontario T37+435 91
Mitchell, Queensland C13-264 111
Mitchell, S. Dakota U48+437 93
Mitchell, Mt., N. Carolina T44+358 97
Mitchell, R., Queensland C47-160 111
Mitchelstown, Ireland, Rep. N50+523 43
Mithankot, Pakistan H28+289 72
Mithi, Pakistan H31+246 70
Mithimna, Greece L23+393 59
Mitho, Vietnam E82+104 69
Mitilini, Lesvos, I., Greece L21+391 59
Mito, Japan C57+364 68
Mitsiz, Gabon M22+008 82
Mittagong, New S. Wales B88-344 109
Mitta Mitta, Victoria C15-365 109
Mittelmark, Germany M10+522 48
Mittelmark, W. Germany M10+522 48
Mitu, Colombia S60+009 104
Mitumba Mts., Zaire L10-016 104
Miyako, Japan C48+397 68
Miyanduab, Iran J83+370 74
Miyazaki, Japan D21+319 68
Mizda, Libya M12+314 81
Mizen Hd., Ireland, Rep. N36+528 43
Mizen Hd., Ireland, Rep. N59+514 43
Mizil, Romania L21+450 58
Mizpah, Montana V01+462 93
Mjölby, Sweden L89+583 47
Mjosa, L., Norway M24+607 47
Mladá Boleslav, Czech. M01+504 48
Mlanje, Mt., See Mulanje Mt.
Mlawa, Poland L58+531 49
Mljet, I., Yugoslavia L75+427 56
Mo, Norway M05+663 46
Moab, Utah V28+386 94
Moama, New South Wales C32-361 109
Mo Ångsåg, Sweden L61+636 46
Moapa, Nevada V59+367 92
Moate, Ireland, Rep. N46+534 43
Moba, Zaire L00+070 82
Mobile & B., Alabama T78+307 97
Mobridge, S. Dakota U63+456 93
Mocajuba, Brazil R26-025 105
Moçambique, Mozambique K26-150 83
Moçâmedes, Angola M16-152 82
Mocha, Yemen K10+133 74
Mocimboa-da-Praia, Mozamb. K28-114 83
Mocksville, N. Carolina T33+358 97
Mocoa, Colombia T10+011 104
Mocorito, Mexico V18+256 100
Moctezuma, Mexico U66+228 100
Moctezuma, Mexico V28+298 100
Modane, France M50+452 55
Modave, Belgium M58+504 44
Modena, Italy M24+446 56
Modesto, California W06+376 92
Modica, Sicily M02+369 57
Modjamboli, Zaire L48+022 82
Mo-duc, Vietnam E66+149 69
Modung, China F50+291 64
Moe, Victoria C22-382 109
Moena, I., Indonesia D75-050 65
Moengo, Surinam R57+056 105
Mofa, Ethiopia K28+106 83
Moffat, Scotland N21+553 41
Mogadiscio (Mogadishu), Somalia J88+020 83
Mogador (Essaouria), Mor. N60+314 80
Mogadouro, Portugal N39+414 52
Mogar, Ethiopia K42+080 83
Mogaung, Burma F48+253 71
Mogilev, Byelorussia K88+539 60
Mogilev Podolskiy, Ukraine L13+485 60
Mogocha, U.S.S.R. E02+537 63
Mogochin, U.S.S.R. G39+577 62
Mogok, Burma F51+229 71
Mogollan Mt., New Mexico V22+336 94
Mogollon Mesa, Arizona V34+344 94
Moguer, Spain N41+372 52
Mogur, Ethiopia K28+050 83
Mohacs, Hungary L68+460 58
Mohako, New Zealand A20-391 112
Mohawk, New York T00+430 96
Mohawk R., New York S88+430 96
Moheli I., Comoro Is. K08-124 83
Moher, Cliffs of, Ireland, Rep. N57+530 43
Mohill, Ireland, Rep. N47+539 42
Moho, China D75+534 63
Mohoro, Tanzania K34-082 83
Moia, Sudan L12+050 81
Moine, L. du, Quebec T18+469 91
Moirang, India F67+245 71
Moisakula, Estonia L29+581 47
Moisie, Quebec S35+503 90
Moissac, France M84+441 55
Mojave, California V79+351 92
Moji, Brazil R09-236 105
Moju & R., Brazil R22-019 105
Mokai, New Zealand A24-385 112
Mokameh, India G24+254 73
Mokolo, Cameroon M08+108 81
Mokpo, Korea D52+348 64
Mokshany, U.S.S.R. K08+534 61
Moldava, Czechoslovakia L54+486 49
Moldavia, Romania L18+467 58
Moldavia, rep., U.S.S.R. L12+474 60
Molde & Fd., Norway M47+628 46
Molepolole, Botswana L26-244 84
Môle St Nicolas, Haiti S80+198 101
Molfetta, Italy L80+412 57
Molina, Chile S67-350 103
Molina, Spain N07+381 53
Molina, Spain N11+409 53
Moline, Illinois U03+414 95
Molino, Florida T74+307 97
Moliro, Zaire K86-084 83
Moll, Belgium M59+512 44
Mollendo, Peru S72-170 104
Mollis, Switzerland M35+471 45
Mollosund, Sweden M21+581 47
Molndal, Sweden M18+577 47
Molong, New South Wales C07-331 109
Molotov. See Perm.
Molotovsk (Severodvinsk) U.S.S.R. K30+645 62
Molucca Pass., Indonesia D58-007 65
Moluccas, Is., Indonesia D45-012 65
Moma, Mozambique K34-166 83
Mombasa, Kenya K32-040 83
Momchilgrad, Bulgaria L28+415 58
Momeik. See Mong-mit.
Momignies, Belgium M65+500 44
Momotombo, Nicaragua T69+125 101
Mompós. Columbia S87+092 104
Møn. I., Denmark M16+550 47
Monä Fd., Finland L48+635 46
Mona, I., Puerto Rico S48+182 101
Mona Pass., West Indies S50+180 101
Monach, Sd. of, Scotland N45+576 40
Monaco, princip., S. Europe M46+437 55
Monadhliath Mts., Scotland N26+571 40
Monaghan & co., Ireland, Rep. N42+542 42
Monango, N.Dakota U52+462 93
Monar L., Scotland N30+574 40
Monaro Ra., New S. Wales C07-364 109
Monasterace Marina, Italy L81+385 57
Monasterevin, Ireland, Rep. N42+531 43
Monastir, Sardinia M36+394 57
Monastir. See Bitola.
Monastir, Tunisia M24+358 81
Monbetsu, Japan C40+443 68
Monbuey, Spain N38+420 52
Mönchengladbach, W. Ger. M52+512 45
Monchique, Portugal N51+373 52
Monclova, Mexico U69+269 100
Moncton, New Brunswick S29+461 90
Mondo, Chad L86+138 81
Mondonedo, Spain N44+434 52
Mondovi, Wisconsin U10+446 93
Mondul, Tanzania K52-032 83
Monemvasia, Greece L42+367 59
Monessen, Pennsylvania T30+402 96
Monetny, U.S.S.R. H85+570 61
Monett, Missouri U24+370 95
Moneva, Spain N05+411 53
Monforte, Portugal N45+390 52
Monforte, Spain N45+425 52
Monga, Zaire L42+040 82
Mongalla, Sudan K80+052 81
Monger, L., W. Australia E17-290 110
Möng-Hsu, Burma F40+218 71
Monghyr, India G21+254 73
Mongka, Burma F33+226 71
Möng Kiang, Burma F40+219 71
Mongkol-borey, Cambodia F12+135 69
Möng Kung, Burma F44+216 71
Möng-Kyet, Burma F39+231 71
Mong-mit, Burma F49+231 71
Mongo, Chad L66+122 81
Mongolia, rep., E. Asia F00+450 31
Mongolia, Inner, China F20+404 64
Mongonu, Nigeria M08+126 81
Mongoumba, Cent. Afr. Rep. L70+036 81
Möng-pai, Burma F48+198 71
Möng Pan, Burma F40+203 71
Möng Pawn, Burma F45+208 71
Möng-Sit, Burma F43+205 71
Mongu, Zambia L42-154 84
Moniaive, Scotland N23+552 41
Moniquira, Colombia S82+059 104
Monivea, Ireland Rep. N52+534 43
Monmouth, Illinois U04+409 95
Monmouth, Wales N16+518 38
Monnikendam, Netherlands M60+525 44
Mono L., California V84+380 92
Monomay I. & Pt., Mass. S60+415 96
Monopoli, Italy L76+409 57
Monovar, Spain N05+385 53
Monreal del Campo, Spain N08+408 53
Monroe, Louisiana U13+325 97
Monroe, Michigan T50+419 91
Monroe, N. Carolina T33+350 97
Monroe, Wisconsin T88+426 95
Monroeville, Alabama T74+315 97
Monrovia, Liberia N64+064 80
Mons, Belgium M66+504 44
Monsanto, Portugal N43+401 52
Monsão, Portugal N50+421 52
Monserrato, Sardinia M35+393 57
Monson, Massachusetts S74+422 96
Monster, Netherlands M65+520 44
Mönsterås, Sweden L81+570 47
Mont, Belgium M55+502 44
Montagne Tremblante Park, Quebec T00+469 91
Montague, Michigan T68+435 91
Montagu I., S. Sandwich Is. P80-580 27
Montaigu, Belgium M60+510 44
Montalbán, Spain N05+408 53
Montana, state, U.S.A. V38+468 94
Montanchez, Spain N37+393 52
Montargis, France M73+480 54
Montauban, France M82+440 55
Montbard, France M64+476 54
Montblanch, Spain M83+414 53
Montbrison, France M66+456 54
Montclair, New Jersey S85+408 96
Montcornet, France M66+497 54
Mont de Marsan, France N03+439 55
Montdidier, France M75+496 54
Mont Dore, le, France M72+456 54
Monte Alegre, Brazil R54-019 105
Monte Alegre, Brazil R24-189 105
Montebello, Quebec T00+457 91
Monte Carlo, Monaco M46+437 55
Monte Caseros, Argentina R77-302 103
Montecollina, S. Australia C60-294 109
Monte Coman, Argentina S47-346 103
Monte Cristi, Dominican Republic S69+199 101
Monte Cristi, Sa. de, Dominican Rep. S64+196 101
Montecristo, I., Italy M28+423 56
Montefrio, Spain N24+373 52
Montego Bay, Jamaica T17+186 101
Montélimar, France M62+446 55
Montello, Wisconsin T86+438 91
Montemorelos, Mexico U59+252 100
Montenegro, Yugoslavia L64+426 58
Montereau, France M72+484 54
Monterey, California W11+366 92

Monterey, Virginia T27+384 97
Monterey, B. of, California W14+367 92
Monteriá, Colombia T05+087 104
Monteros, Argentina S34–272 103
Monterrey, Mexico U61+257 100
Monte San Angelo, Italy L84+417 57
Montes Claros, Brazil Q82–167 105
Montevideo, Minnesota U35+449 93
Montevideo, Uruguay R67–349 103
Monte Vista, Colorado V08+376 94
Montezuma, Georgia T54+324 97
Montfort-sur-Meu, France N12+481 54
Montgomery, Alabama T68+324 97
Montgomery, Missouri U09+390 95
Montgomery, Wales N19+526 38
Monthey, Switzerland M48+463 45
Monticello, Arkansas U10+336 95
Monticello, Georgia T52+333 97
Monticello, Maine S47+463 90
Monticello, New York S88+416 91
Monticello, Utah V26+380 94
Montijo, B. de, Panama T36+076 101
Montilla, Spain N28+375 52
Mont Joli, Quebec S49+486 90
Mont Laurier, Quebec T03+465 91
Montlucon, France M74+464 54
Montmagny, Quebec S63+470 90
Montmédy, France M58+495 54
Montmirail, France M69+489 54
Montmorency, Quebec S67+469 91
Montoursville, Pennsylvania T12+412 96
Montpelier, Idaho V38+423 94
Montpelier, Vermont S76+443 91
Montpellier, France M67+436 55
Montreal, Quebec S82+455 91
Montreal L., Saskatchewan V05+542 88
Montrejeau, France M87+431 55
Montreuil, France M79+505 54
Montreuil Bellay, France N01+471 54
Montreux, Switzerland M48+464 45
Montrose, Colorado V17+384 94
Montrose, Pennsylvania T06+418 96
Montrose, Scotland N15+567 41
Monts, Pt. des, Quebec S44+493 90
Mont-St Jean, Belgium M64+507 44
Mont-St-Michel & B., Fr. N09+487 54
Montserrat, I., Leeward Is. S13+168 101
Monywa, Burma F58+220 71
Monza, Italy M35+456 56
Monze, Zambia L16–162 84
Monzon, Spain M89+419 53
Moolawatana, S. Australia C62–299 109
Moonbi Ra., New S. Wales B84–308 109
Moonta, S. Australia C75–341 109
Moora, W. Australia E24–306 110
Moorcroft, Wyoming V00+443 93
Moore, L., W. Australia E15–294 110
Moorefield, W. Virginia T24+391 96
Moorfoot Hills, Scotland N19+557 41
Moorhead, Minnesota U41+469 93
Moorsel, Belgium M65+509 44
Moorslede, Belgium M72+509 44
Moose L., Manitoba U62+540 88
Moose R., Ontario T42+505 89
Moosehead L., Maine S58+456 90
Moose Jaw, Saskatchewan V04+504 88
Moosic, Mts., Pennsylvania T03+417 96
Moosomin, Saskatchewan U70+501 88
Moosonee, Ontario T34+511 89
Mopti, Mali N24+142 80
Moquegua, Peru S66–172 104
Mora, Ethiopia K54+104 83
Mora, Cameroon M06+110 81
Mora, Minnesota U20+459 93
Mora, Portugal N49+389 52
Mora, Spain N23+397 52
Mora, Sweden M03+610 47
Moradabad, India G67+288 73
Mora de Rubielos, Spain N05+403 53
Moramanga, Madagascar J70-190 83
Morano Calabro, Italy L83+399 57
Morar, India G70+262 73
Morar L., Scotland N34+569 40
Morat. See Murten
Moratalla, Spain N11+382 53
Morava R., Yugoslavia L53+444 58
Moravia, Czechoslovakia L75+493 49
Moravska Trebova, Czech. L79+498 49
Morawhanna, Guyana R88+083 104
Moray Firth, Scotland N22+577 40
Morbihan, dep., France N18+479 54
Morden, Manitoba U50+493 88
Mordialloc, Victoria C29–380 109
Mordova, U.S.S.R. K22+536 61
Mordovskava, aut. rep., U.S.S.R. K10+544 62
Morea, Greece L46+376 59
Moreau R., S. Dakota U72+452 98
Morecambe & B., England N17+451 37
Moreda, Spain N20+374 52
Moree, New South Wales C01–295 109
Moreira, Brazil S21–006 104
Mörel, Switzerland M42+464 45
Morelia, Mexico U67+196 100
Morella, Spain N01+406 53
Morelos, Mexico U65+284 100
Morelos, Mexico V13+267 100
Morelos, state, Mexico U54+186 100
Morena, India G76+261 73
Morena, Sa., Spain N24+383 52
Morenci, Arizona V26+332 94
Morere, New Zealand A13–390 112
Moreton B., Queensland B68–267 111
Morez, France M54+465 54
Morgan, S. Australia C62–340 10
Morgan City, Louisiana U07+297 95
Morganton, N. Carolina T40+357 97
Morgat, France N27+482 54
Morges, Switzerland M51+465 45
Morgins, Switzerland M49+462 45
Moriana, India F64+267 71
Morice L., Brit. Columbia W47+540 88
Morinville, Alberta V52+540 88
Morioka, Japan C53+397 68
Morisset, New South Wales B82–332 109
Morlaix, France N23+485 54
Mormugao, India H07+155 70
Mornington, Victoria C29–382 109
Mornington, I., Chile T02–498 103
Moro G., Philippines D70+069 65
Morobe, Papua New Guinea C15–078 111
Morocco, N.-W. Africa N30+326 80
Morogoro, Tanzania K44–068 83
Morokwen, Cape Province L36–262 84
Moron, Cuba T22+221 101
Morón, Venezuela S49+110 104
Morona, Ecuador T15–028 104
Morondava, Madagascar K04-204 83
Morón de la Frontera, Spain N33+371 52
Morotai, I., Indonesia D40+022 65
Moroto, Uganda K62+026 83
Morpeth, England N10+552 37
Morpeth, New South Wales B81–328 109
Morphou & B., Cyprus K72+352 76
Morrillton, Arkansas U16+352 95
Morrinhos, Brazil R25–178 105
Morrinsville, New Zealand A27–377 112
Morris, Illinois T80+414 95
Morris, Manitoba U45+495 88
Morris, Minnesota U36+456 93
Morrisburg, Ontario T01+449 91
Morris Jesup C., Arctic Oc. Q55+840 26
Morrison, Illinois U00+418 91
Morristown, New Jersey S87+408 96
Morrisville, New York T04+430 91
Morro, Ecuador T32–026 104
Morrosquillo, G. de, Colom. T04+095 104
Mors, Denmark M38+568 47
Morshansk, U.S.S.R. K19+534 61
Mortagne, France M87+485 54
Mortagua, Portugal N49+404 52
Mortain, France N06+486 54
Mortlake, Victoria C43–381 109
Morundah, New S. Wales C22–349 109
Moruya, New S. Wales B89–360 109
Morven, New Zealand A53–448 112
Morven, Queensland C18–264 111
Morvi, India H24+228 70
Morwell, Victoria C22–382 109
Moscow, Idaho V72+467 92
Moscow. See Moskva
Moselle, dep., France M48+489 54
Moselle, R., France M53+489 54
Mosera, I. See Masira I.
Mosgiel, New Zealand A58–458 112
Moshupa, Botswana L28–248 84
Mosjøen, Norway M11+658 46
Moskenesøya, Norway M12+680 46
Moskva, U.S.S.R. K45+558 60
Mosqueiro, Brazil R21–012 105
Mosquera, Colombia T21+024 104
Mosquito Bank, Nicaragua T46+132 101
Moss, Norway M26+595 47
Mossamedes, Angola M16–152 84
Mossburn, New Zealand A70–457 112
Mossel B., Cape Province L46–342 84
Mossendio, Congo M14+030 82
Mossgiel, New South Wales C33–333 109
Mossoro, Brazil Q44–052 105
Mossurize, Mozambique K72+206 84
Moss Vale, New S. Wales B88–346 109
Most, Czechoslovakia M08+505 48
Mostaganem, Algeria N00+358 80
Mostar, Yugoslavia L73+433 58
Mostardas, Brazil R35–310 103
Mosul, Iraq K12+365 74
Mota del Marques, Spain N31+416 52
Motala, Sweden M00+585 47
Motatan, Venezuela S63+094 104
Motherwell, Scotland N24+558 41
Môtier, Switzerland M48+469 45
Môtiers, Switzerland M50+469 45
Motihari, India G30+266 73
Motôt, Switzerland M45+461 45
Motril, Spain N22+367 52
Mott, N. Dakota U75+464 93
Motueka, New Zealand A42–411 112
Motul, Mexico T84+211 100
Moturoa, New Zealand A36–390 112
Moudala, Chad L68+088 81
Moudhros, Greece L29+399 59
Moudon, Switzerland M49+467 45
Mouila, Gabon M24–020 82
Moukden. See Shenyang
Moulamein & R., N.S.W. C36–351 109
Moulins, France M70+466 54
Moulmein, Burma F44+164 71
Moulouya R., Morocco N22+330 80
Moulton, Alabama T74+344 97
Mound City, Illinois T85+370 97
Mountain Grove, Missouri U14+371 97
Mountain Home, Arkansas U15+363 97
Mountain Sheep Bluffs, Montana V03+473 93
Mountain View, Arkansas U13+358 97
Mount Ayr, Iowa U26+407 95
Mount Barker, S. Australia C67–351 109
Mount Bellew, Ireland, Rep. N51+535 43
Mount Carmel, Illinois T76+384 95
Mount Carmel, Pennsylvania T09+408 96
Mount Carroll, Illinois U00+421 91
Mount Clemens, Michigan T47+426 91
Mount Desert I. (Acadia Nat. Park), Maine S50+443 90
Mount Drysdale, N.S.W. C25–312 109
Mount Forest, Ontario T35+440 91
Mount Gambier, S. Aust. C55–379 109
Mount Holly, New Jersey S89+400 96
Mount Hope, N.S.W. C25–329 109
Mount Jewett, Pennsylvania T22+417 96
Mount Lofty Ra., S. Aust. C66–350 109
Mount Magnet, W. Aust. E12–280 110
Mount Manara, N.S.W. C36–324 109
Mountmellick, Ireland, Rep. N44+531 43
Mount Morgan, Queensland C00–237 111
Mount Morris, New York T17+427 96
Mount Murray, Alberta V39+564 88
Mount Olive, Mississippi T88+317 95
Mount Olive, N. Carolina T18+352 97
Mount Pleasant, Iowa U10+409 95
Mount Pleasant, Michigan T59+436 91
Mount Pleasant, Pa. T27+402 96
Mount Pleasant, S. Aust. C66–348 109
Mount Pleasant, Tennessee T75+355 95
Mount Pleasant, Texas U30+332 95
Mount Pleasant, Utah V40+396 94
Mountrath, Ireland, Rep., N45+530 43
Mount Robson Park, B.C. W00+530 88
Mounts B., England N33+500 38
Mount Sterling, Kentucky T54+381 97
Mount Stewart, P.E.I. S17+464 90
Mount Union, Pennsylvania T18+404 96
Mount Vernon, Illinois T84+384 95
Mount Vernon, Indiana T77+380 95
Mount Vernon, Kentucky T57+374 97
Mount Vernon, Virginia T13+387 91
Moura, Brazil S10–016 104
Moura, Portugal N45+381 52
Mourão, Portugal N44+384 52
Mourne Mts., N. Ireland N36+542 42
Mourne R., N. Ireland N45+548 42
Moussoro, Chad L80+136 81
Moutier, Switzerland M46+473 45
Moutohora, New Zealand A14–383 112
Mowlaik, Burma F64+236 71
Mowming, China E54+217 67
Mowping, China D80+374 66
Moy R., Ireland, Rep. N55+541 42
Moyale, Kenya K36+034 83
Moyobamba, Peru T12–062 104
Mozambique, rep., E. Africa K70-200 84
Moehga, U.S.S.R. J45+565 61
Mozyr, Byelorussia L05+520 60
Mpanda, Tanzania K84–064 83
Mporokoso, Zambia K88–094 83
Mstislavl, Byelorussia K80+541 60
Mtakuja, Tanzania K86–072 83
Mtarica, Mozambique K48–128 83
Mtito Andei, Kenya K40–028 83
Mtoko, Zimbabwe K76–174 84
Mtsensk, U.S.S.R. K51+533 60
Mu, R., Burma F57+228 71
Muadhdham, el, Saudi Arabia K43+278 74
Muang Chaiya, Thailand F35+093 69
Muang Chana, Thailand F26+070 69
Muang Langsuan, Thailand F35+100 69
Muang Nan, Thailand F26+188 69
Muang Palien, Thailand F32+073 69
Mubarraz, Saudi Arabia J62+256 74
Mubende, Uganda K82+004 83
Muchinga Mts., Zambia K80–116 83
Muckish, Ireland, Rep. N48+551 42
Muckros Hd., Ireland, Rep. N52+546 42
Mudanya, Turkey L07+404 74
Mudawwara, Jordan K54+294 76
Muddusjarvi, Finland L19+691 46
Mudgee, New S. Wales C02–327 109
Mudhnib, Saudi Arabia K04+259 74
Mugford C., Labrador S13+582 89
Muggendorf, W. Germany M23+498 48
Mugia, Spain N55+431 52
Mugla, Turkey L10+372 74
Muglad, Sudan L14+110 81
Muhamdi, India G58+279 73
Muhammadabad, Iran J05+375 75
Muhammadgarh, India G71+237 73
Muharraq, The Gulf J56+264 75
Mühldorf, W. Germany M15+482 48
Mühlehorn, Switzerland M35+471 45
Mühlhausen, E. Germany M27+512 48
Muhu, Estonia L41+586 47
Muhu Väin, Estonia L40+588 47
Muinak, Uzbek. J06+438 62
Muine Bheag, Ireland, Rep. N42+527 43
Mukalla, Yemen, South J65+146 74
Mukdahan, Thailand F01+164 69
Mukden. See Shenyang
Mukhtuya, U.S.S.R. E30+607 63
Muktinath, Nepal G37+288 73
Muktsar, India H03+305 72
Muktui, Mongolia E80+492 64
Mula, Spain N08+380 53
Mulanje, Mt., Malawi K56-156 83
Mulchen, Chile S73–377 103
Mulege, Mexico V42+268 100
Mulgrave, Nova Scotia S08+456 90
Mulheim, W. Germany M48+510 48
Mulheim, W. Germany M49+515 48
Mulhouse, France M46+477 54
Mulki, India H01+131 70
Mull Hd., Orkney, Scot. N18+594 40
Mull, I., Scotland N36+564 41
Mull, Sd. of, Scotland N35+565 41
Mullaghareirk Mts., Ireland, Rep. N55+523 43
Mullaittivu, Sri Lanka G55+093 70
Mullaley, New South Wales C01–311 109
Muller Peg., Borneo E40+003 65
Mullet L., Michigan T57+455 91
Mullewa, W. Australia E27–284 110
Müllheim, Switzerland M36+476 45
Mullingar, Ireland, Rep. N44+535 43
Mullion Creek, N.S.W. C05–332 109
Muloorina, S. Australia C73–292 109
Muloowurtina, S Australia C60–301 109
Mulroy B., Ireland, Rep. N46+552 42
Multan, Pakistan H21+302 72
Multia, Finland L31+624 46
Mumbondo, Angola M04–104 82
Mumbwa, Zambia L18–150 82
Muna, Indonesia D75+050 65
München, W. Germany M20+482 48
Muncie, Indiana T62+402 91
Mundo Novo, Brazil Q63–118 105
Munfordville, Kentucky T65+373 97
Mungari, Mozambique K68–174 84
Mungindi, N.S.W.-Qnsld. C06–289 109
Munich. See Munchen
Muniesa, Spain N05+410 53
Munising, Michigan T70+464 91
Munkfors, Sweden M09+599 47
Munnerstadt, W. Germany M29+502 48
Munoz Gamero, Pen., Chile S80–526 103
Munroe, Louisiana U12+324 95
Münster, W. Germany M44+520 48
Münster, Switzerland M27+466 45
Münster, Switzerland M41+465 45
Munster, Switzerland M41+472 45
Munster, prov., Ireland, Rep. N52+523 43
Muong Attopeu, Laos E78+149 69
Muong Borikan, Laos F08+186 69
Muong Het, Laos F05+208 69
Muong Hiem, Laos F10+201 69
Muong Saravan, Laos E82+157 69
Muong Sing, Laos F23+212 69
Muonio, R., Swed.-Fin. L39+677 46
Muonionalusta, Sweden L40+679 46
Muotathal, Switzerland M37+470 45
Mur, Yemen K12+156 74
Murakami, Japan C63+382 68
Murat, R., Turkey K28+388 74
Murat Dagh, Turkey L02+389 74
Murbat, Oman J31+171 75
Murça, Portugal N45+414 52
Murcheh Khur, Iran J52+331 75
Murchison, C., N.-W. Terr. S24+636 89
Murchison Falls, see Kabalega Falls
Murchison Mts., N.Z. A76–452 112
Murchison, R., W. Aust. E22–266 110
Murcia, Spain N07+380 53
Murdo, S. Dakota U65+438 93
Muresul (Maros), R., Romania L54+462 58
Murfreesboro, Tennessee T68+358 93
Muri, Switzerland M40+473 45
Murias de Paredes, Spain N37+429 52
Müritz.See, E. Germany M14+534 48
Murjo, mt., Java E55–066 65
Murmansk, U.S.S.R. K70+690 62
Murom, U.S.S.R. K18+555 61
Muroran, Japan C54+423 68
Muros, Spain N54+428 52
Murphy, N. Carolina T54+351 97
Murphysboro, Illinois T86+378 95
Murray, Kentucky T80+366 95
Murray, Utah V42+406 98
Murray, R., N.S.W., etc. C39–352 109
Murray Bridge, S. Australia C65–352 109
Murray Harbour, P.E.I. S15+460 90
Murray River, P.E.I. S16+460 90
Murrayville, Victoria C53–353 109
Murree, Pakistan H10+339 72
Mürren, Switzerland M43+466 45
Murrumbidgee, R., N.S.W. C35–346 109
Murrumburrah & Harden, New South Wales C10–346 109
Murrurundi, New S. Wales B85–318 109
Mursan, India G72+275 72
Murshidabad, India G10+243 73
Mursir, Oman J22+249 75
Murten & See, Switzerland M47+469 45
Murtoa, Victoria C45–367 109
Mururoa I., Tuamotu Arch. X10–215 107
Murwara, India G57+238 73
Murzuq, Libya M06+258 81
Mus, Turkey K21+388 74
Musa Kala, Afghanistan H61+323 75
Musalamiya, Saudi Arabia J65+275 74
Muscat (Masqāt), Oman J09+236 75
Muscat & Oman. See Oman
Muscatine, Iowa U06+414 95
Musemir, Yemen, South K02+134 74
Musgrave Harb., Nfd. R52+495 90
Musgrave Ra., New Guinea C40–063 111
Musgrave Ra., S. Australia D20–260 110
Musheramore, Ireland, Rep. N54+520 43
Mushie, Zaire L78–030 82
Muskeget Chan., Mass. S62+413 96
Muskegon, Michigan T68+432 91
Muskegon R., Michigan T62+440 91
Muskogee, Oklahoma U33+359 95
Muskwaro, L., Quebec S06+506 90
Musmar, Sudan K56+180 81
Musoma, Tanzania K66–016 83
Mussau, I., Pacific Ocean C00–020 106
Musselburgh, Scotland N18+559 41
Mussidan, France M88+450 55
Mussuma, Angola L48–142 82
Mustahil, Ethiopia K02+052 83
Mustajidda, Saudi Arabia K19+266 74
Mustang, Nepal G37+291 73
Mustang I., Texas U43+276 94
Musters, L., Argentina S56–455 103
Muswellbrook, N.S.W. B85–323 109
Mut, Egypt L06+254 81
Mut, Turkey K70+366 74
Mutanda, Zambia L22–124 82
Mutano, Angola M01–166 84
Mutorai, U.S.S.R. F27+615 63
Mutshatsha, Zaire L34–056 82
Mutsu B., Japan C53+411 68
Mutton I., Ireland, Rep. N57+528 43
Mutumbo, Angola L76–134 82
Mutupet, India G66+104 70
Muwale, Tanzania K68–064 83
Muy, le, France M50+435 55
Muya, Japan D02+342 68
Muya, U.S.S.R. E24+563 63
Muy Muy, Nicaragua T63+127 101
Muzaffarabad, Kashmir H09+344 72
Muzaffargarh, Pakistan H23+301 72
Muzaffarnagar, India G74+294 72
Muzaffarpur, India G27+261 73
Muzhi, U.S.S.R. H63+655 62
Muzquiz, Mexico U69+278 100
Muztagh Ata, Sinkiang, China G89+383 72
Mwanza, Tanzania K72–026 83
Mweelrea, Ireland, Rep. N59+536 42
Mweru L., Zaire L08–090 83
Mwinilunga, Zambia L34–120 82
Myanaung, Burma F58+82 71
Myall, L., New S. Wales B77–325 109
Myadaung, Burma F52+238 71
Myaungmya, Burma F60+166 71
Myebon, Burma F69+201 71
Myenmoletkhat, Mt., Burma F37+134 71
Myingyan, Burma F57+214 71
Myitkyina, Burma F45+254 71
Myjava, Czechoslovakia L74+488 49
Mymensingh, Bangladesh F87+248 71
Myohaung, Burma F53+219 71
Myohaung, Burma F71+206 71
Myrdal, Norway M47+607 47
Myrtle Creek, S. Australia C71–304 109
Myrtleford, Victoria C19–366 109
Myslowice, Poland L67+502 49
Mysore. See Karnataka
Mystic, S. Dakota U82+441 93
Mziha, Tanzania K44–058 83
Mzimba, Malawi K68–120 83
Naaf, Bangladesh F75+210 71
Naarden, Netherlands M59+523 44
Naas, Ireland, Rep. N40+532 43
Nabadwip, India G10+234 73
Naband, Iran J43+274 75
Nabatiye, Lebanon K57+334 76
Nabberu, L., W. Australia D87–257 110
Nabha, India G83+304 72
Nablus, Jordan K59+322 76
Nacaome, Honduras T75+136 101
Nachvak B., Labrador S21+592 89
Nacimiento, Mexico U71+279 100
Nackara, S. Australia C65–328 109

Naco, Arizona V30+313 94
Nacogdoches, Texas U28+316 95
Nacozari de Garcia, Mexico V29+305 100
Nadia. See Nabadwip
Nadiad, India H12+226 70
Naerøy, Norway M22+648 46
Naestved, Denmark M20+552 47
Nafels, Switzerland M36+471 45
Naga, Yemen, D.R. J64+149 74
Naga, Philippines D70+136 65
Naga Hills, India F60+262 71
Nagaland, India F64+262 71
Nagambie, Victoria C29–368 109
Nagano, Japan C71+366 68
Nagaoka, Japan C67+374 68
Nagappattinam, India G61+108 70
Nagar, India G77+321 72
Nagar, Kashmir H01+362 72
Nagar Karnul, India G70+164 70
Nagar Parkar, India H25+243 70
Nagasaki, Japan D31+327 68
Nagaur, India H07+270 70
Nagda, India G87+232 70
Nagercoil, India G74+083 70
Nagha Kalat, Pakistan H59+274 70
Nagina, India G69+295 73
Nagoya, Japan C78+351 68
Nagpur, India G65+210 70
Nagu, (Nauvo), Finland L49+602 47
Nagykanizsa, Hungary L78+465 49
Naha, Japan D44+262 68
Nahael Niyeu, Argentina S39–405 103
Nahan, India G76+305 72
Nahariya, Israel K59+330 76
Naibandan, Iran J15+323 75
Naifa, Saudi Arabia J53+199 75
Naifar, Iraq J89+322 74
Naihati, India G09+229 73
Nain, Labrador S11+563 89
Nain, Iran J41+329 75
Naini Tal, India G63+294 73
Nain Sing Ra., Tibet G50+326 70
Nairn, Scotland N23+576 40
Nairobi, Kenya K52–001 83
Naisecho, Kenya K48+018 83
Naismith, Montana V41+484 93
Naivasha, & L., Kenya K52–008 83
Najera, Spain N16+424 53
Najibabad, India G70+296 73
Najira, Saudi Arabia J70+280 74
Nakajo, Japan C64+381 68
Nakatsu, Japan D23+336 68
Nakawn Pathom, Thailand F30+138 69
Nakfa, Ethiopia K40+166 83
Nakhala, Saudi Arabia J53+243 75
Nakhaun Phantom, Thailand F02+174 69
Nakhichevan, U.S.S.R. J85+390 62
Nakhon Ratchasima, Thai. F17+149 69
Nakhon Sawan, Thailand F30+158 69
Nakhon Si Thammarat, Thai. F30+084 69
Nakina, Ontario T70+501 89
Nakl Mubarak, Saudi Arabia K40+243 74
Nakodar, India G87+311 72
Nakuru, Kenya K54–004 83
Nalagarh, India G79+310 72
Nalgonda, India G64+170 70
Nallamalai Hills, India G67+159 70
Nalut, Libya M24+318 81
Namangan, Uzbek. H20+412 62
Namasagali, Uganda K72+010 83
Namatail, Mozambique K32–158 83
Nambala, Zambia L18–152 84
Nambucca, New S. Wales B73–306 109
Namcha Barwa, China F58+295 64
Nam-dinh, Vietnam E83+204 69
Namhoi. See Fatshan
Namib Desert, Namibia M04-250 84
Namibia, S. Africa L76-250 84
Namlea, Buru I., Indonesia D48–034 65
Namling Dzong, Tibet G06+296 71
Nam Mao R., Burma F47+236 71
Namoi, New South Wales B88–310 109
Namonuito, Is., Caroline Is. C00+085 106
Namorona, Madagascar J72–218 83
Nampa, Idaho V70+436 92
Nampula, Mozambique K34–152 83
Nams Vatn, Norway M08+651 46
Namsen, R., Norway M14+647 46
Namsos, Norway M21+645 46
Namtsy, U.S.S.R. D31+627 63
Namtu, Burma F45+229 71
Namur & prov., Belgium M61+503 44
Namutoni, Namibia L78-188 84
Namwala, Zambia L22–158 84
Namyang, China E33+252 67
Nanaimo, Brit. Columbia W34+492 88
Nana Kru, Liberia N52+048 80
Nanan. See Tayu
Nanao, Japan C78+370 68
Nanchang, China E24+286 67
Nancheng (Hanchung), China E78+331 66
Nancheng (Kienchang), China E20+275 67
Nanchung, China E83+308 66
Nancy, France M55+487 54
Nanda Devi, mt., India G60+304 70
Nanded, India G75+192 70
Nandewar Ra., N.S.W. B86–302 109
Nanga Parbat, Kashmir H03+352 72
Nanguar, Mozambique K42–124 83
Nanjangud, India G79+121 70
Nankang. See Tsingtze
Nanking, China E07+320 66
Nannine, W. Australia E10–268 110
Nanning, China E70+228 67
Nanortalik, Greenland Q72+600 26
Nanpara, India G51+278 73
Nanping, China E11+267 67
Nanripo, Mozambique K36–140 83
Nan Shan, China F30+384 62
Nantan, China E74+251 64
Nantes, France N09+472 54
Nanticoke, Pennsylvania T06+412 96
Nantucket, Massachusetts S61+413 91
Nantucket I., Massachusetts S60+412 96
Nantucket Sd., Massachusetts S62+414 96
Nantung, China D85+320 66
Nantwich, England N15+531 37
Nanyang, China E45+330 66
Nanyuki, Kenya K48+001 83
Naoetsu, Japan C70+371 68
Napa, California W14+383 92
Napanee, Ontario T12+442 91
Napas, U.S.S.R. G48+599 62
Napier, New Zealand A18–395 112
Naples. See Napoli
Napoleon, N. Dakota U58+465 93
Napoli, Italy M05+409 57
Napoli, G. di, Italy M07+406 57
Naqb Ashtar, Jordan K57+300 76
Nara, Mali N44+152 80
Nara, Japan C85+347 68
Naracoorte, S. Australia C56–370 109
Naradhan, New S. Wales C22–336 109
Narativat, Thailand F19+064 69
Narayanganj, Bangladesh F82+236 71
Narbada R., India G68+230 73
Narberth, Wales N28+518 38
Narbonne, France M72+432 55
Nares Ld., Greenland R25+820 26
Nari R., Pakistan H43+284 70
Narino. See Japura
Narken, Sweden L44+670 46
Narnaul, India G85+281 72
Narok, Kenya K56–012 83
Narooma, New South Wales B89–363 109
Narovchat, U.S.S.R. K08+538 61
Narowal, Pakistan H01+321 72
Narrabri, New South Wales C01–303 109
Narrabri West, N.S.W. C02–304 109
Narragansett B., Rhode I. S69+414 96
Narran L. & R., N.S.W. C16–296 109
Narranderra, New S. Wales C21–348 109
Narrogin, W. Australia E17–328 110
Narromine, New S. Wales C10–323 109
Narsinghgarh, India G77+238 70
Narsinghpur, India G65+229 73
Naruta, Japan D02+342 68
Narva, Estonia L11+593 47
Narva Laht, Estonia L16+596 47
Narvik, Norway L75+685 46
Narwar, India G73+257 73
Naryan Mar, U.S.S.R. J40+677 62
Narykary, U.S.S.R. H60+634 62
Narym, U.S.S.R. G50+589 62
Naryn, Kirgiz. G84+414 62
Naseby, New Zealand A59–450 112
Nashua and R., N.H. S69+428 96
Nashville, Arkansas U22+339 95
Nashville, Illinois T86+384 95
Nashville, N. Carolina T18+360 97
Nashville, Tennessee T71+361 97
Nasijarvi, Finland L38+616 47
Nasia, Ghana N04+100 80
Nasik, India H07+200 70
Nasirabad, India H01+262 70
Naskaupi R., Labrador S10+542 89
Nassau, Bahamas,The T15+250 101
Nassau, G. de, Chile S46–555 103
Nassau, I., Pacific Ocean Z03–114 106
Nasser, L., Egypt K82+216 81
Nassjo, Sweden M02+577 47
Nata, Panama T33+084 101
Natal, Brazil Q31–058 105
Natal, Brazil S01–068 104
Natal, South Africa L00–286 84
Natal, Sumatra F35+006 65
Natanes Plat., Arizona V26+334 94
Natanya, Israel K61+323 76
Natashquan, Quebec S11+502 90
Natashquan R., Quebec S10+514 89
Natchez, Mississippi U08+316 93
Natimuk, Victoria C48–367 109
National City, California V73+326 92
Natividade, Brazil R16–115 105
Natron L., Tanzania K54–024 83
Nattavaara, Sweden L54+667 46
Naturaliste, C., W. Aust. E30–334 110
Naturawit L., N.-W. Terr. U51+635 88
Naukhas, Namibia L82-236 84
Naumburg, E. Germany M19+512 48
Naumestis, Lithuania L43+548 47
Naumiestis, Lithuania L50+554 47
Nauplia. See Navplion
Naur, Jordan K55+319 76
Nauru, I., Pacific Ocean A78–003 106
Naushahra. See Nowshera
Naushahro, Pakistan H41+268 70
Naushk, U.S.S.R. E84+505 63
Nauta, Peru S81–045 104
Nautla, Mexico U41+202 96
Nauvoo, Illinois T86+406 95
Nava del Rey, Spain N30+414 52
Navajo, Mt., Utah V36+370 94
Navalcarnero, Spain N24+403 52
Navalmoral, Spain N33+399 52
Navan, Ireland, Rep. N40+537 42
Navarino, I., Chile S46–550 99
Navarre, Victoria C42–369 109
Navarre, prov., France N07+433 55
Navojoa, Mexico V26+272 96
Navplion, Greece L43+376 59
Navrongo, Ghana N06+108 80
Navsari, India H12+209 70
Nawa, Syria K54+329 76
Nawabganj, India G47+269 73
Nawabganj, India G53+269 73
Nawada, India G26+249 73
Nawah Basoda, India G70+236 73
Nawahganj, India G62+285 73
Nawai, India G84+264 70
Nawalgarh, India G88+278 72
Naxos, I., Greece L27+370 59
Nayakhan, U.S.S.R. B38+620 63
Nayarit, state, Mexico V00+220 96
Nayarit, Sa. de, Mexico U88+226 96
Nayoro, Japan C44+443 68
Nazaré de Mata, Brazil Q31–077 105
Nazareth, Belgium M69+509 44
Nazareth, Israel K58+327 76
Nazas, Mexico U85+252 96
Nazca, Peru S88–148 104
Naze, The, England M82+519 39
Naze, The (Lindesnes), Nor. M47+580 47
Nazilli, Turkey L10+379 74
Nazimovo, U.S.S.R. F83+595 63
Ncheu, Malawi K62–148 83
Ndala, Tanzania K70–046 83
Ndeni, I., Santa Cruz Is. A82–105 106
N'Djamena, Chad M00+122 81
Ndola, Zambia L08–130 83
Neagh L., N. Ireland N38+546 42
Néapolis, Crete L26+353 59
Near Is., Aleutian Islands A40+517 95
Neath, Wales N23+517 38
Nebikon, Switzerland M42+472 45
Nebit-Dag, Turkmen. J36+392 62
Nebo Mt., Utah V41+398 94
Nebraska, state, U.S.A. U73+416 98
Nebraska City, Nebraska U35+406 95
Necedah, Wisconsin U00+440 91
Neckar, R., W. Germany M36+492 48
Necochea, Argentina R83–386 103
Nederweert, Netherlands M56+513 44
Neede, Netherlands M50+521 44
Needham Market, England M84+522 39
Needles, California V58+348 92
Needles, The, Arizona V55+345 92
Needles, The, England N10+507 39
Neemuch, India H00+245 70
Neenah, Wisconsin T81+442 91
Neerpelt, Belgium M57+512 44
Nefud Des, Saudi Arabia K30+288 74
Negaunee, Michigan T75+465 91
Negocio, Argentina S35–418 103
Negombo, Sri Lanka G61+073 70
Negra Pta., Peru T36–060 104
Negrais, C., Burma F65+160 71
Negro, R., Argentina S30–398 103
Negro, R., Brazil S20–004 104
Negro, R., Uruguay R60–324 103
Negros, I., Philippines D72+100 65
Nehavend, Iran J71+343 74
Nehbandān, Iran J00+315 75
Neilsville, Wisconsin U04+446 91
Neisse. See Nysa,
Neiva, Colombia T02+027 104
Nejd, Saudi Arabia K18+256 74
Neksø, Bornholm I., Den. L89+551 47
Nelia Gaari, New S. Wales C43–321 109
Nelkan, U.S.S.R. C84+577 63
Nelligen, New South Wales B89–356 109
Nellore, India G60+145 70
Nelma, U.S.S.R. C65+475 63
Nelson, Brit. Columbia V73+495 88
Nelson, New Zealand A40–413 112
Nelson, Victoria C54–381 109
Nelson, C., Victoria C51–384 109
Nelson Hd., N.-W. Terr. W10+710 88
Nelson L., Manitoba U63+557 88
Nelson, Mt., Brit. Columbia V68+504 88
Nelson R., Manitoba U25+562 88
Nêma, Mauritania N44+166 80
Nemecke Pravno, Czech. L68+489 49
Nemikiachi L., Quebec S87+475 91
Nemours, (Ghazaouet), Alg. N10+350 80
Nemours, France M74+482 54
Nemunas, R., Lithuania L40+551 47
Nemuro, Japan C26+433 68
Nemuro B., Japan C28+434 68
Nen R., England N03+526 37
Nenagh, Ireland, Rep. N49+528 43
Nendeln, Liechtenstein M33+472 45
Neodesha, Kansas U35+374 95
Neosho, Missouri U26+368 95
Nepa, U.S.S.R. E71+592 63
Nepal, Asia G50+270 30
Nepalganj, Nepal G50+280 73
Nephi, Utah V42+396 94
Nephin, Ireland, Rep. N56+540 42
Nephin Beg, Ireland, Rep. N58+540 43
Nérac, France M88+441 55
Nerchinsk, U.S.S.R. E19+520 63
Nerpio, Spain N14+382 53
Nerriga, New South Wales C00–352 109
Nes, U.S.S.R. K03+667 62
Nesna, Norway M12+662 46
Nespawa, Manitoba U57+503 88
Ness L., Scotland N27+573 40
Ness City, Kansas U60+384 95
Nesset, Norway M42+628 46
Nesslau, Switzerland M35+472 45
Nesthorn, mt., Switzerland M42+464 45
Nesttun, Norway M58+603 47
Netherlands, W. Europe M54+520 50
Nettilling L., N.-W. Terr. S65+662 89
Nettuno, Italy M14+415 57
Neubrandenburg,
E. Germany M10+535 48
Neuburg, W. Germany M23+487 48
Neuchâtel & canton, Switz. M48+470 45
Neuchâtel, L. de, Switz. M49+45
Neufchâteau, Belgium M57+498 44
Neufchâteau, France M56+483 54
Neufchâtel, France M82+498 54
Neufelden, Austria M06+485 48
Neuhausen, Switzerland M38+477 45
Neumünster, W. Germany M30+541 48
Neunkirch, Switzerland M39+477 45
Neuquen, Argentina S49–389 103
Neuse R., N. Carolina T14+353 97
Neusiedler See, Austria L79+477 49
Neuss, W. Germany M50+512 48
Neustadt, W. Germany M25+541 48
Neustettin. See Szczecinek
Neustrelitz, E. Germany M12+533 48
Neu Ulm, W. Germany M30+484 48
Neuva, I., Chile & Argent. S40–552 103
Neuva Esperanza, Bolivia S28–158 104
Neuva Lubeca, Argentina S63–446 103
Neuve Eglise, Belgium M73+508 44
Neuveville, Switzerland M47+471 45
Neuvitas, Cuba T14+215 101
Nevada, Iowa U20+422 95
Nevada, Missouri U26+378 95
Nevada, state, U.S.A. V81+395 98
Nevada, Sa., California W12+411 98
Nevada, Sa., Spain N20+370 52
Nevel, U.S.S.R. L00+560 60
Nevel'sk, U.S.S.R. C48+465 63
Nevers, France M71+470 54
Nevertire, New South Wales C14–319 109
Nevesinje, Yugoslavia L71+433 58
Neveyezhkino, U.S.S.R. K01+512 61
Nevis, I., Leeward Islands S15+172 101
Nevsehir, Turkey K62+386 74
Nevyansk, U.S.S.R. H89+574 61
New Albany, Indiana T65+383 97
New Albany, Mississippi T84+345 95
New Amsterdam,
Guyana R76+061 105
Newark, Delaware T04+397 96
Newark, England N05+531 37
Newark, New Jersey S85+407 96
Newark, Ohio T45+401 91
Newaygo, Michigan T65+434 91
New Bedford, Massachusetts S65+416 96
New Bern, N. Carolina T12+351 97
Newbern, Tennessee T86+362 97
Newberry, Michigan T63+463 91
Newberry, S. Carolina T40+343 97
New Bloomfield, Pa T14+404 96
New Britain, Bismarck
Archipelago B85–060 106
New Britain, Connecticut S76+417 96
New Brunswick, New Jersey S87+405 96
New Brunswick, prov.,
Canada S36+470 89
Newburg, New Brunswick S45+463 90
Newburgh, New York S84+414 96
Newburgh, Scotland N19+563 41
Newbury, England N08+514 39
Newburyport, Massachusetts S65+428 96
Newby Bridge, England N18+543 37
New Caledonia, Pacific Oc. A85–212 106
New Carlisle, Quebec S32+480 90
Newcastle, Delaware T03+397 91
Newcastle, Natal L00–278 84
Newcastle, New Brunswick S34+470 90
New Castle, New Jersey T04+397 96
Newcastle, New South Wales B80–330 109
Newcastle, N. Ireland N35+542 42
New Castle, Pennsylvania T32+411 91
Newcastle, Wyoming U86+439 93
Newcastle Emlyn, Wales N27+520 38
Newcastle-under-Lyme, Eng. N13+530 37
Newcastle-upon-Tyne, Eng. N10+550 37
Newcastle Waters,,
N.T., Australia D09–173 111
Newchwang. See Yingkow.
New City, New York S84+411 96
New Cumberland, W. Va. T34+405 91
New England Ra., N.S.W. B80–306 109
Newfane, Vermont S76+430 96
New Forest, England N10+508 39
Newfoundland, prov., Canada R70+490 89
New Galloway, Scotland N25+551 41
New Georgia, I., Solomon Is. B48–080 105
New Glasgow, Nova Scotia S16+456 90
New Guinea, Pacific Ocean C60–060 31
New Hampshire, state, U.S.A. S70+435 99
New Hampton, Iowa U14+430 95
New Haven, Connecticut S78+413 91
Newhaven, England N00+508 39
New Haven, Missouri U08+386 97
New Hebrides, Is., See Vanuatu
New Iberia, Lousiana U11+300 95
New Ireland, Bismarck Arch. B75–040 106
New Jersey, state, U.S.A. S89+404 99
New Liskeard, Ontario T28+475 91
Newe London, Connecticut S73+413 96
New London, Wisconsin T83+445 91
New Madrid, Missouri T88+366 95
Newmarket, Ireland, Rep. N54+522 43
Newmarket, England M88+522 39
Newmarket, Ontario T27+441 91
New Mexico, state, U.S.A. V20+344 98
Newnes, New South Wales B89–332 109
Newnham, England N16+518 38
New Norfolk, Tasmania C18–428 109
New Orleans, Louisiana U00+300 95
New Plymouth, N.Z. A36–390 112
Newport, Arkansas U08+356 97
Newport, Ireland, Rep. N57+539 42
Newport, I. of W., England N08+507 39
Newport, Kentucky T57+391 91
Newport, New Hampshire S73+434 96
Newport, Quebec S29+483 90
Newport, Rhode Island S68+415 91
Newport, Vermont S73+449 91
Newport, Wales N18+516 38
Newport News, Virginia T08+370 97
Newport-on-Tay, Scotland N18+564 41
New Providence, I.,
Bahamas, The T15+250 101
Newquay, England N30+504 38
New Quay, Wales N26+522 38
New Radnor, Wales N19+522 38
New Richmond, Quebec S35+482 90
New Richmond, Wisconsin U15+452 93
New Rochelle, New York S82+409 96
New Rockford, N. Dakota U55+477 93
New Ross, Ireland, Rep. N42+524 43
Newry & Can., N. Ireland N38+542 42
New Salem, N. Dakota U68+469 93
New Siberian Islands,
See Novosibirskiye Ostrova
New South Wales, state, Aust — 111
Newton, Iowa U18+416 95
Newton, Kansas U44+381 95
Newton, Massachusetts S67+424 96
Newton, New Jersey S89+410 96
Newton-Abbot, England N22+505 38
Newtonmore, Scotland N25+571 40
Newtown Mount Kennedy,
Ireland, Rep. N37+531 43
Newton-Stewart, Scotland N27+550 41
Newtown, Wales N20+525 38
Newtownards, N. Ireland N34+546 42
Newtown Butler, N. Ireland N44+542 42
Newtown Hamilton, N. Ire. N39+542 42
Newtonstewart, N. Ire. N44+547 42
New Ulm, Minnesota U27+443 93
New Waterford, Nova Scotia S00+463 90
New Westminster, B.C. W18+492 88
New World I., Nfd. R59+496 90
New York, New York S84+408 91
New York, state, U.S.A. T20+425 99
New Zealand, Australasia — 112
Nexö. See Neksö,
Neya, U.S.S.R. K06+583 61
Neyriz, Iran J34+296 75
Neyshābūr, Iran J07+362 75
Nezhin, Ukraine K79+511 60
Ngami, L., Botswana L40–210 84
Nganglaring Tso, Tibet G42+315 71
N'Gaoundéré, Cameroon M08+074 81
Ngapara, New Zealand A55–450 112
Ngaruawehia, New Zealand A29–377 112
Ngatik, I., Caroline Islands B47+050 106
Ngauruhoe, Mt., N.Z. A26–391 112
Ngeuni, Sudan L14+060 81
Ngong, Kenya K50–014 83
Ngoring Nor, China F42+348 64
Nguigmi, Niger M12+142 81

Ngulu, I., Pacific Ocean C78+075 106
Ngwasi, Tanzania K46-086 83
Nha-Trang, Vietnam E65+123 69
Nhill, Victoria C50-363 109
Niafounke, Mali N24+160 80
Niagara, Ontario T25+433 91
Niagara Falls, New York T24+431 91
Niagara Falls, Ontario T24+431 91
Niah, Sarawak E38+037 65
Niamey, Niger M78+134 80
Nia Nia, Zaire L14+014 83
Niapa, mt., Borneo E15+017 65
Nias, I., Indonesia F44+011 65
Nicaragua, rep., Cent. Amer. T62+130 101
Nicaragua L., Nicaragua T63+116 101
Nicastro, Italy L82+390 57
Nic Doit Soe Pk., Arizona V36+364 94
Nice, France M47+437 55
Nicobar Is., Indian Ocean F70+085 71
Nicolet, Quebec S76+462 91
Nicoque, Mozambique K36-128 83
Nicosia, Cyprus K70+352 76
Nicoya & Pen., Costa Rica T62+100 101
Nidau, Switzerland M47+471 45
Nidd R., England N10+540 37
Nidzica, Poland L57+533 49
Niedere Tauern, Austria M06+473 48
Niedersachsen, W. Germany M42+528 48
Nielle, Ivory Coast N34+102 80
Niére, Chad L50+142 81
Nieuw Amsterdam, Surinam R60+058 105
Nieuwendijk, Netherlands M61+518 44
Nieuwersluis, Netherlands M60+522 44
Nieuwkoop Netherlands M61+522 44
Nieuw Nickerie, Surinam R73+058 105
Nieuwpoort, Belgium M73+511 44
Nieuwpoort, Netherlands M61+519 44
Nieves, Mexico U78+240 100
Niévre, dep., France M68+471 54
Nigde, Turkey K62+380 74
Niger, rep., W. Africa M30+156 81
Niger R., W. Africa N10+150 80
Nigeria, W. Africa M40+100 80
Nighasan, India G55+282 73
Nigula, Estonia L20+595 47
Niigata, Japan C66+379 68
Niihau, I., Hawaii Y60+220 106
Niitaka Chain, Taiwan D84+240 67
Nijil, Jordan K57+305 76
Nijkerk, Netherlands M58+522 44
Nijmegen, Netherlands M55+518 44
Nikaria. See Ikaria, I.
Nikiforos, Greece L34+412 58
Nikki, Benin M72+098 80
Nikko Nat. Park, Japan C64+368 68
Nikolayevskiy, U.S.S.R. J87+501 61
Nikolayev, Ukraine K78+470 60
Nikolayevsk-na-Amure, U.S.S.R. C56+533 63
Nikolo Kozelsk, Ukraine K71+476 60
Nikolskaya Pestrovka, U.S.S.R. J84+538 61
Nikolsk Berezovka, U.S.S.R. J35+561 61
Nikopol, Ukraine K63+476 60
Niksar, Turkey K48+407 74
Nikšić, Yugoslavia L66+428 58
Nila, I., Indonesia D33-068 65
Nile, R., N. Africa K72+250 81
Niles, Michigan T68+418 91
Nilgiri, India G19+214 71
Nilgiri Hills, India G81+116 70
Nilphamari, Bangladesh G07+259 73
Nimach, (Neemuch), India H00+245 70
Nîmes, France M64+439 55
Nimgiri, Mt., India G39+196 71
Nimmitabel, New S. Wales C05-365 109
Nine de Julio, Argentina S05-354 99
Ninety Mile Beach, Victoria C16-382 109
Nineveh, Iraq K11+366 74
Ningan, China D33+444 64
Ninganpao, China E86+373 66
Ningerh, China F25+231 64
Ninghai, China D81+293 67
Ninghsien, China E37+267 67
Ninghsien. See Ningpo
Ningiang, China E44+283 67
Ningkwo. See Suancheng
Ninglingting. See Kinki
Ningpo, China D80+298 67
Ning-sia. See Yingchwan
Ningteh, China E03+267 67
Ning-wu-fu, China E46+390 66
Ning-yüan chow, China D86+405 66
Ning-yüan-ting, China E44+403 66
Ninh-binh, Vietnam E84+203 69
Ninh Hoa, Vietnam E66+140 65
Ninove, Belgium M66+508 44
Niobrara R., Nebraska U71+424 98
Nioet, mt., Borneo E60+010 65
Nioro, Mali N58+152 80
Niort, France N03+463 54
Nios. See Ios, I.
Nipe, B. de, Cuba T04+208 101
Nipigon, Ontario T80+492 89
Nipigon, L., Ontario T80+500 89
Nipissing, L., Ontario T29+462 91
Nirmal, India G69+191 70
Nis, Yugoslavia L49+433 58
Nisab, Saudi Arabia J81+149 74
Nisehu, Kashmir G65+346 70
Nish. See Nis
Nishapur. See Neyshābūr,
Nishio, Japan C77+348 68
Nisiros, I., Greece L17+366 59
Nissan, Solomon Islands B60-053 106
Nissi, Estonia L34+591 47
Niteroi, Brazil Q79-228 105
Nith, R., Scotland N22+550 41
Nitra, Czechoslovakia L71+483 49
Niue, I. Cook Islands Z30-190 106
Nivala, Finland L30+639 46
Nivelles, Belgium M64+506 44
Nivernais, prov., France M68+471 54
Nizamabad, India G71+187 70
Nizampatnam, India G55+159 70
Nizana, Israel K63+309 76
Nizhne Chirskaya, U.S.S.R. K12+484 61
Nizhne Udinsk, U.S.S.R. F35+549 63
Nizhi Pesha, U.S.S.R. J73+668 62
Nizhniye Serogozy, Ukraine K64+469 60
Nizhniy Kresty, U.S.S.R. B25+687 63
Nizhiy Lomov, U.S.S.R. K02+536 61
Nizhniy Tagil, U.S.S.R. J01+579 61
Nizke Tatry, Czechoslovakia L63+490 49
Njombe, Tanzania K60-094 83
Nkhota-Kota, Malawi K64-130 84
N'Kongsamba, Cameroon M30+050 81
Nmai R., Burma F41+264 71
Noagarh, India G47+204 71
Noakhali. See Sudharam
Noanama, Colombia T13+047 104
Noatak R., Alaska Y60+675 99
Nobber, Ireland, Rep. N40+538 42
Nochistlan, Mexico U44+174 100
Noerbø, Norway M56+587 47
Nogales, Arizona V36+313 94
Nogaro, France N00+438 55
Nogent-le-Rotrou. France M85+483 54
Nogent-sur-Seine, France M69+485 54
Noginsk, U.S.S.R. K40+558 60
Nohar, India H02+292 72
Noirmoutier, I. de, France N14+470 54
Nokhtuysk, U.S.S.R. E11+600 63
Nola, Cent. Afr. Rep. L84+034 82
Nola, Italy M03+409 57
Nome, Alaska Z00+642 99
Nomining Ls., Quebec T00+465 91
Nomoi, Is., Caroline Islands B65+060 106
Nonacho L., N.-W. Terr. V30+614 88
Nonancourt, France M83+488 54
Nong-han, Thailand F11+174 69
Nong Khai, Thailand F13+179 69
Nongoma, Natal K80-280 84
Nong-son, Vietnam E72+156 69
Nonni, R. (Nun), China D64+488 64
Nonno, Ethiopia K46+084 83
Nonoava, Mexico V10+274 100
Nonouti, I., Kiribati A35-005 106
Nõo, Estonia L21+583 47
Noojee, Victoria C24-379 109
Noonthorungee, N.S.W. C46-310 109
Noordeloos, Netherlands M60+519 44
Noordwolde, Netherlands M53+529 44
Nootka I., Brit. Columbia W41+498 88
Nootongoro, Tanzania K62-032 83
Nora, Sweden M00+595 47
Noranda, Quebec T25+482 91
Nord, dep., France M71+505 54
Nord Cap (Horn), Iceland P44+665 46
Norddal, Norway M47+623 46
Nordenshelda, Arkh., U.S.S.R. F55+762 63
Nordhausen, E. Germany M25+515 48
Nordkapp, Norway L25+711 46
Nordkyn Halvøy, Norway L12+709 46
Nördlingen, W. Germany M27+489 48
Nordost Rundingen, Greenland N60+810 26
Nordreisa, Norway L54+698 46
Nordrhein-Westfalen, W. Ger. M48+518 48
Nord Slesvig. See Jylland, South
Nordstrand I., W. Germany M37+545 48
Nordvik, U.S.S.R. E53+739 63
Nore, Norway M36+601 47
Nore R., Ireland, Rep. N42+523 43
Norfolk, Nebraska U44+422 95
Norfolk, Virginia T08+369 97
Norfolk, co., England M84+527 39
Norfolk Broads, England M81+527 39
Norfolk I., Pacific Ocean A72-290 106
Norfolk Res., Arkansas U14+364 95
Norgama, Pakistan H50+286 70
Norheimsund, Norway M53+603 47
Norily, U.S.S.R. G06+694 62
Norman, N.-W. Territories W32+649 88
Norman, Oklahoma U44+352 95
Normandie, prov., France N00+488 54
Normanby I., Papua New Guinea B84-100 111
Normanton, Queensland C53-176 111
Norman Wells, N.-W. Terr. W40+652 88
Norquin, Argentina S64-377 103
Norquinco, Argentina S66-418 103
Norris, L., Tennessee T54+364 97
Norris Arm, Newfoundland R61+491 90
Norristown, Pennsylvania T02+402 96
Norrköping, Sweden L83+586 47
Norrsundet, Sweden L78+610 47
Norrtalje, Sweden L68+598 47
Norseman, W. Australia D80-321 110
Norsholm, Sweden L84+585 47
North C., Antarctica A80-700 27
North C., New Zealand A42-344 112
North, C., Nova Scotia S02+471 90
North Chan., Ontario T50+461 91
North Chan., Scot.-N. Ire. N33+550 42
North Downs, England M87+513 39
North I., New Zealand 112
North Pt., Prince Edward I. S24+471 90
North Sea, W. Europe 34
North Adams, Massachusetts S78+427 96
Northallerton, England N08+543 37
Northam, W. Australia E20-316 110
Northampton, Massachusetts S76+424 96
Northampton, W. Australia E32-282 110
Northampton & co., Eng. N05+523 37
North Bay, Ontario T27+463 91
North Bend, Oregon W25+434 96
North Berwick, Scotland N16+560 41
North Borneo, See Sabah
North Bourke, N.S.W. C24-300 109
Northbridge, Massachusetts S70+422 96
North Carolina, state, U.S.A. T40+358 99
North Creek, New York S84+437 91
North Dakota, state, U.S.A. U78+472 98
Northern Circars, India G50+165 70
Northern Ireland, Brit. Isles N40+544 34
Northern Territory, Aust. 110-111
Northfield, Minnesota U19+445 93
North Land. See Severnaya Zemlya
North Lisbon, Wisconsin U01+439 91
North Little Rock, Arkansas U13+348 99
North Platte, Nebraska U64+411 94
North Pole, Arctic Ocean 26
North Riding, see North Yorkshire
North Ronaldsay, I. & Firth, Orkney, Scotland N14+594 40
North Shields, England N09+550 37
North Sydney, Nova Scotia S02+462 90
North Tonawanday. N.Y. T23+430 96
North Truchas Pk., N. Mex. V04+360 94
Northumberland, co., Eng. N13+553 37
Northumberland, Pa. T11+409 96
Northumberland Str., New Brunswick, etc. S27+465 90
North Vancouver, B.C. W19+494 88
Northville, New York S86+433 91
North West C., W. Aust. E35-218 110
North-West River, Labrador S01+537 89
North-West Territories, Can. 88-89
Northwich, England N15+532 37
Northwood, Iowa U19+434 95
Norton, Kansas U60+398 95
Norton, New Brunswick S34+456 90
Norton Sd., Alaska Z00+636 99
Norwalk, Connecticut S81+411 96
Norwalk, Ohio T46+413 91
Norway, Michigan T77+458 91
Norway, king., N.-W. Europe 46-47
Norwich, Connecticut S72+415 96
Norwich, England M82+526 39
Norwich, New York T03+425 96
Norwood, Massachusetts S67+422 96
Norwood, New York T00+447 91
Noshiro, Japan C60+402 68
Nossegem, Belgium M63+509 44
Nosy Be. I., Madagascar J70-134 83
Noto, Sicily L89+368 57
Noto Pen., Japan C80+372 68
Notodden, Norway M38+595 47
Notre Dame B., Nfd. R60+497 90
Notre Dame Mts., Quebec S60+470 90
Notre Dame-du-Lac, Quebec S53+476 90
Nottawasaga B., Ontario T32+446 91
Nottingham & co., England N07+530 37
Nottingham I., N.-W. Terr. T17+636 89
Nouakchott, Mauritania P06+180 80
Nova Chaves, Angola L52-108 82
Nova Cruz, Brazil Q32-064 105
Nova Gaia, Angola L74-102 82
Nova Goa (Panjim), Goa, Daman & Diu H07+156 70
Nova Lisboa, See Huambo
Novara, Italy M38+454 56
Nova Scotia, prov., Canada S20+450 89
Nova Venecia, Brazil Q63-188 105
Novaya Sibir, Ostrov, U.S.S.R. C10+750 63
Novaya Zemlya, U.S.S.R. J20+730 62
Nova York, Brazil Q84-068 105
Nové Zámky, Czech. L71+480 49
Novgorod, U.S.S.R. K82+586 60
Novi, Yugoslavia M01+451 56
Novi Pazar, Bulgaria L17+434 58
Novi Pazar, Yugoslavia L57+431 58
Novi Sad, Yugoslavia L61+453 58
Novo Alekseyevka, Kasakh. H66+453 62
Novocherkassk, U.S.S.R. K29+474 61
Novokuznetsk, U.S.S.R. G17+538 62
Novo Mesto, Yugoslavia M01+458 56
Novomoskovsk, U.S.S.R. K43+479 60
Novo Moskovsk, Ukraine K58+487 60
Novo Nikolayevskiy, U.S.S.R. K13+510 61
Novo Redondo, Angola M06-114 82
Novorossiysk, U.S.S.R. K44+448 62
Novoshakhtinsk, U.S.S.R. K31+477 61
Novosibirsk, U.S.S.R. G42+550 62
Novosibirskiye Ostrova, U.S.S.R. C60+755 63
Novo Troitsk, U.S.S.R. J21+545 61
Novourgench, Uzbek H86+415 62
Novska, Yugoslavia L78+453 56
Novy Jičin, Czechoslovakia L72+496 49
Novyy Port, U.S.S.R. H12+676 62
Nowa Wilejka, Lithuania L27+547 47
Nowendoc, New S. Wales B80-316 109
Nowgong, India F74+263 71
Nowinga, Victoria C47-346 109
Nowra, New South Wales B87-349 109
Nowshera, Pakistan H18+340 72
Nowy Sacz, Poland L56+496 49
Nowy Targ, Poland L60+495 49
Nowy Tomysl, Poland L83+523 49
Noya, Spain N53+427 52
Nozay, France N10+476 54
Ntungamo, Uganda K86-008 83
Nuanetsi. Zimbabwe K8-214 84
Nueces R., Texas U48+280 94
Nueltin L., N.-W. Terr. U56+602 88
Nueva Imperial, Chile S78-386 103
Nuevo, G., Argentina S28-426 103
Nuevo Laredo, Mexico U57+274 100
Nuevo Leon, state, Mexico U60+262 100
Nûgssuaq, Pen., Greenland R35+700 26
Nuits St Georges, France M60+471 54
Nukuhiva, I., Marquesas Is. X30-100 107
Nukuoro, I., Caroline Is. B60+040 106
Nukus, Uzbek J02+424 62
Nules, Spain N01+398 53
Nullagine, W. Australia E00-218 110
Nullarbor Plain, W. Aust. D40-306 110
Numato, Japan C66+366 68
Numazu, Japan C67+351 68
Numfoor, I., New Guinea D01-010 65
Numurkah, Victoria C27-361 109
Nunchia, Colombia S74+056 104
Nuneaton, England N09+525 37
Nunivak I., Alaska Z15+600 99
Nunkiang, China D59+490 64
Nuoro, Sardinia M34+403 57
Nuqui, Colombia T14+057 104
Nurmes, Finland L05+636 46
Nürnberg, Germany M24+494 48
Nurpur, India G84+323 72
Nurri, Sardinia M35+397 57
Nusaybin, Turkey K23+371 74
Nushki, Pakistan H54+296 70
Nutrias, Venezuela S56+079 104
Nuwara Eliya, Sri Lanka G56+070 70
Nyada, Sweden L72+629 46
Nyah, Victoria C40-352 109
Nyaker, Sweden L64+638 46
Nyala, Sudan L30+120 81
Nyalikungu, Tanzania K70-026 83
Nyamlell, Sudan L18+092 81
Nyandoma, U.S.S.R. K29+617 62
Nyantákara, Tanzania K82-030 83
Nyanza, Rwanda L00-024 83
Nyasa, L., Malawi K64-118 83
Nyasaland, See Malawi
Nyazepetrovsk, U.S.S.R. J03+561 61
Nyda, U.S.S.R. H11+667 62
Nyeri, Kenya K48-004 83
Nyhammar, Sweden M00+603 47
Nyiregyhaza, Hungary L50+479 49
Nykobing, Denmark M19+547 47
Nykøbing, Denmark M37+568 47
Nyköping, Sweden L78+587 47
Nylstroom, Transvaal L10-246 84
Nyamagee, New South Wales C22-321 109
Nymboida & R., N.S.W. B75-299 109
Nyngan, New South Wales C17-316 109
Nyon, Switzerland M53+464 45
Nyonga, Tanzania K78-068 83
Nyons, France M59+444 55
Nysa, Poland L76+505 49
Nysted, Denmark M19+546 47
Nyurba, U.S.S.R. E10+634 63
Nyuya, U.S.S.R. E22+606 63
Nzega, Tanzania K70-042 83
Oababatiya, Israel K58+324 76
Oacoma, S. Dakota U56+438 93
Oahe Res., S. Dakota U62+450 93
Oahu, I., Hawaii Y45+212 107
Oakan, Japan C34+434 68
Oakbank, S. Australia C57-331 109
Oakes, N. Dakota U48+462 93
Oakham, England N04+527 37
Oakland, California W14+378 92
Oakland, Maryland T26+394 91
Oakley, Kansas U66+390 94
Oakville, Ontario T28+435 91
Oamaru, New Zealand A54-451 112
Oates Ld., Antarctica B50-700 27
Oatlands, Tasmania C16-423 109
Oaxaca & state, Mexico U40+170 100
Ob, R., U.S.S.R. H55+665 62
Obama, Japan C85+355 68
Oban, New Zealand A71-469 112
Oban, Scotland N33+564 41
Obatogamau L., Quebec S88+496 90
Obbia, Somalia J68+054 83
Obeh, Afghanistan H71+345 75
Oberammergau, W. Germany M24+476 48
Oberhausen, W. Germany M49+515 48
Oberlin, Kansas U63+398 94
Oberon, New South Wales C01-337 109
Oberriet, Switzerland M33+473 45
Oberwald, Switzerland M40+465 45
Obi, I., Indonesia D44-016 65
Obidos, Brazil R63-018 105
Obidos, Portugal N55+394 52
Obihiro, Japan C40+428 68
Obo, Cent. Afr. Rep. L20+052 81
Oahe Res., S. Dakota U62+448 88
Obock, Djibouti K10+118 83
Oborona, U.S.S.R. K25+521 61
Obrayera, Nicaragua T53+143 101
Obskaya Guba, U.S.S.R. H10+700 62
Ocala, Florida T43+292 97
Ocampo, Mexico U57+229 100
Ocana, Colombia S80+081 104
Ocana, Spain N21+399 52
Occidental, Cord., Colombia T10+050 104
Ocean I., Pacific Ocean A63-012 106
Oceana, W. Virginia T40+377 97
Ocean City, New Jersey S87+393 96
Ochil Hills, Scotland N22+562 41
Ocland, Romania L28+461 58
Ocoa, B. de, Dominican Rep. S64+183 101
Ocona, Peru S78-165 104
Oconto, Wisconsin T77+449 91
Ocos, Guatemala U13+145 100
Ocotal, Nicaragua T68+138 101
Ocumare, Venezuela S41+101 104
Oda, Ghana N06+060 80
Oda, Japan D15+352 68
Odaka, Japan C54+375 68
Odate, Japan C57+403 68
Odawara, Japan C65+352 68
Odemira, Portugal N52+376 52
Odemis, Turkey L12+382 74
Odense, Denmark M28+554 47
Oder R., Germany M04+527 48
Odessa, Texas U74+318 94
Odessa, Ukraine K86+465 60
Odienné, Ivory Coast N46+096 80
Odoorn, Netherlands M49+529 44
Odorhei, Romania L28+463 58
Odra R., Poland M04+527 48
Odzala, Congo M02+006 82
Oedelem, Belgium M70+512 44
Oeiras, Brazil O73-070 105
Oelwein, Iowa U11+426 95
Oetling, Argentina S00-273 103
Of, Turkey K27+410 74
Offaly (Ui Failghe), co., Ireland, Rep. N45+533 43
Offenbach, W. Germany M38+501 48
Ogaki, Japan C79+354 68
Ogallala, Nebraska U70+411 94
Ogden, Utah V42+412 94
Ogdensburg, New York T03+447 91
Ogilvie, Yukon X28+638 88
Ogilvie Ra., Yukon X00+448 88
Ogoja, Nigeria M38+068 80
Ogoki R., Ontario T70+506 89
Ogr, Sudan L16+120 81
Ogulin, Yugoslavia L89+452 56
Ohakune, New Zealand A27-393 112
Ohau, L., New Zealand A61-442 112
Ohey, Belgium M59+504 44
O'Higgins, mt., Chile S80-488 103
Ohio, state, U.S.A. T53+405 99
Ohio R., U.S.A. T68+378 99
Ohrid, Yugoslavia L55+411 58
Ohridsko Jezero, Yugoslavia L56+410 58
Ohura, New Zealand A30-389 112
Oich L., Scotland N29+571 40
Oignies, Belgium M62+500 44
Oil City, Pennsylvania T28+414 96
Oil Springs, Ontario T43+428 91
Oirot Tura, U.S.S.R. G24+518 62
Oirschot, Netherlands M58+515 44
Oise, dep., France M76+494 54
Oise, R., France M76+490 54
Oita, Japan D20+332 68
Ojinaga, Mexico U87+295 100
Ojiya, Japan C67+373 68
Ojocaliente, Mexico U73+225 100
Ojo de Agua, Argentina S23-294 103
Ojo del Toro, Pico, Cuba T14+200 101
Oka R., U.S.S.R. K16+558 61

Okahandja, Namibia L78-220 **84**
Okanagan Lake, B.C. W00+499 **88**
Okanogan R., Washington W00+478 **98**
Okaukweyo, Namibia L86-190 **84**
Okavango, R. & Swamp, Botswana L40-198 **84**
Okayama, Japan D06+346 **68**
Okeechobee, L., Florida T34+269 **97**
Okehampton, England N24+507 **38**
Okha, U.S.S.R. C42+537 **63**
Okhansk, U.S.S.R. J28+576 **61**
Okhotsk, U.S.S.R. C40+593 **63**
Okhotsk, Sea of, U.S.S.R. C10+550 **63**
Okigunto, Japan D12+362 **68**
Okinawa Gunto, Japan D42+265 **68**
Oklahoma, state, U.S.A. U54+357 **98**
Oklahoma City, Oklahoma U45+354 **95**
Okmulgee, Oklahoma U36+356 **95**
Okolona, Mississippi T82+342 **97**
Oktyabrskoy Revolyutsiy, Os., U.S.S.R. F50+790 **63**
Okućani, Yugoslavia L77+453 **56**
Okuru, New Zealand A66-439 **112**
Okushiri I., Japan C63+422 **68**
Okusi Ambeno, Timor D65-094 **110**
Olaine, Latvia L36+568 **47**
Olanchito, Honduras T68+156 **101**
Öland, I., Sweden L80+567 **47**
Olary, S. Australia C58-323 **109**
Olasan, Ethiopia K00+052 **83**
Olavarria, Argentina S02-368 **103**
Olawa, Poland L76+510 **49**
Olbia, Sardinia M33+409 **57**
Olcott, New York T22+433 **96**
Oldcastle, Ireland, Rep. N43+538 **42**
Oldenburg, W. Germany M25+543 **48**
Oldenburg, W. Germany M41+532 **48**
Oldenzaal, Netherlands M48+523 **44**
Old Forge, Pennsylvania T04+413 **96**
Oldham, England N13+535 **37**
Old Orchard, Maine S62+435 **90**
Old Orchard Beach, Maine S62+435 **96**
Oldtown, Maine S52+450 **90**
Olean, New York T21+421 **96**
Olecko, Poland L45+540 **49**
Olekminsk, U.S.S.R. D89+603 **63**
Olenek, U.S.S.R. E45+685 **63**
Olenek, R., U.S.S.R. D80+727 **63**
Olenekskiy Zaliv, U.S.S.R. D85+734 **63**
Oléron, I. d', France N08+460 **54**
Olga, U.S.S.R. C88+436 **63**
Olifants Kloof, Botswana L60-222 **84**
Olimbos. See Olympus.
Oiva de Jerez, Spain N41+383 **52**
Olivares, Spain N15+397 **53**
Olivares, Co. de, Argentina S59-303 **103**
Oliveira, Brazil Q78-122 **105**
Olivenza, Spain N42+387 **52**
Olivone, Switzerland M36+465 **45**
Ollague, Chile S50-212 **103**
Ollague, mt., Bolivia S49-212 **104**
Olmedo, Spain N28+413 **52**
Olney, Illinois T78+387 **95**
Olomouc, Czechoslovakia L77+496 **49**
Olot, Spain M75+422 **53**
Olovyannaya, U.S.S.R. E26+510 **63**
Olpe, W. Germany M43+510 **48**
Olst, Netherlands M53+523 **44**
Olsztyn, Poland L57+538 **49**
Olten, Switzerland M43+473 **45**
Oltu, Turkey K18+406 **74**
Oltul R., Romania L33+458 **58**
Olvera, Spain N31+369 **52**
Olympia, Greece L50+376 **59**
Olympia, Washington W17+470 **92**
Olympic Nat. Park, Wash. W26+476 **98**
Olympus (Olimbos), mts., Greece L46+400 **59**
Olympus, Mt., Washington W23+475 **98**
Olyutorskiy Zaliv, U.S.S.R. A70+600 **63**
Omagh, N. Ireland N44+546 **42**
Omaguas, Peru S80-042 **104**
Omaha, Nebraska U36+412 **95**
Oman, Arabia J26+238 **75**
Oman, G. of, Arabia-Iran J10+248 **75**
Omaruru, Namibia L84-212 **84**
Ombombo, Namibia M06-186 **84**
Omdurman, Sudan K76+156 **81**
Omeo, Victoria C15-371 **109**
Omer, Michigan T53+440 **91**
Ometepec, Mexico U50+166 **100**
Ommen, Netherlands M51+525 **44**
Omoa, Honduras T79+156 **101**
Omsk, U.S.S.R. H10+550 **62**
Omuta, Japan D27+330 **68**
Omutninsk, U.S.S.R. J46+586 **61**
Ona, R., U.S.S.R. F50+570 **63**
Onawa, Iowa U36+420 **95**
Onaway, Michigan T55+453 **91**
Onega & R., U.S.S.R. K39+640 **62**
Onehunga, New Zealand A31-370 **112**
Oneida, New York T04+431 **96**
Oneida L., New York T06+432 **96**
O'Neill, Nebraska U52+424 **95**
Oneonta, New York T00+425 **96**
Onezhskoye Oz., U.S.S.R. K60+618 **62**
Ongole, India G59+156 **70**
Ongudai, U.S.S.R. G23+508 **62**
Onich, Scotland N31+567 **41**
Onipa, Namibia L82-178 **84**
Onitsha, Nigeria M50+062 **80**
Onoto, Venezuela S31+098 **104**
Onotoa, I., Kiribati A30-020 **106**
Onslow, W. Australia E30-217 **110**
Onslow B., N. Carolina T12+343 **97**
Ontario, prov., Canada **89**
Ontario, L., U.S.A.-Canada T20+439 **99**
Onteniente, Spain N04+388 **53**
Ontiñena, Spain N00+417 **53**
Oodnadatta, S. Australia C88-273 **111**
Ooldea, S. Australia D19-305 **110**
Oostburg, Netherlands M69+513 **44**
Oostende (Ostende), Belgium M73+512 **44**
Ooster Schelde, Netherlands M66+516 **44**
Oosterwolde, Netherlands M52+530 **44**
Oosthuizen, Netherlands M60+526 **44**
Oostkamp, Belgium M71+512 **44**
Oostmalle, Belgium M62+513 **44**
Oostyoorne, Netherlands M66+519 **44**
Ootacamund, India G79+114 **70**
Opala, U.S.S.R. B50+520 **63**
Opari, Sudan K78+040 **81**
Opatija, Yugoslavia M04+453 **56**
Opava, Czechoslovakia L73+499 **49**
Opelousas, Louisiana U12+304 **95**
Ophir, Mt., Malaysia F15+024 **69**
Ophoven, Belgium M55+511 **44**
Opis, Iraq K04+339 **74**
Opochka, U.S.S.R. L08+568 **60**
Opodepe, Mexico V34+300 **100**
Opole, Poland L73+507 **49**
Oporto. See Porto
Opotiki, New Zealand A16-380 **112**
Oppa B., Japan C51+386 **68**
Oppeln. See Opole
Opunake, New Zealand A37-394 **112**
Oputo, Mexico V25+300 **100**
Oqair, Saudi Arabia J59+257 **75**
Oradea, Romania L48+470 **58**
Orai, India G63+260 **73**
Oran, Algeria N04+356 **80**
Orange, France M61+442 **55**
Orange, Massachusetts S74+427 **96**
Orange, New South Wales C05-334 **109**
Orange Texas U22+301 **95**
Orange, Virginia T19+382 **97**
Orange R., S. Africa L70-284 **84**
Orange City, Iowa U36+430 **95**
Orangeburg, S. Carolina T35+335 **97**
Orange Free State, S. Africa L20-284 **84**
Orangeville, Ontario T31+439 **91**
Orange Geb., Surinam R60+030 **105**
Oranmore, Ireland, Rep. N53+533 **43**
Oras, Philippines D58+121 **65**
Orăştie, Romania L41+458 **58**
Oravita, Romania L50+451 **58**
Oravská Magura, Czech. L65+493 **49**
Orbe, Switzerland M51+467 **45**
Orbost, Victoria C09-377 **109**
Orcera, Spain N16+383 **53**
Orchha, India G68+253 **73**
Ord, Mt., W. Australia D60-175 **110**
Ordenes, Spain N50+431 **52**
Ord River, W. Australia D37-174 **110**
Ordu, Turkey K42+409 **74**
Ordzhonikidze, U.S.S.R. K02+430 **62**
Ordzhonikidzegrad. See Bezhitsa
Örebro, Sweden L89+593 **47**
Oregon, Illinois T86+419 **95**
Oregon, state, U.S.A. W15+440 **98**
Oregon City, Oregon W16+453 **92**
Öregrund, Sweden L69+603 **47**
Orekhovo Zuyevo, U.S.S.R. K36+558 **60**
Orel, U.S.S.R. K53+530 **60**
Orellana, Peru T01-070 **104**
Orellana, Spain N33+390 **52**
Orenburg, U.S.S.R. J29+517 **61**
Orense, Spain N47+423 **52**
Orepuki, New Zealand Q73-463 **112**
Oresund, Denmark-Sweden M14+560 **47**
Orgaña, Spain M82+422 **53**
Orgaz, Spain N23+396 **52**
Oriental, Cord., Colombia S84+050 **104**
Oriental, Cord., Peru T04-075 **104**
Orihuela, Spain N06+381 **53**
Orillia, Ontario T27+446 **91**
Orinoco, R., Venezuela S20+083 **104**
Orissa, state, India G35+210 **71**
Oristano & G. di, Sardinia M39+399 **57**
Orivesi, Finland L04+623 **46**
Oriximiná, Brazil R65-016 **105**
Orizaba, Mexico U43+188 **100**
Orizare, Bulgaria L14+427 **58**
Orkanger, Norway M31+633 **46**
Orkhon R., Mongolia F08+484 **64**
Orkney Is., Scotland N18+590 **40**
Ørland, Norway M32+637 46
Orlando, Florida T38+285 **97**
Orleanais, prov., France M79+478 **54**
Orleans, France M79+479 **54**
Orleans, I. of, Quebec S66+469 **91**
Orleansville, (El Asnam), Alg. M82+360 **80**
Orman, Syria K49+325 **76**
Ormara, Pakistan H62+251 **70**
Ormondville, New Zealand A22-401 **112**
Ormskirk, England N18+536 **37**
Ornach, Pakistan H53+268 **70**
Orne, dep., France N00+487 **54**
Örnsköldsvik, Sweden L67+633 **46**
Orochen, U.S.S.R. D58+584 **63**
Orocue, Colombia S68+046 **104**
Oroluk, I., Caroline Islands B50+073 **106**
Oron, U.S.S.R. F70+644 **63**
Orono, Maine S52+449 **90**
Oronsay I., Scotland N38+560 **41**
Orontes, R., Syria K52+356 **74**
Orosei, & G. di, Sardinia M32+402 **57**
Orosi, Vol., Costa Rica T62+110 **101**
Orrin R., Scotland N27+576 **40**
Orroroo, S. Australia C68-328 **109**
Orsa, Sweden M02+611 **47**
Orsha, Byelorussia K88+545 **60**
Orsières, Switzerland M47+460 **45**
Orsk, U.S.S.R. J08+512 **61**
Orsova, Romania L45+447 **58**
Ortegal, C., Spain N47+435 **52**
Orthez, France N05+435 **55**
Ortiz, Mexico V03+282 **100**
Ortiz, Venezuela S43+096 **104**
Orugueira, Spain N47+434 **52**
Orulgan, Khrebet, U.S.S.R. D50+677 **63**
Oruro, Bolivia S43-180 **104**
Orust, Sweden M20+582 **47**
Oryekhovo, U.S.S.R. K04+505 **61**
Osa, U.S.S.R. J27+572 **61**
Osage, Iowa U16+412 **95**
Osage City, Kansas U36+386 **95**
Osaka, Japan C87+347 **68**
Osakis, Minnesota U31+459 **93**
Osawatomie, Kansas U30+385 **95**
Osborne, Kansas U52+394 **95**
Oscar II Coast, Antarctica S05-640 **27**
Osceola, Arkansas U00+358 **97**
Osceola, Iowa U22+410 **95**
Oschiri, Sardinia M35+407 **57**
Oscoda, Michigan T50+444 **91**
Osen, Norway M27+643 **46**
Osh, Kirgiz H13+405 **62**
Oshawa, Ontario T23+439 **91**
O Shima, Japan C64+347 **68**
Oshkosh, Wisconsin T81+440 **91**
Oshnoviyeh, Iran K00+370 **74**
Osijek, Yugoslavia L68+455 **58**
Osilo, Sardinia M36+408 **57**
Osipenko, U.S.S.R. C81+525 **63**
Osipovichi, Byelorussia L08+533 **60**
Osire Sud, Namibia L76-212 **84**
Oskaloosa, Iowa U16+412 **95**
Oskarshamn, Sweden L81+573 **47**
Oslo, Norway M25+599 **47**
Oslo Fd., Norway M26+592 **47**
Osmanabad, India G83+180 **70**
Osmancik, Turkey K60+409 **74**
Osnabrück, W. Germany M42+523 **48**
Osorno, Chile S79-405 **103**
Osorno, Spain N26+424 **52**
Osowiec, Poland L44+535 **49**
Oss, Netherlands M57+518 **44**
Ossining, New York S83+412 **96**
Ostavall, Sweden L87+625 **46**
Ostende, Belgium M73+512 **44**
Osterreich, Nieder, prov., Austria L85+486 **49**
Osterreich, Ober, prov., Austria M04+484 **48**
Ostersund, Sweden M02+632 **46**
Osthammar, Sweden L70+603 **47**
Ostrava, Czechoslovakia L70+498 **49**
Ostroda, Poland L60+537 **49**
Ostrołeka, Poland L50+531 **49**
Ostrov, Romania L11+449 **58**
Ostrov, U.S.S.R. L09+574 **60**
Ostrovnoe, U.S.S.R. B00+680 **63**
Ostrowiec, Poland L52+509 **49**
Ostrów Mazowiecka, Poland L49+528 **49**
Ostuni, Italy L75+407 **57**
Østvagøy, Norway M02+683 46
Ösumikaikyō, Japan D24+308 **68**
Osuna, Spain N30+372 **52**
Oswego & R., New York T09+434 **96**
Oswestry, England N18+529 **38**
Otago Peninsula, N.Z. A52-458 **112**
Otaki, New Zealand A29-407 **112**
Otaru & B., Japan C54+432 **68**
Otasuts, Japan C56+433 **68**
Otavalo, Ecuador T19+002 **104**
Otepaa, Estonia L21+580 **47**
Othris, mts., Greece L45+390 **59**
Otira, New Zealand A50-428 **112**
Otis, New Brunswick S43+460 **90**
Otjiwarongo, Namibia L80-204 **84**
Otocac, Yugoslavia L89+449 **56**
Otoineppu, Japan C47+448 **68**
Otorohanga, New Zealand A28-382 **112**
Otpor, (Zabaykal'sk), U.S.S.R. E15+497 **63**
Otranto, Str. of, It.-Albania L66+402 **59**
Otsego, L., New York S89+428 **96**
Otsu, Japan C85+350 **68**
Ottawa, Illinois T83+414 **95**
Ottawa, Kansas U32+386 **95**
Ottawa, Ontario T04+454 **91**
Ottawa Is., N.-W. Terr. T30+596 **89**
Ottawa R., Quebec, etc. T16+462 **91**
Otterlo, Netherlands M55+521 **44**
Otterøy, Norway M49+628 46
Ottignies, Belgium M63+507 **44**
Otting, W. Germany M14+484 **48**
Ottumwa, Iowa U14+410 **95**
Otus, U.S.S.R. K59+450 **60**
Otway, B., Chile S84-535 **103**
Otway, C., Victoria C39-389 **109**
Otwock, Poland L52+521 **49**
Ötz, Austria M25+472 **48**
Otztaler Alpen, Italy M23+470 **56**
Ouachita Mts., Arkansas, etc. U30+345 **99**
Ouachita R., Arkansas U23+340 **99**
Ouagadougou, Upper Volta N08+122 **80**
Ouahigouya, Upper Volta N14+134 **80**
Ouangolodougou, Ivory Coast N30+100 **80**
Ouargla, Algeria M58+316 **80**
Oubangui R., Congo and Zaire L74+004 **82**
Ouddorp, Netherlands M66+518 **44**
Oudekapelle, Belgium M73+510 **44**
Oudenaarde, Belgium M68+508 **44**
Oudenbosch, Netherlands M63+516 **44**
Oudtshoorn, Cape Province L46-336 **84**
Ouessant, I. d', France N30+484 **54**
Ouezzane, Morocco N34+348 **80**
Oughterard, Ireland, Rep. N56+534 **43**
Ouidah, Benin M78+064 **80**
Oukës, Albania L58+411 **58**
Oulu, Finland L27+650 **46**
Oulujärvi, Finland L18+644 **46**
Oulujoki, Finland L23+648 **46**
Oum Chalaouba, Chad L58+158 **81**
Ounasjoki, Finland L32+672 46
Ouricury, Brazil O61-078 **105**
Ourinhos, Brazil R29-230 **105**
Ouro Preto, Brazil Q80-204 **105**
Ouse R., Norfolk, etc., England M88+525 **39**
Ouse R., Yorks, England N07+539 **37**
Outarde B., Quebec S51+490 **90**
Outardes, R. aux, Quebec S54+500 **90**
Outjo, Namibia L84-200 **84**
Outtrim, Victoria C26-385 **109**
Ouyen, Victoria C46-351 **109**
Ovalle, Chile S68-306 **103**
Ovar, Portugal N52+408 **52**
Over Flakkee I., Netherlands M65+517 **44**
Overijssel, prov., Netherlands M51+524 **44**
Overkalix, Sweden L43+663 **46**
Overmark, Finland L51+626 **46**
Overpelt, Belgium M58+512 **44**
Overtornea, Sweden L38+664 **46**
Oviedo, Spain N35+433 **52**
Ovruch, Ukraine L07+512 **60**
Owaka, New Zealand A62-464 **112**
Owasco L., New York T09+428 **96**
Owatonna, Minnesota U18+440 **93**
Owego, New York T08+421 **96**
Owen, Wisconsin U04+450 **91**
Owen's I., Burma F39+110 **71**
Owens L., California V78+364 **92**
Owensboro, Kentucky T73+378 **97**
Owen Sound, Ontario T36+446 **91**
Owen Stanley Ra., Papua New Guinea C14-092 **111**
Owensville, Indiana T77+383 **97**
Owenton, Kentucky T59+386 **97**
Owerri, Nigeria M48+054 **80**
Owl Creek Mts., Wyoming V25+436 **93**
Owo, Nigeria M56+072 **80**
Owosso, Michigan T55+430 **91**
Owyhee R., Oregon V75+432 **92**
Ox Mts., Ireland, Rep. N54+541 **42**
Oxford, Maryland T07+387 **91**
Oxford, Mississippi T87+344 **97**
Oxford, New York T04+424 **91**
Oxford, N. Carolina T21+363 **97**
Oxford & co., England N08+518 **39**
Oxley, New South Wales C35-342 **109**
Oxley's Pk., New S. Wales B88-318 **109**
Oyapock, R., Brazil, etc. R42+034 **105**
Oyem, Gabon M20+016 **82**
Oymyekon, U.S.S.R. C40+630 **63**
Oyo, Nigeria M66+080 **80**
Oyster B., Tasmania C11-423 **109**
Ozark Mts., Ark.-Mo. U20+360 **95**
Ozark Plat., Missouri, etc. U24+364 **99**
Ozarks, L. of the, Missouri U18+382 **95**
Ozd, Hungary L58+482 **49**
Ozerki, U.S.S.R. J87+520 **61**
Ozhogino, U.S.S.R. C16+692 **63**
Ozieri, Sardinia M36+406 **57**
Ozun, Romania L25+458 **58**
Paan, Burma F44+170 **71**
Paan, China F36+299 **64**
Paarl, Cape Province L66-338 **84**
Pabianice, Poland L64+517 **49**
Pabna, Bangladesh G04+240 **73**
Pacaraima, Sa., Brazil, etc. S18+040 **104**
Pacasmayo, Peru T27-074 **104**
Pachbhadra, India H17+260 **70**
Pachow. See Pachung
Pachuca, Mexico U52+200 **100**
Pachung, China E80+318 **66**
Pacific, Missouri U05+385 **97**
Pacific Ocean **102-103**
Paços, Portugal N51+413 **52**
Padam, Kashmir G79+334 **72**
Padang, Sumatra F28-009 **65**
Paderborn, W. Germany M37+517 **48**
Padilla, Bolivia S26-192 **104**
Padova, Italy M19+454 **56**
Padrauna, India G36+269 **73**
Padre I., Texas U44+268 **94**
Padstow, England N30+505 **38**
Padua. See Padova
Paducah, Kentucky T82+370 **97**
Paducah, Texas U61+340 **94**
Padul, Spain N22+370 **52**
Paeroa, New Zealand A26-374 **112**
Pafuri, Mozambique K82-226 **84**
Pagai Is., Indonesia F26-030 **65**
Pagula I., Gulf of Guinea M57+014 82
Pagan, Burma F60+211 **71**
Pagan, I., Mariana Is. C25+170 **106**
Pagasai, G. of, Greece L42+392 **59**
Pago, I., Yugoslavia M00+444 **56**
Pagong L., Kashmir-Tibet G66+336 **70**
Pagosa Springs, Colorado V12+372 **94**
Paharpur, Pakistan H24+321 **72**
Pahiatua, New Zealand A25-404 **112**
Pahlavi Dezh, Iran J33+370 **75**
Pahlevi Bandar-e, Iran J63+375 **74**
Pahsien, China E21+391 **66**
Pahsien. See Chungking
Paide, Estonia L26+589 **47**
Paignton, England N21+504 **38**
Paiho, China E59+328 **66**
Päijänne, L., Finland L27+615 47
Pai-Khoi Khrebet, U.S.S.R. H60+675 **62**
Pailam, India G57+257 **73**
Pailingmiao, China E56+416 **64**
Paimpol, France N18+487 **54**
Painted Des., Arizona V35+360 **98**
Paintsville, Kentucky T47+378 **97**
Paisley, Ontario T38+443 **91**
Paisley, Scotland N26+558 **41**
Paita, Peru T36-051 **104**
Pai Tu Hu, China E17+308 **66**
Paiz do Vinho, Portugal N47+412 **52**
Pajakumbuh, Sumatra F27-001 **65**
Pajala, Sweden L40+672 **46**
Pajares, Spain N34+430 **52**
Pakakku, Burma F59+213 **71**
Pakanbaru, Sumatra F22+006 **65**
Pakaur, India G13+246 **73**
Pakchan, Burma F37+105 **71**
Pak-Loi, China E65+214 **67**
Pakistan, S. Asia H60+280 **70**
Pak-lay, Laos F21+182 **69**
Pakpattan, Pakistan H10+303 **72**
Pakrac, Yugoslavia L77+454 **56**
Paks, Hungary L67+467 **49**
Pakse, Laos E85+151 **69**
Palafrugell, Spain M71+419 **53**
Palaiokhóra, Crete L38+352 **59**
Palamau, India G34+239 **73**
Palamcottah, India G73+087 **70**
Palamós, Spain M71+418 **53**
Palamuse, Estonia L20+587 **47**
Palana, U.S.S.R. B30+590 **63**
Palanpur, India H15+241 **70**
Palatka, Florida T40+296 **97**
Palau Is., Pacific Ocean D02+074 **65**
Palaw, Burma F38+130 **69**
Palawan, I., Phillippines E10+100 **65**
Paldiski, Estonia L35+594 **47**
Palembang, Sumatra F01-030 **65**
Palena, Chile S78-438 **103**
Palenque, Mexico U12+174 **100**
Paleokhorio, Cyprus K71+349 **76**
Palermo, Argentina S25-246 **103**
Palermo, N. Dakota U73+483 **93**
Palermo, Sicily M10+381 **57**
Palestina, Chile S56-240 **103**
Palestine, Texas U34+317 **95**
Palestine, W. Asia K60+320 **74**
Paletwa, Burma F72+213 **71**
Palghat, India G79+108 **70**
Palgrave Pt., Namibia M10-204 **84**
Palgu Tso, Tibet G26+289 **71**
Palhiers, France M80+431 **55**
Palhoca, Brazil R22-278 **103**
Pali, India H10+257 **70**
Palime, Togo M86+068 **80**
Palisade, Nevada V67+406 **92**
Paliseul, Belgium M59+499 **44**
Palizada, Mexico U12+182 **100**
Palk Str., India G60+100 **70**
Palkot, India G32+229 **73**

Palliser B., *New Zealand* A30–415 **112**
Palma, *Balearic Islands* M74+396 **53**
Palma, *Brazil* Q74–212 **105**
Palma, *Brazil* R16–124 **105**
Palma, *Mozambique* K28–110 **83**
Palma, I., *Canary Is* P30+286 **80**
Palmaras, *Brazil* R33–303 **103**
Palmas, *Brazil* R42–265 **103**
Palmas, B., *Mexico* V28+237 **100**
Palmas C., *Liberia* N46+044 **80**
Palmas, G. of, *Sardinia* M39+390 **57**
Palm Beach, *Florida* T30+267 **97**
Palmeira, *Brazil* R50–279 **103**
Palmer Land, *Antarctica* S24–725 **27**
Palmerston, *Ontario* T35+439 **91**
Palmerston I., *Cook Islands* Y80–158 **106**
Palmerston North, *N.Z.* A26–403 **112**
Palmerston South, *N.Z.* A56–454 **112**
Palmira, *Colombia* T08+037 **104**
Palms, *Michigan* T47+436 **91**
Palmyra, *Missouri* U07+398 **95**
Palmyra, *Syria* K41+346 **74**
Palmyra I., *Pacific Ocean* Y72+060 **106**
Palni Hills, *India* G76+104 **70**
Paloh, *Borneo* E64+016 **65**
Paloich, *Sudan* K74+104 **81**
Palo Santo, *Argentina* R86–255 **103**
Palpa, *Nepal* G38+279 **73**
Palu, *Turkey* K30+388 **74**
Palwal, *India* G76+281 **72**
Pambon Chan., *India* G66+092 **70**
Pamekasan, *Indonesia* E39–070 **65**
Pamir, mts., *U.S.S.R.* H15+374 **62**
Pamlico Sd., *N. Carolina* T06+352 **97**
Pampa, *Texas* U66+356 **94**
Pampas, *Peru* S89–122 **104**
Pamplona, *Colombia* S76+076 **104**
Pamplona, *Spain* N10+428 **53**
Panache L., *Ontario* T38+462 **91**
Panagyurishte, *Bulgaria* L35+425 **58**
Panaji, *Goa, Daman & Diu* H07+156 **70**
Panama & rep.,
Central America T27+090 **101**
Panama Can., *Panama* T28+080 **89**
Panama, G. of, *Panama* T26+080 **101**
Panama City, *Florida* T64+302 **97**
Panarea, I., *Italy* M00+386 **57**
Panat, *Thailand* F23+134 **69**
Panay, I., *Philippines* D75+112 **65**
Pancevo, *Yugoslavia* L56+449 **58**
Panciu, *Romania* L17+459 **58**
Pandan, *Philippines* D77+116 **65**
Pan de Azucar, *Chile* S64–261 **103**
Pandharpur, *India* G88+177 **70**
Pando, *Uruguay* R66–347 **103**
Paneviys, *Lithuania* L34+558 **47**
Panfilov, *Kazakh.* G59+441 **62**
Panfilovo, *U.S.S.R.* K12+503 **61**
Pangala, *Congo* M02–034 **82**
Pangbourne, *England* N07+515 **39**
Pangkiang, *China* E41+426 **64**
Panguitch, *Utah* V45+378 **94**
Pania Mutombo, *Zaire* L36–054 **82**
Panipat, *India* G78+294 **72**
Panja, *China* F82+400 **64**
Panjim, *See* Panaji
Panjnad R., *Pakistan* H25+290 **72**
Pannerden, *Netherlands* M54+519 **44**
Panruti, *India* G62+118 **70**
Pantanaw, *Burma* F58+169 **71**
Pantar, I., *Indonesia* D66–084 **65**
Pantelleria, I., *Medit. Sea* M18+368 **57**
Pánuco, *Mexico* U67+266 **100**
Pao-an-chow, *China* E29+403 **66**
Paochang, *China* E26+420 **66**
Pão de Assucar, *Brazil* Q45–097 **105**
Pão dos Ferros, *Brazil* Q49–061 **105**
Paoking. *See* Shaoyang
Paola, *Italy* L84+394 **57**
Paola, *Kansas* U30+386 **95**
Paoli, *Indiana* T69+385 **97**
Paoning. *See* Langchung
Paosham, *China* F36+252 **64**
Paoting, *China* E27+389 **66**
Pao-tow, *China* E60+406 **66**
Papakura, *New Zealand* A30–371 **112**
Papantla, *Mexico* U44+205 **100**
Papa Stour I., *Scotland* N10+603 **40**
Papa Westray, I., *Scotland* N17+594 **40**
Papenburg, *W. Germany* M46+531 **48**
Papendrecht, *Netherlands* M62+518 **44**
Paphos, *Cyprus* K76+347 **76**
Paposo, *Chile* S63–250 **103**
Papua, G. of, *Papua New Guinea*
C30–086 **111**
Papua New Guinea
Pacific Ocean C60–060 **31**
Papun, *Burma* F45+181 **71**
Pará, *Brazil* R21–014 **105**
Para, R., *Brazil* R20–010 **105**
Paracatu, *Brazil* R11–172 **105**
Paracel Is & Reefs,
S. China Sea E50+165 **69**
Parachilna, *S. Australia* C70–311 **109**
Parachinar, *Pakistan* H29+339 **72**
Paracin, *Yugoslavia* L52+439 **58**
Paracuro, *Brazil* Q54–034 **105**
Parag, *Iran* H86+255 **75**
Paragould, *Arkansas* U03+361 **99**
Paraguari, *Paraguay* R73–256 **103**
Paraguay, rep., *S. America* — **103**
Paraguay, R., *Argent., etc.* R80–267 **103**
Parah, *Afghanistan* H79+342 **75**
Parakes, *Botswana* L48–186 **84**
Parakou, *Benin* M74+094 **80**
Paramaribo, *Surinam* R62+057 **105**
Paramonga, *Peru* T17–107 **104**
Paramoshiri, *U.S.S.R.* B55+505 **63**
Parana, *Argentina* S03–318 **103**
Parana, R., *Argentina* R86–292 **103**
Paranagua, *Brazil* R21–255 **103**
Paranáiba & R., *Brazil* R37–197 **105**
Parang, *Philippines* D84+059 **65**
Paranga, *Uganda* K72+024 **83**
Parapola I., *Greece* L39+369 **59**
Parattah, *Tasmania* C16–424 **109**
Parbati R., *India* G78+235 **70**
Parbhani, *India* G79+193 **70**
Parchim, *E. Germany* M19+534 **48**
Pardubice, *Czechoslovakia* L84+500 **49**
Parecis, *Brazil* R72–140 **105**
Parecis, Sa. dos, *Brazil* S10–119 **104**
Paren, *U.S.S.R.* B10+624 **63**
Parent, *Quebec* S88+480 **90**
Pareora, *New Zealand* A52–445 **112**
Pariaguan, *Venezuela* S28+088 **104**
Parika, *Guyana* R81+068 **104**
Parinari, *Peru* S87–044 **104**
Paringa, *S. Australia* C55–342 **109**
Parintins, *Brazil* R69–025 **105**
Paris, *France* M76+488 **54**
Paris, *Illinois* T76+396 **95**
Paris, *Kentucky* T55+382 **97**
Paris, *Ontario* T33+432 **91**
Paris, *Tennessee* T80+362 **95**
Paris, *Texas* U34+336 **95**
Parita, B. de, *Panama* T32+081 **101**
Pariz, *Iran* J26+299 **75**
Park Ra., *Colorado* V08+400 **94**
Park Ra., *Wyoming* V14+413 **98**
Parker, *S. Dakota* U42+434 **93**
Parker, C., *N.-W. Terr.* T25+750 **89**
Parker Dam, *Arizona* V55+342 **98**
Parkersburg, *W. Virginia* T39+393 **91**
Parkes, *New South Wales* C11–332 **109**
Park Falls, *Wisconsin* U03+459 **91**
Park Rapids, *Minnesota* U30+469 **93**
Parkston, *S. Dakota* U48+434 **93**
Parma, *Italy* M28+448 **56**
Parmele, *N. Carolina* T13+358 **93**
Parnagua, *Brazil* Q86–103 **105**
Parnahyba, *Brazil* Q71–029 **105**
Parnaiba, R., *Brazil* Q76–037 **105**
Parnu & G., *Estonia* L33+583 **47**
Paro, *Bhutan* G04+274 **73**
Paron, *India* G78+249 **70**
Paroo, R., *New South Wales* C34–300 **109**
Páros, I., *Greece* L29+371 **59**
Parowan, *Utah* V48+388 **94**
Parral, *Chile* S71–361 **103**
Parral, *Mexico* V04+269 **100**
Parramatta, *New S. Wales* B85–338 **109**
Parras, *Mexico* U73+255 **100**
Parrett R., *England* N18+511 **38**
Parry I., *Ontario* T31+453 **91**
Parry Is., *N.-W. Terr.* V30+762 **88**
Parry Sound, *Ontario* T30+454 **91**
Parsa, *India* G30+259 **73**
Parsnip R., *Brit. Columbia* W20+556 **88**
Parsons, *Kansas* U32+374 **95**
Parsons, *W. Virginia* T28+391 **96**
Partabgarh, *India* H01+239 **70**
Partabgarh, *India* G48+259 **73**
Partabpur, *India* G40+234 **73**
Parthenay, *France* N01+466 **54**
Partinico, *Sicily* M11+381 **57**
Partridge L., *Tibet* G20+330 **71**
Partry Mts., *Ireland, Rep.* N57+537 **42**
Pas, The, *Manitoba* U68+540 **88**
Pasadena, *California* V79+341 **92**
Pasargadae, *Iran* J42+302 **75**
Pascagoula, *Mississippi* T81+304 **97**
Pas-de-Calais, dep., *France* M76+505 **54**
Paseagoula & R., *Mississippi* T81+304 **95**
Paskuh, *Iran* H80+276 **75**
Pasley, C., *W. Australia* D69–340 **110**
Pasni, *Pakistan* H70+252 **70**
Paso de Indios, *Argentina* S54–438 **103**
Paso de los Libres, *Argent.* R72–297 **103**
Paso de los Toros, *Uruguay* S39–326 **103**
Paso Limay, *Argentina* S63–405 **103**
Paso Robles, *California* W05+356 **92**
Paspebiac, *Quebec* S31+481 **90**
Pasrur, *Pakistan* H02+322 **72**
Passamaquoddy B., *N.B.* S42+451 **90**
Passau, *W. Germany* M09+486 **48**
Passendale, *Belgium* M72+509 **44**
Passero C., *Sicily* L89+367 **57**
Passiac, *New Jersey* S85+408 **96**
Passo Fundo, *Brazil* R44–281 **103**
Passos, *Brazil* R10–206 **105**
Pasto, *Colombia* T14+012 **104**
Pastrana, *Spain* N18+404 **52**
Pasvik Elv, *Norway* L04+693 **46**
Pásztó, *Hungary* L62+479 **49**
Patan, *India* H16+238 **70**
Patan, *India* H07+174 **70**
Patan, *Nepal* G28+276 **73**
Pataudi, *India* G79+283 **72**
Pataz, *Peru* T16–076 **104**
Patchewollock, *Victoria* C47–354 **109**
Patchogue, *New York* S78+407 **96**
Patea, *New Zealand* A33–397 **112**
Patencia, *Spain* N28+420 **52**
Paterno, *Sicily* M01+375 **57**
Paterson, *New Jersey* S85+409 **96**
Pathankot, *India* G86+323 **72**
Pathari, *India* G71+239 **73**
Pathfinder Res., *Wyoming* V11+424 **93**
Patiala, *India* G81+303 **72**
Pa-tiao, mt., *Laos* F15+193 **69**
Patkai Hills, *Burma* F55+268 **71**
Pátmos, I., *Greece* L20+373 **59**
Patna, *India* G41+207 **71**
Patna, *India* G28+256 **73**
Patos, *Brazil* Q43–070 **105**
Patos, L. dos, *Brazil* R40–314 **103**
Patquia, *Argentina* S41–301 **103**
Pátrai, *Greece* L49+383 **59**
Pátrai, G. of, *Greece* L50+383 **59**
Patras. *See* Pátrai.
Patrasayar, *India* G15+232 **73**
Patricio Lynch, I., *Chile* T02–485 **103**
Patrocinio, *Brazil* R12–190 **105**
Pattani, *Thailand* F22+068 **69**
Patten, *Maine* S51+460 **90**
Patterson, *Louisiana* U08+297 **97**
Patti, *Sicily* M00+381 **57**
Patutahi, *New Zealand* A12–386 **112**
Patzcuaro, *Mexico* U69+194 **100**
Pau, *France* N02+433 **55**
Pau d'Arco, *Brazil* R26–079 **105**
Paul, L., *N.-W. Territories* V30+651 **88**
Paulista, *Brazil* Q67–082 **105**
Paul's Valley, *Oklahoma* U42+347 **95**
Paungde, *Burma* F57+183 **71**
Pauni, *India* G62+208 **70**
Pautrask, *Sweden* L75+648 **46**
Pavia, *Italy* M35+452 **56**
Pāvilosta, *Latvia* L53+569 **47**
Pavlodar, *Kazakh.* G79+522 **62**
Pavlograd, *Ukraine* K55+486 **60**
Pavlovka, *U.S.S.R.* K10+519 **61**
Pavlovo, *U.S.S.R.* K11+560 **61**
Pavlovsk, *U.S.S.R.* K29+504 **61**
Pavlovski, *U.S.S.R.* K38+558 **60**
Pawnee City, *Nebraska* U37+402 **95**
Paw Paw, *Michigan* T65+422 **91**
Pawtucket, *Rhode Island* S69+419 **96**
Paxoi, I., *Greece* L59+392 **59**
Paxton, *Illinois* T78+405 **95**
Payerne, *Switzerland* M48+468 **45**
Payne L., *Quebec* S75+598 **89**
Payne R., *Quebec* S70+601 **89**
Paynesville, *Minnesota* U29+454 **93**
Payo Obispo. *See* Ciudad Chetumal
Paysandu, *Uruguay* R79–322 **103**
Payson, *Utah* V41+401 **94**
Paz, R., *El Salvador* U00+138 **101**
Pazardzhik, *Bulgaria* L34+422 **58**
Pazaung, *Burma* F46+190 **71**
Peace R., *Brit. Columbia* W20+560 **88**
Peace River, *Alberta* V75+560 **88**
Peak, The, *England* N11+534 **37**
Peak Hill, *New S. Wales* C10–328 **109**
Peak Hill, *W. Australia* E08–257 **110**
Peale, Mt., *Utah* V26+384 **94**
Pearce Point, *N.-W. Terr.* W17+690 **88**
Pearl R., *Mississippi* T88+306 **95**
Pearl Harbor, *Hawaii* Y45+212 **107**
Pearsall, *Texas* U54+290 **94**
Peary Ld., *Greenland* Q35+830 **26**
Pebane, *Mozambique* K40–168 **83**
Pebble I., *Falkland Islands* R88–512 **103**
Pébo, *Cent. Afr. Rep.* L68+080 **81**
Pec, *Yugoslavia* L58+427 **58**
Pechenga, *U.S.S.R.* K84+696 **62**
Pechora, *U.S.S.R.* J14+648 **62**
Pechora, R., *U.S.S.R.* J47+660 **62**
Pecos, *New Mexico* V04+356 **94**
Pecos, *Texas* U82+314 **94**
Pecos R., *Texas, etc.* U72+310 **94**
Pecs, *Hungary* L71+461 **58**
Pedernales, *Venezuela* S13+098 **104**
Pedhoulas, *Cyprus* K73+350 **76**
Pedregal, *Panama* T44+084 **101**
Pedro Pt., *Sri Lanka* G58+198 **70**
Pedro Juan Caballero, *Para.* R64–224 **103**
Pedroll, *Brazil* Q69–045 **105**
Pedro Luro, *Argentina* S16–396 **103**
Pedrotallagalla, mt., *Sri Lanka* G56+071 **70**
Peebinga, *S. Australia* C54–349 **109**
Peebles, *Scotland* N19+556 **41**
Peekskill, *New York* S83+413 **96**
Peel R., *Yukon* X05+658 **88**
Peenemünde, *E. Germany* M07+541 **48**
Peery L., *New S. Wales* C38–308 **109**
Peetri, *Estonia* L25+589 **47**
Pegasus, & B., *New Zealand* A41–432 **112**
Pega Yoma, *Burma* F55+190 **71**
Pegu, *Burma* F51+173 **71**
Pegunungan Maoke,
New Guinea C80–038 **65**
Pehan, *China* D52+482 **64**
Pehowa, *India* G80+299 **72**
Pehuajó, *Argentina* S11–357 **103**
Peineta, mt., *Chile* S81–503 **103**
Peiping. *See* Peking
Peipus, L., *See* Chudskoye Oz.
Peixe, *Brazil* R21–120 **105**
Pekan, *Malaysia* F10+036 **69**
Pekin, *Illinois* T88+406 **91**
Peking, *China* E21+400 **66**
Pelagie Is., *Medit. Sea* M13+355 **81**
Pélagos, I., *Greece* L36+393 **59**
Peledui, *U.S.S.R.* E42+597 **63**
Pelée I., *Ontario* T46+418 **91**
Peleng, I., *Indonesia* D70–014 **65**
Peljesac Pen., *Yugoslavia* L76+430 **57**
Pelkosenniemi, *Finland* L15+670 **46**
Pella, *Greece* L48+409 **59**
Pella, *Iowa* U18+414 **95**
Pellegrini, *Argentina* S19–362 **103**
Pellworn I., *W. Germany* M38+545 **48**
Pelly Pt., *N.-W. Terr.* U66+701 **88**
Pelly Ra., *Yukon* W70+612 **88**
Pelly R., *Yukon* W83+618 **88**
Peloncillo Ra., *Arizona* V25+326 **94**
Peloponnisos, *Greece* L48+370 **59**
Pelotas, *Brazil* R45–318 **103**
Pemba Is., *E. Africa* K32–052 **83**
Pembroke, *Ontario* T13+458 **91**
Pembroke, *Wales* N30+517 **38**
Pembroke, C., *Falkland Is.* R76–516 **103**
Pembroke, C., *N.-W. Terr.* T35+635 **89**
Penafiel, *Portugal* N50+412 **52**
Peñafiel, *Spain* N25+413 **52**
Penalva, *Brazil* R00–031 **105**
Penambo Ra., *Sarawak* E30+030 **65**
Peña Negra, Sa. de, *Spain* N37+421 **52**
Penápolis, *Brazil* R30–215 **105**
Peñaranda de Bracamonte,
Spain N31+409 **52**
Peñarroya, *Spain* N28+383 **52**
Penarth, *Wales* N19+514 **38**
Penas, G. de, *Chile* T00–472 **103**
Pendembu, *Sierra Leone* N64+082 **80**
Pendleton, *Arkansas* U09+340 **97**
Pendleton, *Oregon* V83+457 **92**
Pend Oreille, L., *Idaho* V70+480 **98**
Penedo, *Brazil* Q39–103 **105**
Penedono, *Portugal* N45+410 **52**
Penggaram, *Malaysia* F13+019 **69**
Penghu, Is., *China* E03+234 **67**
Penglai, *China* D85+378 **66**
Pengpu, *China* E15+328 **64**
Penguin, *Tasmania* C24–411 **109**
Penhalonga, *Zimbabwe* K74–188 **84**
Peniche, *Portugal* N56+394 **52**
Penicuik, *Scotland* N19+558 **41**
Peñiscola, *Spain* M88+404 **53**
Penn, *N. Dakota* U54+483 **93**
Pennfield, *New Brunswick* S40+451 **90**
Pennine, Alpi, *Switzerland* M46+460 **45**
Pennine Chain, *England* N14+540 **37**
Penns Grove, *New Jersey* T03+397 **96**
Pennsylvania, state, *U.S.A.* T25+408 **99**
Penn Yan, *New York* T12+427 **96**
Penobscot B., *Maine* S54+441 **90**
Penola, *S. Australia* C55–374 **109**
Penong, *S. Australia* D12–318 **110**
Penonome, *Panama* T32+082 **101**
Penrith, *England* N17+547 **37**
Penrith, *New South Wales* B86–338 **109**
Pensacola, *Florida* T73+304 **93**
Penshurst, *Victoria* C46–379 **109**
Pentland Firth, *Scotland* N20+587 **40**
Pentland Hills, *Scotland* N21+558 **41**
Pentwater, *Michigan* T68+438 **91**
Penza, *U.S.S.R.* K00+532 **61**
Penzance, *England* N33+501 **38**
Penzhino, *U.S.S.R.* A71+633 **63**
Penzhinskaya Guba, *U.S.S.R.* B20+610 **63**
Peoria, *Illinois* T88+407 **95**
Peperga, *Netherlands* M54+528 **44**
Pepinster, *Belgium* M55+506 **44**
Peqin, *Albania* L62+411 **58**
Perak, *Malaysia* F28+054 **69**
Peralta, *Spain* N11+424 **53**
Perce, *Quebec* S26+485 **90**
Perdido, Mte., *Spain* M87+427 **53**
Pereira, *Colombia* T04+048 **104**
Perello, *Spain* M86+409 **53**
Perez, *Chile* S60–260 **103**
Pergamno, *Argentina* S04–338 **103**
Perho, *Finland* L33+632 **46**
Peribonca R., *Quebec* S68+510 **90**
Perico, *Argentina* S31–244 **103**
Perigueux, *France* M85+452 **55**
Perija, Sa. de, *Venezuela* S76+100 **104**
Perim I., *Red Sea* K09+127 **74**
Peripery, *Brazil* Q71–042 **105**
Peristéra, I., *Greece* L36+392 **59**
Perlas & Lag. de las, *Nic.* T52+124 **101**
Perlas, Arch. de las, *Pan.* T26+084 **101**
Perm, *U.S.S.R.* J23+580 **61**
Pernambuco (Recife), *Braz.* Q30–080 **105**
Peronne, *France* M72+499 **54**
Péronnes, *Belgium* M65+504 **44**
Perpignan, *France* M73+427 **55**
Perranporth, *England* N31+503 **38**
Perrot I., *Quebec* S84+454 **91**
Perry, *Iowa* U24+418 **95**
Perry, *New York* T18+428 **96**
Perry, *Oklahoma* U44+362 **95**
Perry R., *N.-W. Terr.* U80+666 **88**
Perryville, *Missouri* T89+377 **97**
Persepolis, *Iran* J42+300 **75**
Persia. *See* Iran
Persian Gulf, *See* The Gulf
Perth, *New Brunswick* S46+467 **90**
Perth, *Ontario* T08+449 **91**
Perth, *W. Australia* E25–319 **110**
Perth, *Scotland* N21+564 **41**
Perth Amboy, *New Jersey* S86+405 **96**
Peru, *Indiana* T67+407 **91**
Peru, rep., *S. America* **104**
Perufune, *Japan* C40+424 **68**
Perugia, *Italy* M20+431 **56**
Peruibe, *Brazil* R12–242 **105**
Peruwelz, *Belgium* M68+505 **44**
Pervijze, *Belgium* M73+511 **44**
Pervomaisk, *Ukraine* K85+481 **60**
Perwez, *Belgium* M61+506 **44**
Pesaro, *Italy* M12+439 **56**
Pescadores Is. *See* Penghu Is.
Pescara, *Italy* M05+425 **56**
Peschici, *Italy* L84+419 **57**
Peshawar, *Pakistan* H20+340 **72**
Peshtigo R., *Wisconsin* T80+455 **91**
Pesqueira, *Brazil* Q40–084 **105**
Pestravka, *U.S.S.R.* J60+524 **61**
Petah Tiqva, *Israel* K61+321 **76**
Petalioi, G. of, *Greece* L35+379 **59**
Patalioi, I., *Greece* L34+380 **59**
Pataluma, *California* W16+383 **92**
Peterborough, *England* N03+526 **37**
Peterborough, *Ontario* T20+443 **91**
Peterborough, *S. Australia* C67–329 **109**
Peter I. Øy, *Antarctica* U05–690 **27**
Peterhead, *Scotland* N11+575 **40**
Peterlee, *England* N08+548 **37**
Petermann Fd., *Greenland* S05+810 **26**
Petermann Pk., *Greenland* Q00+730 **26**
Petermann Ra., *W. Aust.* D35–250 **110**
Peter Pond L., *Sask.* V22+558 **88**
Petersburg, *Alaska* W75+568 **99**
Petersburg, *Virginia* T15+372 **97**
Pēterupe, *Latvia* L33+573 **47**
Petit Bois I., *Alabama* T80+302 **95**
Petit Francois, *Fr. Guiana* R44+031 **105**
Petit Nord Pen., *Nfd.* R70+509 **90**
Petitot R., *Brit. Columbia* W08+598 **88**
Petitsikapau L., *Labrador* S40+544 **89**
Peto, *Mexico* T82+201 **100**
Petone, *New Zealand* A31–412 **112**
Petoroa, *Chile* S66–321 **103**
Petoskey, *Michigan* T60+454 **91**
Petra, *Jordan* K57+303 **76**
Petra Velikogo Zaliv, *U.S.S.R.* D18+428 **63**
Petrich, *Bulgaria* L41+414 **58**
Petrified Forest Nat. Mon.,
Arizona V28+348 **94**
Petrinja, *Yugoslavia* L82+454 **56**
Petrodvorets, *U.S.S.R.* L02+598 **60**
Petrolia, *Ontario* T43+429 **91**
Petrolina, *Brazil* Q63–094 **105**
Petropavlovsk, *Kazakh.* H35+549 **62**
Petropavlovsk, *U.S.S.R.* B36+530 **63**
Petropolis, *Brazil* Q80–225 **105**
Petrovac, *Yugoslavia* L51+444 **58**
Petrovsk, *U.S.S.R.* J22+536 **61**
Petrovsk, *U.S.S.R.* E66+513 **63**
Petrovsk, *U.S.S.R.* J88+523 **61**
Petrozavodsk, *U.S.S.R.* K65+618 **62**
Petsamo. *See* Pechenga
Pettigoe, *Ireland, Rep.* N47+545 **42**
Pevas, *Peru* S71–032 **104**
Pewsey, *England* N11+513 **39**
Pézenas, *France* M70+435 **55**
Pforzheim, *W. Germany* M38+489 **48**
Phagwara, *India* G85+312 **72**
Phalodi, *India* H16+270 **70**
Phanom Dang Rae,
Thailand F16+143 **69**
Phan Rang, *Vietnam* E65+116 **69**
Phan-Thiet & B. of,
Vietnam E71+110 **69**
Phaphund, *India* G63+266 **73**
Phatthalung, *Thailand* F29+076 **69**
Phenix City, *Alabama* T60+325 **97**
Phet Buri, *Thailand* F31+132 **69**
Philadelphia, *Pennsylvania* T01+400 **91**
Philip, *S. Dakota* U70+441 **93**
Philippeville, *Belgium* M63+502 **44**

Philippeville & G. of, (Skikda), Algeria M48+366 80
Philippi, W. Virginia T30+391 91
Philippi, L., Queensland C66-244 111
Philippines, Is., Pacific Oc. 65
Philippopolis. See Plovdiv
Philaur, India G85+310 72
Phillip I., Victoria C28-384 109
Phillip Edward I., Ontario T38+459 91
Phillips, Maine S62+448 90
Phillips, Wisconsin U03+457 91
Phillipsburg, Kansas U56+398 95
Phillipsburg, New Jersey T01+406 96
Philomena, Alberta V39+551 88
Phitsanulok Muang, Thailand F29+170 69
Phnom-Penh, Khmer F00+115 69
Phoenix, Arizona V43+334 94
Phoenix I., Phoenix Is. Z36-040 106
Phoenix Is., Pacific Ocean Z40-040 106
Phoenixville, Pennsylvania T03+401 96
Pho-mo-chang-thang Tso, Tibet F87+286 71
Phu-dien, N. Vietnam E86+190 69
Phulji, Pakistan H43+270 70
Phulpur, India G47+255 73
Phu-Quoc, I., Khmer F06+102 69
Phu-yen, S. Vietnam E65+134 69
Piacenza, Italy M32+450 56
Pian, R., New S. Wales C06-302 109
Piangil, Victoria C41-351 109
Pianosa, I., Italy M29+426 56
Pias, Portugal N45+380 52
Piatra Neamt, Romania L22+469 58
Piazza Armerina, Sicily M04+373 57
Piazzi, I., Chile S84-518 103
Pibor Post, Sudan K72+068 81
Picardie, prov., France M78+500 54
Piceno. See Ascoli.
Pichanal, Argentina S26-233 103
Picher, Oklahoma U30+370 95
Pichilemu, Chile S71-344 103
Pickens, Mississippi U00+329 97
Pickering, England N05+542 37
Pickwick L., Tennessee, etc. T78+349 95
Picola, Victoria C29-360 109
Picos, Brazil Q85-059 105
Picton, New South Wales B87-342 109
Picton, New Zealand A36-413 112
Picton, Ontario T13+440 91
Picton, Mt., Tasmania C21-432 109
Pictou, Nova Scotia S15+458 90
Pictou I., Nova Scotia S17+457 90
Picun Leufu, Argentina S55-395 103
Pidark, Pakistan H71+257 70
Piedad, La, Mexico U73+203 100
Piedmont, Missouri U05+371 97
Piedmont, Quebec S84+459 91
Piedmont, S. Carolina T45+347 97
Piedmont, S. Dakota U81+442 93
Piedrahita, Spain N32+405 52
Piedras Negras, Mexico U63+288 100
Piedra Sola, Uruguay R67-320 103
Pieksämäki, Finland L17+623 46
Pielinen, Finland L04+633 46
Pieman R., Tasmania C30-417 109
Piemonte, dep., Italy M44+450 56
Pierre, S. Dakota U62+444 93
Pierreville, Quebec S77+461 91
Pietarsaari (Jakobstad), Fin. L44+637 46
Pietermaritzburg, Natal K88-296 84
Pietersburg, Transvaal L04-238 84
Piggot, Arkansas U02+364 95
Pigue, Argentina S15-376 103
Pihtipudas, Finland L26+634 46
Pikes Pk., Colorado V00+388 94
Pikeville, Kentucky T45+374 97
Pila, Argentina R80-360 103
Pila, Poland L80+532 49
Pilao Arcado, Brazil Q75-102 105
Pilar, Argentina S07-314 103
Pilar, Brazil R28-147 105
Pilar, Paraguay R80-269 103
Pilar, C., Chile S88-528 103
Pilcaniyeu, Argentina S64-410 103
Pilibhit, India G61+286 73
Pillau, Lithuania L60+547 47
Pilliga, New South Wales C07-304 109
Pillinger, Tasmania C27-424 109
Pilos, Greece L50+369 59
Pilot, The, New S. Wales C11-368 109
Pilot Knob, Missouri U04+374 97
Pilsen. See Plzen.
Piltene, Latvia L50+572 47
Pi Mai, Thailand F15+152 69
Pimentel, Peru T29-067 104
Pina, Spain N03+415 53
Pinaki I., Tuamotu Arch. X20-195 107
Pinaleno Ra., Arizona V30+326 94
Pinang I., Malaya F28+051 69
Pinarbasi, Turkey K52+387 74
Pinar del Rio, Cuba T52+224 101
Pinckneyville, Illinois T87+381 97
Pind Dadan Khan, Pakistan H12+326 72
Pindhos, mts., Greece L50+393 59
Pindi Gheb, Pakistan H16+332 72
Pine I., Florida T43+266 97
Pine Mts., Kentucky T52+369 97
Pine Bluff, Arkansas U12+342 97
Pine City, Minnesota U18+458 93
Pine Creek, N. Territory, Australia D18-138 110
Pinedale, Wyoming V28+429 93
Pinehurst, N. Carolina T27+352 97
Pineola, N. Carolina T42+362 97
Pine River, Minnesota U26+467 93
Pinetown, Natal K86-298 84
Pineville, Kentucky T52+367 97
Pineville, Missouri U26+366 95
Pineville, W. Virginia T38+376 97
Piney Buttes, Montana V12+475 93
Ping-chuan-chow, China E07+410 66
Pingelap, I., Caroline Is. B25+045 106
Pingelly, W. Australia E18-324 110
Pingkiang, China E38+285 67
Pingliang, China E80+354 66
Pinglo, China E55+246 67
Pingrup, W. Australia E07-333 110
Ping-ting-chow, China E39+378 66
Pingwu, China F02+323 66
Pingyang. See Linfen.
Pingyüan, China E21+371 66
Pinhel, Portugal N42+408 52
Pini, I., Indonesia F38+002 65
Pinjarra, W. Australia E25-326 110
Pinnacles, New South Wales C52-321 109
Pinnaroo, S. Australia C55-353 109
Pinos, Mexico U69+228 100
Pinos, I. de, Cuba T47+216 101
Pinos, Mt., California V85+348 92
Pinrang, Celebes E02-038 65
Pinsk, Belorussia L24+521 60
Pintados, Chile S58-207 103
Pinto, Argentina S16-292 103
Pioneer, Os., U.S.S.R. F80+800 63
Piotrkow, Poland L62+509 49
Pipar, India H08+264 70
Pipestone, Minnesota U36+440 98
Pipinas, Argentina R74-355 103
Pipmuacan L., Quebec S62+496 90
Pippli, India G15+216 71
Piqua, Ohio T56+401 91
Piracuruca, Brazil Q70-039 105
Piraeus. See Piraievs.
Piraievs, Greece L38+379 59
Piramide, mt., Chile S81-490 103
Piranhas, Brazil Q47-095 105
Pirapora, Brazil R00-173 105
Piratini, Brazil R49-314 103
Piray, Argentina R59-266 103
Pirgos, Greece L45+366 59
Pirgos, Greece L51+377 59
Pirgos, Crete L29+350 59
Pirin Planina, Bulgaria-Greece L40+415 58
Piritu, Venezuela S30+101 104
Pirmasens, W. Germany M45+492 48
Pirna, E. Germany M06+510 48
Pirot, Yugoslavia L45+431 58
Pir Panjal Ra., Kashmir H04+340 72
Pisa, Italy M28+437 56
Pisagua, Chile S62-196 103
Pisco, Peru T08-136 104
Pisek, Czechoslovakia M05+493 48
Pishin, Pakistan H48+305 70
Pishin, Iran H79+261 75
Pisticci, Italy L80+404 57
Pitanguy, Brazil Q89-198 105
Pitarpunga L., N.S.W. C40-344 109
Pitcairn I., Pacific Ocean W60-254 107
Pite Älv, Sweden L64+660 46
Piteå, Sweden L51+653 46
Piterka, U.S.S.R. J75+506 61
Piteşti, Romania L31+449 58
Pithiviers, France M77+482 54
Pithoria, India G69+241 73
Pitlochry, Scotland N22+567 41
Pitt, Mt., Oregon W14+424 92
Pitt R., California W11+409 92
Pittsboro, N. Carolina T25+357 93
Pittsburg, Kansas U28+371 99
Pittsburgh, Pennsylvania T30+405 91
Pittsfield, Illinois U05+396 95
Pittsfield, Maine S56+448 90
Pittsfield, Massachusetts S79+425 91
Pittston, Pennsylvania T05+413 96
Piua-Petri, Romania L13+446 58
Piaura, Peru T34-052 104
Piza, Latvia L48+576 47
Placentia B., Newfoundland R58+468 90
Placer Guadalupe, Mexico V02+292 100
Plainfield, New Jersey S87+406 91
Plainview, Nebraska U49+424 95
Plainview, Texas U70+342 94
Plainwell, Michigan T64+425 91
Pláka B., Crete L34+352 59
Plakoti C., Cyprus K65+355 76
Plana, Czechoslovakia M13+498 48
Planaltina, Brazil R16-156 105
Planina, Yugoslavia M05+458 56
Plant City, Florida T43+280 97
Plascenia, Spain N36+401 52
Plaški, Yugoslavia L88+450 56
Plassen, Norway M15+611 47
Plaster Rock, N.B. S44+470 90
Plastun, U.S.S.R. C82+446 63
Plata, R. de la, Argent., etc. R70-350 103
Platamon, Greece L44+400 59
Plati, Greece L45+405 59
Platres, Cyprus K73+349 76
Platt Nat. Park, Oklahoma U42+345 98
Platte R., Nebraska U60+408 95
Platteville, Wisconsin U03+428 95
Plattsburg, Missouri U27+396 95
Plattsburg, New York S81+447 91
Plattsmouth, Nebraska U36+410 95
Plauen, E. Germany M17+505 48
Plav, Yugoslavia L60+426 58
Plavnica, Yugoslavia L65+423 58
Playas L., New Mexico V23+317 98
Plaza Huincul, Argentina S55-389 103
Pleasant B., Maine S47+445 90
Pleasant Grove, Utah V41+404 94
Pleasantville, New Jersey S87+394 96
Pleiku, S. Vietnam E72+140 65
Plenty, B. of, New Zealand A18-378 112
Plentywood, Montana U88+488 93
Plessisville, Quebec S70+462 91
Plettenberg B., Cape Prov. L38-342 84
Pleven, Bulgaria L33+434 58
Pljevlja, Yugoslavia L64+434 58
Płock, Poland L61+525 49
Ploiesti, Romania L24+449 58
Plomarion, Greece L22+389 59
Plomosa Mts., Arizona V53+338 92
Plon, W. Germany M28+541 48
Plonge, Lac la, Saskatchewan V13+552 88
Plonsk, Poland L58+526 49
Plovdiv, Bulgaria L32+421 58
Plumtree, Rhodesia L12-206 84
Plymouth, Indiana T68+414 91
Plymouth, Massachusetts S64+420 91
Plymouth, New Hampshire S70+437 91
Plymouth, N. Carolina T10+359 97
Plymouth, Pennsylvania T06+413 96
Plymouth, Wisconsin T78+438 91
Plymouth & Sd., England N25+504 38
Plynlimmon, Wales N22+525 38
Plzeň, Czechoslovakia M10+492 48
Poai, China E41+352 66
Pobedy, Pik, mt., China, etc. G60+420 62
Pobla de Segur, Spain M84+422 53
Pocahontas, Arkansas U06+362 95
Pocahontas, Virginia T36+373 97
Pocatello, Idaho V45+428 94
Pochinki, U.S.S.R. K01+547 61
Pochutla, Mexico U39+158 100
Pocklington, England N05+539 37
Podkagernaya, U.S.S.R. B19+604 63
Podkamennaya Tunguska, U.S.S.R. G00+616 63
Podlubovo, U.S.S.R. J25+543 61
Podolsk, U.S.S.R. K45+554 60
Pogamasing, Ontario T41+469 91
Pohai, G. of, China E06+385 66
Pohai, Str. of, China D84+385 66
Point L., N.-W. Territories V50+652 88
Pointe à Pitre, Leeward Is. S08+164 101
Pointe du Chene, N.B. S27+462 90
Poitiers, France M88+466 54
Poitou, prov., France N02+465 54
Poix, Belgium M58+500 44
Poix, France M78+498 54
Pokaakku, I., Pacific Ocean A65+140 106
Pokaran, India H20+268 70
Pokataroo, New S. Wales C08-296 109
Pokemouche, N.B. S29+477 90
Pokhara, Nepal G36+282 73
Pokka, Finland L26+681 46
Pokrovsk, U.S.S.R. K14+531 61
Pokrovsk, U.S.S.R. K36+474 61
Pokrovsk. See Engels.
Pokrovskoe, U.S.S.R. D34+613 63
Pola. See Pula.
Pola de Siero, Spain N34+434 52
Poland, rep., Cent. Europe L72+520 51
Polesk, U.S.S.R. L53+548 47
Polevskoi, U.S.S.R. H89+564 61
Polgahawela, Sri Lanka G58+074 70
Polgar, Hungary L53+478 49
Poli, Cameroun M10+084 81
Poliaigos, I., Greece L32+368 59
Policastro, G. di, Italy L86+400 57
Poligny, France M56+468 54
Polillo Is., Philippines D78+148 65
Pólinos. See Poliaigos, I.
Polis, Cyprus K75+350 76
Pollensa, Balearic Islands M71+399 53
Polotsk, Belorussia L08+555 60
Polson, Montana V55+477 92
Poltava, Ukraine K62+496 60
Poluostrov Buzachi, Kazakh. J50+448 62
Põlva, Estonia L18+580 47
Polynesia, Pacific Oc. Z30-100 106
Poman, Argentina S37-283 103
Pomaro, Mexico U75+184 100
Pombal, Brazil Q47-067 105
Pombal, Portugal N52+399 52
Pombets, Japan C38+431 68
Pomene, Mozambique K56-230 84
Pomeroy, N. Ireland N41+546 42
Pommersche B., E. Germany M04+542 48
Pomorie, Bulgaria L15+426 58
Pomorze, Poland L72+536 49
Pomos Pt., Cyprus K75+352 76
Pompey's Pillar, Montana V17+460 93
Ponape, I., Caroline Islands B45+070 106
Ponca City, Oklahoma U42+366 95
Ponce, Puerto Rico S39+180 101
Pondicherry, India G61+120 70
Ponente, Riviera di, Italy M40+437 56
Ponferrada, Spain N39+425 52
Ponoi, U.S.S.R. K24+670 62
Pons, France N03+456 54
Pons, Spain M83+419 53
Ponta Grossa, Brazil R31-252 103
Pontardawe, Wales N23+517 38
Pont-Audemer, France M87+494 54
Pontchartrain, L., Louisiana U00+302 95
Pont Chateau, France N12+474 54
Pont d'Ain, France M58+461 54
Ponte, Switzerland M30+466 45
Ponte Boa, Brazil S36-026 104
Ponte da Barca, Portugal N51+418 52
Ponte de Sôr, Portugal N48+392 52
Pontefract, England N08+537 37
Ponte Nova, Brazil Q78-204 105
Pontevedra, Spain N52+424 52
Pontiac, Illinois T82+409 91
Pontiac, Michigan T50+427 91
Pontianak, Borneo E64-002 65
Pontivy, France N18+481 54
Pontoise, France M77+491 54
Pontotoc, Mississippi T84+342 97
Pontresina, Switzerland M31+465 45
Ponts, les, Switzerland M50+470 45
Pontypool, Wales N18+517 38
Pontypool, Ontario T22+441 91
Pontypridd, Wales N20+516 38
Ponza, I., Italy M12+410 57
Poole, England N12+507 39
Poole, Mt., New S. Wales C50-297 109
Poolewe, Scotland N34+578 40
Poona, India H06+186 70
Pooncarie, New South Wales C46-334 109
Poopelloe, L., New S. Wales C36-316 109
Poopo, Bolivia S42-184 104
Poopo, L., Bolivia S43-188 104
Popa Mt., Burma F58+209 71
Popakai, Surinam R62+032 105
Popayan, Colombia T09+025 104
Poperinge, Belgium M74+508 44
Poplar, Montana V01+481 93
Poplar R., Manitoba U37+528 88
Poplar Bluff, Missouri U02+368 97
Poplarville, Mississippi T87+308 97
Popocatepetl, mt., Mexico U52+192 100
Popovača, Yugoslavia L80+456 56
Poppel, Belgium M60+514 44
Porahat, India G27+226 73
Porbandar, India H33+216 70
Porcupine R., Alaska X40+698 99
Poreč, Yugoslavia M08+452 56
Pori, Finland L50+615 47
Porjus, Sweden L61+670 46
Porkhov, U.S.S.R. L03+578 60
Porkkala, Finland L34+600 47
Porlamar, Margarita I., Venezuela S23+109 104
Pornic, France N13+471 54
Poronaysk, U.S.S.R. C42+492 63
Póros I., Greece L39+375 59
Poro Tso, Tibet G38+310 71
Porsanger Fd., Norway L28+704 46
Porsanger-halvøya, Norway L36+700 46
Porsgrund, Norway M32+591 47
Portachuela, Bolivia S20-171 104
Port Adelaide, S. Australia C69-349 109
Portadown, N. Ireland N39+544 42
Portaferry, N. Ireland N33+544 42
Portage, Wisconsin T87+436 91
Portage I., New Brunswick S30+472 90
Portage la Prairie, Manitoba U50+500 88
Portage River, N. B. S30+474 90
Portageville, New York T18+426 96
Portal, N. Dakota U75+490 93
Portal, N. Saskatchewan U76+491 88
Port Albert, Victoria C20-386 109
Portalegre, Portugal N45+393 52
Portales, New Mexico U80+341 94
Port Alfred, Quebec S65+484 90
Port Allen, Louisiana U07+304 97
Port Antonio, Jamaica T08+182 101
Portarlington, Ireland, Rep. N43+532 43
Port Arthur. See Lushun
Port Arthur, Tasmania C13-432 109
Port Arthur, Texas U23+299 95
Port Augusta, S. Australia C74-325 109
Port au Port B., Nfd. R84+490 90
Port au Prince, Haiti S73+186 101
Port aux Basques, Nfd. R85+476 90
Port Blandford, Nfd. R55+484 90
Port Borden, Pr. Edward I. S22+462 90
Port Broughton, South Australia C73-336 109
Port Campbell, Victoria C42-386 109
Port Chalmers, N.Z. A56-457 112
Port Chester, New York S81+410 96
Port Clinton, Ohio T48+415 91
Port Cornwallis, Andaman Islands F72+134 71
Port Dalhousie, Ontario T26+432 91
Port Daniel Quebec S29+482 90
Port Darwin, Falkland Is. R84-518 103
Port Davey, Tasmánia C24-434 109
Port de Paix, Haiti S76+199 101
Port Dickson, Malaya F19+02 69
Port Douglas, Queensland C28-164 111
Port Dover, Ontario T31+428 91
Portel, Brazil R34-019 105
Port Elgin, Ontario T38+445 91
Port Elizabeth, Cape Prov. L26-340 84
Port Ellen, Scotland N37+556 41
Port Etienne, Mauritania P12+210 80
Port Eynon, Wales N25+516 38
Port Fairy, Victoria C47-384 109
Port Germein, S. Australia C72-330 109
Port Gibson, Mississippi U06+320 95
Port Glasgow, Scotland N27+559 41
Porglenone, N. Ireland N39+549 42
Portgordon, Scotland N18+577 40
Port Harcourt, Nigeria M48+048 80
Port Hedland, W. Australia E08-205 110
Porthmadog, Wales N25+529 38
Port Hope, Michigan T46+440 91
Port Hope, Ontario T20+439 91
Port Huron, Michigan T45+430 91
Portimão, Portugal N51+371 52
Port Jackson, New S. Wales B83-339 109
Port Jervis, New York S88+414 96
Port Joli, Nova Scotia S29+439 90
Port Kelang, Malaya F22+030 69
Port Kembla, New S. Wales B85-345 109
Portland, Arkansas U09+332 97
Portland, Maine S62+437 90
Portland, New South Wales C00-334 109
Portland, Oregon W16+455 92
Portland, Victoria C51-383 109
Portland C., Tasmania C13-407 407 109
Portland Harb. & I., Eng. N14+506 38
Portland Point, Jamaica T13+178 101
Portland Prom., Quebec T20+590 89
Port Laoise, Ireland, Rep. N44+530 43
Port Lavaca, Texas U40+286 94
Portlaw, Ireland, Rep. N44+522 43
Port Lincoln, S. Australia C85-347 111
Port Loko, Sierra Leone N76+088 80
Port Lyautey. See Kenitra N40+344 80
Port M'Donnell, S. Aust. C56-380 109
Port M'Nicoll, Ontario T29+448 91
Port Macquarie, N.S.W. B73-314 109
Port Medway, Nova Scotia S27+441 90
Port Menier, Anticosti I., Que. S26+498 90
Port Moresby, Papua New Guinea C17-094 111
Portnacroish, Scotland N32+566 41
Port Nelson (abandoned), Manitoba U18+567 89
Portneuf, Quebec S71+467 91
Port Nolloth, Cape Province L78-292 84
Port Norris, New Jersey T00+392 91
Porto, Portugal N52+411 52
Porto Acre, Brazil S46-097 104
Porto Alegre, Brazil Q57-180 105
Porto Alegre, Brazil R37-300 103
Porto Alegre, Brazil Q74-034 105
Porto Alexandre, Angola M18-158 84
Porto Amelia, Mozambique K26-130 83
Porto Barreirão, Brazil R20-126 105
Portobelo, Panama T28+096 101
Porto Botte, Sardinia M39+391 57
Porto Camargo, Brazil R53-234 105
Porto Civitanova, Italy M08+433 56
Porto d'Ascoli, Italy M07+429 56
Porto de Moz, Brazil R42-018 105
Porto de Moz, Portugal N53+394 52
Porto do Jeronymo, Brazil R31-186 105
Porto Empedocle, Sicily M09+373 57
Porto Esperanca, Brazil R74-197 105
Porto Espiridião, Brazil R79-158 104
Porto Franco, Brazil R26-086 105
Porto Franco, Brazil R13-099 105
Porto Franco, Brazil R14-064 105
Port of Spain, Trinidad S08+107 104
Porto Guaira, Brazil R55-240 105
Port Okha, India H36+223 70
Portola, California W03+398 92
Porto Lucena, Brazil R60-277 103
Porto Mendes, Brazil R56-244 105
Porto Nacional, Brazil R20-108 105
Porto Novo, Benin M74+064 80
Porto Novo, India G62+116 70

Port Ontario, New York T07+435 96
Porto Seguro, Brazil Q54-163 105
Porto Torres, Sardinia M40+408 57
Porto Vecchio, Corsica M35+416 57
Porto Velho, Brazil S23-088 104
Portoviejo, Ecuador T32-010 104
Port Patrick, Scotland N31+548 41
Port Pegasus, New Zealand A73-472 112
Port Phillip B., Victoria C31-382 109
Port Pirie, S. Australia C72-332 109
Port Pleasant, New Jersey S85+401 91
Port Radium, N.-W. Terr. V75+659 88
Portree, Scotland N37+574 40
Port Rowan, Ontario T33+427 91
Port Royal, Jamaica T11+179 101
Port Royal, S. Carolina T34+324 97
Portrush, N. Ireland N40+552 42
Port Safaga, Egypt K66+261 81
Port Said, Egypt K76+312 81
Port St John's, Cape Prov. L02-318 84
Portsalon, Ireland, Rep. N46+552 42
Port Shepstone, Natal K88-308 84
Port Simpson, B.C. W63+546 88
Portsmouth, England N07+508 39
Portsmouth, New Hampshire S65+431 90
Portsmouth, Ohio T48+387 91
Portsmouth, Virginia T08+368 97
Portsonachan, Scotland N31+563 41
Portsoy, Scotland N16+577 40
Port Stanley, Ontario T37+427 91
Port Stephens, N.S.W. B78-328 109
Port Sudan, Sudan K46+196 81
Port Talbot, Wales N23+516 38
Port Tampa City, Florida T45+278 97
Port Taufiq, Egypt K74+300 81
Portugal, W. Europe N48+400 50
Portugalia, Angola L56-074 82
Portuguese Guinea, See Guinea-Bissau
Portumna, Ireland, Rep. N49+531 43
Port Vendres, France M71+425 55
Port Victoria, Kenya K66+002 83
Port Wakefield, S. Aust. C71-342 109
Port Washington, Wisconsin T77+434 91
Port Weller, Ontario T25+432 91
Porvenir, Chile S62-533 103
Porvoo, (Borga) Finland L26+604 47
Posadas, Argentina R66-273 103
Posadowsky B., Antarctica G05-670 27
Poschiavo, Switzerland M30+463 45
Poseh, China E81+239 67
Posen. See Poznan
Poshan, China E13+365 66
Posht-i-kuh, Iran J84+336 74
Poso, Celebes D86-014 65
Poso Danau, Celebes. D87-018 65
Possession I., Antarctica A50-720 27
Post, Texas U68+332 94
Posušje, Yugoslavia L76+435 56
Potapovo, U.S.S.R. G21+687 62
Potchefstroom, Transvaal L16-266 84
Poteau, Oklahoma U28+350 95
Potemkino, U.S.S.R. J84+504 61
Potenza, Italy L85+407 57
Poti, Gruzinskaya, U.S.S.R. K20+422 62
Potiskum, Nigeria M24+116 81
Potomac R., Maryland, etc. T20+396 96
Potosi, Bolivia S34-197 104
Potosi, Missouri U05+379 97
Potrerillos, Chile S57-265 103
Potsdam, E. Germany M12+524 48
Pottstown, Pennsylvania T04+403 91
Pottsville, Pennsylvania T07+407 91
Pouce Coupe, B.C. W00+554 88
Poughkeepsie, New York S83+417 91
Pouso Alegre, Brazil R72-118 104
Pouso Alegre, Brazil R06-212 105
Povenets, Karelskaya K62+628 62
Poverty B., New Zealand A12-388 112
Povoa de Varzim, Portugal N53+414 52
Povorina, U.S.S.R. K16+512 61
Povungnituk, Quebec T25+602 89
Povungnituk R., Quebec T05+602 89
Powder R., Montana V04+453 98
Powder River Ra., Montana V00+454 93
Powderville, Montana V01+458 93
Powell, L., Utah V36+370 98
Powell Mts., Pa.-Va. T49+366 97
Powell Creek, N.-T. Aust. D09-179 111
Powys, co., Wales N23+523 38
Poyang, China E20+290 67
Poyang Hu, China E22+290 67
Poza de la sal, Spain N21+427 52
Požarevac, Yugoslavia L53+446 58
Požega, Yugoslavia L74+453 58
Poznan, Poland L78+524 49
Pozo Almonte, Chile S58-203 103
Pozoblanco, Spain N29+384 52
Prachim Buri, Thailand F22+140 69
Prado, Brazil Q56-173 105
Praga, Poland L54+523 49
Prague. See Praha
Praha, Czechoslovakia M04+501 48
Praid, Romania L29+466 58
Prainha, Brazil S02-072 104
Prairie, Queensland C32-209 111
Prairie du Chien, Wisconsin U06+430 95
Prairie du Sac, Wisconsin T89+433 91
Pratapgarth, India G48+259 73
Prato, Italy M24+439 56
Pratt, Kansas U53+376 95
Pratt City, Alabama T71+335 97
Pravia, Spain N37+434 52
Pregolya, R., U.S.S.R. L51+546 47
Prenay, Lithuania L36+546 47
Prentice, Wisconsin U02+455 91
Přerov, Czechoslovakia L75+495 49
Prescott, Arizona V45+345 92
Prescott, Ontario T03+447 91
President R. Sáenz-Pena, Argentina S02-266 103
Presidente Hermes, Brazil S11-113 104
Presidente Penna, Brazil S11-108 104
Prešov, Czechoslovakia L53+490 49
Prespansko Jezero, Albania, etc. L54+409 59
Presque Isle, Maine S48+466 90
Pressburg. See Bratislava
Přeštice, Czechoslovakia M10+495 48
Preston, England N16+538 37
Preston, Idaho V41+421 94
Preston, Minnesota U13+437 93
Prestonpans, Scotland N18+560 41
Prestonsburg, Kentucky T47+377 97
Prestwick, Scotland N28+555 41
Pretoria, Transvaal L10-258 84
Pretty Boy L., Maryland T10+396 96
Préveza, Greece L56+390 59
Pribilof Is. Bering Sea Z30+568 99
Příbram, Czechoslovakia M06+497 48
Price and R., Utah V34+396 94
Priego, Spain N25+374 52
Prieska, Cape Province L44-296 84
Prignitz, E. Germany M18+531 48
Prijedor, Yugoslavia L80+450 56
Prijepolje, Yugoslavia L62+434 58
Prilep, Yugoslavia L51+414 58
Priluki, Ukraine K76+506 60
Prim Pt., Prince Edward I. S19+461 90
Primrose L., Saskatchewan V28+549 88
Prince Albert, Cape Province L48-332 84
Prince Albert, Saskatchewan V05+534 88
Prince Albert Mts., Antarc. B25-770 27
Prince Albert Park, Sask. V00+540 88
Prince Albert Pen., N.-W. T. V60+718 88
Prince Albert Sd., N.-W. T. V55+704 88
Prince Alfred, C., N.-W. T. W29+734 88
Prince Charles I., N.W.T. T10+672 89
Prince Edward I., Canada S20+464 89
Prince Edward Is., Indian Oc. K40-460 77
Prince Edwad Pen., Ont. T14+440 91
Prince George, B.C. W17+541 88
Prince Harald Ld., Antarc. K80-710 27
Prince of Wales, C., Alaska Z15+653 99
Prince of Wales I., Alaska W75+556 99
Prince of Wales I., N.-W. T. U60+720 88
Prince of Wales I., Qnsld. C47-107 111
Prince of Wales Str., N.-W. T. V80+724 88
Prince Patrick I., N.-W. T. W00+756 88
Prince Regent Inl., N.-W. T. U00+728 89
Prince Rupert, B.C. W61+543 88
Princes Lake, Ontario T18+454 91
Princess Astrid Ld., Antarc. M30-710 27
Princess Charlotte B., Queensland C36-142 111
Princess Elizabeth Ld., Antartica G70-720 27
Princess Ragnhild Ld., Antartica L00-710 27
Princess Royal I., B.C. W52+530 88
Princeton, Illinois T87+414 95
Princeton, Indiana T76+384 95
Princeton, Kentucky T77+372 95
Princeton, Maine S46+452 90
Princeton, Wisconsin T85+438 91
Princetown, England N24+505 38
Princetown, Pr. Edward I. S22+465 90
Prince William Sd., Alaska X70+600 99
Principe I., G. of Guinea M46+016 82
Principe da Beira, Brazil S27-124 104
Pringles, Argentina S23-404 103
Prins Karl's Forland, Arctic Ocean M25+785 62
Prinzapolca, Nicaragua T51+134 101
Pripyat (Pripet) Marshes, Byelorussia L18+520 60
Pripyat (Pripet), R., Byelorussia L03+518 60
Pristina, Yugoslavia L53+427 58
Pritzwalk, E. Germany M17+532 48
Privalnoye, U.S.S.R. J83+509 61
Prizren, Yugoslavia L56+422 58
Prizzi, Sicily M09+377 57
Progreso, Mexico 188-212 100
Prokop'yevsk, U.S.S.R. G20+541 62
Prokuplie, Yugoslavia L51+433 58
Prome, Burma F58+188 71
Prong, Ghana N06+080 80
Propria, Brazil Q41-103 105
Proskurov, Ukraine L18+494 60
Provence, prov., France M54+438 55
Providence, Kentucky T78+373 97
Providence, N.-W. Terr. V75+611 88
Providence, Rhode Island S68+418 91
Providence, C., N.-W. Terr. V45+736 88
Providence I., Indian Ocean J50-090 77
Provins, France M70+485 54
Provo, Utah V40+402 94
Prozor, Yugoslavia L74+438 56
Prudentopolis, Brazil R36-253 103
Prudhoe Ld., Greenland S45+780 26
Prüm, W. Germany M51+502 48
Prut, R. U.S.S.R., etc. L11+468 58
Przasnysz, Poland L55+530 49
Przemysl, Poland L43+498 49
Przhevalsk, Kirgiz. G70+425 62
Psará, I., Greece L26+386 59
Pskov, U.S.S.R. L10+578 60
Pskovskoye Oz., U.S.S.R. Estonia L12+580 60
Ptuj, Yugoslavia L85+464 56
Puan, Argentina S17-376 103
Pucacuro, Peru T04-028 104
Pucallpa, Peru S87-086 104
Puchezh, U.S.S.R. K11+570 61
Puchow. See Yungtsi
Puck, Poland L69+547 49
Pudasjärvi, Finland L19+654 46
Pudukkottai, India G68+104 70
Puebla & state, Mexico U49+188 100
Puebla Bonito, New Mexico V17+360 99
Puebla de Alcocer, Spain N31+390 52
Puebla de Sanabria, Spain N40+420 52
Puebla de Trives, Spain N44+425 52
Pueblo, Colorado U88+383 94
Pueblo Hundido, Chile S60-263 103
Puelches, Argentina S35-382 103
Puente Caldelas, Spain N51+423 52
Puentedeume, Spain N49+432 52
Puerco, R., Arizona V28+350 94
Puerhken, Mongolia F87+460 63
Puerto Armuelles, Panama T47+084 101
Puerto Asis, Colombia T09+005 104
Puerto Ayacucho, Venezuela S46+057 104
Puerto Aysen, Chile S78-453 103
Puerto Barrios, Guatemala T80+158 100
Puerto Bermudez, Peru S89-102 104
Puerto Berrio, Colombia S87+065 104
Puerto Cabello, Venezuela S48+105 104
Puerto Cabezas, Nicaragua T50+140 101
Puerto Carreno, Colombia S44+060 104
Puerto Casado, Paraguay R77-223 103
Puerto Chicama, Peru T27-078 104
Puerto Colombia, Colombia T00+109 104
Puerto Cordoba, Colombia S59-014 104
Puerto Cortes, Honduras T78+157 101
Puerto Coyle, Argentina S56-508 103
Puerto Cumarebo, Venez. S56+114 104
Puerto de Carrizal, Chile S67-281 103
Puerto de Chanaral, Chile S64-263 103
Puerto de Santa Maria, Spain N37+366 52
Puerto Deseado, Argentina S36-476 103
Puerto Eten, Peru T29-068 104
Puerto Harberton, Argent. S44-548 103
Puerto Heath, Bolivia S52-124 104
Puerto Ichilo, Bolivia S26-170 104
Puerto Isabel, Mexico V59+317 100
Puerto Leguisamo, Colombia S88-003 104
Puerto Libertad, El Salvador T86+134 101
Puertollano, Spain N25+387 52
Puerto Lobos, Argentina S31-420 103
Puerto Lomas, Peru S89-155 104
Puerto Madryn, Argentina S30-427 103
Puerto Maldonado, Peru S56-126 104
Puerto Mexico, Mexico U27+180 100
Puerto Montt, Chile S78-413 103
Puerto Morelos, Mexico T70+209 100
Puerto Natales, Chile S76-516 103
Puerto Patillos, Chile S61-208 103
Puerto Pirámide, Argentina S26-426 103
Puerto Plata, Dom. Rep. S64+198 101
Puerto Princesa, Phil. E08+097 65
Puerto Principe, Colombia S85+004 104
Puerto Quellen, Chile S81-428 103
Puerto Quijarro, Bolivia R77-178 104
Puerto Raso, Argentina S32-444 103
Puerto Rico, I., West Indies S38+183 101
Puerto Suarez, Bolivia R77-190 104
Puerto Sucre, Bolivia S32-108 104
Puerto Toledo, Bolivia S16-175 104
Puerto Varas, Chile S78-413 103
Puerto Victoria, Peru T00-098 104
Puerto Villamizar, Colombia S75+082 104
Puerto Visser, Argentina S43-454 103
Puerto Wilches, Colombia S83+073 104
Pueyrredón, L., Argentina S71-476 103
Pugachev, U.S.S.R. J67+520 61
Pugal, India H14+286 72
Puget, France M49+440 55
Puget Sd., Washington W18+474 98
Puglia, dep. Italy L80+409 57
Pühalepa, Estonia L42+589 47
Puimro, Brazil R58+010 105
Pukaki, L., New Zealand A59-441 112
Pukapaka I., Tuamotu Arch. X22-150 107
Pukapuka I., Pacific Ocean Z06-108 106
Pukchong, Korea D39+404 64
Pukekohe, New Zealand A31-372 112
Puket, Thailand F40+079 69
Pukow, China E08+321 66
Pula, Yugoslavia M07+449 56
Pulacayo, Bolivia S40-204 104
Pulap, I., Caroline Islands C25+073 106
Pulaski, New York T07+436 91
Pulaski, Tennessee T72+352 97
Pulaski, Virginia T35+371 97
Pulicat L., India G59+140 70
Pulkkila, Finland L25+643 46
Pullen I. (Richards I.), N.-W. Territories X00+686 88
Pullen, Ontario T40+494 89
Pultneyville, New York T13+432 96
Puma, Tanzania K62-050 83
Puna, I., Ecuador T31-030 104
Punakha, Bhutan G01+276 73
Punch, Kashmir H05+338 72
Pundri, India G80+298 72
Punjab, India G84+305 72
Puno, Peru S60-159 104
Punta Alta, Argentina S12-388 103
Punta Arenas, Chile S66-532 103
Punta Colorado, Chile S66-292 103
Punta del Faro, Sicily L87+383 57
Punta de Pedras, Brazil R23-014 105
Punta Gorda, Belize T83+162 101
Puntarenas, Costa Rica T58+100 101
Punta Salinas, Venezuela S61+117 104
Punxsutawney, Pennsylvania T24+409 96
Puolanka, Finland L14+649 46
Purang Chaka, Tibet G47+329 71
Purbeck Downs, England N15+507 38
Purgatoire R., Colorado U82+376 94
Puri, India G24+198 71
Purificacion, Colombia T00+038 104
Purna, India G76+192 70
Purnea, India G15+258 73
Pursat, Cambodia F06+125 69
Purulia, India G21+233 73
Purus, R., Brazil, etc. S32-074 104
Purvis, Mississippi T86+311 97
Purwa, India G55+265 73
Pusan, Korea D36+351 64
Pu-san, mt., Laos F11+198 69
Pushchino, U.S.S.R. E62+580 63
Pust-i-Badam, Iran J27+328 75
Putao, Burma F43+274 71
Putbus, W. Germany M09+543 48
Putien, China E05+255 67
Putignano, Italy L77+408 57
Putnam, Connecticut S71+419 96
Putnok, Hungary L58+483 49
Putorana, Gory, U.S.S.R. F60+690 63
Puttalam, Sri Lanka G61+081 70
Putte, Belgium M64+514 44
Putte, Belgium M62+511 44
Putten, Netherlands M56+522 44
Putumayo, R., Colombia, etc. S88-006 104
Putussibau, Borneo E42+008 65
Puula Vesi, Finland L20+617 47
Puurs, Belgium M64+511 44
Puy, le, France M67+450 55
Puyallup, Washington W14+472 92
Puy-de-Dôme, dep., France M70+456 54
Pwllheli, Wales N27+529 38
Pyapon, Burma F56+162 71
Pyatistennoe, U.S.S.R. B20+680 63
Pyevyek, U.S.S.R. A53+698 63
Pyhäjärvi, Finland L24+636 46
Pyhäjärvi, Finland L46+610 47
Pyhäntä, Finland L22+641 46
Pyinmana, Burma F52+197 71
Pyŏngyang, Korea D54+393 64
Pyramid L., Nevada V87+400 92
Pyramid Pk., California W01+389 92
Pyramid Hill, Victoria C35-361 109
Pyrénées, Mt., France-Spain 53
Pyrénées-Orientales dep., France M76+425 55
Pyrzyce, Poland M01+531 48
Pyu, Burma F51+185 71
Pyzdry, Poland L74+522 49
Qafar, Saudi Arabia K19+274 74
Qaiya, Saudi Arabia J88+241 74
Qala, Afghanistan H14+369 75
Qala Mashiz, Iran J20+299 75
Qal'at al Akhdhar, Saudi Arabia K45+281 74
Qal'at Dar al Hamra, Saudi Arabia K42+275 74
Qal'at ed Dab'a, Jordan K54+316 76
Qal'at el Marqan, Syria K54+352 76
Qal'at el Mudiq, Syria K51+355 74
Qal'at Uneiza, Jordan K55+305 76
Qalqiliya, Jordan K60+322 76
Qamr B., Yemen, South J44+160 75
Qara, Egypt L20+298 81
Qardaha, Syria K54+355 76
Qartaba, Lebanon K55+341 76
Qasim, Saudi Arabia K21+272 74
Qasr Amij, Iraq K19+334 74
Qasr el Azraq, Jordan K49+319 76
Qasr e Qand, Iran H85+262 75
Qasr Haiyaniya, Saudi Arabia K14+286 74
Qasr ibn Aliya, Saudi Arabia K10+291 74
Qasr-i-Shirin, Iran J86+346 74
Qa'taba, Yemen K01+139 74
Qatana, Syria K53+334 76
Qatar, The Gulf J52+250 75
Qatif, Saudi Arabia J60+267 74
Qayen, Iran J05+338 75
Qena, Egypt K74+262 81
Qeshm I., Iran J26+267 75
Qeys, I., Iran J36+265 75
Qishn, Yemen, D.R. J50+155 75
Qishran, I., Saudi Arabia K30+202 74
Qizan, Saudi Arabia K14+169 74
Qom, Iran J55+347 75
Qotur, Iran K04+385 74
Qoz Bal 'Air, Saudi Arabia K21+192 74
Quabbin Res., Massachusetts S74+424 96
Quadda, Cent. Afr. Rep. L46+082 81
Quakenbruck, W. Germany M42+527 48
Quambatook, Victoria C39-359 109
Quambone, New S. Wales C13-309 109
Quang Tri, Vietnam E77+168 65
Quantock Hills, England N19+511 38
Quarai, Brazil R69-304 103
Quatre Bras, Belgium M63+506 44
Qubeiyat, Lebanon K52+346 76
Quchan, Iran J10+371 75
Queanbeyan, New S. Wales C04-354 109
Quebec, Quebec S67+468 91
Quebec, prov., Canada 89
Queen Alexandra Ra., Antarctica B20-840 27
Queen Anne, Maryland T06+388 96
Queen Charlotte B. Falkland Islands S04-517 103
Queen Charlotte Is., B.C. W75+530 88
Queen Charlotte Sd., B.C. W50+514 88
Queen Charlotte Str., B.C.W45+508 88
Queen Elizabeth Is., N.-W.T. V40+770 88
Queen Mary Ld., Antarctica F65-670 27
Queen Maud G., N.-W. Territories U60+676 88
Queen Maud Ld., Antarc. L60-720 27
Queen Maud Ra., Antarc. Y50-870 27
Queen's Chan., N. Terr., Australia D33-147 110
Queenscliff, Victoria C32-383 109
Queenscliffe, S. Australia C74-356 109
Queensland, state, Australia 111
Queenstown, Cape Province L18-320 84
Queenstown, New Zealand A68-450 112
Queenstown. See Cobh
Queenstown, Tasmania C27-421 109
Queimadas, Brazil Q58-110 105
Quelimane, Mozambique K48-178 84
Quemu Quemú, Argentina S21-360 103
Quequen, Argentina R82-385 103
Queretaro, Mexico U62+206 100
Quesnel, Brit. Columbia W15+532 88
Quesnel L., Brit. Columbia W08+528 88
Quetta, Pakistan H48+302 70
Quetzalapa, Mexico U49+170 100
Quezaltenango, Guatemala U09+148 100
Quezon City, Philippines D83+149 65
Quibdo, Colombia T10+057 104
Quiberon B. de., France N18+475 54
Quievrain, Belgium M68+504 44
Quila, Mexico V13+245 100
Quilca, Peru S75-166 104
Quilino, Argentina S28-301 103
Quillabamba, Peru S77-128 104
Quillan, France M77+429 55
Quillota, Chile S68-328 103
Quilon (Kollam), India G90+111 70
Quilpie, Queensland C35-266 111
Quimper, France N25+480 54
Quimperle, France N21+479 54
Quincy, Illinois U08+399 95
Quincy, Massachusetts S66+423 91
Quincy, Michigan T59+420 91
Quines, Argentina S34-321 103
Quinnimont, W. Virginia T36+378 97
Quintana de la Serena, Sp. N34+388 52
Quintanar de la Orden, Sp. N19+396 52
Quintana Roo, state, Mexico T78+194 100
Quipapa, Brazil Q36-087 105
Quirindi, New South Wales B86-316 109
Quiriquite, Venezuela S18+100 104
Quiroga, Spain N43+424 52
Quissanga, Mozambique K28-124 83
Quissico, Mozambique K62-248 84
Quitapa, Angola L70-106 82
Quito, Ecuador T21-002 104
Quixada, Brazil Q55-050 105
Quixeramobim, Brazil Q56-052 105
Qunsuliye, Saudi Arabia K13+221 74
Quoich L., Scotland N32+571 40
Quorn, S. Australia C72-323 109
Quryat, Oman J07+233 75
Qus, Egypt K74+260 81
Qusayar, Yemen, South J58+150 75

Quseir, *Egypt* K64+260 **81**
Qusuriya, *Saudi Arabia* K03+238 **74**
Quteife, *Syria* K50+337 **76**
Quyon, *Quebec* T08+455 **91**
Raahe, *Finland* L33+646 **46**
Raasay & Sd. of, *Scotland* N37+574 **40**
Rab., I., *Yugoslavia* M02+448 **56**
Raba, *Sumbawa, I., Indon.* E07-085 **65**
Rabat, *Morocco* N42+340 **80**
Rabat Kerim, *Iran* J53+355 **75**
Rabigh, *Saudi Arabia* K36+228 **74**
Rabkob. *See* Dharmjaygarh
Race, C., *Newfoundland* R49+466 **90**
Race, The, *Conn.-New York* S73+412 **96**
Rach-zhia, *Vietnam* E89+100 **69**
Raciborz, *Poland* L71+501 **49**
Racine, *Wisconsin* T77+427 **91**
Rada, *Yemen* K01+146 **74**
Radak Chain, *Marshall Is.* A40+100 **106**
Rădăuti, *Romania* L24+479 **60**
Radford, *Virginia* T33+371 **97**
Radhanpur, *India* H21+238 **70**
Radhwa, Jebel, *Saudi Arabia* K41+245 **74**
Radnevo, *Bulgaria* L24+423 **58**
Radnor, *See* Powys
Radnor Forest, *Wales* N20+522 **38**
Radom, *Poland* L53+504 **49**
Radomir, *Bulgaria* L42+425 **58**
Radomsko, *Poland* L64+511 **49**
Radstadt, *Austria* M09+474 **48**
Radviliškis, *Lithuania* L39+558 **47**
Radzyn, *Poland* L44+518 **49**
Rae, *N.-W. Territories* V65+633 **88**
Rae Isthmus, *N.-W. Terr.* T70+666 **89**
Rae R., *N.-W. Territories* V70+676 **88**
Rae Bareli, *India* G53+263 **73**
Raeside, L., *W. Australia* D82-290 **110**
Raetihi, *New Zealand* A28-394 **112**
Rafaela, *Argentina* S09-312 **103**
Rafah, *Egypt* K65+313 **76**
Rafsinjan, *Iran* J25+305 **75**
Raga, *Sudan* L26+084 **81**
Ragaine, *Lithuania* L48+550 **47**
Ragaz Bad, *Switzerland* M33+470 **45**
Raghugarh, *India* G77+244 **73**
Raghunathpur, *India* G20+235 **73**
Raglan, *New Zealand* A31-378 **112**
Raglan Ra., *New Zealand* A41-420 **112**
Ragunda, *Sweden* L81+631 **46**
Ragusa. *See* Dubrovnik
Ragusa, *Sicily* M02+369 **57**
Rahaeng. *See* Tak
Raheita, *Ethiopia* K12+126 **83**
Rahhyut, *Oman* J40+168 **75**
Raiatea, I., *Society Islands* Y10-168 **107**
Raichur, *India* G76+162 **70**
Raida, *Yemen, South* J74+148 **74**
Raida, *Yemen, South* J57+151 **75**
Raiganj, *India* G11+256 **73**
Raikot, *India* G86+306 **72**
Rainbow, *Victoria* C48-359 **109**
Raingarh, *India* G73+311 **72**
Rainier, Mt., *Washington* W10+468 **92**
Rainy L., *Ontario* U18+488 **89**
Raipur, *India* G50+213 **70**
Raivavae, I., *Austral Is.* X75-245 **107**
Raiwind, *Pakistan* H05+312 **72**
Raja, mt., *Borneo* E44-008 **65**
Rajahmundry, *India* G48+170 **70**
Rajakhera, *India* G71+269 **73**
Rajang, R., *Sarawak* E46+020 **65**
Rajanpur, *Pakistan* H28+291 **72**
Rajapalaiyam, *India* G74+095 **70**
Rajasthan, *India* H10+270 **70**
Rajburi, *Thailand* F32+136 **69**
Rajgarh, *India* G88+286 **72**
Rajkot, *India* H25+222 **70**
Rajmahal, *India* G13+250 **73**
Rajmahal Hills, *India* G24+245 **73**
Rajpura, *India* G80+305 **72**
Rajshahi, *Bangladesh* G08+243 **73**
Rajura, *India* G64+197 **70**
Rakahanga, I., *Pacific Oc.* Y66-100 **106**
Rakaposhi, mt., *Kashmir* H03+361 **72**
Raka Tsangpo, R., *Tibet* G20+296 **71**
Rakvere, *Estonia* L22+593 **47**
Raleigh, *New South Wales* B73-305 **109**
Raleigh, *N. Carolina* T22+356 **99**
Raleigh B., *N. Carolina* T06+348 **97**
Ralik Chain, *Marshall Is.* A70+080 **106**
Ram, *Jordan* K57+296 **76**
Rama, *Ethiopia* K30+124 **83**
Rama, *Israel* K58+329 **76**
Ramadi, *Iraq* K10+334 **74**
Ramallah, *Jordan* K59+319 **76**
Ramallo, *Argentina* S00-335 **103**
Ramanthapuran, *India* G67+094 **70**
Rambouillet, *France* M79+487 **54**
Ramee, *Burma* F66+192 **71**
Rathmelton, *Ireland, Rep.* N46+550 **42**
Rameswaram, *India* G64+092 **70**
Ramgarh, *India* H00+281 **72**
Ramgarh, *India* G54+228 **73**
Ramgarh, *India* G26+236 **73**
Ram Hormuz, *Iran* J63+312 **74**
Ramishk, *Iran* J06+269 **75**
Ramkola, *India* G42+236 **73**
Ramle, *Israel* K61+319 **76**
Ramnagar, *India* G57+226 **73**
Ramnagar, *Kashmir* G88+328 **72**
Ramnagar, *Pakistan* H07+323 **72**
Râmnicul Sărat, *Romania* L18+454 **58**
Râmnicu Valcea, *Romania* L34+451 **58**
Ramore, *Ontario* T32+484 **91**
Ramoutsa, *Botswana* L26-248 **84**
Rampart House, *Yukon* X35+671 **88**
Rampur, *India* G33+210 **71**
Rampur, *India* G74+315 **72**
Rampur, *India* G66+288 **73**
Ramsay, *Ontario* T44+474 **91**
Ramsbottom, *England* N14+537 **37**
Ramsele, *Sweden* L81+635 **46**
Ramsey, *Isle of Man* N26+543 **37**
Ramsey I., *Wales* N32+519 **38**
Ramsgate, *England* M82+513 **39**
Ramsgate, *Tasmania* C19-435 **109**
Ramsjö, *Sweden* L86+621 **47**
Ramskapelle, *Belgium* M73+511 **44**
Ramtha, *Jordan* K54+326 **76**
Ramtok, *India* G63+215 **70**
Rana, Fd., *Norway* M12+662 **46**
Ranaghat, *India* G09+231 **73**
Rancagua, *Chile* S65-341 **103**
Rance, *Belgium* M64+501 **44**
Ranchi, *India* G28+234 **73**
Ranchito, *Mexico* U71+233 **100**
Rand, *New South Wales* C21-356 **109**
Randalstown, *N. Ireland* N38+547 **42**
Randazzo, *Sicily* M00+379 **57**
Randers, *Denmark* M30+564 **47**
Randolph, *Vermont* S76+439 **91**
Random I., *Newfoundland* R52+481 **90**
Randsfjord, *Norway* M27+603 **47**
Ranenburg, *U.S.S.R.* K30+532 **61**
Ranfurly, *New Zealand* A59-451 **112**
Rangamati, *Bangladesh* F77+227 **71**
Rangeley, *Maine* S64+450 **90**
Rangeley Ls., *Maine* S65+449 **90**
Rangemore, *New S. Wales* C34-354 **109**
Ranger, *Texas* U52+322 **98**
Rangiora, *New Zealand* A44-433 **112**
Rangitaiki, R., *New Zealand* A20-385 **112**
Rangitikei, R., *New Zealand* A27-401 **112**
Rangitoto Ra., *New Zealand* A26-385 **112**
Rangoon & R., *Burma* F53+168 **71**
Rangpur, *Bangladesh* G04+257 **73**
Rania, *India* H01+295 **72**
Ranibennur, *India* G86+147 **70**
Raniganj, *India* G12+259 **73**
Raniganj, *India* G17+236 **73**
Ranikhet, *India* G63+296 **73**
Rankin Inl., *N.-W. Terr.* U15+632 **89**
Rankins Springs, *N.S.W.* C22-339 **109**
Rannoch, L., *Scotland* N26+567 **41**
Rannoch Moor, *Scotland* N28+566 **41**
Ranong, *Thailand* F39+100 **65**
Rantauparapat, *Sumatra* F31+021 **65**
Rantekombola, mt., *Celebes* E00-034 **65**
Rantsila, *Finland* L26+645 **46**
Ranua, *Finland* L21+659 **46**
Rapa, I., *Austral Islands* X65-275 **107**
Rapadama, *Upper Volta* N06+122 **80**
Raphoe, *Ireland, Rep.* N45+549 **42**
Rapid City, *S. Dakota* U80+441 **93**
Rapla, *Estonia* L31+590 **47**
Rappahannock R., *Virginia* T10+381 **97**
Rapperswil, *Switzerland* M37+472 **45**
Raqqa, *Syria* K36+359 **74**
Rarotonga, I., *Cook Islands* Y60-210 **106**
Ras al Had, *Oman* J01+225 **75**
Ras al Khaymah, *U.A.E.* J24+259 **75**
Rashad, *Sudan* K84+118 **81**
Rashadiya, *Jordan* K56+307 **76**
Rasheiye, *Lebanon* K55+335 **76**
Rashin, *Korea* D28+420 **64**
Rashm, *Iran* J34+352 **75**
Rasht, *Iran* J62+373 **74**
Raška, *Yugoslavia* L56+433 **58**
Ras Lanuf, *Libya* L67+304 **81**
Rason, L., *W. Australia* D64-286 **110**
Rasova, *Romania* L12+442 **58**
Rasskazovo, *U.S.S.R.* K19+526 **61**
Ratangarh, *India* H02+280 **72**
Rat Buri, *Thailand* F32+136 **69**
Rathdrum, *Ireland, Rep.* N37+529 **43**
Rathfriland, *N. Ireland* N37+542 **42**
Ratheale, *Ireland, Rep.* N54+525 **43**
Rathlin I., *N. Ireland* N37+553 **42**
Rathnew, *Ireland, Rep.* N36+530 **43**
Ratibor. *See* Raciborz.
Ratnagiri, *India* H10+170 **70**
Raton, *New Mexico* U87+369 **94**
Rattlesnake Ra., *Wyoming* V14+428 **93**
Rattray Hd., *Scotland* N11+576 **40**
Rättvik, *Sweden* L89+609 **47**
Rauch, *Argentina* R85-367 **103**
Raudha, *Yemen* K05+155 **74**
Raukumara Ra., *N.Z.* A12-380 **112**
Rauma, *Finland* L51+611 **47**
Rautas, *Sweden* L61+680 **46**
Rautavaara, *Finland* L10+635 **46**
Rautio, *Finland* L35+641 **46**
Rauwaq, Jebel er, *Syria* K48+341 **74**
Ravar, *Iran* J20+314 **75**
Ravenna, *Italy* M17+444 **56**
Ravi R., *Pakistan* H03+317 **72**
Rawaidha, *Saudi Arabia* K02+239 **74**
Rawalpindi, *Pakistan* H11+336 **72**
Rawandiz, *Iraq* K30+367 **74**
Rawatsar, *India* H04+292 **72**
Rawene, *New Zealand* A39-354 **112**
Rawlinna, *W. Australia* D58-309 **110**
Rawlins, *Wyoming* V14+418 **93**
Rawson, *Argentina* S31-433 **103**
Ray, C., *Newfoundland* R86+476 **90**
Rayadrug, *India* G79+148 **70**
Raymond, *Alberta* V47+495 **88**
Raymondville, *Texas* U46+266 **94**
Rayon, *Mexico* U58+218 **100**
Rayon, *Mexico* V34+296 **100**
Rays Hill, *Pennsylvania* T20+398 **96**
Razelm L., *Romania* L06+448 **58**
Razgrad, *Bulgaria* L21+435 **58**
Razmak, *Pakistan* H31+327 **72**
Ré, I. de, *France* N08+462 **54**
Reading, *England* N06+514 **39**
Reading, *Pennsylvania* T05+404 **91**
Real, Cord., *Bolivia* S50-162 **104**
Real, Cord., *Ecuador, etc.* T24-020 **104**
Real Castillo, *Mexico* V67+320 **100**
Realico, *Argentina* S25-351 **103**
Realp, *Switzerland* M39+466 **45**
Reata, *Mexico* U67+262 **100**
Rebun, I., *Japan* C54+454 **68**
Recalde, *Argentina* S07-365 **103**
Recherche Arch., *W. Aust.* D73-346 **110**
Rechna Doab, *Pakistan* H15+310 **72**
Recht, *Belgium* M54+503 **44**
Recife, *Brazil* Q30-080 **105**
Reconquista, *Argentina* R88-291 **103**
Recreio, *Brazil* R77-080 **105**
Red Des., *Wyoming* V18+420 **93**
Red L., *Minnesota* U30+480 **93**
Red R., *Louisiana, etc.* U12+313 **95**
Red R., *Minn. Man.* U42+479 **88**
Red R. *See* Song-koi.
Red Sea, *Africa-Arabia* K50+200 **30**
Redbank, *New Jersey* S85+403 **96**
Red Bluff Res., *New Mex.-Texas* U84+320 **94**
Redby, *Minnesota* U29+479 **93**
Red Cliffs, *Victoria* C47-344 **109**
Red Deer, *Alberta* V53+520 **88**
Red Deer R., *Alberta* V38+510 **88**
Redding, *California* W14+406 **92**
Redditch, *England* N12+523 **37**
Redempção, *Brazil* R65-106 **105**
Redfield, *Arkansas* U13+344 **97**
Redfield, *S. Dakota* U55+449 **93**
Red Hill, *S. Australia* C71-336 **109**
Red Hill, *Victoria* C30-384 **109**
Red Indian L., *Nfd.* R70+488 **90**
Redlands, *California* V73+341 **92**
Red Lodge, *Montana* V26+452 **93**
Red Oak, *Iowa* U31+410 **95**
Redon, *France* N13+477 **54**
Redondeta, *Spain* N51+422 **52**
Red Pine, *New Brunswick* S34+474 **90**
Redruth, *England* N31+502 **38**
Redruth, *Michigan* T79+466 **91**
Red Salt L., *Tibet* G18+338 **71**
Red Wing, *Minnesota* U15+446 **93**
Redwood Falls, *Minnesota* U31+445 **93**
Ree L., *Ireland, Rep.* N48+535 **43**
Reed City, *Michigan* T63+439 **91**
Reedsburg, *Wisconsin* U00+435 **91**
Reefton, *New Zealand* A49-421 **112**
Reelfoot, L., *Tennessee* T86+364 **95**
Refresco, *Chile* S59-254 **103**
Regensburg, *Germany* M17+490 **48**
Reggan, *Algeria* M88+264 **80**
Reggio, *Italy* L86+381 **57**
Reggio nell'Emilia, *Italy* M26+447 **56**
Reghin, *Romania* L32+468 **58**
Regina, *Saskatchewan* U87+504 **88**
Registro do Araguaia, *Brazil* R41-157 **105**
Regua, *Portugal* N47+412 **52**
Rehoboth, *Namibia* L78-232 **84**
Rehovo, *Israel* K61+319 **76**
Reichenbach, *E. Germany* M16+506 **48**
Reidsville, *N. Carolina* T28+364 **97**
Reigate, *England* N01+512 **39**
Reigi, *Estonia* L45+589 **47**
Reims, *France* M66+493 **54**
Reina Adelaide, Arch. de la, *Chile* T00-522 **103**
Reindeer L., *Saskatchewan* U75+570 **88**
Reinosa, *Spain* N25+430 **52**
Reitan, *Norway* M22+629 **46**
Reitz, *Orange Free State* L10-278 **84**
Rekinniki, *U.S.S.R.* B07+608 **63**
Relizane, (Ighil-Izane), *Alg.* M86+356 **80**
Remanso, *Brazil* Q73-096 **105**
Remarkable, Mt., *S. Aust.* C71-328 **109**
Rembang, *Java* E52-067 **65**
Remedios, *Cuba* T27+225 **101**
Remedios, *Panama* T40+083 **101**
Remiremont, *France* M51+480 **54**
Remoulins, *France* M63+440 **55**
Remscheid, *W. Germany* M47+512 **48**
Remüs, *Switzerland* M28+468 **45**
Rena, *Norway* M22+611 **47**
Renaix, *Belgium* M68+507 **44**
Renca, *Argentina* S32-327 **103**
Rendsburg, *Germany* M32+543 **48**
Renfrew, *Ontario* T10+455 **91**
Renfrew, *Scotland* N26+559 **41**
Rengat, *Sumatra* F14-006 **65**
Reni, *India* H00+287 **72**
Renigunta, *India* G63+138 **70**
Renk, *Sudan* K72+118 **81**
Renkum, *Netherlands* M56+520 **44**
Renmark, *S. Australia* C56-342 **109**
Rennell, I., *Solomon Islands* B29-120 **106**
Rennes, *France* N10+481 **54**
Reno, *Nevada* V89+395 **92**
Renovo, *Pennsylvania* T16+413 **91**
Rensselaer, *New York* S82+426 **91**
Renswoude, *Netherlands* M57+521 **44**
Renville, *Minnesota* U32+448 **93**
Reo, *Flores I., Indonesia* D87-083 **65**
Réole la, *France* N00+445 **55**
Reparticão, *Brazil* R67-048 **105**
Republic Dominican, *W.I.* S64+190 **101**
Republican R., *Nebraska* U54+400 **95**
Repulse B., *N.-W. Terr.* T66+662 **89**
Repulse B., *Queensland* C05-206 **111**
Requena, *Peru* S81-049 **104**
Requena, *Spain* N07+395 **53**
Resita, *Romania* L49+453 **58**
Resistencia, *Argentina* R84-274 **103**
Resolution, *New Zealand* A80-457 **112**
Resolution, *N.-W. Terr.* V52+609 **88**
Resolution I., *N.-W. Terr.* S30+614 **89**
Rethel, *France* M64+495 **54**
Réthimnon, *Crete* L33+354 **59**
Retie, *Belgium* M61+513 **44**
Réunion, I., *Indian Ocean* J30-210 **77**
Reusel, *Netherlands* M59+514 **44**
Reutlingen, *W. Germany* M35+485 **48**
Reutte, *Austria* M26+475 **48**
Revda, *U.S.S.R.* J00+568 **61**
Revel. *See* Tallinn
Revelstoke, *B.C.* V79+509 **88**
Revilla Gigedo Is., *Mexico* V42+190 **100**
Revivum, *Israel* K61+310 **76**
Rewa, *India* G52+245 **73**
Rewari, *India* G80+282 **72**
Rey, I. del, *Panama* T25+084 **101**
Reydharfjord, *Iceland* N81+650 **46**
Reyes, *Mexico* U74+196 **100**
Reykjavik, *Iceland* P41+641 **46**
Reynosa, *Mexico* U50+260 **100**
Rezā'iyeh, *Iran* K00+376 **74**
Rēzēkne, *Latvia* L16+565 **47**
Rhatikon, mts., *Switzerland-Austria* M32+470 **45**
Rhayader, *Wales* N21+523 **38**
Rheden, *Netherlands* M54+520 **44**
Rhein R., *Germany, etc.* M46+506 **48**
Rheine, *W. Germany* M46+523 **48**
Rheinland-Pfalz, *W. Germany* M48+502 **48**
Rhenen, *Netherlands* M57+520 **44**
Rheydt, *W. Germany* M51+512 **48**
Rhine, R. *N.-W. Europe* M50+510 **50**
Rhinelander, *Wisconsin* T87+457 **91**
Rhode I., *Rhode Island* S68+415 **96**
Rhode Island, state, *U.S.A.* S70+416 **99**
Rhodes. *See* Rodhos, I.
Rhodesia, N. *See* Zambia
Rhodesia, *See* Zimbabwe
Rhon Geb., *W. Germany* M30+504 **48**
Rhondda, *Wales* N21+516 **38**
Rhône, dep., *France* M62+459 **54**
Rhône, R.,*France, etc.* M62+445 **55**
Rhyl, *Wales* N21+533 **38**
Riaño, *Spain* N30+430 **52**
Riau, Kep., arch., *Indon.* F04+004 **65**
Riaza, *Spain* N21+413 **52**
Ribabesella, *Spain* N30+434 **52**
Ribadeo, *Spain* N42+433 **52**
Ribble R., *England* N14+539 **37**
Ribe, *Denmark* M38+553 **47**
Ribeirão Preto, *Brazil* R17-212 **105**
Ribera, *Sicily* M11+375 **57**
Riberalta, *Bolivia* S36-110 **104**
Riccall, *England* N06+538 **37**
Riccarton, *New Zealand* A44-435 **112**
Rice Lake, *Wisconsin* U10+455 **93**
Richards C., *Arctic Ocean* T30+830 **26**
Richardson Mts., *N.Z.* A68-448 **112**
Richardton, *N. Dakota* U74+469 **93**
Richey, *Montana* U89+477 **93**
Richfield, *Utah* V43+388 **92**
Richibucto, *New Brunswick* S29+467 **90**
Richland, *Missouri* U14+379 **97**
Richland, *Washington* V86+463 **92**
Richland Center, *Wisconsin* U02+433 **91**
Richmond, *California* W15+379 **92**
Richmond, *Cape Province* L38-314 **84**
Richmond, *England* N10+544 **37**
Richmond, *England* N02+514 **39**
Richmond, *Indiana* T59+399 **91**
Richmond, *Kentucky* T56+378 **97**
Richmond, *Maine* S59+441 **90**
Richmond, *New South Wales* B86-336 **109**
Richmond, *New York* S85+406 **91**
Richmond, *New Zealand* A41-413 **112**
Richmond, *Quebec* S73+457 **91**
Richmond, *Queensland* C41-208 **111**
Richmond, *Utah* V41+419 **94**
Richmond, *Virginia* T15+375 **97**
Richmond R., *New S. Wales* B70-289 **109**
Richwood, *Minnesota* U35+469 **93**
Richwood, *W. Virginia* T33+382 **97**
Rickmansworth, *England* N03+516 **39**
Ricla, *Spain* N09+415 **53**
Riddes, *Switzerland* M47+462 **45**
Ridgetown, *Ontario* T41+425 **91**
Ridgway, *Pennsylvania* T22+414 **91**
Ridi, *Nepal* G39+280 **73**
Riding Mount Park, *Man.* U60+506 **88**
Ridout, *Ontario* T48+476 **91**
Riesa, *E. Germany* M10+513 **48**
Rietavas, *Lithuania* L48+557 **47**
Rieti, *Italy* M13+424 **56**
Rifle, *Colorado* V17+395 **94**
Riga, *Latvia* L35+569 **47**
Riga, G. of *Latvia* L36+577 **47**
Rigan, *Iran* J06+286 **75**
Rigmati, *Iran* J11+276 **75**
Rignasco, *Switzerland* M38+463 **45**
Rigolet, *Labrador* R80+542 **89**
Rihand Dam, *India* G43+241 **73**
Rijeka, *Yugoslavia* M04+453 **56**
Rijswijk, *Netherlands* M64+521 **44**
Rimatara, I., *Austral Is.* Y20-230 **107**
Rimini, *Italy* M15+440 **56**
Rimouski, *Quebec* S51+484 **90**
Rincon, *Cuba* T44+230 **101**
Rincon, *New Mexico* V12+326 **98**
Rindal, *Norway* M35+631 **46**
Rineanna, *Ireland, Rep.* N53+527 **43**
Ringarooma B., *Tasmania* C14-408 **109**
Ringelspitz, mt., *Switz.* M34+469 **45**
Ringkøbing, *Denmark* M40+561 **47**
Ringvassøy, I., *Norway* L66+700 **46**
Ringwood, *Victoria* C29-378 **109**
Rinihue, *Chile* S75-397 **103**
Riobamba, *Ecuador* T22-018 **104**
Rio Branco, *Brazil* R27-251 **103**
Rio Branco, *Brazil* S48-100 **104**
Rio Branco, R., *Brazil* S09+015 **104**
Rio Branco, *Uruguay* R51-325 **103**
Rio Bueno, *Chile* S78-404 **103**
Rio Chico, *Argentina* S52-498 **103**
Rio Chico, *Venezuela* S35+103 **104**
Rio Colorado, *Argentina* S25-389 **103**
Rio Conchos, *Mexico* V00+292 **94**
Rio Cuarto, *Argentina* S26-332 **103**
Rio de Janeiro, *Brazil* Q80-229 **105**
Rio dè Oro, *Colombia* S80+084 **104**
Rio-de-Oro, *Morocco* N80+250 **80**
Rio Fenix, *Argentina* S66-464 **103**
Rio Florido, *Mexico* V01+265 **100**
Rio Gallegos & R., *Argent.* S56+516 **103**
Rio Grande, *Argentina* S47-538 **103**
Rio Grande, *Brazil* R43-320 **103**
Rio Grande, *Mexico, etc.* U84+300 **94**
Rio Grande City, *Texas* U53+264 **94**
Rio Grande del Norte, *Mexico-U.S.A.* V02+308 **100**
Rio Hacha, *Colombia* S77+115 **104**
Rio Hondo, *Argentina* S29-275 **103**
Rio Muerto, *Argentina* S10-262 **103**
Rio Mulato, *Bolivia* S41-196 **104**
Rio Muni, *W. Africa* M30+016 **82**
Rio Negro, *Brazil* R29-261 **103**
Rionero in Vulture, *Italy* L86+409 **57**
Rio Pardo, *Brazil* R53-203 **105**
Rio Verde, *Brazil* R35-178 **105**
Rio Verde, *Ecuador* T26+010 **104**
Rio Verde, *Mexico* U60+220 **100**
Rioz, *France* M54+475 **54**
Riozinho, *Brazil* S41-094 **104**
Ripats, *Sweden* L56+669 **46**
Ripley, *California* V59+335 **92**
Ripley, *England* N09+531 **37**
Ripley, *Mississippi* T84+347 **97**
Ripley, *New York* T28+422 **96**
Ripley, *Tennessee* T88+358 **97**
Ripley, *W. Virginia* T40+388 **91**
Ripon, *England* N09+541 **37**
Ripon, *Quebec* T01+459 **91**
Ripon, *Wisconsin* T83+439 **91**
Risafe, *Syria* K37+357 **74**
Risalpur, *Pakistan* H18+341 **72**
Risbäck, *Sweden* L59+673 **46**
Rishiri, I., *Japan* C53+452 **68**
Rishon-le-Zion, *Israel* K61+320 **76**
Risør, *Norway* M34+587 **47**
Ristijarvi, *Finland* L10+645 **46**
Risut, *Oman* J36+170 **75**
Ritchie's Arch., *Andaman Is.* F70+122 **71**

Rivadavia, Argentina S18-241 103
Rivas, Nicaragua T65+115 101
Rivera, Argentina S20-371 103
Rivera, Uruguay R64-310 103
Riverhead, New York S76+409 91
Rivero, I., Chile S86-456 103
Riversdale, New Zealand A67-459 112
Riverside, California V74+340 92
Riverside Mt., California V57+340 92
Riverton, New Zealand A71-463 112
Riverton, S. Australia C67-342 109
Riverton, Wyoming V20+430 93
Riviera di Levante, Italy M34+440 54
Riviera di Ponente, Italy M42+438 54
Rivière a Pièrre, Quebec S73+470 91
Rivière du Loup, Quebec S57+479 90
Riyadh (Ar Riyād), Saudi Arabia J80+246 74
Riyaq, Lebanon K54+339 76
Rizaiyeh. See Rezā'īveh
Rize, Turkey K25+413 74
Rizokarpaso, Cyprus K64+356 76
Rizzuto C., Italy L77+389 57
Roa, Spain N24+417 52
Roanne, France M66+461 54
Roanoke, Alabama T62+332 97
Roanoke, Virginia T30+373 97
Roanoke R., N. Carolina T18+366 97
Roaringwater B., Ireland, Rep. N57+515 43
Roatan I., Honduras T69+164 101
Robat Thana, Pakistan H84+298 70
Robbins I., Tasmania C30-407 109
Robe, S. Australia C62-372 109
Robe, Mt., New S. Wales C53-316 109
Robe R., Ireland, Rep. N55+536 42
Roberts, Montana V25+454 93
Robertsfors, Sweden L55+642 46
Robertsganj, India G41+247 73
Robertsport, Liberia N68+068 80
Robertstown, Ireland, Rep. N41+532 43
Robertstown, S. Australia C66-340 109
Roberval, Quebec S73+485 90
Robeson Ch., Arctic Ocean S00+820 26
Robinson, Illinois T76+390 95
Robinson Crusoe, I., Chile T25-335 107
Robinson's, Newfoundland R83+483 90
Robinvale, Victoria C43-345 109
Robore, Bolivia R87-183 104
Robson, Mt., B.C. V84+533 88
Robstown, Texas U46+278 94
Roca, la, Spain N40+391 52
Rocha, Uruguay R55-344 103
Rochdale, England N13+536 37
Rochefort, Belgium M59+502 44
Rochefort, France N06+459 54
Rochester, England M87+514 39
Rochester, Michigan T49+427 91
Rochester, Minnesota U15+441 93
Rochester, New Hampshire S66+433 91
Rochester, New York T16+432 91
Rochester, Victoria C32-364 109
Roche-sur-Yon, la, France N09+467 54
Rock Pt., New Zealand A47-409 112
Rock, The, New S. Wales C18-353 109
Rockall, I., Atlantic Ocean N82+575 34
Rockefeller Plateau, Antarc. X40-800 27
Rockford, Alabama T68+329 97
Rockford, Illinois T85+423 91
Rockhampton, Queensland B86-232 111
Rock Hill, S. Carolina T36+349 97
Rockingham, N. Carolina T29+349 97
Rock Island, Illinois U04+415 91
Rockland, Maine S55+441 90
Rockland, Massachusetts S65+421 96
Rockland, Ontario T02+455 91
Rockport, Indiana T72+379 97
Rockport, Missouri U34+404 95
Rock Springs, Wyoming V26+416 93
Rockstone, Guyana R81+058 104
Rockville, Maryland T13+391 96
Rockwell City, Iowa U28+424 95
Rockwood, Tennessee T58+358 97
Rocky Mts., N. America V30+550 88
Rockyford, Colorado U82+381 94
Rocky Mount, N. Carolina T16+360 97
Rockymount, Virginia T29+370 97
Rocky Mt. Nat. Park, Colo. V09+406 98
Rocroi, France M63+499 54
Rødby, Denmark M22+547 47
Rodez, France M75+443 55
Rodhopi, Greece L28+412 58
Rodhos, Greece L14+364 59
Rodhos, I., Greece L12+362 59
Rodkhan, Pakistan H64+261 70
Rodney, Mississippi U07+319 97
Rodopi Planina, Bulg.-Greece L36+415 59
Rodosto. See Tekirdag
Rodriguez, I., Indian Ocean H70-195 77
Roe R., N. Ireland N42+551 42
Roebourne, W. Australia E17-208 110
Roermond, Netherlands M54+512 44
Roesbrugge, Belgium M74+509 44
Roeselare, Belgium M71+509 44
Roes Welcome Sound, N.-W. Territories T70+650 89
Roeulx, Belgium M65+505 44
Rogachev, Byelorussia L00+531 60
Rogers City, Michigan T53+455 91
Rogersville, New Brunswick S33+468 90
Rogersville, Tennessee T48+364 97
Rogliano, Corsica M33+374 55
Rohri, Pakistan H36+276 70
Rohtak, India G80+289 72
Roi Et, Thailand F08+161 69
Roisin, Belgium M68+503 44
Rojas, Argentina S04-342 103
Rokishkis, Lithuania L25+560 47
Rolde, Netherlands M50+530 44
Rolla, Missouri U11+380 97
Rolle, Switzerland M52+465 45
Rolvsøya, Norway L36+709 46
Roma, Queensland C07-265 111
Roma, Sweden L69+575 47
Roma, Italy M15+419 57
Romang I., Indonesia D46-077 65
Romaine, Quebec S04+502 90
Romaine R., Quebec S21+514 90
Roman, Romania L19+469 58
Romania, S.-E. Eur. L24+460 51
Romans, France M60+451 55
Romanshorn, Switzerland M34+476 45
Romanzof, C., Alaska Z10+618 99
Rome, Georgia T61+342 97
Rome, New York T03+432 91
Rome. See Roma.
Romerée, Belgium M62+501 44
Romford, England M89+516 39
Romney, W. Virginia T23+393 91
Romney Marsh, England M85+511 39
Romny, Ukraine K69+508 60
Rømø, I., Denmark M39+551 47
Romodanovo, U.S.S.R. J88+544 61
Romont, Switzerland M48+467 45
Romsdalshorn, Norway M43+625 46
Romsey, England N09+510 39
Ron, Vietnam E81+178 69
Ronda, Kashmir G89+355 72
Ronda, Spain N31+367 52
Rondeau, Ontario T42+423 91
Rondonia, state, Brazil S31-118 104
Ronge Lac la, Sask. V00+552 88
Rønne, Bornholm, I., Den. M01+551 47
Ronneby, Sweden L88+562 47
Ronne Entrance, Antarctica T00-720 27
Ronne Ice Shelf, Antarctica S00-770 27
Ronse, Belgium M68+507 44
Roosendaal, Netherlands M63+515 44
Roosevelt, I., Antarctica Y65-800 27
Roosevelt Res., Arizona V33+340 98
Rooseveltown, New York S88+450 91
Roosky, Ireland, Rep. N47+538 42
Roper, R., N. Terr., Aust. D00-154 111
Roquefort, France N02+440 55
Rora Hd., Orkney N21+589 40
Rori, India G89+297 72
Røros, Norway M21+626 46
Rorschach, Switzerland M33+475 45
Røs Vatn, Norway M06+658 46
Rosa, la, Switzerland M30+464 45
Rosa, Monte, Switz.-Italy M43+459 45
Rosablanche, mt., Switz. M46+461 45
Rosarinho, Brazil R85-036 104
Rosario, Argentina S04-329 103
Rosario, Brazil Q86-029 105
Rosario, Chile S60-243 103
Rosario, Mexico V03+263 100
Rosario, Mexico V64+301 100
Rosario, Mexico V05+229 100
Rosario de la Frontera, Argentina S30-258 103
Rosario Oeste, Brazil R68-148 105
Rosario Tala, Argentina R85-323 103
Rosas, Spain M71+423 53
Rosas, G. of, Spain M70+422 53
Roscommon, Michigan T58+445 91
Roscommon & co., Ireland, Rep. N49+536 42
Roscrea, Ireland, Rep. N47+529 43
Rose, I., Samoa Z18-150 106
Roseau, Minnesota U34+488 93
Rosebery, Tasmania C27-418 109
Rosebud, S. Dakota U65+432 93
Roseburg, Oregon W20+432 92
Rosedale, Mississippi U06+338 97
Roseires, Sudan K64+118 81
Rosenheim, W.Germany M17+478 48
Rosetown, Saskatchewan V16+514 88
Rosetta (Rashid), Egypt K88+314 81
Rosier, C., Quebec S25+489 90
Rosignano Marittamo, Italy M27+433 56
Rosignol, Guyana R76+063 104
Roslavl, U.S.S.R. K73+540 60
Rosport, Luxembourg M51+498 44
Ross, England N16+519 38
Ross, New Zealand A55-429 112
Ross, Tasmania C15-420 109
Ross Ice Shelf, Antarctica Z80-810 27
Ross, I., Antarctica A70-770 27
Ross I., Burma F42+122 71
Ross R., Yukon W70+618 88
Ross Sea, Antarctica Z30-750 27
Rossa, Switzerland M35+464 45
Ross & Cromarty, co., See Highland
Rossano, Italy L80+396 57
Rosscarberry, Ireland, Rep. N54+516 43
Rosseau L., Ontario T28+452 91
Rossel I., Papua New Guinea B66-114 111
Rossignol, Belgium M57+497 44
Rossignol L., Nova Scotia S31+442 90
Rossland, British Columbia V78+492 88
Rosslare Harb, Ireland, Rep. N38+523 43
Rosslyn, Virginia T13+389 96
Rosta, Norway L61+690 46
Rosthern, Saskatchewan V09+529 88
Rostock, E. Germany M18+541 48
Rostov, U.S.S.R. K32+472 61
Rostov, U.S.S.R. K34+572 60
Roswell, New Mexico U87+334 94
Rosyth, Scotland N21+560 41
Rota, I., Mariana Islands C27+148 106
Rothenburg, Germany M29+494 48
Rotherham, England N08+534 37
Rothesay, Scotland N30+558 41
Roti, I., Indonesia D72-108 65
Roto, New South Wales C27-331 109
Rotorua, New Zealand A22-381 112
Rotterdam, Netherlands M63+519 44
Rotuma, I., Fiji A17-130 106
Roubaix, France M71+507 54
Rouen, France M84+495 54
Rõuge, Estonia L18+577 47
Roulers, Belgium M71+509 44
Round Mt., New S. Wales B77-304 109
Roundup, Montana V22+464 93
Roura, Fr. Guiana R44+046 105
Rous, Pen., Chile S55-555 103
Rousay I., Orkney, Scotland N18+592 40
Rouse's Point, New York S80+450 91
Rousseau, S. Dakota U61+443 93
Roussillon, prov., France M74+427 55
Rouveen, Netherlands M53+526 44
Rouyn, Quebec T25+482 91
Rovaniemi, Finland L26+665 46
Roveredo, Switzerland M35+462 45
Rovigo, Italy M19+451 56
Rovinari, Romania L41+449 58
Rovno, Ukraine L22+506 60
Rowena, New South Wales C07-298 109
Roxburgh, New Zealand A64-457 112
Roxburgh, Scotland N15+556 41
Roxbury, New York S87+423 96
Royal Canal, Ireland, Rep. N38-534 43
Royale, I., Michigan T84+480 91
Royan, France N06+456 54
Rozet, Wyoming V02+443 93
Rožňava, Czechoslovakia L57+485 49
Rtishchevo, U.S.S.R. K07+523 61
Ruabon, Wales N18+530 38
Ruahine Ra., New Zealand A24-400 112
Ruapehu, Mt., New Zealand A26-393 112
Rubtsovsk, U.S.S.R. G53+513 62
Ruby, Alaska Y30+645 99
Rucava, Latvia L53+561 47
Rudauli, India G49+267 73
Rudbar, Afghanistan H74+301 75
Ruddervoorde, Belgium M71+511 44
Rudkøbing, Denmark M26+549 47
Rudnaya Pristan, U.S.S.R. C84+442 63
Rudok, Tibet G62+334 70
Rudolf L., Kenya K54+034 83
Rueiba, Sudan L08+156 81
Ruel, Ontario T39+472 91
Ruffec, France M89+460 54
Rufino, Argentina S16-342 103
Rugby, England N08+524 37
Rugby, N. Dakota U60+484 93
Rugeley, England N12+528 37
Rügen, I., E. Germany M10+544 48
Rui Khaf, Iran H89+346 75
Rūjiena, Latvia L28+579 47
Ruk, Pakistan H38+278 70
Rukumkot, Nepal G44+286 73
Rukwa L., Tanzania K76-080 83
Rumania. See Romania.
Rum, I., Scotland N38+570 40
Rumbek, Sudan L02+068 81
Rumburk, Czechoslovakia M03+509 48
Rumegies, France M70+505 44
Rumford Falls, Maine S63+445 90
Rumigny, France M66+498 44
Rumillies, Belgium M69+506 44
Rum Jungle, N. Terr., Aust. D24-123 110
Rumoi, Japan C50+439 68
Rumuruti, Kenya K50+002 83
Runanga, New Zealand A52-424 112
Runcorn, England N16+533 37
Rungwa, Tanzania K68-070 83
Rungwe Mt., Tanzania K66-092 83
Rupar, India G81+309 72
Rupbas, India G75+270 73
Rupert, Idaho V54+426 94
Rurrenabaque, Bolivia S45-145 104
Rurutu I., Tubuai Islands X60-250 107
Rusape, Zimbabwe K78-186 84
Ruse (Ruschuk), Bulgaria L24+438 58
Ruseifa, Jordan K54+320 76
Rusele, Sweden L72+648 46
Rushworth, Victoria C30-366 109
Rusne, R., Lithuania L51+552 47
Russas, Brazil Q48-049 105
Russel, C., N.-W. Terr. V75+753 88
Russelkonda, India G32+200 71
Russell, Kansas U54+388 95
Russell, New Zealand A35-353 112
Russell Pt., N.-W. Terr. V62+729 88
Russellville, Alabama T76+345 95
Russellville, Kentucky T72+368 97
Russian Soc. Federated Soviet Reps. (Russia), U.S.S.R. 62-63
Russkoye Ustye, U.S.S.R. C07+713 63
Russo, Switzerland M38+462 45
Rustak, Afghanistan H31+371 75
Rustburg, Virginia T25+372 97
Ruston, Louisiana U16+326 95
Rutba, Iraq K29+329 74
Rutherfordton, N. Carolina T42+353 97
Ruthi, Switzerland M33+473 45
Ruthin, Wales N20+531 38
Rutland, Vermont S78+436 91
Rutland, co., See Leicester & co.
Rutland I., Andaman Is. F74+114 71
Ruurlo, Netherlands M51+521 44
Ruvuma R., Mozambique K30-108 83
Ruwenzori, Mts., Uganda L00+004 83
Ružomberok, Czechoslovakia L64+491 49
Rwanda, Central Africa L00-025 83
Ryan, L., Scotland N30+550 41
Ryazan, U.S.S.R. K32+546 60
Ryazhsk, U.S.S.R. K30+537 60
Rybachiy, Pol., U.S.S.R. K75+694 62
Rybinsk, U.S.S.R. K37+580 60
Rybinskoye Res., U.S.S.R. K40+586 60
Rybnoe, U.S.S.R. E85+729 63
Ryde, I. of W., England N07+507 39
Rye, England M86+510 39
Rye Patch Res., Nevada V80+406 92
Rylstone, New South Wales C00-328 109
Rymarov, Czechoslovakia L77+499 49
Rypin, Poland L64+531 49
Ryukyu Retto, Japan D50+250 64
Rzeszów, Poland L48+501 49
Rzhev, U.S.S.R. K64+563 60
Saalfeld, E. Germany M22+506 48
Saanen, Switzerland M46+465 45
Saarbrücken, W. Germany M48+492 48
Saaremaa, I., Estonia L44+584 47
Saariselkä, Finland L12+682 46
Saarland, W. Germany M46+493 48
Saarlouis, W. Germany M50+493 48
Saas Grund, Switzerland M42+461 45
Saavedra, Argentina S15-378 103
Saavedra, Chile S80-387 99
Saba, Iran J69+308 74
Sabac, Yugoslavia L62+448 58
Sabah (N. Borneo), Borneo 65
Sabalgarh, India G78+262 70
Sabana, Arch. de, Cuba T30+232 101
Sabanalarga, Colombia T00+106 104
Sabancuy, Mexico U06+190 100
Sab Biyar, Syria K44+338 76
Sabile, Latvia L44+570 47
Sabiñanigo, Spain N03+425 53
Sabine and L., Texas U23+296 95
Sabine R., Texas U22+300 95
Sabine Mt., Antarctica A65-720 27
Sable, France N02+478 54
Sable, C., Florida T37+252 99
Sable, C., Nova Scotia S33+435 90
Sable I., Nova Scotia S00+439 90
Sables d'Olonne, les, France N10+465 54
Sabrina Coast, Antarctica E45-660 27
Sabzawar (Shindand), Afghan. H77+334 75
Sabzawar, Iran J14+362 75
Sacandaga Res. & R., New York S85+431 96
Sac City, Iowa U30+424 95
Sacedon, Spain N17+405 53
Sachigo R., Ontario U05+546 89
Sachsen-Anhalt, W. Germany M22+520 48
Sackets Harbor, New York T07+439 91
Sackville, New Brunswick S26+459 90
Saco, Maine S63+435 90
Saco, Montana V14+485 93
Sacramento, Brazil R14-199 105
Sacramento, California W09+385 92
Sacramento Mts., New Mex. V03+332 94
Sacramento R., California W12+392 92
Sada, Yemen K07+169 74
Sádaba, Spain N07+423 53
Sadabad, India G72+274 73
Sada Bandeira, Angola M08-148 82
Sadad, Syria K48+343 76
Saddleback Mt., Maine S63+449 90
Sadhaura, India G77+304 72
Sadij, Iran J07+257 75
Sadiya, India F56+278 71
Sa'diya, Jebel, Saudi Arabia K29+207 74
Sadmarda, Afghanistan H47+356 75
Sado, I., Japan C70+380 68
Sadra, India H13+233 70
Saduan, Saudi Arabia K11+192 74
Saeki, Japan D19+330 68
Safad, (Zefat), Israel K57+330 76
Safed Koh Ra., Afghan.-Pak. H26+340 72
Saffuriya, Israel K58+327 76
Safi, Morocco N56+320 80
Safidabeh, Iran H87+308 75
Safif, Saudi Arabia J53+214 75
Safita, Syria K53+348 76
Safranbolu, Turkey K73+412 74
Saga, Japan D28+332 68
Sagaing, Burma F54+218 71
Sagami B., Japan C64+352 68
Sagar, India G67+238 73
Sagar I., India G10+217 73
Sagata, Ethiopia K60+058 83
Sagauli, India G31+267 73
Sage Plains, Oregon W06+437 92
Saginaw, Michigan T54+435 91
Saginaw B., Michigan T52+440 91
Sagone, G. de, Corsica M39+421 56
Sagres, Portugal N53+370 52
Sagua la Grande, Cuba T30+228 101
Saguenay R., Quebec S64+483 90
Sagunto, Spain N01+397 53
Saham, Oman J19+242 75
Sahambavany, Madagascar J60-142 83
Sahand, mt., Iran J82+376 74
Sahara Desert, Africa 80-81
Saharanpur, India G74+297 72
Saharien Atlas Mts., Algeria M80+334 80
Sahaswan, India G67+281 73
Sahiadriparvat Ra., India G85+206 70
Sahibganj, India G14+252 73
Sahiwal, Pakistan H11+307 72
Sahuajo, Mexico U76+200 100
Sahuaripa, Mexico V24+288 100
Sahugun, Spain N30+423 52
Sahun, Yemen, South J72+141 74
Sahy, Czechoslovakia L66+481 49
Sahyadri Mts., India H03+150 70
Saibai, I., Papua New Guinea C44-095 111
Saida. See Sidon
Saidabad, Iran J26+295 75
Saidapet, India G58+130 70
Said Bundas, Sudan L32+084 81
Saidpur, India G41+256 73
Saidu, Pakistan H16+348 70
Saignelégier, Switzerland M48+473 45
Saigon, Vietnam E80+108 69
Saihut, Yemen, South J53+153 75
Sailana, India H00+235 70
Saimaa Kanal, Fin.-U.S.S.R. L10+610 47
Saimaa, L., Finland L12+613 47
St Abb's Hd., Scotland N13+559 41
St Affrique, France M73+440 55
St Agatha, Maine S50+472 90
St Agrève, France M64+450 55
St Albans, England N02+517 39
St Albans, Vermont S79+448 91
St Amour, France M58+464 54
St Andre, Quebec S58+477 90
St André C., Madagascar K04-164 83
St Andrews, New Brunswick S42+451 90
St Andrews, New Zealand A53-445 112
St Andrews, Scotland N17+563 41
Ste Anne, Quebec S60+474 90
Ste Anne de Beaupré, Quebec S66+470 91
Ste Anne de la Pérage, Que. S73+466 91
Ste Anne des Monts, Quebec S39+491 90
St Anns Bay, Jamaica T13+185 101
St Anthonis, Netherlands M55+516 44
St Anthony, Idaho V41+440 98
St Antönien, Switzerland M31+470 45
St Arnaud, Victoria C41-367 109
St Asaph, Wales N21+532 38
St Augustin, C. de, Madagascar K10-238 83
St Augustine, Florida T38+299 97
St Austell & B., England N29+503 38
Ste Barbara, Venezuela S22+096 104
St Barthélemy, I., Leeward Is. S17+179 101
St Béat, France M86+429 55
St Bečej, Yugoslavia L60+456 58
St Bernard Pass, Gd., Switzerland-Italy M46+457 56
St Boniface, Manitoba U40+500 88
St Bride's B., Wales N32+518 38
St Brieuc, France N17+485 54
St Calais, France M86+480 54
St Catherines, Ontario T25+432 91
Ste Cécile, Quebec S66+457 91
St Chamond, France M63+455 54
St Charles, Michigan T55+433 91
St Charles, C., Labrador R64+524 89
St Chély d'Apcher, France M70+448 55
St Christopher, I. (St Kitts), Leeward Islands S16+173 101
St Clair, Michigan T45+429 91
St Clair, L., Mich.-Ont. T46+425 91
St Clair L., Tasmania C23-421 109
St Cloud, Minnesota U25+456 93
Ste Croix, Switzerland M51+468 45
St Croix, R., Wisconsin U16+457 99

St Davids & Hd., *Wales* N32+519 **38**
St Denis, *France* M76+489 **54**
St di Nova Siri, *Italy* L80+402 **57**
St Dizier, *France* M60+486 **54**
St Elias Mt., *Alaska* X40+604 **99**
St Elias Ra., *Yukon* X30+602 **88**
Saintes, *France* N04+457 **54**
St Etienne, *France* M64+454 **54**
St Eustatius, I., *Leeward Is.* S17+175 **101**
St Fabien, *Quebec* S53+483 **90**
St Fargeau, *France* M72+477 **54**
St Felicien, *Quebec* S74+486 **90**
Saintfield, *N. Ireland* N35+545 **42**
St Filipsland, *Netherlands* M65+516 **44**
St Fillans, *Scotland* N25+564 **41**
St Finans B., *Ireland, Rep.* N58+518 **43**
St Florent & G. de, *Corsica* M35+428 **56**
St Florentin, *France* M68+480 **54**
St Flour, *France* M72+450 **55**
St Francis, *Maine* S54+472 **90**
St Francis B., *Namibia* M02-252 **84**
St Francis, L., *Quebec* S67+459 **91**
St Francis, L., *Quebec* S86+452 **91**
St Francis R., *Arkansas* U03+358 **97**
St Francis R., *Quebec* S76+459 **91**
St Fulgent, *France* N07+469 **54**
St Gabriel de Brandon, *Que.* S80+463 **91**
St Gallen & canton, *Switz.* M34+474 **45**
St Gaudens, *France* M86+431 **55**
St Gédéon, *Quebec* S70+485 **90**
Ste Genevieve, *Missouri* U00+380 **97**
St George, *New Brunswick* S41+452 **90**
St George Hd., *N.S.W.* B86-352 **109**
St George I., *Bering Sea* Z29+564 **99**
St Georges, *Fr. Guiana* R41+037 **105**
St George's B., *Nfd.* R86+483 **90**
St George's Chan., *Ire.-Wales* N34+520 **38**
St Georges de Beauce, *Que.* S64+461 **90**
St Gérard, *Belgium* M62+502 **44**
St Germain, *France* M77+488 **54**
St German, *Puerto Rico* S42+181 **101**
St Gheorghe I., *Romania* L03+450 **58**
St Ghislain, *Belgium* M67+504 **44**
St Gilgen, *Austria* M10+477 **48**
St Gilles, *France* M64+437 **55**
St Gillis, *Belgium* M65+510 **44**
St Gillis-Waas, *Belgium* M65+512 **44**
St Gingolph, *Switzerland* M49+464 **45**
St Girons, *France* M83+430 **55**
St Gotthard, pass, *Switz.* M38+466 **45**
St Guenolé, *France* N26+478 **54**
St Helena, *Atlantic Ocean* N36-158 **85**
St Helena B.,*Cape Province* L72-328 **84**
St Helens, *England* N17+535 **37**
St Helens, Mt., *Washington* W12+461 **92**
St Hilaire, *New Brunswick* S51+473 **90**
St Hubert, *Belgium* M58+500 **44**
St Hyacinthe, *Quebec* S78+457 **91**
St Ignace, *Michigan* T59+459 **91**
St Imier, *Switzerland* M48+472 **45**
St Irénée, *Quebec* S61+476 **91**
St Ives, *England* N01+524 **37**
St Ives & B., *England* N33+502 **38**
St Jacques, *New Brunswick* S51+475 **90**
St James, *Minnesota* U28+440 **93**
St James, C., *B.C.* W67+518 **88**
St Jan, *Belgium* M73+509 **44**
St Jean, *France* M52+453 **54**
St Jean, *Quebec* S79+453 **91**
St Jean d'Angély, *France* N03+459 **54**
St Jean de Luz, *France* N10+434 **55**
St Jérôme, *Quebec* S84+458 **91**
St Joachim, *Quebec* S65+471 **91**
St John, *New Brunswick* S36+453 **90**
St John, West, *N.B.* S37+452 **90**
St John B., *Newfoundland* R76+509 **90**
St John, L., *Quebec* S72+486 **90**
St John, Mt., *Quebec* S22+504 **90**
St Johns, *Arizona* V27+345 **94**
St John's, Michigan T57+430 **91**
St Johns, *Newfoundland* R46+475 **90**
St John's Pt., *Ireland, Rep.* N51+546 **42**
St John's Pt., *N. Ireland* N34+542 **42**
St Johns R., *Florida* T39+300 **97**
St Johnsbury, *Vermont* S72+445 **91**
St Joseph, *Louisiana* U07+319 **97**
St Joseph, *Michigan* T68+422 **91**
St Joseph, *Missouri* U30+398 **95**
St Joseph, *Quebec* S65+463 **90**
St Joseph I., *Ontario* T54+462 **91**
St Joseph I., *Texas* V42+280 **94**
St Joseph L., *Ontario* U02+510 **89**
Ste Justine, *Quebec* S62+464 **91**
St Kilda, Is., *Scotland* N51+578 **40**
St Kitts, I., *West Indies* S16+173 **101**
St Laurent, *Fr. Guiana* R55+054 **105**
St Lawrence, *Queensland* C03-222 **111**
St Lawrence, G. of, *Canada* S12+486 **90**
St Lawrence I., *Alaska* Z30+632 **99**
St Lawrence, R., *Quebec* S62+474 **89**
St Lawrence Seaway,
N. America T01+448 **91**
St Leger, *Belgium* M56+496 **44**
St Léonard, *France* M81+458 **54**
St Leonard, *New Brunswick* S47+472 **90**
St Leonards, *England* M87+509 **39**
St Lewis, C., *Labrador* R64+528 **89**
St Lin, *Quebec* S83+458 **91**
St Lô, *France* N06+491 **54**
St Louis, *Mauritania* P10+160 **80**
St Louis, *Michigan* T58+434 **91**
St Louis, *Missouri* U02+386 **97**
St Louis, L., *Quebec* S83+454 **91**
St Louis de Kent, *N.B.* S30+467 **90**
St Lucia C., *Natal* K74-284 **84**
St Lucia, I., *Windward Is.* S05+140 **101**
St Lucia L., *Natal* K76-280 **84**
St Luke's I., *Burma* F41+102 **71**
St Maartensdijk, *Netherlands* M66+515 **44**
St Magnus B., *Scotland* N09+604 **40**
St Maixent, *France* N01+464 **54**
St Malo & Gulf, *France* N12+487 **54**
St Marc, *Haiti* S76+192 **101**
St Mard, *Belgium* M57+496 **44**
Ste Marie C., *Madagascar* J88-256 **83**
Ste Marie I., *Madagascar* J60-170 **83**
St Marks, *Florida* T55+302 **97**
St Martin, I., *Leeward Is.* S18+181 **101**
St Martins, *New Brunswick* S33+454 **90**
St Mary B., *Nova Scotia* S37+442 **90**
St Mary Is., *India* H03+135 **70**
St Mary's, *Ontario* T37+433 **91**
St Marys, *Pennsylvania* T22+414 **96**
St Marys, *Tasmania* C11-416 **109**
St Mary's B., *Newfoundland* R53+467 **90**
St Mary's L., *Scotland* N19+555 **41**
St Mary's Pk., *S. Australia* C65-315 **111**
St Matthew I., *Alaska* Z45+603 **99**
St Matthew's I., *Burma* F41+100 **71**
St Maurice, *Switzerland* M48+462 **45**
St Maurice R., *Quebec* S77+475 **91**
St Mazimin, *France* M55+435 **55**
St Meen, *France* N13+482 **54**
St Michael, *Alaska* Y70+631 **99**
St Michaels, *Maryland* T05+389 **91**
St Moritz, *Switzerland* M31+465 **45**
St Nazaire, *France* N15+473 **54**
St Neots, *England* N02+522 **37**
St Nicolaasga, *Netherlands* M56+529 **44**
St Nicolas. *See* St Niklaas
St Niklaas, *Belgium* M65+512 **44**
St Niklau, *Switzerland* M43+462 **45**
St Odilienberg, *Netherlands* M54+512 **44**
St Omer, *France* M77+508 **54**
Saintonge, prov., *France* N02+454 **54**
St Paul, *Minnesota* U19+450 **93**
St Paul I., *Bering Sea* Z32+570 **99**
St Paul, I., *Indian Ocean* G76-386 **77**
St Paul de Fenouillet, *France* M75+428 **55**
St Peter, *Minnesota* U24+443 **93**
St Peter, *Prince Edward I.* S15+464 **90**
St Peter, L., *Quebec* S78+461 **91**
St Petersburg, *Florida* T46+278 **97**
St Petersburg, *Pennsylvania* T28+412 **96**
St Pierre, *Martinique, W.I.* S06+147 **101**
St Pierre, I., *Quebec* S64+469 **91**
St Pierre, I., *Atlantic Ocean* R67+468 **90**
St Pol, *France* M76+504 **54**
St Polten, *Austria* L87+482 **49**
St Pons, *France* M73+435 **55**
St Pourçain, *France* M70+463 **54**
St Quentin, *France* M70+499 **54**
St Raymond, *Quebec* S71+469 **91**
St Rémi d'Amherst, *Quebec* S89+461 **91**
St Roch, *Quebec* S61+473 **90**
St Sébastien C., *Madagascar* J68-124 **83**
St Sernin-sur-Rance, *France* M75+439 **55**
St Servan, *France* N12+486 **54**
St Sever, *France* N03+438 **55**
St Simeon, *Quebec* S59+478 **91**
St Simon, *Quebec* S54+482 **90**
St Stephen, *New Brunswick* S44+452 **90**
St Thecle, *Quebec* S75+469 **91**
Ste Thérèse, L., *N.-W. Terr.* W07+646 **88**
St Thomas, *Ontario* T37+428 **91**
St Thomas, I., *Virgin Is.* S30+184 **101**
St Tronde. *See* St Truiden
St Tropez, *France* M50+433 **55**
St Truiden, *Belgium* M59+508 **44**
St Valery, *France* M80+502 **54**
St Valery-en-Caux, *France* M86+499 **54**
St Veit, *Austria* M04+468 **48**
St Vincent, *Windward Is.* S07+132 **101**
St Vincent C., *Madagascar* K10-220 **83**
St Vincent, G., *S. Australia* C72-346 **109**
St Vith, *Belgium* M53+503 **44**
St Xavier, *Montana* V16+454 **93**
Saipan, I., *Mariana Is.* C25+152 **106**
Saiping, *China* E36+326 **64**
Saiun, *Yemen, South* J66+160 **74**
Saivomuotka, *Sweden* L41+681 **46**
Saiyidwala, *Pakistan* H09+311 **72**
Saka Dzong, *Tibet* G28+295 **71**
Sakai, *Japan* C87+346 **68**
Sakaka, *Saudi Arabia* K29+299 **74**
Sakakawea, L., *N. Dakota* U74+476 **93**
Sakania, *Zaire* L08-128 **83**
Sakaria, R., *Turkey* K86+400 **74**
Sakata, *Japan* C61+389 **68**
Sakesar, *Pakistan* H17+324 **72**
Sakha, *Saudi Arabia* K08+232 **74**
Sakhalin, *U.S.S.R.* C40+510 **63**
Sakhalinskiy Zaliv, *U.S.S.R.* C55+539 **63**
Saki, *U.S.S.R.* K68+451 **60**
Šakiai, *Lithuania* L42+549 **47**
Sakishima Gunto, *Japan* D66+244 **68**
Sakr, *Yemen, D.R.* J48+156 **75**
Sakti, *India* G42+220 **73**
Säkylä, *Finland* L46+610 **47**
Šala, *Czechoslovakia* L73+482 **49**
Sala, *Sweden* L80+599 **47**
Salatsgriva, *Latvia* L34+578 **47**
Salada, L., *Mexico* V63+322 **100**
Salado, R., *Argentina* S14-292 **103**
Salado, R., *Texas* U58+270 **94**
Salaga, *Ghana* N04+086 **80**
Salahiye, *Syria* K26+348 **74**
Salala, *Oman* J35+171 **75**
Salama, *Guatemala* U02+151 **100**
Salamanca, *Mexico* U67+206 **100**
Salamanca, *New York* T22+422 **91**
Salamanca, *Spain* N34+409 **52**
Salamaua, *Papua New Guinea* C18-072 **111**
Salamina, *Colombia* T03+054 **104**
Salamis & I., *Greece* L39+379 **59**
Salangen, *Norway* L74+690 **46**
Salas, *Spain* N38+434 **52**
Salas de los Infantes, *Spain* N19+420 **52**
Salaverry, *Peru* T24-083 **104**
Sala-y-Gomez I., *Pacific Oc.* V00-258 **107**
Salbris, *France* M78+474 **54**
Saldana, *Spain* N29+425 **52**
Saldus, *Latvia* L45+567 **47**
Sale, *Victoria* C18-381 **109**
Salekhard, *U.S.S.R.* H51+664 **62**
Salem, *Illinois* T84+386 **95**
Salem, *India* G71+118 **70**
Salem, *Massachusetts* S65+425 **91**
Salem, *Missouri* U10+376 **97**
Salem, *New Jersey* T03+396 **91**
Salem, *Oregon* W18+449 **92**
Salem, *Virginia* T31+373 **97**
Salemi, *Sicily* M13+378 **57**
Sälen, *Sweden* M11+612 **47**
Salerno, *Italy* M02+407 **57**
Salerno, G. di, *Italy* M02+405 **57**
Salford, *England* N14+535 **37**
Salida, *Colorado* V06+386 **94**
Salina, *Kansas* U46+388 **95**
Salina, *Malawi* K64-136 **83**
Salina, *Utah* V41+390 **94**
Salina, I., *Italy* M01+386 **57**
Salina Cruz, *Mexico* U32+162 **100**
Salinas, *California* W10+366 **92**
Salinas, *Ecuador* T35-022 **104**
Salinas, *Mexico* U70+226 **100**
Salinas, *Mexico* U61+259 **100**
Salinas Pk., *New Mexico* V09+334 **94**
Salinas R., *California* W09+364 **92**
Saline R., *Kansas* U58+391 **98**
Salinitas, *Chile* S60-250 **103**
Salinópolis, *Brazil* R15-007 **105**
Salisbury, *England* N11+511 **39**
Salisbury, *Maryland* T03+385 **99**
Salisbury, *New Brunswick* S30+460 **90**
Salisbury, *N. Carolina* T33+356 **97**
Salisbury, *Zimbabwe* K84-178 **84**
Salisbury, *S. Australia* C68-348 **109**
Salisbury I., *N.-W. Terr.* T12+639 **89**
Salisbury L., *Uganda* K66+016 **83**
Salisbury Plain, *England* N11+512 **39**
Salkhad, *Syria* K50+325 **76**
Salyan, *Nepal* G47+284 **71**
Salmon R., *Idaho* V62+452 **92**
Salmon River Mts., *Idaho* V58+444 **92**
Salo, *Finland* L41+604 **47**
Salon, *France* M60+436 **55**
Salon, *India* G51+260 **73**
Salonica. *See* Thessaloniki
Salonta, *Romania* L50+469 **58**
Salop, co., *England* N16+544 **37**
Salqin, *Syria* K51+361 **76**
Salsette I., *India* H13+192 **70**
Salt Fd., *Norway* M06+672 **46**
Salt L., *Utah* V46+392 **94**
Salt L., *W. Australia* E37-240 **110**
Salt Ls., *W. Australia* D40-290 **110**
Salt Ra., *Pakistan* H18+326 **70**
Salt R., *Arizona* V34+338 **94**
Salta, *Argentina* S33+248 **103**
Saltash, *England* N25+504 **38**
Saltcoats, *Scotland* N29+556 **41**
Saltdal, *Norway* L87+671 **46**
Saltee, Is., *Ireland, Rep.* N40+521 **43**
Saltillo, *Mexico* U65+255 **100**
Salt Lake City, *Utah* V42+408 **94**
Salto, *Argentina* S02-343 **103**
Salto, *Uruguay* R78-314 **103**
Salto Grande, *Brazil* Q60-160 **105**
Salton Sea, *California* V66+334 **92**
Salt Plains Res., *Oklahoma* U50+368 **95**
Saltrou, *Haiti* S71+183 **101**
Salt Sulphur Springs, *W.Va.* T34+376 **97**
Saltville, *Virginia* T41+369 **97**
Saluda, *Virginia* T09+377 **97**
Salûm & G. of, *Egypt* L30+316 **81**
Salur, *India* G40+186 **71**
Salut, Is. du, *Fr. Guiana* R46+054 **105**
Saluzzo, *Italy* M45+446 **56**
Salvador (Bahia), *Brazil* Q51-130 **105**
Salvador, L., *Louisiana* U01+296 **95**
Salvador, El, rep., *Cent Amer.* T84+136 **101**
Salvaterra, *Portugal* N53+390 **52**
Salvatierra, *Mexico* U65+202 **100**
Salzburg, *Austria* M12+478 **48**
Salzwedel, *E. Germany* M23+528 **48**
Samahala, *Botswana* L38-196 **84**
Samalut, *Egypt* K86+282 **81**
Samana & B. de, *Dom. Rep.* S56+192 **101**
Samar, I., *Philippines* D60+117 **65**
Samarai, *Papua New Guinea* B87-107 **111**
Samarinda, *Borneo* E17-006 **65**
Samarkand, *Uzbek.* H48+395 **62**
Samarra Balad, *Iraq* K06+342 **74**
Samastipur, *India* G25+259 **73**
Samawa, *Iraq* J89+312 **74**
Sambalpur, *India* G35+214 **71**
Sambeek, *Netherlands* M54+516 **44**
Sambhal, *India* G69+285 **73**
Sambhar, *India* G88+268 **70**
Sambor, *Ukraine* L40+496 **60**
Samborombón, B., *Argent.* R70-359 **103**
Sambre, R., *Belgium* M64+504 **44**
Same, *Japan* C51+405 **68**
Samedan, *Switzerland* M31+465 **45**
Sami, *Pakistan* H70+260 **70**
Samira, *Saudi Arabia* K17+264 **74**
Sam Ka, *Burma* F48+202 **71**
Sam-nua, *Laos* F05+204 **69**
Samoa Is., *Pacific Ocean* Z40-150 **106**
Samokov, *Bulgaria* L39+423 **58**
Samorogan, *Upper Volta* N30+114 **80**
Samos, I., *Greece* L19+337 **59**
Samothrace. *See* Samothraki I.
Samothráki I., *Greece* L27+405 **59**
Sampacho, *Argentina* S28-334 **103**
Sampit, *Borneo* E41-028 **65**
Samrée, *Belgium* M56+502 **44**
Samsat, *Turkey* K39+376 **74**
Samshui, *China* E42+232 **67**
Samsø, I., *Denmark* M26+558 **47**
Samsu, *Korea* D42+413 **64**
Samsun, *Turkey* K52+414 **74**
Samthar, *India* G67+258 **73**
Samuie Str., *Thailand* F30+092 **69**
San, *Mali* N28+130 **80**
San'a, *Yemen* K05+154 **74**
Sanam, Jebel, *Iraq* J75+301 **74**
San Ambrosio I., *Pacific Oc.* T30-250 **107**
Sanandaj, *Iran* J77+354 **74**
San Andres Mts., *New Mex.* V08+330 **94**
San Angelo, *Texas* U61+313 **98**
San Antioco, I., *Sardinia* M40+390 **57**
San Antonio, *Chile* S56-233 **103**
San Antonio *Chile* S70-336 **103**
San Antonio, *Mexico* V30+238 **100**
San Antonio, *Texas* U51+294 **95**
San Antonio, C. *Argentina* R70-366 **103**
San Antonio, C,, *Cuba* T59+218 **101**
San Antonio Pk., *New Mex.* V06+368 **94**
San Antonio R. & B., *Texas* U44+286 **94**
San Antonio Oeste, *Argent.* S30-408 **103**
San Bartolomeu de Nessines,
Portugal N50+372 **52**
San Benedetto del Tronto, *It.* M07+430 **56**
San Benito, *Mexico* U14+147 **100**
San Benito, *Texas* U46+261 **94**
San Benito Is., *Mexico* V64+282 **100**
San Bernardino, *California* V74+341 **92**
San Bernardino Ra., *Cal.* V66+340 **92**
San Bernardo, *Chile* S64-335 **103**
San Blas, *Argentina* S14-405 **103**
San Blas, *Mexico* V02+215 **100**
San Blas, *Mexico* V22+262 **100**
San Blas, C., *Florida* T62+297 **99**
San Blas, G. de, *Panama* T23+096 **101**
San Borja, *Mexico* V52+288 **100**
Sanborn, *N. Dakota* U49+469 **93**
San Carlos, *Argentina* S35-260 **103**
San Carlos, *Argentina* S55-337 **103**
San Carlos, *Argentina* S31-312 **103**
San Carlos, *Chile* S71-363 **103**
San Carlos, *Mexico* U53+244 **100**
San Carlos, *Nicaragua* T58+111 **101**
San Carlos,
Amazonas, Venez. S42+019 **104**
San Carlos, *Cojedes, Venez.* S52+097 **104**
San Carlos, L. *Arizona* V32+332 **94**
San Carlos de Bariloche,
Argentina S68-411 **103**
San Carlos del Zulia, *Venz.* S70+090 **104**
Sanchez, *Dominican Rep.* S58+192 **101**
San Clemente, *Spain* N15+394 **53**
San Cosme, *Paraguay* R68-272 **103**
San Cristobal, *Argentina* S07-303 **103**
San Cristobal, *Mexico* U15+168 **100**
San Cristobal, *Venezuela* S73+078 **104**
San Cristobal I., *Galapagos Is.* U00-007 **107**
San Cristobal, I., *Solomon Is.* B20-110 **106**
Sancti Spiritus, *Cuba* T27+218 **101**
Sand, *Norway* M52+595 **47**
Sandakan, *Sabah* E11+059 **65**
Sanday I. & Sd., *Orkney, Scot.* N15+592 **40**
Sandbach, *England* N14+532 **37**
Sandefjord, *Norway* M29+591 **47**
Sandefjord B., *Antarctica* G80-700 **27**
Sanders, *Arizona* V26+352 **94**
Sandgate, *England* M83+511 **39**
Sandgate, *Queensland* B72-272 **111**
Sandhornøy, *Norway* M06+671 **46**
Sandia, *Peru* S57-143 **104**
San Diego, *California* V73+327 **92**
San Diego, *Texas* U50+277 **94**
San Diego, C., *Argentina* S31-547 **99**
San Diego de Cabrutica,
Venezuela S28+084 **104**
Sandikli, *Turkey* K88+384 **74**
Sandila, *India* G56+270 **73**
San Dimas, *Mexico* V04+241 **100**
Sandnes, *Norway* M56+589 **47**
Sandoa, *Zaire* L44-098 **82**
San Domingos, *Portugal* N45+377 **52**
Sandoway, *Burma* F63+185 **71**
Sandown, *I. of Wight, Eng.* N07+507 **39**
Sandpoint, *Idaho* V70+480 **98**
Sandringham, *England* M87+528 **39**
Sandstone, *Minnesota* U17+461 **93**
Sandstone, *W. Australia* E05-279 **110**
Sandträsk, *Sweden* L52+661 **46**
Sandusky, *Michigan* T47+434 **91**
Sandusky, *Ohio* T46+414 **91**
Sandvig, *Bornholm, I., Den.* M01+553 **47**
Sandwich, *England* M82+513 **39**
Sandwich, *Ontario* T48+423 **91**
Sandy C., *Queensland* B70-246 **111**
Sandy L., *Manitoba* U68+598 **88**
Sandy L., *Ontario* U18+531 **89**
San Esteban de Formaz,
Spain N19+415 **52**
San Felipe, *Chile* S65-327 **103**
San Felipe, *Guatemala* U10+146 **100**
San Felipe, *Mexico* U01+179 **100**
San Felipe, *Mexico* U67+215 **100**
San Felipe, *Venezuela* S52+104 **104**
San Feliu de Guixals, *Spain* M72+418 **53**
San Feliu de Llobregat, *Sp.* M78+414 **53**
San Félix, *Venezuela* S16+083 **104**
San Felix I., *Pacific Ocean* U05-250 **107**
San Fernando, *Chile* S66-344 **103**
San Fernando, *Mexico* U49+248 **100**
San Fernando, *Mexico* V63+300 **100**
San Fernando, *Philippines* D88+166 **65**
San Fernando, *Trinidad* S08+103 **104**
San Fernando de Apure,
Venezuela S45+077 **104**
San Fernando de Atabapo,
Venezuela S47+040 **104**
Sanford, *Florida* T38+288 **97**
Sanford, *Maine* S65+435 **90**
Sanford, *N. Carolina* T25+355 **97**
Sanford, Mt., *Alaska* X60+620 **99**
San Francisco, *Argentina* S13-314 **103**
San Francisco, *California* W15+378 **92**
San Francisco Mts., *Arizona* V42+354 **94**
San Francisco Pk., *Arizona* V40+355 **98**
Sanga, *Angola* L88-114 **82**
Sangareddipet, *India* G71+176 **70**
Sanger, *N. Dakota* U66+472 **93**
Sanggau, *Borneo* E56+002 **65**
Sangihe Kep., *Indonesia* D58+027 **65**
San Giovanni in Fiore, *Italy* L80+393 **57**
Sangkulirang, *Borneo* E12+010 **65**
Sangla Hill, *Pakistan* H09+316 **72**
Sangre de Cristo Mts., *Colo.-*
New Mexico V01+370 **94**
Sangre Grande Town,
Trinidad S06+106 **104**
Sangrur, *India* G85+302 **72**
Sangwin, *Liberia* N56+054 **80**
San Ignacio, *Bolivia* S33-150 **104**
San Ignacio, *Bolivia* S05-162 **104**
San Ignacio, *Mexico* V07+241 **100**
San Ignacio, *Mexico* V48+271 **100**
San Ignacio, *Paraguay* R72-269 **103**
Sanish, *N. Dakota* U75+480 **93**
San Javier, *Argentina* S00-305 **103**
San Javier, *Chile* S70-356 **103**
San João, *Portugal* N44+412 **52**
San Joaquim, *Bolivia* S29-132 **104**
San Jorge, G., *Argentina* S40-460 **103**
San José, *Bolivia* S04-176 **104**
San José, *California* W12+373 **92**
San José, *Colombia* S71+025 **104**
San José, *Costa Rica* T54+099 **101**
San José, *Guatemala* U05+139 **100**
San José, *Uruguay* R70-342 **103**
San José, G., *Argentina* S26-422 **103**
San José, I., *Mexico* V34+250 **100**
San José Carpizo, *Mexico* U03+194 **100**
San José de Amacuro, *Venez.* S03+085 **104**
San José de Feliciano, *Argent.* R83-303 **103**
San José del Cabo, *Mexico* V28+230 **100**
San José da Ocune, *Colombia* S61+041 **104**
San Juan, *Bolivia* R88-177 **104**
San Juan, *Puerto Rico* S36+185 **101**

San Juan, *Venezuela* S50+111 **104**
San Juan & R., *Argentina* S51-316 **103**
San Juan, C., *Argentina* S22-548 **103**
San Juan Mts., *Colorado* V12+374 **94**
San Juan, R., *Mexico* U32+181 **100**
San Juan, R., *Nicaragua* T54+108 **101**
San Juan R., *Utah, etc.* V30+372 **94**
San Juan de Camarones, *Mexico* V06+250 **100**
San Juan de Guadalupe, *Mexico* U77+245 **100**
San Juan del Norte, *Nic.* T52+110 **101**
San Juan de los Lagos, *Mex.* U73+213 **100**
San Juan del Rio, *Mexico* U59+204 **100**
San Juan del Sur, *Niçaragua* T65+114 **101**
San Juan Sabinas, *Mexico* U68+278 **100**
San Julian, *Argentina* S47-493 **103**
San Justo, *Argentina* S03-307 **103**
Sankuri Post, *Kenya* K32-004 **83**
San Lazaro, C., *Mexico* V43+247 **100**
San Leandro, *California* W13+377 **92**
San Lorenzo, *Argentina* S04-327 **103**
San Lorenzo, *Ecuador* T23+013 **104**
San Lorenzo, *Honduras* T74+134 **101**
San Lorenzo, *Mexico* V35+306 **100**
San Lorenzo, *Peru* S56-115 **104**
San Lorenzo Is., *Mexico* V46+286 **100**
San Lorenzo del Escorial, *Sp.* N25+406 **52**
Sanlucar la Mayor, *Spain* N37+374 **52**
San Lucas, *Bolivia* S31-200 **104**
San Lucas, C., *Mexico* V29+229 **100**
San Luis, *Argentina* R81-276 **103**
San Luis, *Argentina* S39-332 **103**
San Luis, *Cuba* T02+203 **101**
San Luis de la Paz, *Mexico* U61+212 **100**
San Luis Obispo, *California* W04+353 **92**
San Luis Potosi & state, *Mexico* U65+222 **100**
Sanluri, *Sardinia* M37+396 **57**
San Marcos, *Colombia* T01+086 **104**
San Marino, rep., *Italy* M15+441 **56**
San Martin, *Argentina* S64-440 **103**
San Martin, *Colombia* S82+038 **104**
San Martin, L., *Chile-Argent.* S76-489 **103**
San Martin de los Andes, *Argentina* S68-402 **103**
San Martin de Valdeiglesais, *Spain* N26+403 **52**
San Martinho, *Portugal* N55+395 **52**
San Mateo, *Florida* T39+296 **97**
San Mateo, *Spain* M89+404 **53**
San Mateo Pk., *New Mexico* V15+339 **94**
San Matias, *Bolivia* R79-164 **104**
San Matias, G., *Argentina* S26-414 **103**
San Maura. *See* Levkás I.
San Miguel, *Bolivia* S05-166 **104**
San Miguel, *Mexico* U65+209 **100**
San Miguel, *Peru* S83-130 **104**
San Miguel, *El Salvador* T79+135 **101**
San Miguel. *See* Rey, I. del
San Miguel, B. de, *Panama* T19+084 **101**
San Miguel I., *California* W02+341 **92**
San Miguel, R., *Bolivia* S20-160 **104**
San Miguel de Tucuman, *Argentina* S32-268 **103**
San Nicolás, *Argentina* S01-334 **103**
Sano Nocera, *Italy* M02+407 **57**
San Pablo, *Bolivia* S40-216 **104**
San Pablo, C., *Argentina* S40-543 **103**
San Pedro, *Argentina* R87-338 **103**
San Pedro, *Bolivia* S37-181 **104**
San Pedro, *Belize* T78+180 **101**
San Pedro, *California* V80+337 **92**
San Pedro, *Ivory Coast* N40+048 **80**
San Pedro, *Mexico* U78+259 **100**
San Pedro, *Paraguay* R72-240 **103**
San Pedro Chan, *California* V87+336 **92**
San Pedro R., *Arizona* V32+326 **94**
San Pedro de Arimena, *Colombia* S70+044 **104**
San Pedro del Gallo, *Mexico* U87+256 **100**
San Pedro de Lloc, *Peru* T26-076 **104**
San Pedro de Macoris, *Dominican Rep.* S56+186 **101**
San Pedro do Sul, *Portugal* N48+407 **52**
San Pedro Soloma, *Guat.* U08+157 **100**
San Pedro Sula, *Honduras* T78+155 **101**
San Pietro I., *Sardinia* M40+392 **56**
San Quintin & B., *Mexico* V66+304 **100**
San Rafael, *Argentina* S50-346 **103**
San Rafael, *California* W15+379 **92**
San Rafael, *New Mexico* V18+352 **98**
San Ramon, *Mexico* V66+308 **100**
San Ramon, *Peru* T01-111 **104**
San Remo, *Italy* M43+438 **56**
San Roque, *Argentina* R82-286 **103**
San Salvador, *Angola* M04-062 **82**
San Salvador, *Bahamas, The* S88+240 **101**
San Salvador, *El Salvador* T86+137 **101**
Sansanne Mango, *Togo* M86+104 **80**
San Sebastian, *Spain* N12+433 **53**
San Sebastian & B. de, *Argentina* S51-533 **103**
San Severo, *Italy* L88+417 **57**
Sans Souci, *Ontario* T29+451 **91**
Santa, *Peru* T22-090 **104**
Santa Ana, *Bolivia* S34-138 **104**
Santa Ana, *Bolivia* R82-186 **104**
Santa Ana, *California* V77+337 **92**
Santa Ana, *Ecuador* T32-012 **104**
Santa Ana, *Mexico* V35+305 **100**
Santa Ana, *Peru* S77-129 **104**
Santa Ana, *El Salvador* T87+140 **101**
Santa Anna (Bananal), I. de, *Brazil* R32-114 **105**
Santa Antonio da Gloria, *Brazil* Q50-093 **105**
Santa Barbara, *California* V88+344 **92**
Santa Barbara, *Honduras* T80+149 **101**
Santa Barbara Chan., *Cal.* W06+343 **92**
Santa Barbara Is., *California* W00+340 **98**
Santa Barbara de Samana, *Dominican Rep.* S56+192 **101**
Santa Carolina, *Brazil* S44-077 **104**
Santa Catalina, *Chile* S58-252 **103**
Santa Catalina I., *California* V80+334 **92**
Santa Catalina, I., *Mexico* V34+257 **100**
Santa Catalina, mt., *Mexico* V63+309 **100**
Santa Catalina Ra., *Arizona* V34+324 **94**
Santa Catarina, *Mexico* V28+231 **100**
Santa Catarina, I., *Brazil* R21-276 **103**
Santa Clara, *Brazil* S58-028 **104**
Santa Clara, *Cuba* T30+224 **101**
Santa Clara, Sa., *Mexico* V54+273 **100**
Santa Coloma de Farnes, *Sp.* M74+418 **53**
Santa Cruz, *Argentina* S52-500 **103**
Santa Cruz, *Bolivia* S20-177 **104**
Santa Cruz, *Brazil* Q61-200 **105**
Santa Cruz, *Brazil* S75-059 **104**
Santa Cruz, *California* W12+370 **92**
Santa Cruz, *Chile* S68-346 **103**
Santa Cruz, *Mexico* V02+258 **100**
Santa Cruz, *Mexico* V34+312 **100**
Santa Cruz, *Nicaragua* T66+134 **101**
Santa Cruz, *Peru* T05-056 **104**
Santa Cruz, *Philippines* D81+140 **65**
Santa Cruz Chan. & I., *Cal.* V89+340 **92**
Santa Cruz, I., *West Indies* S28+178 **101**
Santa Cruz Is., *Pacific Ocean* A80-112 **106**
Santa Cruz, R., *Argentina* S66-502 **103**
Santa Cruz de Bravo, *Mex.* T76+196 **100**
Santa Cruz de la Zarza, *Sp.* N20+400 **52**
Santa Cruz del Sur, *Cuba* T19+208 **101**
Santa Cruz de Tenerife, *Canary Is.* P08+284 **80**
Santa Elena, *Ecuador* T35-023 **104**
Santa Eufemia, G. di, *Italy* L84+389 **57**
Santa Fé, *Argentina* S05-316 **103**
Santa Fé, *Cuba* T46+217 **101**
Santa Fé, *New Mexico* V06+356 **94**
Santa Helena, *Brazil* R56-249 **103**
Santa Helena, *Brazil* R02-024 **105**
Santai, *China* F00+311 **66**
Santa Innes, B., *Mexico* V41+269 **100**
Santa Isabel, *Argentina* S41-362 **103**
Santa Isabel, *See* Macias Nguema
Santalnes, I., *Chile* S76-539 **103**
Santa Lucia, *Cuba* T06+210 **101**
Santa Luzia, *Brazil* R18-162 **105**
Santa Margarita, I., *Mexico* V41+244 **100**
Santa Maria, *Argentina* S36-266 **103**
Santa Maria, *Brazil* R52-297 **103**
Santa Maria, *California* W03+349 **92**
Santa Maria, I., *Atlantic Oc.* P61+372 **80**
Santa Maria, I., *Chile* S81-370 **103**
Santa Maria, mt., *Argentina* S56-362 **103**
Santa Maria del Rio, *Mex.* U64+218 **100**
Santa Maria di Leuea C., *It.* L70+398 **57**
Santa Maria la Real de Nieva, *Spain* N26+411 **52**
Santa Maria Nova, *Brazil* R28-092 **105**
Santa Marta, *Colombia* S85+112 **104**
Santa Monica, *California* V81+341 **92**
Santa Monica B., *California* V88+338 **92**
Santander, *Colombia* T08+030 **104**
Santander, *Spain* N23+434 **52**
Santa Paula, *California* V84+342 **92**
Santa Philomena, *Brazil* R04-091 **105**
Santa Quiteria, *Brazil* Q76-034 **105**
Santarem, *Brazil* Q55-137 **105**
Santarem, *Portugal* N52+392 **52**
Santa Rita, *Venezuela* S68+104
Santa Rosa, *Argentina* S31-323 **103**
Santa Rosa, *Argentina* S49-331 **103**
Santa Rosa, *Bolivia* S07-170 **104**
Santa Rosa, *Brazil* R57-278 **103**
Santa Rosa, *California* W16+384 **92**
Santa Rosa, *Honduras* T84+147 **101**
Santa Rosa, *New Mexico* U88+348 **94**
Santa Rosa, *Uruguay* R76-303 **103**
Santa Rosa I., *California* W01+340 **92**
Santa Rosa de Toay, *Argent.* S25-365 **103**
Santa Rosalia, *Mexico* V44+272 **100**
Santa Vitoria do Palmar, *Brazil* R50-336 **103**
Santerem, *Brazil* R58-024 **105**
Santiago, *Brazil* R59-291 **103**
Santiago, *Chile* S64-334 **103**
Santiago, *Mexico* V28+236 **100**
Santiago, *Mexico* V01+217 **100**
Santiago, *Panama* T35+081 **101**
Santiago, *Dominican Rep.* S64+194 **101**
Santiago Mts., *Texas* U81+300 **94**
Santiago de Compostela, *Sp.* N51+429 **52**
Santiago, Cerro, *Panama* T40+087 **101**
Santiago, Sa. de, *Bolivia* S00-183 **104**
Santiago de Cuba, *Cuba* T05+201 **101**
Santiago del Estero, *Argent.* S26-278 **103**
Santiago Papasquiaro, *Mex.* V02+248 **100**
Santillana, *Spain* N24+433 **52**
Santipur, *India* G08+232 **73**
Santis, mt., *Switzerland* M34+472 **45**
Santo Angelo, *Brazil* R56-283 **103**
Santo Antonio, *Brazil* S24-089 **104**
Santo Antonio, *Brazil* S21-124 **104**
Santo Antonio, *Brazil* R43-009 **105**
Santo Antonio do Zaire, *Angola* M16-064 **82**
Santo Corazon, *Bolivia* R82-179 **104**
Santo Domingo, *Cuba* T31+226 **101**
Santo Domingo, *Domin. Rep.* S59+186 **101**
Santo Domingo, *Mexico* V65+307 **100**
San Tomé, *Venezuela* S24+091 **104**
Santorini, *See* Thira, I.
Santos, *Brazil* R08-238 **105**
Santo Thome, *Argentina* R67-285 **103**
Santo Tomas, *Mexico* V68+315 **100**
Santo Tomas, *Peru* S74-144 **104**
Santvliet, *Belgium* M64+513 **44**
San Urbano, *Argentina* S09-336 **103**
San Vicente, *El Salvador* T82+136 **101**
San Vito C., *Italy* L77+404 **57**
São Anna do Livramento, *Brazil* R63-309 **103**
São Antonio de Balsas, *Brazil* R06-076 **105**
São Antonio do Ica, *Brazil* S48-031 **104**
São Benedicto, *Brazil* S10-002 **104**
São Bento do Norte, *Brazil* Q36-051 **105**
São Borja, *Brazil* R66-287 **103**
São Carlos, *Brazil* R17-221 **105**
São Christovão, *Brazil* Q44-110 **105**
São Domingos, *Brazil* R07-135 **105**
São Domingos, *Brazil* R17-016 **105**
São Felippe, *Brazil* S59-065 **104**
São Felippe, *Brazil* S44+004 **104**
São Felix, *Brazil* R44-065 **105**
São Francisco, *Brazil* Q58-038 **105**
São Francisco, *Brazil* Q77-063 **105**
São Francisco, *Brazil* Q89-160 **105**
São Francisco, *Brazil* R56-046 **105**
São Francisco do Sul & I. de, *Brazil* R22-263 **103**
São Francisco, R., *Brazil* Q56-089 **105**
Sao Hill, *Tanzania* K60-084 **83**
São Jeronimo, *Brazil* R36-237 **105**
São Jeronymo, *Brazil* R40-299 **103**
São Joao da Barra, *Brazil* Q66-216 **105**
São Joao da Boa Vista, *Brazil* R11-218 **105**
São Joao del Rei, *Brazil* Q85-210 **105**
São João do Araguaya, *Brazil* R22-053 **105**
São João do Piauhy, *Brazil* Q74-084 **105**
São Joaquim, *Brazil* S44 000 **104**
São Joaquin, *Brazil* R66-048 **105**
São José, *Brazil* R42-320 **103**
São José, *Brazil* R22-276 **103**
São José, *Brazil* S38-003 **104**
São José do Duro, *Brazil* R08-113 **105**
São José do Mipibu, *Brazil* Q31-061 **105**
São José dos Martyrios, *Brazil* R20-063 **105**
São Jose do Rio Prêto, *Brazil* R26-207 **105**
São José dos Mattoes, *Brazil* Q79-054 **105**
São José do Tocantins, *Brazil* R21-144 **105**
São Lourenco & R., *Brazil* R61-165 **105**
São Luis, *Brazil* Q86-026 **105**
São Luis, I. de, *Brazil* Q86-025 **105**
São Luiz do Caceres, *Brazil* R76-162 **105**
São Luiz Gonzaga, *Brazil* R60-283 **103**
São Marcello, *Brazil* R01-110 **105**
São Mateus do Sul, *Brazil* R32-260 **103**
São Matheus, *Brazil* Q59-188 **105**
São Miguel, *Brazil* R14-016 **105**
São Miguel, I., *Atlantic Oc.* P64+380 **80**
Saona, I. *Dominican Rep.* S52+182 **101**
Saône, R., *France* M60+463 **54**
Saône-et-Loire, dep., *France* M61+466 **54**
Sao Paulo, *Brazil* R10-234 **105**
Sao Paulo de Olivenca, *Brazil* S53-035 104
São Raymundo Nonato, *Brazil* Q76-090 **105**
São Sebastião & I. da, *Brazil* R02-238 **105**
São Simão, *Brazil* R15-214 **105**
São Thomé I., *G. of Guinea* M50+002 **82**
Saoura, *Algeria* N24+278 **80**
São Vicente, *Brazil* R09-238 **105**
São Vicente, *Brazil* R19-058 **105**
Sapaya, *Ecuador* T24+008 **104**
Sapiéntza I., *Greece* L50+367 **59**
Saposoa, *Peru* T10-070 **104**
Sapporo, *Japan* C52+430 **68**
Sapri, *Italy* L86+400 **57**
Sapulpa, *Oklahoma* U37+360 **95**
Saqqez, *Iran* J82+363 **74**
Saragossa (Zaragoza), *Spain* N05+416 **53**
Saraikela, *India* G24+227 **73**
Sarajevo, *Yugoslavia* L70+438 **58**
Sarala, *U.S.S.R.* G04+550 **62**
Saranac Lake, *New York* S85+444 **91**
Saranda, *India* G28+222 **73**
Sarandi del Yi, *Uruguay* R64-333 **103**
Sarangarh, *India* G41+215 **71**
Saranovo, *Bulgaria* L35+422 **58**
Saransk, *U.S.S.R.* J89+542 **61**
Sarapul, *U.S.S.R.* J38+565 **61**
Sarasota, *Florida* T45+273 **97**
Saratoga, *Wyoming* V11+415 **93**
Saratoga L., *New York* S82+430 **96**
Saratoga Springs, *New York* S82+431 **91**
Saratov, *U.S.S.R.* J84+515 **61**
Saratsi-ting, *China* E53+407 **66**
Sarawak, *Borneo* E54+013 **65**
Sarbaz, *Iran* H82+266 **75**
Sárbogárd, *Hungary* L68+469 **49**
Sarco, *Chile* S69-288 **103**
Sardarshahr, *India* H03+285 **103**
Sardasht, *Iran* J87+361 **74**
Sardegna, I., *Italy* M36+400 **57**
Sardhana, *India* G74+291 **72**
Sardinia. *See* Sardegna.
Sardis, *Mississippi* T89+344 **97**
Sardis Res., *Mississippi* T88+345 **95**
Sardoal, *Portugal* N49+396 **52**
Sareks Nat. Park, *Sweden* L76+673 **46**
Sargans, *Switzerland* M33+471 **45**
Sarh, *Chad* L70+092 81
Sari, *Iran* J42+366 **75**
Sarikamis, *Turkey* K15+404 **74**
Sarina, *Queensland* C04-215 **111**
Sariñena, *Spain* N01+418 **53**
Sar-i-Pul, *Afghanistan* H54+361 **75**
Sar-i-Pul, *Iran* J85+345 **74**
Sarir, *Libya* L46+276 **81**
Sark, I., *Channel Islands* N14+494 **54**
Sarkad, *Hungary* L52+468 **49**
Sarlat, *France* M83+449 **55**
Sarles, *N. Dakota* U54+490 **93**
Sarmi, *New Guinea* C68-019 **65**
Sarmiento, mt., *Chile* S65-545 **103**
Sarna, *Sweden* M11+617 **47**
Sarnen, *Switzerland* M40+469 **45**
Sarnia, *Ontario* T44+430 **91**
Saronic G., *Greece* L38+376 **59**
Saronno, *Italy* M35+456 **56**
Sarpsborg, *Norway* M23+593 **47**
Sarpul, *Iran* J58+371 **75**
Sarrebourg, *France* M48+487 **54**
Sarreguemines, *France* M48+491 **54**
Sarre Union, *France* M47+489 **54**
Sarria, *Spain* N44+428 **52**
Sart, *Belgium* M54+505 **44**
Sartene, *Corsica* M36+416 **57**
Sarthe R. & dep., *France* M89+480 **54**
Sarufutso, *Japan* C48+452 **68**
Sarur, *Saudi Arabia* J12+233 **75**
Saruru, *Japan* C40+421 **68**
Sarvar, *Hungary* L79+472 **49**
Sasa Baneh, *Ethiopia* K08+078 **83**
Sasaram, *India* G35+249 **73**
Sasawara, *Tanzania* K48-116 **83**
Sasebo, *Japan* D32+331 **68**
Saskatchewan, prov., *Canada* **88**
Saskatchewan R. N., *Sask.* V30+509 **88**
Saskatchewan R. S., *Sask.* V20+530 **88**
Saskatoon, *Saskatchewan* V19+518 **88**
Saskylakh, *U.S.S.R.* E36+720 **63**
Sasmaka, *Latvia* L44+573 **47**
Sasovo, *U.S.S.R.* K18+543 **61**
Sassandra & R., *Ivory Coast* N36+050 **80**
Sassari, *Sardinia* M39+407 **57**
Sassnitz, *E. Germany* M08+545 **48**
Sastre, *Argentina* S11-318 **103**
Sas-van-Gent, *Netherlands* M67+512 **44**
Satadougou, *Mali* N68+126 **80**
Satara, *India* H05+178 **70**
Säter, *Sweden* L86+603 **47**
Satevo, *Mexico* V06+279 **100**
Satins, *France* M55+470 **54**
Satka, *U.S.S.R.* J06+550 **61**
Satkhira, *Bangladesh* G05+227 **73**
Satoraljaujhely, *Hungary* L50+484 **49**
Satpura Ra., *India* H05+217 **70**
Satul, *Thailand* F30+066 **69**
Satu Mare, *Romania* L43+478 **49**
Sauda, *Norway* M52+597 **47**
Saudhárkrókur, *Iceland* P28+657 **46**
Saudi Arabia, *S.-W. Asia* **74**
Saugeen Pen., *Ontario* T38+451 **91**
Saugerties, *New York* S84+421 **91**
Sauk Center, *Minnesota* U30+457 **93**
Sauk Rapids, *Minnesota* U25+456 **93**
Saulieu, *France* M65+473 **54**
Sault Ste Marie, *Michigan* T56+465 **91**
Sault Ste Marie, *Ontario* T56+465 **91**
Saumur, *France* N01+473 **54**
Saunders, I., *S. Sandwich Is.* P80-570 **27**
Sauqira B., *Oman* J16+185 **75**
Saurashtra, *India* H25+220 **70**
Sava, R., *Yugoslavia* L61+447 **58**
Savai'i, I., *Samoa Islands* Z45-140 **106**
Savalan, mt., *Iran* J73+383 **74**
Savanna, *Illinois* U01+421 **91**
Savannah, *Georgia* T37+321 **97**
Savannah, *Missouri* U30+399 **95**
Savannah R., *Georgia-S. Car.* T46+340 **97**
Savannakhet, *Laos* F02+166 **69**
Savanna la Mar, *Jamaica* T19+183 **101**
Savantvadi, *India* H07+160 **70**
Savanur, *India* G87+150 **70**
Save, *Benin* M76+080 **80**
Save R., *Mozambique* K60-210 **84**
Saveh, *Iran* J58+352 **75**
Savenay, *France* N12+473 **54**
Savoie, dep., *France* M49+455 **54**
Savoie, prov., *France* M53+457 **54**
Savona, *Italy* M39+443 **56**
Savonlinna, *Finland* L07+619 **46**
Savu Sea, *Indonesia* D80-096 **65**
Savukoski, *Finland* L11+673 **46**
Sawa, *Yemen, South* J74+159 74
Sawatch Mts., *Colorado* V10+388 **94**
Sawel, *N. Ireland* N42+548 **42**
Saxmundham, *England* M81+522 **39**
Saxnäs, *Sweden* L88+649 **46**
Saxton, *Pennsylvania* T20+402 **96**
Saya, *Syria* K54+351 **76**
Sayan, *Peru* T13-110 **104**
Sayan, Vostochnya, *U.S.S.R.* F30+525 **63**
Sayan, Zapadnyy, *U.S.S.R.* F60+535 **63**
Sayre, *Oklahoma* U56+354 **95**
Sayre, *Pennsylvania* T09+420 **96**
Sayula, *Mexico* U82+198 **100**
Scafell Pike, *England* N19+544 **37**
Scalea, *Italy* L85+398 **57**
Scanteia, *Romania* L15+470 **58**
Scapa Flow, *Orkney, Scot.* N18+589 **40**
Scarba, I., *Scotland* N34+562 **41**
Scarboro, *Maine* S62+436 **90**
Scarborough, *England* N02+543 **37**
Scariff I., *Ireland, Rep.* N62+517 **43**
Scărisoara, *Romania* L43+465 **58**
Scatari I., *Nova Scotia* R88+460 **90**
Schafer, *N. Dakota* U79+478 **93**
Schaffhausen & canton, *Switzerland* M38+477 **45**
Schelde, Ooster & Wester, *Netherlands* M66+515 **44**
Schenectady, *New York* S83+428 **91**
Scheveningen, *Netherlands* M64+521 **44**
Schiedam, *Netherlands* M64+519 **44**
Schiermonnikoog I, *Netherlands* M53+535 **44**
Schiphol, *Netherlands* M61+523 **44**
Schleins, *Switzerland* M27+469 **45**
Schleswig, *W. Germany* M33+545 **48**
Schleswig-Holstein, *Germany* M33+540 **48**
Schneidemühl. *See* Piła.
Schoharie, *New York* S86+427 **96**
Schönbuhl, *Switzerland* M45+470 **45**
Schonebeck, *E. Germany* M20+520 **48**
Schongau, *W. Germany* M25+478 **48**
Schoonhoven, *Netherlands* M61+519 **44**
Schötz, *Switzerland* M42+472 **45**
Schouten, I., *Tasmania* C11-424 **109**
Schouwen I., *Netherlands* M67+517 **44**
Schuchinsk, *Kazakh* H28+530 **62**
Schull, *Ireland, Rep.* N57+515 **43**
Schuls, *Switzerland* M28+468 **45**
Schüpfheim, *Switzerland* M42+470 **45**
Schuyler, *Nebraska* U42+414 **95**
Schwabach, *W. Germany* M24+493 **48**
Schwägalp, *Switzerland* M34+473 **45**
Schwandorf, *W. Germany* M17+493 **48**
Schwaner, Peg., *Borneo* E46-011 **65**
Schwarzhorn, mt., *Switz.* M43+462 **45**
Schwarzwald, *W. Germany* M38+486 **48**
Schwedt, *E. Germany* M04+531 **48**
Schweidnitz. *See* Swidnica
Schweinfurt, *W. Germany* M29+501 **48**
Schwerin, *E. Germany* M22+536 **48**
Schwyz & canton, *Switz.* M38+470 **45**
Sciacca, *Sicily* M12+375 **57**
Scilly, Is. of, *England* N38+500 **38**
Scituate, *Massachusetts* S64+422 **96**
Scobey, *Montana* V02+488 **93**
Scone, *New South Wales* B85-320 **109**
Scone, *Scotland* N20+564 **41**
Scoresby, C., *N.-W. Terr.* U20+714 **89**
Scoresby Ld., *Greenland* P85+730 **26**
Scoresby Sd., *Greenland* P38+700 **26**
Scotia, *Ontario* T26+455 **91**
Scotia Sea, *Antarctica* R90-580 **27**
Scotland, *Great Britain* N24+560 **34**
Scotland, *S. Dakota* U46+431 **93**
Scott, C., *Brit. Columbia* W51+507 **88**
Scott Inl., *N.-W. Territories* S65+710 **89**
Scott I., *Antarctica* A02-670 **27**
Scott, Mt., *Oregon* W12+432 **98**
Scott City, *Kansas* U66+384 **94**
Scottsbluff, *Nebraska* U82+416 **98**
Scottsdale, *Tasmania* C16-412 **109**
Scourie, *Scotland* N31+584 **40**
Scranton, *Pennsylvania* T04+414 **91**
Scridain, L., *Scotland* N37+563 **41**
Scugog L., *Ontario* T23+442 **91**
Scunthorpe, *England* N04+536 **37**

Scutari (Shkodër), *Albania* L63+421 **58**
Scutari (Uskudaı), *Turkey* L06+411 **74**
Seaford, *Delaware* T04+386 **91**
Seahorse Pt., *N.-W. Terr.* T30+641 **89**
Sea Isle City, *New Jersey* S88+392 **91**
Scal R., *Manitoba* U40+590 **88**
Sea Lake, *Victoria* C43-356 **109**
Sea Lion Is., *Falkland Is.* R84-524 **103**
Searcy, *Arkansas* U10+352 **95**
Seattle, *Washington* W14+476 **92**
Sebago L., *Maine* S63+439 **90**
Sebastián Vizcaino B. de, *Mexico* V58+282 **100**
Sebenico. *See* Sibenik
Sebewaing, *Michigan* T50+437 **91**
Sebha, (Sabhah), *Libya* M04+270 **81**
Sebin Karahisar, *Turkey* K40+403 **74**
Sebree, *Kentucky* T75+376 **97**
Sečovce, *Czechoslovakia* L50+487 **49**
Secretary I., *New Zealand* A78-452 **112**
Secunderabad, *India* G68+175 **70**
Seda, *Lithuania* L47+561 **47**
Sedalia, *Missouri* U20+389 **99**
Sedan, *France* M60+497 **54**
Sedan, *S. Australia* C64-346 **109**
Sedano, *Spain* N23+427 **52**
Sedbergh, *England* N15+543 **37**
Seddon, *New Zealand* A35-417 **112**
Seddonville, *New Zealand* A48-415 **112**
Sedhiou, *Senegal* P04+128 **80**
Sedom, *Israel* K57+311 **76**
Sedrun, *Switzerland* M37+467 **45**
Seeheim, *Namibia* L72-270 **84**
Seelisberg, *Switzerland* M38+470 **45**
Sées, *France* M89+486 **54**
Seewis, *Switzerland* M32+470 **45**
Sefrou, *Morocco* N30+340 **80**
Sefton, *New Zealand* A41-432 **112**
Sefton, Mt., *New Zealand* A59-437 **112**
Segorbe, *Spain* N03+398 **53**
Ségou, *Mali* N38+132 **80**
Segovia, *Spain* N25+409 **52**
Segovia, R., *Nicaragua* I54+147 **101**
Seguela, *Ivory Coast* N42+080 **80**
Sehkukeh, *Iran* H81+307 **75**
Sehwan, *Pakistan* H43+264 **70**
Seibo, *Dominican Rep.* S54+190 **101**
Seiland, *Norway* L40+704 **46**
Seine, R., *France* M87+495 **54**
Seine-et-Marne, dep., *France* M73+487 **54**
Seine-et-Oise, dep., *France* M79+488 **54**
Seine-Maritime, dep., *Fr.* M86+497 **54**
Seitler, *U.S.S.R.* K61+454 **60**
Seiyala, *Egypt* K74+226 **81**
Sejal, *Colombia* S48+026 **104**
Sekenke, *Tanzania* K66-044 **83**
Seki, *Japan* C78+354 **68**
Sekieshan I., *China* D76+303 **67**
Sekondi, *Ghana* N10+050 **80**
Sektyakh, *U.S.S.R.* D60+700 **63**
Selby, *England* N06+538 **37**
Selby, *S. Dakota* U60+454 **93**
Selemiya, *Syria* K48+350 **76**
Selenga, R., *Mong.-U.S.S.R.* E80+515 **63**
Selima Oasis, *Sudan* L04+212 **81**
Selinsgrove, *Pennsylvania* T11+408 **96**
Selkirk, *Manitoba* U42+502 **88**
Selkirk, *Yukon* X14+631 **88**
Selkirk, *Scotland* N17+555 **41**
Selkirk Mts., *Brit. Columbia* V70+500 **88**
Selle, Sa. de la, *Haiti* S72+184 **101**
Selles, *France* M81+473 **54**
Selma, *Alabama* T72+324 **97**
Selma, *N. Carolina* T20+355 **97**
Selous Mt., *Yukon* W68+634 **88**
Selva, *Argentina* S13-297 **103**
Selwyn, *Queensland* C56-215 **111**
Selwyn Ra., *Queensland* C60-214 **111**
Selwyn Ra., *Yukon* W60+634 **88**
Selzaete, *Belgium* M67+512 **44**
Sem, *Norway* M28+593 **47**
Semarang, *Java* E58-070 **65**
Semawe, Jeb., *Israel* K62+304 **76**
Seminoe Res., *Wyoming* V11+420 **93**
Semipalatinsk, *Kazakh* G59+505 **62**
Semnan, *Iran* J40+356 **75**
Senador Pompeu, *Brazil* Q56-055 **105**
Senatobia, *Mississippi* U00+346 **97**
Sendai, *Japan* C53+383 **68**
Seneca L., *New York* T11+427 **91**
Seneca Falls, *New York* T11+429 **96**
Sénégal, rep., *W. Africa* P00+146 **80**
Sénégal, R., *W. Africa* N80+150 **80**
Senev, *Michigan* T66+463 **91**
Senga Hill, *Zambia* K82-094 **83**
Sengilei, *U.S.S.R.* J67+540 **61**
Senise, *Italy* L82+402 **57**
Senj, *Yugoslavia* M01+450 **56**
Senja, *Norway* L76+693 **46**
Senna Madureira, *Brazil* S53-092 **104**
Senneterre, *Quebec* T14+484 **91**
Sens, *France* M70+482 **54**
Senta, *Yugoslavia* L59+459 **58**
Sentinel Ra., *Antarctica* T80-770 **27**
Seondha, *India* G67+262 **73**
Seoni, *India* G63+221 **73**
Seoni-Malwa, *India* G75+225 **73**
Seoul (Sŏul), *Korea* D48+377 **64**
Separation Pt., *New Zealand* A42-407 **112**
Seperior, *Nebraska* U48+400 **95**
Sepólno, *Poland* L74+535 **49**
Sepulveda, *Spain* N22+413 **52**
Sequeros, *Spain* N36+405 **52**
Sequoia Nat. Park., *Cal.* V83+365 **92**
Serai, *Syria* K54+358 **76**
Serakhs, *Turkmen* H83+365 **62**
Seram I., *Indonesia* D40-030 **65**
Serampore, *India* G10+228 **73**
Serbia, *Yugoslavia* L52+430 **58**
Serdeles, *Libya* M26+258 **81**
Serdobol, *Karelia* K86+617 **46**
Serdobsk, *U.S.S.R.* K04+525 **61**
Serengeti Nat. Pk., *Tanzania* K60-020 **83**
Sergach, *U.S.S.R.* J88+556 **61**
Sergiyevsk, *U.S.S.R.* J53+540 **61**
Serifos, I., *Greece* L33+372 **59**
Sermata, I., *Indonesia* D36-085 **65**
Serov, *U.S.S.R.* H88+599 **62**
Serowe, *Botswana* L20-224 **84**
Serpa, *Portugal* N45+379 **52**
Serpins, *Portugal* N49+402 **52**
Serpukhov, *U.S.S.R.* K46+549 **60**
Sérrai, *Greece* L39+411 **58**
Serra San Bruno, *Italy* L82+386 **57**
Serrezuela, *Argentina* S32-306 **103**
Sertã, *Portugal* N49+398 **52**
Sertig, *Switzerland* M31+467 **45**
Sérvia, *Greece* L48+401 **59**
Serviceton, *Victoria* C54-364 **109**
Sesheke, *Zambia* L30-174 **84**
Sete, *France* M68+434 **55**
Sete Lagoas, *Brazil* Q85-194 **105**
Setif, *Algeria* M58+360 **80**
Setubal, *Portugal* N53+385 **52**
Seul, Lac, *Ontario* U15+502 **89**
Sevan, Oz., *Armyan, U.S.S.R.* K00+403 **62**
Sevastopol, *U.S.S.R.* K68+446 **60**
Sevelen, *Switzerland* M33+471 **45**
Seven Islands (Sept-Iles), *Quebec* S38+503 **90**
Sevenoaks, *England* M89+513 **39**
Severac-le-Château, *France* M72+443 **55**
Severn, *Cape Province* L42-268 **84**
Severn, *Ontario* T77+558 **89**
Severn R., *England* N15+526 **37**
Severn, R., *Ontario* T88+543 **89**
Severnaya Dvina, *U.S.S.R.* K10+628 **62**
Severnaya Zemlya, *U.S.S.R.* F50+800 **63**
Sevier L., *Utah* V49+390 **92**
Sevier R., *Utah* V44+394 **94**
Sevilla, *Spain* N36+374 **52**
Seville. *See* Sevilla
Seward, *Alaska* X86+602 **99**
Seward Pen., *Alaska* Y80+651 **99**
Seybaplaya, *Mexico* U04+196 **100**
Seychelles, Is., *Indian Ocean* J30-050 **77**
Seydhisfjördhur, *Iceland* N84+653 **46**
Seymchan, *U.S.S.R.* B76+630 **63**
Seymour, *Indiana* T66+390 **91**
Seymour, *Victoria* C29-370 **109**
Seyne, *France* M51+444 **55**
Sezanne, *France* M68+487 **54**
Sfakia. *See* Khóra Sfakion.
Sfântu Gheorghe, *Romania* L25+459 **58**
Sfax, *Tunisia* M26+348 **81**
Sfira, *Syria* K46+361 **76**
Sgurr Mor., *Scotland* N30+577 **40**
Shaam, *U.A.E.* J23+260 **75**
Shaba, *Zaire* L50+100 **82**
Shadegan, *Iran* J68+306 **74**
Shadrinsk, *U.S.S.R.* H69+560 **61**
Shaduela, *Ethiopia* K18+134 **83**
Shadwan, I., *Egypt* K66+274 **81**
Shafa Amr, *Israel* K59+328 **76**
Shaftesbury, *England* N13+510 **39**
Shag Rocks, *Atlantic Ocean* Q85-540 **27**
Shahabad, *India* G79+302 **72**
Shahabad, *India* G60+276 **73**
Shah Abdul Azim, *Iran* J52+356 **75**
Shahba, *Syria* K50+328 **76**
Shahbandar, *Pakistan* H43+241 **70**
Shah Dad, *Iran* J14+306 **75**
Shahdadkot, *Pakistan* H42+278 **70**
Shahdadpur, *Pakistan* H38+258 **70**
Shahdara, *India* G76+287 **72**
Shadheri, *Pakistan* H12+337 **72**
Shahdol, *India* G51+230 **73**
Shahganj, *India* G44+260 **73**
Shahi, *Iran* J43+365 **75**
Shahin, *Iran* J81+367 **74**
Shahjahanpur, *India* G61+278 **73**
Shahjui, *Afghanistan* H44+325 **75**
Shahpur, *Pakistan* H15+323 **72**
Shāhpūr, *Iran* K02+382 **74**
Shahpura, *India* H01+257 **70**
Shah Rakht, *Iran* J00+338 **75**
Shahr-i-Babak, *Iran* J30+320 **75**
Shahriza, *Iran* J49+320 **75**
Shahr-i-Zabul, *Iran* H81+310 **75**
Shahrud, *Iran* J30+364 **75**
Shahsien, *China* E14+264 **67**
Shaiba, *Saudi Arabia* K12+280 **74**
Shajara, *Saudi Arabia* J84+223 **74**
Shakhty, *U.S.S.R.* K28+476 **61**
Shakopee, *Minnesota* U21+448 **93**
Shakubetsueki, *Japan* C37+428 **68**
Shala L., *Ethiopia* K38+074 **83**
Shalasha, *Sudan* L20+106 **81**
Shamil, *Iran* J20+274 **75**
Shammar, Jebel, *Saudi Arabia* K24+277 **74**
Shamokin, *Pennsylvania* T10+408 **91**
Shanghai, *China* D81+312 **66**
Shangjao, *China* E12+285 **67**
Shangkiu, *China* E26+345 **66**
Shangtung Pen., *China* D86+370 **64**
Shangyiu, *China* E32+260 **67**
Shan-hai-kwan. *See* Linyu.
Shansien, *China* E53+347 **66**
Shanklin, I. of W., *England* N07+506 **39**
Shanna, *Saudi Arabia* J54+190 **75**
Shannon, *New Zealand* A27-405 **112**
Shannon, I., *Greenland* P25+750 **26**
Shannon, R. & Airport, *Ireland, Rep.* N52+527 **43**
Shansi, *China* E48+380 **66**
Shantarskiye Os., *U.S.S.R.* C73+550 **63**
Shantung, prov., *China* E12+360 **66**
Shaohing, *China* D86+300 **67**
Shaowu, *China* E15+273 **67**
Shaoyang, *China* E51+272 **67**
Shap, *England* N16+545 **37**
Shapinsay, I., *Orkney Is., Scot.* N17+590 **40**
Shaqa, *Qatar, Saudi Arabia* K25+198 **74**
Shaqiq, *Saudi Arabia* J51+257 **75**
Shaqra, *Saudi Arabia* J89+252 **74**
Sharakpur, *Pakistan* H05+315 **72**
Sharjah, *U.A.E.* J72+254 **75**
Shark B., *W. Australia* E40-254 **110**
Sharon, *Pennsylvania* T33+413 **91**
Sharqi, Jeb, esh, *Leb.-Syria* K52+340 **76**
Sharr, Jebel el, *Saudi Arabia* K55+276 **74**
Sharya, *U.S.S.R.* J87+584 **61**
Shasi, *China* E46+302 **67**
Shasta, *California* W15+407 **92**
Shasta, Mt., *California* W13+415 **92**
Shasta Res., *California* W12+408 **92**
Shatra, *Iraq* J84+314 **74**
Shatt-al-Arab, *Iraq* J73+307 **74**
Shaubek, *Jordan* K57+305 **76**
Shawano, *Wisconsin* T82+448 **91**
Shawinigan Falls, *Quebec* S77+465 **91**
Shawnee, *Oklahoma* U42+353 **95**
Shawneetown, *Illinois* T79+377 **97**
Shchors, *Ukraine* K78+518 **60**
Sheboygan, *Wisconsin* T76+438 **91**
Shediac, *New Brunswick* S27+462 **90**
Sheelin L., *Ireland, Rep.* N44+538 **42**
Sheenjik R., *Alaska* X55+673 **80**
Sheep Haven, *Ireland, Rep.* N48+552 **42**
Sheep's Hd., *Ireland, Rep.* N59+515 **43**
Sheerness, *England* M85+514 **39**
Sheffield, *Alabama* T76+348 **95**
Sheffield, *England* N09+534 **37**
Sheffield, *New Zealand* A48-434 **112**
Sheffield, *Tasmania* C22-414 **109**
Sheikh, Jeb. esh, *Syria* K55+334 **76**
Sheikh 'Abd er Rahman. *See* Arka.
Sheikh Miskin, *Syria* K53+328 **76**
Sheik 'Othman, *Yemen, South* K00+129 **74**
Sheik Seraq, *Syria* K46+330 **76**
Shekha, *Yemen, South* J64+151 **74**
Shekhupura, *Pakistan* H05+317 **72**
Sheklung, *China* E36+231 **67**
Shelburne, *Nova Scotia* S32+438 **90**
Shelburne, *Ontario* T31+441 **91**
Shelby, *Michigan* T68+436 **91**
Shelby, *Montana* V41+485 **93**
Shelby, *N. Carolina* T38+352 **97**
Shelbyville, *Illinois* T84+394 **95**
Shelbyville, *Kentucky* T61+382 **97**
Shelbyville, *Tennessee* T69+356 **97**
Sheldon, *Iowa* U35+412 **95**
Shelikhova Zaliv, *U.S.S.R.* B45+600 **63**
Shellharbour, *New South Wales* B85-346 **109**
Shelter I., *New York* S74+411 **96**
Shenandoah, *Iowa* U32+408 **95**
Shenandoah, *Pennsylvania* T07+409 **91**
Shenandoah R., *Virginia* T18+392 **96**
Shenandoah Junct., *W. Va.* T17+394 **96**
Shenandoah Nat. Park, *Va.* T20+384 **97**
Shenchow. *See* Yuanling.
Shendam, *Nigeria* M34+088 **81**
Shendi, *Sudan* K70+166 **81**
Shëngjin, *Albania* L63+418 **58**
Shenkursk, *U.S.S.R.* K12+623 **62**
Shensi, prov., *China* E66+350 **66**
Shenyang, *China* D70+418 **66**
Sheopur, *India* G80+256 **70**
Shepetovka, *Ukraine* L17+502 **60**
Shepparton, *Victoria* C27+364 **109**
Sheppey, I. of, *England* M85+514 **39**
Sherada, *Ethiopia* K52+072 **83**
Sherard Osborn Fd., *Greenland* R30+820 **26**
Sherbro I., *Sierra Leone* N76+078 **80**
Sherbrooke, *Quebec* S72+454 **91**
Sheridan, *Wyoming* V12+448 **93**
Sheridan, Mt., *Wyoming* V34+443 **93**
Sherman, *Texas* U40+336 **95**
Sherpur, *Bangladesh* G03+246 **73**
Sherridon, *Manitoba* U66+551 **88**
Shetland (Zetland), *Scotland* N06+604 **40**
Shevaroy Hills, *India* G68+119 **70**
Sheyenne, *N. Dakota* U55+479 **93**
Shiant Is. & Sd. of, *Scotland* N38+579 **40**
Shibam, *Yemen, South* J68+159 **74**
Shibarghan, *Afghanistan* H55+366 **75**
Shibata, *Japan* C64+379 **68**
Shibin el Kom, *Egypt* K84+306 **81**
Shickshock Mts., *Quebec* S44+488 **90**
Shiel, L., *Scotland* N34+568 **41**
Shieldaig, *Scotland* N34+575 **40**
Shigatse, *Tibet* G07+293 **71**
Shihnan. *See* Enshih.
Shih Pao Shan, *China* E64+294 **64**
Shihshow, *China* E45+296 **67**
Shihtao, *China* D76+369 **66**
Shihtsien, *China* E70+275 **67**
Shikarpur, *Pakistan* H38+278 **70**
Shikohabad, *India* G68+271 **73**
Shikoku, I., *Japan* D06+340 **68**
Shilka & R., *U.S.S.R.* E23+519 **63**
Shillelagh, *Ireland, Rep.* N39+527 **43**
Shillong, *India* F79+255 **71**
Shiloh, *Tennessee* T80+350 **97**
Shilongol, *China* E24+434 **64**
Shimoga, *India* G86+140 **70**
Shimoni, *Kenya* K34-046 **83**
Shimonoseki, *Japan* D24+340 **68**
Shimoshima, *Japan* D29+324 **68**
Shimshal & Pass, *Kashmir* G88+364 **72**
Shin, L., *Scotland* N27+581 **40**
Shinas, *Oman* J22+247 **75**
Shinghar, *Pakistan* H31+317 **72**
Shingu, *Japan* C84+337 **68**
Shinjo, *Japan* C58+388 **68**
Shinshar, *Syria* K49+346 **76**
Shinyanga, *Tanzania* K70-036 **83**
Shipets, *Japan* C29+436 **68**
Shippigan, *New Brunswick* S28+477 **90**
Shippigan I., *New Brunswick* S28+478 **90**
Shiraishi, *Japan* C56+380 **68**
Shiraz, *Iran* J45+296 **75**
Shireza, *Pakistan* H56+277 **70**
Shirley, *Montana* V04+466 **93**
Shirley Mts., *Wyoming* V09+422 **93**
Shirokaya, *U.S.S.R.* B47+619 **63**
Shisur, *Saudi Arabia* J39+182 **75**
Shiuhing. *See* Koyiu.
Shiukwan, *China* E38+248 **67**
Shivpuri, *India* G74+254 **73**
Shizugawa, *Japan* C51+387 **68**
Shizuoka, *Japan* C69+350 **68**
Shklov, *U.S.S.R.* K88+542 **60**
Shkoder, *Albania* L63+421 **58**
Shoal Harbour, *Newfoundland* R54+482 **90**
Shoalhaven R., *N.S.W.* B86-348 **109**
Shoeburyness, *England* M85+515 **39**
Shoka, *Taiwan* D86+241 **67**
Sholapur, *India* G84+176 **70**
Shonai. *See* Tsuruoka.
Shorkot, *Pakistan* H17+308 **72**
Short, *Missouri* U06+368 **97**
Short Mts., *W. Virginia* T22+392 **96**
Short Pine Hills, *S. Dakota* U80+453 **93**
Shoshone Falls, *Idaho* V57+424 **97**
Shoshone Mts., *Wyoming* V28+442 **93**
Shoshone Res., *Wyoming* V25+442 **98**
Shovo Tso, *Tibet* G40+313 **71**
Shreveport, *Louisiana* U22+325 **95**
Shrewsbury, *England* N17+527 **37**
Shropshire (Salop), *See* Salop
Shtora, *Lebanon* K55+338 **76**
Shubuta, *Mississippi* T82+318 **97**
Shuikow, *China* E07+263 **67**
Shujabad, *Pakistan* H22+299 **72**
Shumagin Is., *Alaska* Y60+549 **99**
Shumaisa, *Saudi Arabia* J87+249 **74**
Shumen, *Bulgaria* L19+433 **58**
Shumerlya, *U.S.S.R.* J81+555 **61**
Shunking. *See* Nanchung.
Shunteh. *See* Singtai.
Shuqra, *Yemen, South* J86+134 **74**
Shurab, *Iran* J21+338 **75**
Shurma, *Saudi Arabia* K18+232 **74**
Shuru Tso, *Tibet* G22+302 **71**
Shushal, *Kashmir* G68+335 **70**
Shushtar, *Iran* J67+321 **74**
Shusp, *Iran* J00+317 **75**
Shuttleton, *New S. Wales* C24-322 **109**
Shuya, *U.S.S.R.* K21+568 **61**
Shuyang, *China* E07+342 **66**
Shwebo, *Burma* F56+225 **71**
Shwedaung, *Burma* F59+186 **71**
Shwegyin, *Burma* F48+180 **71**
Sialkot, *Pakistan* H03+325 **72**
Siam. *See* Thailand.
Siam, G. of, *Thailand, etc.* F20+110 **69**
Sian, *China* E66+342 **66**
Siangtan, *China* E43+279 **67**
Siangyang, *China* E47+320 **66**
Siangyin, *China* E42+286 **67**
Siao Hingan Ling, *China* D42+488 **64**
Siapu, *China* E00+269 **67**
Siargao, I., *Philippines* D54+100 **65**
Siaton, *Philippines* D72+091 **65**
Siauliai, *Lithuania* L40+559 **47**
Sib, *Oman* J11+237 **75**
Sibenik, *Yugoslavia* L85+437 **56**
Siberut, I., *Indonesia* F36-014 **65**
Sibi, *Pakistan* H42+296 **70**
Sibiu, *Romania* L35+458 **58**
Sibolga, *Sumatra* F37+018 **65**
Sibsagar, *India* F61+270 **71**
Sibu, *Sarawak* E49+022 **65**
Sicasica, *Bolivia* S46-174 **104**
Sichang, *China* F16+278 **64**
Sicie C., *France* M55+430 **55**
Sicilia, I., *Italy* M06+380 **57**
Sicilian Channel, *Mediterranean Sea* M18+373 **57**
Sicily. *See* Sicilia, I.
Sicuani, *Peru* S67-143 **104**
Sid, *Yugoslavia* L65+452 **58**
Sidaka, *Iraq* K02+369 **74**
Sideby (Siipyy), *Finland* L52+621 **47**
Siderno Marina, *Italy* L82+383 **57**
Sidhout, *India* G66+145 **70**
Sidi Barrani, *Egypt* L24+316 **81**
Sidi Beben, *Libya* L70+306 **81**
Sidi-bel-Abbes, *Algeria* N04+352 **80**
Sidi Ifni, *Ifni, N.-W. Africa* N69+288 **80**
Sidlaw Hills, *Scotland* N19+565 **41**
Sidnaw, *Michigan* T82+465 **91**
Sidney, *Montana* U86+477 **93**
Sidney, *Nebraska* U78+412 **94**
Sidney, *New York* T02+423 **91**
Sidon (Saida), *Lebanon* K58+336 **76**
Sidra, Gulf of, *Libya* L70+316 **81**
Siedlce, *Poland* L47+522 **49**
Siegen, *W. Germany* M42+509 **48**
Siem-Reap, *Cambodia* F06+133 **69**
Siena, *Italy* M26+433 **56**
Sieradz, *Poland* L68+516 **49**
Sierra Colorada, *Argentina* S46-406 **103**
Sierra Grande, *Argentina* S32-414 **103**
Sierra Leone, *W. Africa* N70+088 **80**
Sierra Mojada, *Mexico* U82+273 **100**
Sierra Rosaria, *Argentina* S48-427 **103**
Sifnos, I., *Greece* L32+370 **59**
Sigean, *France* M72+430 **55**
Sighet, *Romania* L37+479 **49**
Sighisoara, *Romania* L31+462 **58**
Siglufjördhur, *Iceland* P23+662 **46**
Sigmaringen, *W. Germany* M35+481 **48**
Sigourney, *Iowa* U14+412 **95**
Sigsig, *Ecuador* T23-030 **104**
Sigüenza, *Spain* N16+411 **53**
Siguiri, *Guinea* N56+114 **80**
Sigulda, *Latvia, U.S.S.R.* L31+572 **47**
Sihl See, *Switzerland* M37+471 **45**
Sihsien, *China* E09+288 **67**
Siilinjärvi, *Finland* L14+630 **46**
Sikandarabad, *India* G74+285 **72**
Sikandra Rao, *India* G70+277 **73**
Sikar, *India* G89+275 **72**
Sikasso, *Mali* N34+112 **80**
Si Kiang, R., *China* E54+232 **64**
Siking. *See* Sian
Sikinos, I., *Greece* L29+367 **59**
Sikkim, *India* G09+275 **73**
Sila, La., *Italy* L81+392 **57**
Silairsk, *U.S.S.R.* J14+523 **61**
Silao, *Mexico* U69+209 **100**
Silchar, *India* F73+248 **71**
Silenen, *Switzerland* M38+468 **45**
Silenrieux, *Belgium* M64+502 **44**
Silesia, *Montana* V23+455 **93**
Silgarhi, *Nepal* G54+293 **73**
Silifke, *Turkey* K67+364 **74**
Silistra, *Bulgaria* L16+441 **58**
Siljan, L., *Sweden* M02+609 **47**
Silkeborg, *Denmark* M33+561 **47**
Silloth, *England* N20+549 **37**
Sils, *Switzerland* M31+464 **45**
Silvaplana, *Switzerland* M31+465 **45**
Silva Porto, *Angola* L78-124 **82**
Silver L., *Oregon* W06+431 **92**
Silver City, *New Mexico* V20+328 **94**
Silverton, *Colorado* V17+378 **94**
Silverton, *New S. Wales* C53-320 **109**
Silves, *Brazil* R80-027 **104**
Silves, *Portugal* N50+372 **52**
Silvretta, mts., *Austria-Switzerland* M30+469 **48**
Simand, L., *Quebec* T22+477 **91**
Simcoe, *Ontario* T32+429 **91**
Simcoe, L., *Ontario* T26+444 **91**
Simeulue, I., *Indonesia* F54+025 **65**
Simferopol, *U.S.S.R.* K66+450 **60**
Simi, I., *Greece* L13+366 **59**
Simla, *India* G77+310 **72**
Simleul Silvaniei, *Romania* L43+472 **49**
Simo, *Finland* L31+657 **46**
Simola, *Finland* L11+609 **47**
Simon, L., *Quebec* T01+460 **91**
Simpelveld, *Netherlands* M54+508 **44**

Index

Simplon and Pass, Switzerland M42+462 45
Simpson, Fort, N.-W. Terr. W11+614 88
Simpson, C., Alaska Y25+709 88
Simpson Des., Australia C80-254 111
Simpson, I., Chile S83-459 103
Simuna, Estonia L22+590 47
Sinai, pen., Egypt K70+290 81
Sinaloa, state, Mexico V12+250 100
Sinaloa & R., Mexico V20+260 100
Sinamaica, Venezuela S71+110 104
Sinbo, Burma F48+247 71
Sinchang, China D84+295 67
Sin-chow, China E43+385 66
Sind, Pakistan H40+255 70
Sindel, Bulgaria L15+431 58
Sindhuli Garhi, Nepal G25+272 73
Sind Sagar Doab, Pakistan H21+311 72
Sines, Portugal N53+379 52
Singa, Sudan K66+132 81
Singapore & Str., S. Asia F07+012 69
Singaraja, Bali I., Indon. E29-081 65
Singen, W. Germany M38+477 48
Singhbhum, India G27+224 73
Singida, Tanzania K62-046 83
Singitic G., Greece L36+402 59
Singkawang, Borneo E66+010 65
Singkep, I., Riouw Arch., Indon. F04-006 65
Singleton, New South Wales B83-326 109
Singora. See Songkhla
Singsingsia, China F58+418 64
Singtai, China E33+371 66
Sinho, China E28+375 66
Sinhsien, China E44+384 64
Sinhwa, China E52+277 67
Sining, China F18+363 64
Siniscola, Sardinia M32+406 57
Sinj, Yugoslavia L80+437 56
Sinjar, & Jebel, Iraq K18+364 74
Sinjil, Israel K58+320 76
Sinkiang, China G30+400 30
Sin-min-fu, China D74+420 66
Sinnamary, Fr. Guiana R47+053 105
Sinning, China E55+266 67
Sinoe L., Romania L06+446 58
Sinoia, Zimbabwe K88-172 84
Sinop, Turkey K58+420 74
Sinton, Texas U44+280 94
Sintra, Portugal N56+388 52
Sinuiju, N. Korea D64+401 64
Sinyang, China E35+322 66
Sion, Switzerland M46+462 45
Sioux City, Iowa U38+426 95
Sioux Falls, S. Dakota U40+435 93
Sioux Lookout, Ontario U11+502 89
Siparia, Trinidad S09+102 104
Sipolilo, Zimbabwe K86-166 84
Sipora, I., Indonesia F32-022 65
Siquisique, Venezuela S58+106 104
Sira, India G78+138 70
Sira. See Siros, I.
Siracusa, Sicily M88+371 57
Sirajganj, Bangladesh G01+245 73
Sir Douglas, Mt., Alberta V60+505 88
Sir Edward Pellew Group, N. Territory, Australia C77-157 111
Siretul, R., Romania L18+462 58
Sirhind, India G81+306 72
Siri, Ethiopia K36+080 83
Sirjan, Iran J28+296 75
Sirna, I., Greece L20+363 59
Sironcha, India G60+188 70
Sironj, India G74+241 73
Siros, I., Greece L30+374 59
Sirsa, India H00+295 72
Sirsi, India G68+286 73
Sirsi, India H00+146 70
Sirte (Surt), Libya L80+312 81
Sisak, Yugoslavia L82+454 56
Sisaket, Thailand F04+150 69
Sisal, Mexico U00+211 100
Sisi, Botswana L16-218 84
Sisopon, Cambodia F12+136 69
Sister I., E., Tasmania C13-397 109
Sister I., W., Tasmania C14-397 109
Sisteron, France M54+442 55
Sitamarhi, India G27+266 73
Sitamau, India G87+240 70
Sitapur, India G56+275 73
Sitara, Saudi Arabia J83+227 74
Sithonia, Greece L37+401 59
Sitia, Crete L23+352 59
Sitka, Alaska X04+569 99
Sitpur, Pakistan H25+292 72
Sittang, Burma F49+174 71
Sittang, R., Burma F51+192 71
Sittard, Netherlands M55+510 44
Sitten. See Sion
Sivand, Iran J42+301 75
Sivas, Turkey K48+398 74
Siverek, Turkey K34+378 74
Sivrihisar, Turkey K81+395 74
Sivry, Belgium M65+502 44
Siwa, Egypt L28+292 81
Siwalik Hills, India G73+304 70
Siwan, India G34+262 73
Sixmilebridge, Ireland, Rep. N53+527 43
Sixteen, Montana V36+462 93
Sjælland, Denmark M18+556 47
Sjötorp, Sweden M06+588 47
Skadarsko Jezero, Yugosl.-Alb. L64+422 58
Skagafjord, Iceland P28+660 46
Skagen, Denmark M26+577 47
Skagerrak, Norway-Denmark M42+573 47
Skagway, Alaska X00+592 99
Skaneateles, L., New York T08+428 96
Skara, Sweden M09+584 47
Skardu, Kashmir G86+353 72
Skarnes, Norway M20+602 47
Skeena R., Brit. Columbia W52+546 88
Skegness, England M88+531 37
Skellefte Alv, Sweden L66+654 46
Skellefteå, Sweden L54+647 46
Skiathos, I., Greece L39+392 59
Skibbereen, Ireland, Rep. N56+515 43
Skiddaw, mt., England N19+546 37
Skien, Norway M32+592 47
Skierniewice, Poland L59+520 49
Skiftet Kihti, Finland L54+600 47
Skipton, England N12+540 37
Skiros, I., Greece L32+389 59
Skive, Denmark M36+566 47
Skofja Loka, Yugoslavia M04+462 56
Skópelos, I., Greece L36+391 59
Skopin, U.S.S.R. K33+538 60
Skopje, Yugoslavia L51+420 58
Skövde, Sweden M07+584 47
Skovorodino, U.S.S.R. D67+540 63
Skowhegan, Maine S58+448 90
Skradin, Yugoslavia L85+438 56
Skrunda, Latvia L48+567 47
Skudenshamn, Norway M58+592 47
Skuodas, Lithuania L51+562 47
Skye, I., Scotland N38+574 40
Slagelse, Denmark M22+554 47
Slamet, mt., Java E66-072 65
Slammannon, New S. Wales C38-320 109
Slane, Ireland, Rep. N39+537 42
Slaney R., Ireland, Rep. N39+524 43
Slapin, L., Scotland N36+571 40
Slatina, Yugoslavia L74+457 58
Slatina, Romania L34+444 58
Slatington, Pennsylvania T03+407 96
Slave R., N.-W. Territories V48+604 88
Slăveni, Romania L33+441 58
Slavgorod, U.S.S.R. G70+532 62
Slavonia, Yugoslavia L72+454 58
Slavonski Brod, Yugoslavia L72+452 56
Slavyansk, Ukraine K44+488 60
Slea Hd., Ireland, Rep. N63+521 43
Sleaford, England N02+530 37
Sleat, Sd. of, Scotland N35+571 40
Sleepers, The, N.-W. Terr. T36+572 89
Sleydinge, Belgium M68+511 44
Slide Mt., New York S86+420 91
Sliedrecht, Netherlands M61+518 44
Slievanea, Ireland, Rep. N61+522 43
Slieve Anierin, Ireland, Rep. N48+541 42
Slieve Aughty, Mts., Ireland, Rep. N51+531 43
Slieve Bernagh, Ireland, Rep. N51+528 43
Slieve Bloom Mts., Ireland, Rep. N45+530 43
Slieve Car, Ireland, Rep. N58+541 42
Slieve Donard, N. Ireland N35+542 42
Slievefelim Mts., Ireland, Rep. N50+527 43
Slieve Gamph Mts., Ireland, Rep. N54+541 42
Slieve League, Ireland, Rep. N52+546 42
Slieve Mish, mts., Ireland, Rep. N59+522 43
Slieve Miskish, Ireland, Rep. N60+516 43
Slievemore, Ireland, Rep. N60+540 42
Slievenakilla, Ireland, Rep. N48+542 42
Slievenamon, Ireland, Rep. N45+524 43
Slieve Snaght, Ireland, Rep. N44+552 42
Slieve Tooey, Ireland, Rep. N52+548 42
Sligo & co., Ireland, Rep. N51+542 42
Sligo B., Ireland, Rep. N53+543 42
Slite, Sweden L67+577 47
Sliven, Bulgaria L22+427 58
Slobodskoy, U.S.S.R. J58+587 61
Sloka, Latvia L38+569 47
Slonim, Byelorussia L28+530 60
Sloten, Netherlands M56+529 44
Slough, England N04+515 39
Slovakia, Czechoslovakia L60+485 49
Slovenija, Yugoslavia M00+459 56
Slovensko, Czechoslovakia L60+488 49
Sluis, Netherlands M70+513 44
Sluiskil, Netherlands M67+513 44
Slunj, Yugoslavia L86+451 56
Słupsk, Poland L78+545 49
Slussfors, Sweden L82+655 46
Slutsk, Byelorussia L15+530 60
Slyne Hd., Ireland, Rep. N61+534 43
Slyudyanka, U.S.S.R. F08+516 63
Smerwick Harb., Ireland, Rep N62+522 43
Smethport, Pennsylvania T21+418 96
Smilde, Netherlands M51+530 44
Smiltene, Latvia L25+574 47
Smith, Alberta V54+551 88
Smith B., N.-W. Territories T20+770 89
Smith B., Gt. Bear L., N.-W. Territories W15+661 88
Smith I., Quebec T24+606 89
Smith I., South Shetlands S12-630 27
Smithers, British Columbia W42+548 88
Smithfield, N. Carolina T20+355 97
Smithfield, Virginia T11+370 97
Smithfield, Utah V41+418 94
Smithland, Kentucky T80+371 97
Smiths Falls, Ontario T06+449 91
Smithton, Tasmania C29-409 109
Smoky R., Alberta V78+552 88
Smoky Hill R., Kansas U65+388 98
Smøla, Norway M42+634 46
Smolensk, U.S.S.R. K78+548 60
Smoothstone L., Sask. V13+542 88
Smyrna. See Izmir
Snaefell, Isle of Man N27+543 37
Snake, R. & Canyon, Washington, etc. V83+464 92
Snake R., Yukon W77+657 88
Snares Is., New Zealand A81-481 112
Snåsa, Norway M16+642 46
Snåsa Vatn, Norway M18+642 46
Sneek, Netherlands M56+530 44
Sneen, Ireland, Rep. N59+518 43
Snizort, L., Scotland N39+576 40
Snøhetta, mt., Norway M34+623 46
Snow Flake, Arizona V31+345 94
Snow Lake, Manitoba U60+548 88
Snow Pk., Wyoming V09+414 98
Snowdon, mt., Wales N24+530 38
Snowtown, S. Australia C71-338 109
Snow Water L., Nevada V60+406 94
Snowy Mts., Vict.-N.S.W. C12-366 109
Snowy R., Victoria C11-386 109
Snyder, Texas U66+326 94
Soanzano, Italy L80+403 57
Soazza, Switzerland M35+463 45
Sobakin, U.S.S.R. J71+538 61
Soboko, Cent. Afr. Rep. L30+068 81
Sobrado, Brazil R49-055 105
Sobral, Brazil Q62-037 105
Sobrance, Czechoslovakia L47+487 49
Sobraon, India H00+311 72
Sochi, U.S.S.R. K34+438 62
Social Circle, Georgia T52+336 97
Society Is., Pacific Ocean Y20-150 107
Socorro, Colombia S80+064 104
Socorro, New Mexico V12+341 94
Socorro I., Mexico V36+188 100
Socotra, I., Indian Ocean J36+124 83
Soc-trang, Vietnam E84+096 69
Sodankylä, Finland L20+674 46
Soda Springs, Idaho V40+426 94
Söderfors, Sweden L77+604 47
Söderhamn, Sweden L78+613 47
Söderköping, Sweden L82+585 47
Södertälje, Sweden L74+592 47
Sodiri, Sudan L06+142 81
Sodus, New York T12+432 96
Sodus Pt., New York T12+432 96
Soela (Sulu) Eiln, Indonesia D58-018 65
Soemba (Sumba), I., Indon. E00-100 65
Soembawa (Sumbawa), I., Indonesia E10-088 65
Soerabaja, See Surabaya
Soest, W. Germany M41+516 48
Soest, Netherlands M58+522 44
Sofala, Mozambique K62-202 84
Sofala, New South Wales C02-331 109
Sofiya (Sofia), Bulgaria L40+427 58
Sogamosa, Colombia S77+057 104
Sogndal, Norway M52+583 47
Sogne Fd., Norway M54+611 47
Sögut, Turkey K89+401 74
Sohag, Egypt K80+266 81
Sohagpur, India G51+233 73
Sohan R., Pakistan H16+330 72
Sohar, Oman J20+244 75
Sohawal, India G55+246 73
Soheb, Yemen, South J79+139 74
Sohna, India G77+283 72
Soignies, Belgium M66+506 506 44
Soissons, France M70+494 54
Soke, England N02+526 37
Soke, Turkey L16+378 74
Sok Gomba, Tibet F68+320 64
Sok Karmalinsk, U.S.S.R. J45+541 61
Sokki, Chad L68+112 81
Sokode, Togo M84+090 80
Sokol, U.S.S.R. K29+594 60
Sokolo, Mali N36+146 80
Sokota, Ethiopia K36+126 83
Sokoto, Nigeria M58+128 80
Sola Consilina, Italy L87+404 57
Solai, Kenya K52+001 83
Solbad Hall, Austria M21+473 48
Soledad, Venezuela S21+082 104
Soledade, Brazil S55-066 104
Solent, The, England N08+508 39
Solenzara, Corsica M34+418 57
Sol Iletsk, U.S.S.R. J29+511 61
Solimoes (Amazonas), R., Brazil S40-020 104
Solingen, W. Germany M48+512 48
Sollefteå, Sweden L76+632 46
Sollum, see Salûm,
Solok, Sumatra F25-007 65
Solomon Is., Pacific Ocean B30-060 106
Solomon R., Kansas U59+396 98
Solon, India G77+309 72
Solothurn & canton, Switz. M45+472 45
Solsona, Spain M81+420 53
Solstad, Norway M17+651 46
Soltau, W. Germany M31+530 48
Solund, I., Norway M60+611 47
Solway, Minnesota U31+475 93
Solway Firth, Eng.-Scot. N22+548 37
Solwezi, Zambia L22-122 82
Soma, Turkey L14+392 74
Somalia, E. Africa K00+050 83
Sombor, Yugoslavia L66+458 58
Sombreiro Chan., Nicobar Is. F70+076 71
Sombrerete, Mexico U81+238 100
Sombrero, I., Leeward Is. S21+187 101
Somcuta Mare, Romania L39+475 49
Someren, Netherlands M56+514 44
Somerset, Kentucky T58+371 97
Somerset, Pennsylvania T24+400 91
Somerset, Queensland C45-108 111
Somerset, co., England N18+510 38
Somerset I., N.-W. Terr. U20+730 89
Somerset Res., Vermont S77+430 96
Somerville, New Jersey S88+405 96
Somerville, Tennessee T86+353 97
Somme, Belgium M58+503 44
Somme, dep., France M76+500 54
Somme, R., France M79+502 54
Sommieres, France M66+438 55
Somoto, Nicaragua T70+136 101
Somovit, Bulgaria L31+437 58
Somzee, Belgium M63+503 44
Son R., India G32+253 73
Sonamukhi, India G16+232 73
Sonbarsa, India G18+253 73
Sönderborg, Denmark M31+549 47
Sonepat, India G78+290 72
Song-Cau, Vietnam E65+135 69
Songea, Tanzania K56-108 83
Songkhla, Thailand F27+071 69
Song-koi, R., Vietnam F10+229 69
Sonhat, India G45+235 73
Sonkajärvi, Finland L15+637 46
Sonkovo, U.S.S.R. K47+578 60
Sonmiani, Pakistan H50+258 70
Sonneberg, E. Germany M23+503 48
Sonogno, Switzerland M37+463 45
Sonora, state & R., Mexico V38+288 100
Sonoyta, Mexico V47+319 100
Sonpur, India G36+208 71
Sonpur, India G29+257 73
Sonson, Colombia T01+057 104
Soochow, China D86+313 66
Soping. See Yuyu
Sopley, England N11+508 39
Soppero, Sweden L50+681 46
Sopron, Hungary L80+476 56
Sopur, Kashmir H03+343 72
Sora, Italy M08+417 57
Sorata, Bolivia S52-158 104
Sorbas, Spain N11+371 53
Sorell, Tasmania C15-428 109
Sörenberg, Switzerland M42+468 45
Sørfold, Norway L87+675 46
Sorgono, Sardinia M35+400 57
Soria, Spain N15+418 53
Soriano, Uruguay R80-336 103
Sornico, Switzerland M38+464 45
Sorocaba, Brazil R15-234 105
Soroki, Moldavia L10+482 60
Sorol, I., Caroline Is. C55+075 106
Soromesis, Botswana L46-194 84
Soron, India G67+279 73
Sorong, New Guinea D22-008 65
Sororoca, Brazil S09+008 104
Soroti, Uganda K68+016 83
Sørøya I., Norway L44+705 46
Sorrento, Italy M04+406 57
Sorsele, Sweden L75+655 46
Sortavala, Karelia K86+617 46
Sosnovka, U.S.S.R. K21+532 61
Sosnovo Ozerskoye, U.S.S.R. E50+526 63
Sosnowiec, Poland L66+504 49
Sosva, U.S.S.R. H80+592 62
Soto la Marina, Mexico U49+237 100
Sotra, I., Norway M60+603 47
Sotuta, Mexico T83+205 100
Souanke, Congo M06+020 82
Soudan, N. Terr. Aust. C77-200 111
Souflion, Greece L23+411 58
Souillac, France M81+449 55
Sŏul. See Seoul
Soure, Brazil R21-007 105
Soure, Portugal N52+401 52
Souris, Manitoba U62+497 88
Souris, Prince Edward I. S13+464 90
Sousse, Tunisia M26+358 81
Souterraine, la, France M81+462 54
South Africa, rep., Africa L30-280 84
South Downs, England N04+507 39
South I., New Zealand 112
Southampton, England N08+509 39
Southampton, New York S74+409 91
Southampton, Ontario T38+445 91
Southampton, C., N.-W. Terr. T52+618 89
Southampton I., N.-W. Terr. T60+646 89
South Australia, state, Aust. 110-111
South Bend, Indiana T68+417 91
South Bend, Washington W23+467 92
Southbridge, Massachusetts S72+422 96
Southbridge, New Zealand A46-438 112
South Boston, Virginia T24+367 97
South Carolina, state, U.S.A. T40+341 99
South China Sea, Asia E60+100 31
South Dakota, state, U.S.A. U78+448 98
South-East C., Tasmania C19-436 109
South-East C., Victoria C22-390 109
Southend-on-Sea, England M86+515 39
Southern Alps, New Zealand A60-436 112
Southern Cross, W. Australia E04-311 110
South Foreland, England M83+511 39
South Georgia, I., Atlant. Oc. Q40-540 27
South Hadley Falls, Mass. S76+422 96
South Haven, Michigan T68+424 91
South Indian L., Manitoba U52+568 88
South Jacksonville, Florida T40+303 97
South Milwaukee, Wisconsin T77+430 91
South Nahanni R., N.-W. Territories W40+616 88
South Orkneys, Is., Atlantic Ocean R00-610 27
South Paris, Maine S63+443 90
South Pittsburg, Tennessee T64+350 97
South Polar Plateau, Antarc. B30-870 27
South Pole, Antarctica 27
Southport, England N18+536 37
Southport, Prince Edward I. S18+463 90
Southport, Queensland B70-279 111
South River, New Jersey S87+404 96
South Ronaldsay I., Scot. N18+588 40
South Sandwich Is., Atl. Oc. P80-570 27
South Shetland Is., Antarc. S00-630 27
South Shields, England N08+550 37
South-West C., Tasmania C23-435 109
South-West Africa, See Namibia
South Yemen, Asia J80+150 74
South Yorkshire, co., Eng. N08+535 37
Souza, Brazil Q49-067 105
Souzel, Brazil R44-024 105
Souzel, Portugal N46+389 52
Sovetsk, U.S.S.R. L48+551 47
Sovetsk, U.S.S.R. J66+576 61
Sovetskaya Gavan, U.S.S.R. C57+488 63
Soy, Kenya K58+008 83
Soya & B., Japan C50+454 68
Soya Misaki, Japan C49+455 68
Soyopa, Mexico V26+290 100
Spa, Belgium M55+505 44
Spain, W. Europe N24+400 50
Spalato. See Split
Spalding, England N01+528 37
Spalding, S. Australia C68-334 109
Spandau, W. Berlin M11+525 48
Spanish, Ontario T44+462 91
Spanish Fork, Utah V40+401 94
Spanish Town, Jamaica T12+180 101
Sparks, Nevada V89+395 92
Sparta, Illinois T88+382 95
Sparta, N. Carolina T37+365 97
Sparta, Wisconsin U05+439 91
Sparta (Sparti), Greece L46+371 59
Spartanburg, S. Carolina T42+350 97
Spartivento C., Italy L83+379 57
Spask, U.S.S.R. J64+550 61
Spask, U.S.S.R. K11+538 61
Spassk, U.S.S.R. D13+447 63
Spencer, Iowa U30+432 95
Spencer, S. Dakota U46+437 93
Spencer G., S. Australia C78-340 111
Spenser Mts., New Zealand A44-420 112
Sperrin Mts., N. Ireland N42+548 42
Spetsai I., Greece L41+372 59
Spey, R., Scotland N19+576 40
Speyer, W. Germany M39+493 48
Spezand, Pakistan H48+299 70
Spezia, La, Italy M31+441 56
Sphinx, Montana V36+452 93
Spilsby, England M89+532 37
Spinazzola, Italy L83+410 57
Spiringen, Switzerland M38+469 45
Spirit Lake, Iowa U30+434 95
Spitsbergen, Arctic Ocean L40+800 62
Spitsbergen, Vest, Arctic Ocean L80+790 62
Spittal, Austria M09+468 48
Split, Yugoslavia L81+435 56
Split L., Manitoba U38+560 88
Splügen, Switzerland M34+466 45
Splügen Pass, Switzerland-Italy M30+465 45
Spofford, Texas U62+292 94
Spokane, Washington V75+476 92
Spoleto, Italy M14+428 56
Spontin, Belgium M60+503 44
Sporadhes, Aegean Sea L18+370 59

Sporadhes, Voriai, Aegean Sea L32+392 59
Spotsylvania, Virginia T16+382 97
Spree R., E. Germany M06+523 48
Spremberg, E. Germany M04+516 48
Sprimont, Belgium M56+505 44
Springbok, Cape Province L72-296 84
Spring City, Tennessee T59+356 97
Springdale, Arkansas U24+362 93
Springdale, Montana V32+457 93
Springer, New Mexico U88+364 94
Springerville, Arizona V26+342 94
Springfield, Colorado U76+374 94
Springfield, Georgia T38+323 97
Springfield, Illinois T88+398 91
Springfield, Massachusetts S75+421 91
Springfield, Missouri U20+372 95
Springfield, Ohio T53+399 91
Springfield, Vermont S75+433 96
Springfontein, Orange Free State L26-304 84
Springhill, Nova Scotia S24+456 90
Spring Hope, N. Carolina T19+360 97
Springlands, Guyana R73+058 105
Spring Place, Georgia T59+348 97
Springsure, Queensland C12-239 111
Springville, New York T22+425 91
Springville, Utah V40+402 94
Spruce Brook, Newfoundland R79+488 90
Spruce Knob, W. Virginia T28+387 96
Spruga, Switzerland M39+462 45
Squillace, G. di, Italy L78+387 57
Srbija (Serbia), Yugoslavia L58+435 58
Srebrenica, Yugoslavia L65+441 58
Sredinnyy Khrebet, U.S.S.R. B30+570 63
Sredne Kamchatsk, U.S.S.R. B31+555 63
Sredne Kolyma, U.S.S.R. B80+670 63
Sredne Vilyuysk, U.S.S.R. D70+639 63
Srem, Poland L78+521 49
Srepok, R., Cambodia E78+136 65
Sretensk, U.S.S.R. E12+524 63
Srikakulam, India G36+183 71
Sri Lanka, S. Asia G55+076 70
Sri Madhopur, India G86+274 72
Srinagar, Kashmir H01+341 72
Srirangapatnam, India G79+124 70
Srivilliputtur, India G74+095 70
Srnetica, Yugoslavia L81+445 56
Sroda, Poland L76+522 49
Stackpool, Ontario T41+479 91
Stack's Mts., Ireland, Rep. N57+523 43
Stadacona, Quebec S73+474 91
Staden, Belgium M72+510 44
Staffa, I., Scotland N38+564 41
Stafford, Arizona V28+328 94
Stafford, England N13+528 37
Stafford, Kansas U52+379 95
Stafford, Virginia T15+384 97
Stafford, co., England N12+529 37
Staines, England N03+514 39
Stambaugh, Michigan T81+461 91
Stamford, Connecticut S81+411 91
Stamford, England N03+526 37
Stamprooi, Netherlands M56+512 44
Stanberry, Missouri U28+403 95
Stanchik, U.S.S.R. B89+710 63
Standerton, Transvaal L04-270 84
Standish, Michigan T54+439 91
Stange, Norway M23+607 47
Stanislav, Ukraine L34+490 49
Stanley, Falkland Is. R78-516 99
Stanley, Tasmania C28-408 109
Stanley Falls, See Boyoma Falls
Stanleyville. See Kisangani L28+006 82
Stann Creek, Belize T80+170 101
Stanovoy Khrebet, U.S.S.R. D60+557 63
Stans, Switzerland M40+470 45
Stansmore Ra., W. Australia D45-214 110
Stanthorpe, Queensland B78-285 111
Stanton, Michigan T61+433 91
Stanton, N. Dakota U69+473 93
Staphorst, Netherlands M53+526 44
Staples, Minnesota U29+463 93
Stara Planina, Bulgaria L30+427 59
Staraya Russa, U.S.S.R. K80+580 60
Stara Zagora, Bulgaria L26+424 58
Starbuck, I., Pacific Ocean Y32-055 107
Star City, Arkansas U11+340 97
Stargard, Poland L90+533 48
Starkville, Mississippi T84+334 95
Starkweather, N. Dakota U53+485 93
Starobel'sk, Ukraine K36+492 60
Starodub, U.S.S.R. K73+526 60
Starogard, Poland L69+540 49
Staro Konstantinov, Ukraine L16+498 60
Staryy Oskol, U.S.S.R. K43+512 60
Staten I., Argentina. See Estados, I. de los
Staten I., New York S85+406 96
Statesville, N. Carolina T35+357 97
Stattlandet, Norway M58+622 46
Staunton, Virginia T25+382 97
Stavanger, Norway M56+590 47
Stavelot, Belgium M54+504 44
Stavenisse, Netherlands M66+516 44
Stavern, Norway M30+590 47
Staveren, Netherlands M58+529 44
Stavropol, U.S.S.R. K20+450 62
Stawell, Victoria C43-371 109
Steckborn, Switzerland M36+477 45
Steele, N. Dakota U60+469 93
Steelton, Pennsylvania T11+402 96
Steelville, Missouri U08+380 95
Steenbergen, Netherlands M64+516 44
Steensel, Netherlands M58+514 44
Steenwijk, Netherlands M53+528 44
Stefanie L., Ethiopia K48+046 83
Steiermark, prov., Austria M00+472 48
Stein, Switzerland M37+477 45
Steinkjer, Norway M21+640 46
Stekene, Belgium M66+512 44
Stellarton, Nova Scotia S16+456 90
Stenay, France M59+495 54
Stendal, E. Germany M19+526 48
Stenness, L. of, Orkney, Scot. N19+590 40
Stenträsk, Sweden L61+663 46
Stephenson, Michigan T76+454 91
Stephenville, Newfoundland R81+485 90
Stepnoy, U.S.S.R. K05+465 62
Stepnyak, Kazakh. H25+531 62
Sterea, Greece L48+387 59
Sterling, Colorado U79+406 94
Sterling, Illinois T88+418 95
Sterlitamak, U.S.S.R. J24+536 61
Šternberk, Czechoslovakia L77+497 49
Sterrebeek, Belgium M63+509 44
Stettin. See Szczecin
Stettler, Alberta V45+520 88
Steubenville, Ohio T34+404 91
Stevens Point, Wisconsin T88+445 91
Stewart, Brit. Columbia W60+557 88
Stewart River, Yukon X26+636 88
Stewart, I., Chile S68-548 103
Stewart Is., New Zealand A73-470 112
Stewart R., Yukon X05+640 88
Stewart Sd., Andaman Is. F72+130 71
Steyr, Austria M04+480 48
Stia, Italy M20+438 56
Stikine R., Brit. Columbia W70+568 88
Stillwater, Minnesota U17+451 93
Stillwater, Oklahoma U42+362 95
Stimlje, Yugoslavia L54+424 58
Štip, Yugoslavia L47+417 58
Stirling, Scotland N24+561 41
Stirling Ra., W. Australia E10-342 110
Stjernøya, Norway L44+703 46
Stockholm, Sweden L72+594 47
Stockinbingal, New South Wales C13-346 109
Stockport, England N13+534 37
Stockton, California W08+379 92
Stockton, Kansas U56+394 95
Stockton, New South Wales B80-329 109
Stockton-on-Tees, England N08+546 37
Stoer, Pt. of, Scotland N32+583 40
Stoke-on-Trent, England N13+530 37
Stolbovaya, U.S.S.R. B69+645 63
Stolp. See Słupsk
Ston, Yugoslavia L74+428 56
Stonehaven, Scotland N13+569 40
Stony L., Ontario T19+445 91
Stony Crossing, New South Wales C39-351 109
Stony Stratford, England N06+520 39
Stor Sjön, Sweden M04+633 46
Stora Lulevatten, Sweden L64+672 46
Stora Sjöfallets Nat. Park, Sweden L74+676 46
Storavan, Sweden L70+657 46
Stord, I., Norway M58+598 47
Støren, Norway M28+631 46
Storforshei, Norway M03+664 46
Storlien, Sweden M17+634 46
Storm B., Tasmania C15-432 109
Storm Lake, Iowa U31+426 95
Stornoway, Scotland N38+582 40
Storsund, Sweden L56+656 46
Storuman, Sweden L77+650 46
Storvik, Sweden L82+606 47
Stour, R., England M84+520 39
Stourbridge, England N13+525 37
Stourport, England N14+524 37
Stowmarket, England M84+522 39
Strabane, N. Ireland N45+548 42
Strachan, Quebec T00+480 91
Strachan I., Papua N. Guin., C47-090 111
Stradbally, Ireland, Rep. N43+530 43
Strahan, Tasmania C28-422 109
Stralsund, E. Germany M12+543 48
Strand, Norway M54+590 47
Stranda, Norway M48+623 46
Strangford, N. Ireland N33+544 42
Strangford L., N. Ireland N33+545 42
Strangways Springs, South Australia C80-289 111
Stranorlar, Ireland, Rep. N46+548 42
Stranraer, Scotland N30+549 41
Strasbourg, France M43+485 54
Strasburg, Virginia T20+390 96
Stråssa, Sweden L89+598 47
Stratford, Connecticut S78+412 96
Stratford, Michigan T60+445 91
Stratford, New Zealand A34-393 112
Stratford, Ontario T36+434 91
Stratford, Victoria C18-379 109
Stratford-upon-Avon, England N10+522 37
Strathalbyn, S. Australia C67-352 109
Strathclyde, reg., Scotland N32+558 41
Strathcona Park, B.C. W35+498 88
Strathpeffer, Scotland N27+576 40
Strathroy, Ontario T40+430 91
Strathy Pt., Scotland N24+586 40
Strathyre, Scotland N26+563 41
Straubing, W. Germany M15+489 48
Štrba, Czech. L60+491 49
Streaky B., S. Australia D05-324 111
Streator, Illinois T83+411 95
Strelka, U.S.S.R. B79+618 63
Strelka, U.S.S.R. F14+617 63
Strelka, U.S.S.R. F70+581 63
Strencis, Latvia L26+576 47
Stribro, Czechoslovakia M12+497 48
Strijbeek, Netherlands M61+515 44
Strijen, Netherlands M63+517 44
Strimón, G. of, Greece L36+406 59
Strokestown, Ireland, Rep. N48+538 42
Stroma, I., Scotland N19+586 40
Stromboli, I., Italy L89+388 57
Stromeferry, Scotland N33+573 40
Stromness, Orkney, Scot. N20+590 40
Strömsberg, Sweden L75+604 47
Strömsbruk, Sweden L76+619 47
Strömstad, Sweden M23+590 47
Strömsund, Sweden L86+639 46
Ströms Vattudal, Sweden M04+644 46
Strömtorp, Sweden M03+593 47
Strongoli, Italy L78+393 57
Stronsay I., & Firth, Scot. N15+591 40
Stroud, England N13+517 39
Stroudsburg, Pennsylvania T01+410 96
Struga, Yugoslavia L56+412 58
Strule, R., N. Ireland N44+547 42
Struma, R., Bulgaria-Greece L42+418 58
Strumica, Yugoslavia L44+414 58
Stryy, Ukraine L37+493 60
Strzelecki Pk., Tasmania C13-402 109
Strzelin, Poland L78+508 49
Stuart, Florida T32+272 97
Stuart, Virginia T32+366 97
Stuart Ra., S. Australia D05-290 111
Stuart Highway, N.T., Aust. D06-186 111
Stugun, Sweden L86+632 46
Stung-Treng, Cambodia E84+135 69
Sturgeon Bay, Wisconsin T75+449 91
Sturgeon Falls, Ontario T30+464 91
Sturgis, S. Dakota U82+444 93
Sturt Des., S. Australia, etc. C54-282 111
Sturt, Mt., New S. Wales C50-296 109
Stuttgart, Arkansas U10+345 97
Stuttgart, W. Germany M35+488 48
Suakin, Sudan K46+196 81
Suancheng, China E07+309 66
Süan-hwa, China E29+406 66
Suaqui, Mexico V27+286 100
Subeimanieh, Iran J54+358 75
Subh, Jebel, Saudi Arabia K36+237 74
Subotica, Yugoslavia L62+461 58
Sucha, Poland L62+498 49
Suchan, U.S.S.R. D11+430 63
Süchow (Tungshan), China E15+343 66
Suck R., Ireland, Rep. N49+533 43
Sucre, Bolivia S32-192 104
Sudan, rep. Africa — 81
Sudbury, England M86+520 39
Sudbury, Ontario T36+465 91
Suddie, Guyana R81+070 104
Sudety, mts., Czech., etc. L84+507 49
Sudharam, Bangladesh F83+228 71
Suez, Egypt K74+300 81
Suez Canal, Egypt K75+310 81
Suez, Gulf of, Egypt K72+286 81
Suffolk, Virginia T09+367 97
Suffolk, co., England M84+523 39
Suggsville, Alabama T76+316 97
Suhl, E. Germany M26+506 48
Suifu. See Ipin
Suihwa, China D47+466 64
Suining, China E12+339 66
Suipacha, Bolivia S33-215 104
Suir R., Ireland, Rep. N43+523 43
Suiteh, China E59+374 66
Sujangarh, India H02+277 72
Sujanpur, India G86+323 72
Sujanpur, India G81+318 72
Sujica, Yugoslavia L77+438 56
Sukarnapura. See Djajapura
Sukarno, Pk. See Puntjak Djaja
Sukhumi, Gruzinskaya K25+430 62
Sukkur, Pakistan H37+276 70
Suklek B., Labrador S20+588 89
Sukow, China E45+375 66
Sukumo, Japan D13+330 68
Sulaiman Ra., Pakistan H30+310 70
Sulaimiya, Saudi Arabia J75+242 74
Sulaiyil, Saudi Arabia J87+204 74
Sulaymānīya, Iraq J87+356 74
Sulecin, Poland L87+521 49
Sulgen, Switzerland M35+475 45
Sulina, Romania L02+451 58
Sulitelma, mt., Norway L82+671 46
Sullana, Peru T34-049 104
Sullivan, Illinois T82+396 95
Sullivan, Indiana T74+390 95
Sullivan, Missouri U07+382 97
Sulmona, Italy M07+419 57
Sulphur Springs, Texas U34+332 95
Sultan Bulak, Iran J65+358 74
Sultan Dagh, Turkey K84+383 74
Sultan Hamud, Kenya K46-020 83
Sultaniyeh, Iran J67+365 74
Sultanpur, India G47+262 73
Sultanpur, India H00+312 72
Sulu Arch., Philippines D82+055 65
Sulu Kep., Indonesia D58-018 65
Sulu Sea, Philippines E00+081 65
Sumagawa, Japan C48+434 68
Sumatra, I., Indonesia F30+005 65
Sumba, I., Indonesia E00-100 65
Sumbawa, I., Indonesia E10-088 65
Sumbur, Mongolia E68+465 64
Sumburgh Hd., Scotland N08+599 40
Sümeg, Hungary L77+470 49
Sumiswald, Switzerland M44+470 45
Summerside, Pr. Edward I. S22+464 90
Summit, S. Dakota U42+453 93
Sumperk, Czechoslovakia L79+500 49
Sumprabum, Burma F44+266 71
Sumter, S. Carolina T32+339 97
Sumy, Ukraine K61+509 60
Suna, Tanzania K62-056 83
Sunapee, New Hampshire S72+434 96
Sunart L., Scotland N34+567 41
Sunbury, Pennsylvania T11+409 91
Suncho Corral, Argentina S21-279 103
Sunchow. See Kweiping
Suncook, New Hampshire S69+431 91
Sunda Str., Indonesia F00-064 65
Sundance, Wyoming U86+444 93
Sundargarh, India G35+221 73
Sunderland, England N08+549 37
Sundridge, Ontario T27+458 91
Sundsvall, Sweden L76+624 46
Sungari Res., China D50+430 64
Sungari R., China D60+456 64
Sungkiang, China D81+311 66
Sunndal, Norway M38+627 46
Sunnyside, Utah V32+395 94
Suntar, U.S.S.R. E14+622 63
Sunyani, Ghana N14+074 80
Suonnejoki, Finland L17+625 46
Supaul, India G20+261 73
Superior, Wisconsin U12+467 93
Superior L., U.S.A.-Canada T80+475 99
Supiori, I., New Guinea, Indonesia C87-006 65
Suq ash Shuyukh, Iraq J81+309 74
Sur, Oman J03+226 75
Sur (Tyre), Lebanon K59+333 76
Sura R., U.S.S.R. J81+551 61
Surab, Pakistan H52+283 70
Surabaya, Java E43-072 65
Surajgarh, India G85+283 72
Surakarta, Java E55-075 65
Suran, Syria K49+353 76
Surapur, India G79+166 70
Surat, India H12+211 70
Suratgarh, India H06+293 72
Surat, Thani, Thailand F34+091 69
Surendranagar, India H20+227 70
Surgères, France N05+461 54
Surgut, U.S.S.R. G70+613 62
Suri, India G15+239 73
Surigao Str., Philippines D60+092 65
Surin, Thailand F09+148 69
Surinam (Dutch Guiana) S. America R70+040 105
Suriname, R., Surinam R63+042 105
Suriya, Yemen, South J84+135 74
Surling, Mt., Vietnam E73+115 69
Surrey, co., England N03+513 39
Sursee, Switzerland M41+472 45
Sursk, Ukraine K61+484 60
Süs (Susch), Switzerland M30+468 45
Susa, Iran J70+323 74
Susak, Yugoslavia M03+447 56
Susquehanna R., Pa., etc. T08+398 91
Sussex, New Brunswick S33+457 90
Sussex, E. & W., co., England N01+510 39
Susteren, Netherlands M55+511 44
Sutherland, Cape Province L56-324 84
Sutherland, co., See Highland
Suting. See Tahsien.
Sutlej R., Pakistan H12+302 72
Sutsien, China E10+339 66
Sutton, Ontario T26+443 91
Suure Jaani, Estonia L27+585 47
Suvavesi, Finland L11+626 46
Suvorov, I., Pacific Ocean Y80-138 106
Suwair, Saudi Arabia K28+301 74
Suwałki, Poland L43+541 49
Suwayh, Oman J02+222 75
Suwayq, Oman J15+239 75
Suweilih, Jordan K55+320 76
Suwo Nada, Japan D21+338 68
Svalbard, Arctic Ocean L60+790 62
Svanstein, Sweden L37+666 46
Svappavaara, Sweden L54+677 46
Svørholt-halvøya, Norway L24+704 46
Svartenhuk Pen., Greenland R38+720 26
Svartisen, Norway M06+666 46
Svartvik, Sweden L76+623 46
Šveksna, Lithuania L50+556 47
Svendborg, Denmark M26+551 47
Sventoji, Lithuania L53+560 47
Sverdlovsk, U.S.S.R. H86+568 61
Sverdrup Is., N.-W. Terr. U30+778 88
Sverdrup, Os., U.S.S.R. G64+745 62
Svishtov, Bulgaria L28+436 58
Svitavy, Czechoslovakia L80+497 49
Svobodny, U.S.S.R. D41+514 63
Svolvaer, Norway M02+682 46
Swabi, Pakistan H15+341 72
Swakopmund, Namibia M02-226 84
Swale R., England N09+543 37
Swan, R., W. Australia E22-314 110
Swan Hill, Victoria C39-354 109
Swan Reach, S. Australia C62-346 109
Swan River, Manitoba U66+524 88
Swansea, Tasmania C12-422 109
Swansea & B., Wales N24+516 38
Swanton, Vermont S79+449 91
Swarzewo, Poland L70+547 49
Swastika, Ontario T31+481 91
Swat & R., Pakistan H15+350 72
Swatow, China E20+234 67
Swaziland, S. Africa K80-264 84
Sweden, N.-W. Europe 46-47
Sweet Grass Hills, Montana V37+489 93
Sweetwater, Texas U62+324 94
Swellendam, Cape Province L58-340 84
Swidnica, Poland L81+509 49
Swietochlowice, Poland L67+503 49
Swift Current, Saskatchewan V17+502 88
Swilly L., Ireland, Rep. N45+552 42
Swinburne, C., N.-W. Terr. U54+710 88
Swindon, England N11+515 39
Swinemünde. See Swinioujscie
Swinford, Ireland, Rep. N54+539 42
Swinoujście, Poland M04+539 48
Switzerland, Central Europe M42+470 50
Swords, Ireland, Rep. N37+534 43
Syasstroy, U.S.S.R. K75+602 60
Sybil Pt., Ireland, Rep. N63+522 43
Sycamore, Illinois T82+420 91
Sydney, New South Wales B83-339 109
Sydney, Nova Scotia S01+461 90
Sydney Mines, Nova Scotia S01+463 90
Syeti Vrach, Bulgaria L40+416 58
Syktyvkar, U.S.S.R. J56+616 62
Sylhet, Bangladesh F78+250 71
Sylt, I., W. Germany M40+549 48
Sylte, Norway M46+623 46
Syracuse, Kansas U70+380 94
Syracuse, New York T06+430 96
Syracuse, Sicily M88+371 57
Syr Darya, Kazakh. H50+440 62
Syria, W. Asia K40+350 74
Syrian Des., Iraq, etc. K30+323 74
Sysert, U.S.S.R. H86+566 61
Syurkum, U.S.S.R. C57+500 63
Syzran, U.S.S.R. J68+532 68
Szarvas, Hungary L56+469 49
Szczecin, Poland M03+534 48
Szczecinek, Poland L80+537 49
Szczecinski Zalew, E. Germany-Poland M04+537 48
Szczytno, Poland L54+536 49
Szechwan, prov., China E84+308 66
Szeged, Hungary L59+463 58
Székesféheryar, Hungary L69+472 49
Szekszard, Hungary L68+463 58
Szemao, China F23+227 64
Szenan, China E69+279 67
Szengen, China E72+235 67
Szentes, Hungary L58+467 49
Szolnok, Hungary L59+472 49
Szombathely, Hungary L80+472 56
Szreńsk, Poland L59+530 49
Szrotawa, Poland L87+516 49
Taba, Saudi Arabia K16+269 74
Tabab, Saudi Arabia K15+187 74
Tabala, Saudi Arabia K15+197 74
Tabas, Iran J19+337 75
Tabasara, Sierra de, Panama T36+086 101
Tabasco, state, Mexico U20+180 100
Tabas Sunnikhane, Iran H89+327 75
Tabatinga, Brazil R22-216 105
Tabatinga, Brazil S60-045 104
Tabelbala, Algeria N20+292 80
Table B. & Mt., Cape Prov. L69-339 84
Taboieiro, Brazil R81-052 104
Tábor, Czechoslovakia M02+494 48
Tabora, Tanzania K74-050 83
Tabriz, Iran J82+381 74
Tabu, Ivory Coast N44+046 80
Tabuk, Saudi Arabia K49+285 74
Tabut, Yemen South J47+159 75
Tacambaro, Mexico U67+190 100

Tache, L., N.-W. Territories W03+642 88
Tacloban, Philippines D60+111 65
Tacna, Peru S62-180 104
Taco, Argentina S20-256 103
Tacoma, Washington W15+473 92
Taconic Mts., N.Y.-Mass. S80+425 96
Tacuarembo, Uruguay R66-317 103
Tadcaster, England N08+539 37
Tadjoura & G. of, Djibouti K12+116 83
Tadoussac, Quebec S58+481 90
Tadzhikskaya, rep., U.S.S.R. H30+390 62
Taegu, Korea D38+358 64
Taejŏn, Korea D44+363 64
Taf R., Wales N27+518 38
Tafalla, Spain N10+425 53
Taff R., Wales N20+515 38
Tafila, Jordan K56+309 76
Taft, Iran J34+318 75
Taftville, Connecticut S72+415 96
Taganrog & G., U.S.S.R. K36+473 61
Taga Zong, Bhutan G00+270 71
Tagish, Yukon W86+602 88
Tagula, I., Papua New Guinea B70-115 111
Tagus, N. Dakota U72+484 93
Tagus, R. See Tajo R.
Tahakopa, New Zealand A63+465 112
Tahat Mt., Algeria M56+230 80
Tahcheng, China G42+467 62
Ta Hingan Ling, China D84+480 64
Tahiti, I., Society Islands X82-180 107
Tahoe, L., California W00+391 92
Tahora, New Zealand A31-390 112
Tahoua, Niger M58+148 80
Tahsien, China E75+313 66
Tahta, Egypt K82+268 81
Tahuna, Indonesia D58+037 65
Tai-an, China E17+362 66
Taichow. See Linhai.
Taichung, Taiwan D86+242 67
Taieri, R., New Zealand A58-456 112
Taïf, Saudi Arabia K28+211 74
Tai-hang-shan, China E36+370 66
Taihape, New Zealand A25-396 112
Taihsien, China E00+325 66
Taihsien, China E43+391 66
Tai Hu, China D88+312 66
Taiku, China E46+374 66
Tailem Bend, S. Australia C63-353 109
Taima, Saudi Arabia K36+277 74
Tainan, Taiwan D88+230 67
Taipale, Finland L04+627 46
Taipei, Taiwan D82+250 67
Taiping. See Tsungtso.
Taiping, Malaysia F26+049 69
Taiping. See Tangtu.
Taipingchwan, China D72+444 64
Taipinghs. See Wanyuan.
Taira, Japan C54+371 68
Tairadate Str., Japan C56+411 68
Taishan I., China D77+303 67
Taishet, U.S.S.R. F41+560 63
Taishun, China E01+275 67
Taitao, Pen. de. Chile S88-462 103
Taiwan, I., China D84+240 67
Taiwan Hai Hsai, China E06+240 67
Taiwara, Afghanistan H63+335 75
Taiyetos, mts., Greece L46+370 59
Taiyiba, Jordan K57+303 76
Taiyuan, China E45+378 66
Ta'izz, Yemen K06+136 74
Tajan, Borneo E59-001 65
Tajo, R., Spain-Portugal N44+397 52
Tajrish, Iran J52+358 75
Tajumulco, mt., Guatemala U11+151 100
Tak, Thailand F35+169 69
Takada, Japan C70+371 68
Takahashi, Japan D08+348 68
Takaka, New Zealand A43-409 112
Takamatsu, Japan D06+343 68
Takao. See Kaohsiung.
Takaoka, Japan C78+368 68
Takapuna, New Zealand A31-368 112
Takasaki, Japan C66+363 68
Takaungu, Kenya K30-038 83
Takayama, Japan C76+362 68
Takefu, Japan C83+358 68
Takhta Bazar, Turkmen H74+360 62
Takht-i-Sulaiman, Pakistan H30+316 72
Takingeun, Sumatra F49+047 65
Takla L., British Columbia W35+554 88
Takla Makan, des., Sinkiang, China G40+380 30
Takoradi, Ghana N12+050 80
Ta-ku, China E14+389 66
Takuapa, Thailand F40+088 69
Talagang, Pakistan H15+329 72
Talaimanar, Sri Lanka G62+091 70
Talasski Ala Tau, Kirgiz. H20+423 62
Talar Ra., Pakistan H64+254 70
Talara, Peru T38-045 104
Talavera de la Reina, Spain N29+399 52
Talca, Chile S70-354 103
Talcahuano, Chile S79-367 103
Tali, China E61+348 66
Tali, China F30+257 64
Taliabu, I., Indonesia D60-018 65
Taliwang, Sumbawa I., Indonesia E19-088 65
Talladega, Alabama T67+334 97
Tallahassee, Florida T56+304 97
Tallangatta, Victoria C16-362 109
Tallata-Mafara, Nigeria M54+124 80
Tallinn, Estonia L31+595 47
Tallow, Ireland, Rep. N48+521 43
Tallulah, Louisiana U07+324 95
Tallulah Falls, Georgia T50+347 97
Talmenka, U.S.S.R. G39+538 62
Talou Shan, China E82+280 64
Talsi, Latvia L45+572 47
Taltal, Chile S63-254 103
Tamale, Ghana N04+094 80
Tamanrasset, Algeria M58+226 80
Tamaqua, Pennsylvania T06+408 96
Tamar R., England N25+505 38
Tamar R., Tasmania C19-412 109
Tamarite de Litera, Spain M87+419 53
Tamási, Hungary L71+467 49
Tamatave, Madagascar J64-182 83
Tamaulipas, state, Mexico U53+235 100
Tamaya, Chile S69-305 103
Tamba, Zimbabwe L02-214 84
Tambach, Kenya K56+006 83
Tambacounda, Senegal N82+138 80
Tambo de Mora, Peru T07-135 104
Tambohorano, Madagascar K06-176 83
Tamboril, Brazil Q63-048 105
Tambov, U.S.S.R. K22+527 61
Tambura, Sudan L14+056 81
Tame, Colombia S71+066 104
Tamel Aiken, Argentina S66-482 103
Tamiahua & L., Mexico U46+212 100
Tamil Nadu, state, India G70+114 70
Tamins, Switzerland M33+468 45
Tamluk, India G12+223 73
Tammisaari (Ekenäs), Finland L39+600 47
Tammu, Burma F54+242 71
Tampa, Florida T45+280 97
Tampa B., Florida T46+278 99
Tampere, Finland L37+615 47
Tampico, Mexico U48+222 100
Tamra, Saudi Arabia J88+204 74
Tamsalu, Estonia L23+591 47
Tamtsak Bulak, Mongolia E13+470 64
Tamworth, England N10+526 37
Tamworth, New S. Wales B85-311 109
Tana Fd., Norway L10+707 46
Tana, I., Vanuatu A65-195 106
Tana L., Ethiopia K46+118 83
Tana, R., Norway L23+698 46
Tanabe, Japan C88+338 68
Tanabu, Japan C52+413 68
Tanaga I., Aleutian Is. Z80+512 99
Tanah Merah, Malaysia F17+057 69
Tanahmerah, New Guinea C60-062 65
Tanami, N. Terr., Australia D32-200 110
Tanana, Alaska Y10+652 99
Tanana, R., Alaska X60+635 99
Tananarive (Antananarivo), Madagascar J76-190 83
Tancanhuitz, Mexico U54+216 100
Tancheng, China E09+346 66
Tanda, India G44+266 73
Tanda Urmar, India G86+316 72
Tandil, Argentina R85-372 103
Tandou L., New S. Wales C47-326 109
Taneatua, New Zealand A18-380 112
Tanega Shima, Japan D24+306 68
Tanen-taung-gyi Mts., Thailand-Burma F42+191 69
Tanga, Tanzania K36-050 83
Tanganyika. See Tanzania
Tanganyika, L., E. Cent. Afr. L00-050 83
Tangen, Norway M22+606 47
Tangermünde, E. Germany M18+526 48
Tangier, (Tanger), Morocco N34+356 80
Tang-shan, China E11+396 66
Tangshan, China E21+344 66
Tangtu, China E09+316 66
Tangui, U.S.S.R. F24+555 63
Tanimbar Kep., Indon. D22-074 65
Tanjungpandan, Billiton I., Indonesia E74-027 65
Tanjungperiuk, Java, Indon. E78+060 65
Tanjungredeb, Borneo E16+021 65
Tanjungselor, Borneo E16+028 65
Tank, Pakistan H27+322 72
Tankapirtti, Finland L16+682 46
Tankse, Kashmir G70+340 70
Tännäs, Sweden M14+625 46
Tanta, Egypt K84+308 81
Tantung, China D63+401 66
Tanuf, Oman J17+230 75
Tanzania, E. Africa K60-050 83
Tao, Burma F71+228 71
Taoan, China D73+454 64
Taochow. See Lintan
Taofu, China F23+310 64
Taormina, Sicily L88+378 57
Taos, New Mexico V04+364 94
Tapa, Estonia L24+592 47
Tapachula, Mexico U13+149 100
Tapah, Malaysia F22+042 69
Tapajos, R., Brazil R63-040 105
Tapalque, Argentina S00-362 103
Tapan, Sumatra F24-021 65
Tapanui, New Zealand A64-459 112
Tapa Shan, China E67+320 66
Tapauá, Brazil S26-057 104
Tapera do Retiro, Brazil S11-099 104
Taplang Dzong, Nepal G14+274 73
Tappahannock, Virginia T11+381 97
Tapti R., India G78+216 70
Tapuaenuku, mt., N.Z. A38-420 112
Taqa, Oman J33+171 75
Taquanalsinho, Brazil R80-092 104
Taquara, Brazil R35-297 103
Taquaretinga, Brazil Q36-079 105
Tara, U.S.S.R. H05+567 62
Tārabulus esh Shām, (Tripoli), Lebanon K55+344 76
Taradale, New Zealand A18-395 112
Tarago, New South Wales C02-351 109
Tarahumare, Sa., Mexico V16+280 100
Tarakan, Borneo E14+034 65
Tarakli, Turkey K87+404 74
Taralga, New South Wales C01-344 109
Tarana, New South Wales C01-336 109
Taranaki Bight, N., N.Z. A36-388 112
Taranaki Bight, S., N.Z. A38-397 112
Tarancón, Spain N18+400 52
Taranto, Italy L76+404 57
Taranto, G. di, Italy L77+400 57
Tarapoto, Peru T08-065 104
Taraqua, Brazil S49-002 104
Tararua Ra., New Zealand A28-409 112
Tarascon, France M80+428 55
Tarasp, Switzerland M28+468 45
Tarata, Peru S61-177 104
Tarauaca, Brazil S65-084 104
Tarawa, I., Kiribati A40+020 106
Tarawera, New Zealand A20-390 112
Tarazona, Spain N10+419 53
Tarazona de la Mancha, Sp. N12+392 53
Tarbagatai Khrebet, Kazakh G40+470 62
Tarbat Ness, Scotland N23+579 40
Tarbert, Ireland, Rep. N56+526 43
Tarbert, Scotland N32+558 41
Tarbert, Scotland N41+579 40
Tarbes, France N00+432 55
Tarboro, N. Carolina T15+359 97
Tarchan, Tibet G52+310 70
Tarcoola, S. Australia D02-307 111
Tarcoon, New South Wales C20-303 109
Tarcutta, New South Wales C14-353 109
Taree, New South Wales B76-320 109
Tärendö, Sweden L44+672 46
Târgoviste, Romania L27+449 58
Târgu Mures, Romania L33+466 58
Târgul Ocna, Romania L20+463 58
Tarija, Bolivia S29-214 104
Tarim, Basin & R., Sinkiang G30+400 30
Tarlac, Philippines D87+156 65
Tarma, Peru T05-114 104
Tarn, dep. & R., France M77+438 55
Tärna, Sweden L88+657 46
Tarn-et-Garonne, dep., Fr. M81+442 55
Tarnobrzeg, Poland L50+506 49
Tarnów, Poland L54+500 49
Tarnowskie Gory, Poland L67+505 49
Tarn Taran, India H00+314 72
Tarnu Măgurele, Romania L31+437 58
Taroudant, Morocco N54+304 80
Tarragona, Spain M82+411 53
Tarran Hills, New S. Wales C23-326 109
Tarrega, Spain M83+416 53
Tarsale, U.S.S.R. G70+648 62
Tarso Muri, mt., Libya L68+212 81
Tarsus, Turkey K61+370 74
Tartagal, Argentina S22-227 103
Tartas, France N05+438 55
Tartna Point, New S. Wales C45-330 109
Tartu, Estonia L19+583 47
Tartus, Syria K55+349 76
Tarum, Iran J26+281 75
Taseevo, U.S.S.R. F61+573 63
Taseko Ls., Brit. Columbia W22+514 88
Tashi Bhup Tso, Tibet G30+322 71
Tashihto, China F82+438 64
Tashkent, Uzbek. H34+415 62
Tashkurghan, Afghanistan H43+367 75
Tash Kurghan, China G88+377 72
Tashmalik, China G86+392 72
Tasil, Syria K54+328 76
Taskan, U.S.S.R. B89+630 63
Tasköprü, Turkey K62+416 74
Tasman B., New Zealand A40-410 112
Tasman, Mt., New Zealand A58-435 112
Tasman Mts., New Zealand A45-410 112
Tasman Pen., Tasmania C13-431 109
Tasmania I. & state, Aust. C20-420 111
Tassgong, Bhutan F80+272 71
Tata, Hungary L70+478 49
Tatakoto, Tuamotu Arch X20-175 107
Tatarsk, U.S.S.R. G84+552 62
Tatarskaya, aut. rep., U.S.S.R. J60+553 62
Tatarskiy Proliv, U.S.S.R. C50+500 63
Tathlina, L., N.-W. Terr. V75+604 88
Tating, China E86+271 67
Tatinnai L., N.-W. Terr. U47+606 88
Tatnam C., Manitoba U05+578 89
Tatong, Victoria C24-367 109
Tatranská Lomnica, Czech. L59+491 49
Tatry, mts., Poland-Czech. L60+493 49
Tatta, Pakistan H43+247 70
Tatu R., China F22+320 64
Tatuhy, Brazil R16-232 105
Ta-tung, China E41+401 66
Tatung Ho, China F14+370 64
Tauapeçaçú, Brazil S06-025 104
Taubate, Brazil R03-230 105
Tauha, Brazil Q62-060 105
Taumarunui, New Zealand A28-388 112
Taungdwingyi, Burma F56+200 71
Taunggyi, Burma F48+209 71
Taungup, Burma F64+189 71
Taunton, England N18+510 38
Taunton, Massachusetts S67+419 91
Taunus, mts., W. Germany M40+503 48
Taupo & L., New Zealand A24-387 112
Taurage, Lithuania L46+552 47
Tauranga & Harb., N.Z. A23-377 112
Tauste, Spain N07+419 53
Tauysk, U.S.S.R. C03+598 63
Tavda, U.S.S.R. H57+581 62
Taverne, Switzerland M36+461 45
Tavistock, England N25+505 38
Tavolara, I., Sardinia M32+409 57
Tavoy & R., Burma F41+140 71
Tavoy I., Burma F40+130 71
Tavsanli, Turkey L03+396 74
Tawang, India F78+276 71
Tawas City, Michigan T51+443 91
Tawau, Sabah E12+043 65
Tawitawi, I., Philippines E00+052 65
Taxco, Mexico U57+184 100
Tay, Firth of & R., Scotland N19+564 41
Tay, L., Scotland N25+565 41
Tayga, U.S.S.R. G27+558 62
Taylor, Mt., New Mexico V18+352 94
Taylorsville, Alabama T69+345 97
Taylorsville, N. Carolina T37+359 97
Taymyr, Ozero, U.S.S.R. F15+746 63
Tayport, Scotland N17+564 41
Tayside, reg., Scotland N23+567 41
Taytay, Philippines E04+108 65
Tayü, China E34+255 67
Tayung, China E57+292 67
Taza, Morocco N24+342 80
Tazewell, Virginia T39+371 97
Tazovskaya G., U.S.S.R. G85+692 62
Tbilisi, Gruzinskaya, U.S.S.R. K01+418 62
Tchad. See Chad
Tchaourou, Benin M76+088 80
Tczew, Poland L67+541 49
Te Anau, L., New Zealand A73-452 112
Teano Ra., W. Australia E10-245 110
Teapa, Mexico U18+174 100
Te Aroha, New Zealand A26-376 112
Te Awamutu, New Zealand A28-380 112
Teboursouk, Tunisia M34+364 81
Tebyulyakh, U.S.S.R. C31+648 63
Tecamachalco, Mexico U46+188 100
Tecka & R., Argentina S65-434 103
Tecolutla, Mexico U43+205 100
Tecoripe, Mexico V28+290 100
Tecpan, Mexico U62+172 100
Tecuniseh, Michigan T54+420 91
Tedzhen, Turkmen. H87+373 62
Tegerhi, Libya M04+240 81
Tegucigalpa, Honduras T72+141 101
Teheruak L., N.-W. Terr. U72+663 88
Tehpao, China E80+233 67
Tehran, Iran J52+357 75
Tehri, India G69+304 70
Tehsien, China E22+375 66
Tehuacan, Mexico U44+185 100
Tehucan, Mexico U44+185 100
Tehuantepec, Mexico U32+164 100
Tehuantepec, G. of, Mexico U30+158 100
Tehauntepec, Isth. of, Mex., U28+172 100
Teian. See Anlu
Teifi, R., Wales N26+520 38
Teign, R., England N22+506 38
Teignmouth, England N21+505 38
Teith, R., Scotland N24+561 41
Tekapo, L., New Zealand A57-439 112
Te Karaka, New Zealand A13-384 112
Tekari, India G31+250 73
Tekirdag, Turkey L15+410 74
Te Kuiti, New Zealand A29-383 112
Tela, Honduras T75+158 101
Tel-Aviv-Yafo, Israel K62+321 76
Telegraph Creek, B.C. W67+581 88
Telford, England N15+527 37
Telichie, S. Australia C61-317 109
Telkalakh, Syria K52+347 76
Tel Kochek, Syria K17+370 74
Tell Bise, Syria K49+348 76
Tell Ejine, Syria K48+358 76
Tell el Milh, Israel K60+312 76
Tellicherry, India G87+118 70
Teloloapan, Mexico U60+182 100
Tel Or, Israel K56+326 76
Telpos-iz, U.S.S.R. J05+637 62
Telsen, Argentina S41-424 103
Tel'shyay, Lithuania L46+560 47
Telukbetung, Sumatra, Indon. E89-054 65
Teluk Cenarawasih, New Guinea D00-024 65
Tembeling, Malaysia F16+040 69
Temblador, Venezuela S17+090 104
Teme R., England N15+523 37
Temesvar. See Timisoara
Temir, Kazakh. J18+491 62
Temir Tau, U.S.S.R. G16+532 62
Temiscouata, L., Quebec S53+476 90
Temma, Tasmania C31-413 109
Temnikov, U.S.S.R. K10+546 61
Temora, New South Wales C15-345 109
Temosachic, Mexico V15+288 100
Tempe, Arizona V41+334 94
Tempio, Sardinia M35+409 57
Temple, Texas U44+310 95
Templemore, Ireland, Rep. N47+528 43
Temse, Belgium M65+511 44
Temta, U.S.S.R. J84+575 61
Temuco, Chile S76-386 103
Temuka, New Zealand A52-440 112
Tenanzingo, Mexico U57+189 100
Tenasique, Mexico U09+174 100
Tenasserim, Burma F36+120 71
Tenasserim R., Burma F37+136 71
Tenby, Wales N28+517 38
Ten Degree Chan., Andaman Islands F75+098 71
Tenerife, I., Canary Is. P10+282 80
Ténès, Algeria M84+362 80
Tengchow. See Penglai
Tengiz, Oz., Kazakh. H35+504 62
Tennant's Creek, N. Territory, Australia D05-195 111
Tennessee, state, U.S.A. T80+357 99
Tennessee Pass, Colorado V07+394 98
Tennessee R., Kentucky, etc. T79+368 97
Tenterfield, New S. Wales B78-290 109
Ten Thousand Is., Florida T37+256 99
Ten Thousand Smokes, Val. of, Alaska Y35+578 99
Teocaltiche, Mexico U77+215 100
Teocuitatlan, Mexico U80+200 100
Téophilo Otoni, Brazil Q69-178 105
Tepatitlan, Mexico U77+208 100
Tepehuanes, Mexico V05+254 100
Tepelene, Albania L60+403 59
Tepic, Mexico U89+215 100
Teramo, Italy M08+426 56
Terang, Victoria C43-383 109
Ter Apel, Netherlands M48+529 44
Terban, Jebel, Saudi Arabia K18+197 74
Terborg, Netherlands M52+519 44
Terenceville, Newfoundland R58+477 90
Teresina, Brazil Q77-050 105
Teressa I., Nicobar Is F71+083 71
Terewah L., New South Wales C16-296 109
Terezin, Czechoslovakia M05+505 48
Teri, Pakistan H23+332 72
Teri Nam Tso, Tibet G26+310 71
Termez, Uzbek. H47+370 62
Termini Imerese, Sicily M08+380 57
Termoli, Italy M00+420 57
Termonde, Belgium M65+510 44
Ternate, Halmahera I. D46+008 65
Terneuzen, Netherlands M67+513 44
Terni, Italy M14+426 56
Ternopol, Ukraine L27+496 60
Terowie, S. Australia C67-331 109
Terpeniya, Zal, U.S.S.R. C40+485 63
Terracina, Italy M10+413 57
Terralba, Sardinia M38+397 57
Terra Nova, Newfoundland R55+485 90
Terra Santa, Brazil R69-019 105
Terrazas, Mexico V17+303 100
Terrebonne B., Louisiana U04+292 95
Terre Haute, Indiana T74+395 91
Terrel, Texas U38+327 95
Terrel, Mt., Utah V40+386 94
Terror Mt., Antarctica B30-790 27
Terry, Montana V02+468 93
Terschelling I., Netherlands M58+534 44
Teruel, Spain N07+404 53
Tervola, Finland L31+661 46
Tervuren, Belgium M63+508 44
Teshekpuk, L., Alaska Y20+705 88
Tesin, Mongolia F44+492 64
Tesio, Japan C50+459 68
Teslin, Yukon W76+602 88
Teslin L., Yukon W75+600 88
Teslin R., Yukon W84+609 88
Tessaoua, Niger M40+134 80
Tessenderlo, Belgium M59+511 44
Tete, Mozambique K68-162 84
Teton Ra., Wyoming V36+436 93
Tetouan (Tetuan), Morocco N32+356 80
Tetyukhe, U.S.S.R. See Rudnaya Pristan
Tetyushi, U.S.S.R. J67+549 61
Teulada, Sardinia M37+390 57
Teulada C., Sardinia M38+389 57
Teutoburger Wald, W. Germany M41+521 48

Tevere. See Tiber
Teviot, R., Scotland N15+555 41
Tevriz, U.S.S.R. H16+573 62
Te Waewae B., N.Z. A76-463 112
Texarkana, Arkansas U24+334 95
Texas, state, U.S.A. U67+318 98
Texcoco, Mexico U53+195 100
Texel I., Netherlands M61+531 44
Texoma, L., Oklahoma U40+340 95
Tezpur, India F73+266 71
Thachap Kangri, Tibet G46+334 70
Thadiq, Saudi Arabia J86+252 74
Thailand, S.-E. Asia F30+160 69
Thakhek, Laos F01+174 69
Thal, Pakistan H26+334 72
Thale Sap, L., Thailand F28+075 69
Thalkirch, Switzerland M34+466 45
Thames, New Zealand A27-372 112
Thames, Firth of, N.Z. A28-370 112
Thames R., Connecticut S73+414 96
Thames, R., England N00+515 39
Thana, India H12+194 70
Thanesar, India G79+299 72
Thanh-hoa, Vietnam E86+198 69
Thanjavur, India G65+108 70
Thann, France M47+478 54
Thar Des., India H27+257 70
Tharrawaddy, Burma F55+176 71
Tharsis, Spain N42+376 52
Thásos I., Greece L32+407 59
Thásos Str., Greece L32+408 59
Thatcher, Arizona V28+328 94
Thaton, Burma F46+169 71
Thaungdut, Burma F62+244 71
Thayer, Missouri U10+365 97
Thayetmyo, Burma F59+193 71
Thazi, Burma F53+208 71
The Gulf, Arabia, etc. 74-75
Thelon R., N.-W. Territories U84+645 88
Theodore, Queensland B89-250 111
Theodore Roosevelt L., Ariz. V37+337 94
Thérmai, G. of, Greece L43+402 59
Thérmiá, See Kithnos, I.
Thermopolis, Wyoming V19+437 93
Thesprotia, Greece L58+395 59
Thessalia, Greece L46+395 59
Thessaloniki, Greece L42+406 59
Thetford, England M85+524 39
Thetford Mines, Quebec S67+461 91
Theux, Belgium M55+505 44
Thibodaux, Louisiana U04+298 95
Thief River Falls, Minnesota U38+482 93
Thielsen, Mt., Oregon W12+432 92
Thielt, Belgium M70+510 44
Thies, Senegal P12+148 80
Thimbu, Bhutan G06+275 73
Thingvalla vatn, Iceland P37+642 46
Thio, Ethiopia K24+146 83
Thionville, France M53+494 54
Thira, I., Greece L27+364 59
Thirsk, England N08+542 37
Thirtyone Mile L., Quebec T15+461 91
Thisted, Denmark M38+570 47
Thistilfjord, Iceland P02+663 46
Thityabin, Burma F56+233 71
Thiviers, France M84+455 54
Thjórsá, R., Iceland P23+645 46
Thok Jalung, Tibet G51+323 70
Tholen & I., Netherlands M65+515 44
Thomaston, Georgia T56+329 97
Thomastown, Ireland, Rep. N43+525 43
Thomasville, Georgia T54+308 97
Thompsonville, Connecticut S76+420 96
Thomson Ville, Michigan T65+445 91
Thongwa, Burma F51+167 71
Thorn. See Torun
Thornhill, Scotland N23+552 41
Thórshavn, Faeröe Is. N41+618 34
Thórshöfn, Iceland P01+662 46
Thouars, France N01+469 54
Thourout. See Torhout
Thousand Isles, New York T06+443 91
Thousand Lake Mt., Utah V39+384 94
Thraki, Dhitiki, Greece L24+412 58
Three Hummock I., Tasmania C30+404 109
Three Kings Is., N.Z. A47-341 112
Three Points C., Ghana N14+048 80
Three Rivers, Michigan T64+420 91
Three Rivers (Trois Rivières), Quebec S76+464 89
Throssel Ra., W. Australia D80-220 110
Thueyts, France M65+447 55
Thuin, Belgium M64+503 44
Thule, Greenland S58+760 26
Thule I. South Sandwich Is. P80-590 27
Thumail, Iraq K13+331 74
Thun, Switzerland M44+468 45
Thunder B., Michigan T50+450 91
Thunder Bay, Ontario T86+486 89
Thuner See, Switzerland M44+467 45
Thur, R., Switzerland M37+476 45
Thurgau, canton, Switz. M36+476 45
Thüringen, W. Germany M24+507 48
Thüringer Wald, E. Germany M24+505 48
Thurles, Ireland, Rep. N47+527 43
Thurloo Downs, N.S.W. C40-293 109
Thursday I., Queensland C47-105 111
Thurso & R., Scotland N21+586 40
Thusis, Switzerland M33+467 45
Tia, New South Wales B80-312 109
Tiaret, Algeria M82+354 80
Tiassale, Ivory Coast N30+060 80
Tibati, Cameroon M16+064 81
Tiber (Tevere), R., Italy M15+420 57
Tiberias & L., Israel K56+328 76
Tibet, China G30+325 30
Tibnin, Lebanon K58+332 76
Tibooburra, New S. Wales C48-293 109
Tiburón, Haiti S86+184 101
Tiburon I., Mexico V45+289 100
Ticino, canton, Switzerland M38+463 45
Ticonderoga, New York S80+439 91
Ticul, Mexico T87+204 100
Tidjikja, Mauritania N70+184 80
Tidworth, England N10+512 39
Tiebissou, Ivory Coast N30+072 80
Tiefencastel, Switzerland M32+467 45
Tieh-ling, China D67+423 66
Tiel, Netherlands M57+519 44
Tielt, Belgium M70+510 44
Tien Chih, China F14+246 64
Tien-chwang-tai, China D78+409 66
Tienen (Tirlemont), Belgium M61+508 44
Tienpaoshan, China E15+419 66
Tiensha Pass, China E79+341 66
Tien Shan, Central Asia G70+430 30
Tienshui, China E84+344 66
Tientsin (Tienching), China E17+391 66
Tiermas, Spain N06+426 53
Tierra del Fuego, Chile-Argentina S50-540 103
Tiffin, Ohio T49+411 91
Tifton, Georgia T51+314 97
Tiganesti, Romania L23+447 58
Tighina. See Bendery.
Tighnabruaich, Scotland N31+559 41
Tigil, U.S.S.R. B37+577 63
Tignish, Prince Edward I. S24+470 90
Tigris, R., Iraq J86+325 74
Tihwa, China G14+437 62
Tijuana, Mexico V74+324 100
Tikhvin, U.S.S.R. K70+596 60
Tikrit, Iraq K08+346 74
Tiksi, U.S.S.R. D36+716 63
Tilburg, Netherlands M60+516 44
Tilbury, England M88+514 39
Tilcara, Argentina S32-236 103
Tilichiki, U.S.S.R. A83+605 63
Tilamook, Oregon W23+454 92
Tillangchong I., Nicobar Is. F68+085 71
Tillsonburg, Ontario T34+429 91
Tilos, I., Greece L16+364 59
Tilpa, New South Wales C33-310 109
Tilsit. See Sovetsk.
Timanski Kryazh, U.S.S.R. J60+650 62
Timaru, New Zealand A52-444 112
Timbalier B., Louisiana U02+292 95
Timber Lake, S. Dakota U66+454 93
Timboon, Victoria C42-385 109
Timbuktu. See Tombouctou.
Timiskaming, Quebec T25+467 91
Timisoara, Romania L53+458 58
Timmins, Ontario T38+485 91
Timor, I. & Sea, Indonesia D60-100 65
Timote, Argentina S14-354 103
Tinaca Pt., Philippines D58+056 65
Tinahely, Ireland, Rep. N39+528 43
Tindouf, Algeria N46+274 80
Tineo, Spain N39+433 52
Tingchow. See Changting.
Tingha, New South Wales B83-300 109
Tinghsien, China E29+385 66
Tingnan, China E31+246 67
Tingo Maria, Peru T05-091 104
Tingri Dzong, Tibet G20+285 71
Tinian, I., Mariana Is. C26+140 106
Tinkhannock, Pennsylvania T06+415 96
Tinnevelly. See Tirunelveli.
Tinogasta, Argentina S46-281 103
Tinos, I., Greece L29+376 59
Tinsukia, India F57+274 71
Tintigny, Belgium M57+497 44
Tintina, Argentina S16-270 103
Tintinara, S. Australia C59-358 109
Tinwald, New Zealand A49-439 112
Tioman, Pulau, I., Malaysia F05+028 69
Tionesta, Pennsylvania T27+415 96
Tipperary & co., Ireland, Rep. N49+525 43
Tipton, Iowa U06+418 95
Tiracumba, Sa. de, Brazil R10-036 105
Tiran, I., Saudi Arabia K63+280 74
Tirana. See Tiranë.
Tiranë, Albania L62+413 58
Tiraspol, Moldavia L02+468 60
Tire, Turkey L14+380 74
Tireboli, Turkey K37+409 74
Tiree, I., Scotland N41+565 41
Tirgu Jiu, Romania L40+450 58
Tirich Mir, Pakistan H19+363 72
Tirlemont, Belgium M60+508 44
Tirlyanski, U.S.S.R. J08+542 61
Tirnavos, Greece L46+397 59
Tirol, Austria M22+471 48
Tiruchirapalli, India G68+107 70
Tiruchendur, India G71+084 70
Tiru Kona Malai. See Trincomalee.
Tirunelveli, India G73+088 70
Tirupati, India G64+136 70
Tiruvannamalai, India G65+123 70
Tisiye, Syria K51+324 76
Tissa, Nigeria M28+074 81
Tisza (Tisa), R., Hungary-Yugoslavia L56+475 51
Titalyah, Bangladesh G09+265 73
Titicaca, L., Bolivia-Peru S56-158 104
Titisee, W. Germany M41+479 48
Titograd, Yugoslavia L65+424 58
Titovo Uzice, Yugoslavia L61+439 58
Titu, Romania L27+447 58
Titusville, Pennsylvania T28+417 91
Tiverton, England N21+509 38
Tiwi, Oman J04+228 75
Tixkokob, Mexico T85+210 100
Tixtla, Mexico U55+176 100
Tizimin, Mexico T77+211 100
Tizi Ouzou, Algeria M66+366 80
Tjalang, See Calang
Tjilatjap, See Cilacap
Tjirebon, See Cirebon
Tjörn, I., Sweden M20+580 47
Tlacotalpan, Mexico U34+186 100
Tlaltenango, Mexico U80+218 100
Tlapa, Mexico U51+176 100
Tlaxcala & state, Mexico U50+193 100
Tlaxiaco, Mexico U46+173 100
Tlemcen, Algeria N08+350 80
Tmèssa, Libya L86+264 81
Toay, Argentina S26+368 103
Toba, Japan C79+345 68
Tobago, I., Trinidad S04+112 101
Toba Meer, Sumatra F37+026 65
Tobarro, Spain N10+386 53
Tobel, Switzerland M36+475 45
Tobelo, Halmahera I., Indon. D42+016 65
Tobermory, Ontario T40+452 91
Tobermory, Scotland N36+566 41
Toboali, Bangka I., Indonesia E81-030 65
Toboli, Celebes, D89-008 65
Tobolsk, U.S.S.R. H39+581 62
Tobruq (Tobruk), Libya L36+320 81
Toccoa, Georgia T50+346 97
Toco, Chile S58-220 103
Tocopilla, Chile S62-220 103
Tocumwal, New S. Wales C28-359 109
Tocuyo, Venezuela S59+098 104
Todenyang, Kenya K54+044 83
Todmorden, England N13+537 37
Todos Santos, Mexico V31+235 100
Todos Santos, B., Mexico V71+317 100
Toe Hd., Ireland, Rep. N55+515 43
Togarakaikyo, Japan D28+301 68
Toghraqbulaq, China F68+404 64
Togo, rep., W. Africa M88+080 80
To Huping Tso, Tibet G41+342 71
Tojo, Japan D11+348 68
Tokanga, U.S.S.R. K33+680 62
Tokanui, New Zealand A66-465 112
Tokar, Sudan K44+182 83
Tokara Retto, Japan D32+296 68
Tokat, Turkey K50+403 74
Tokatidake, Japan C42+434 68
Tokelau Is., Pacific Ocean Z45-090 106
Tokmak, Kirgiz. G88+429 62
Tokomaru, New Zealand A10-382 112
Tokoto, China E53+403 66
Tokushima, Japan D03+341 68
Tokuyama, Japan D19+340 68
Tōkyō & B., Japan C62+357 68
Tolaga Bay, New Zealand A10-384 112
Tolbukhin, Bulgaria L13+435 58
Toledo, Chile S63-273 103
Toledo, Ohio T51+417 91
Toledo, Spain N24+399 52
Toledo, Mtes. de, Spain N26+397 52
Tolmin, Yugoslavia M08+462 56
Tolo, G. of, Celebes, D76-022 65
Tolsta Hd., Scotland N37+583 40
Toluca, Mexico U58+193 100
Toluca, Montana V17+457 93
Tolun, China E22+423 66
Tölz, Bad, Germany M21+478 48
Tomah, Wisconsin U03+440 91
Tomahawk, Wisconsin T88+455 91
Tomar, Portugal N51+396 52
Tomari, U.S.S.R. C46+477 63
Tomaszów Mazowiecki, Pol. L60+515 49
Tomatin, Scotland N24+573 40
Tomatumari, Guyana R84+053 104
Tombigbee R., Alabama T77+315 99
Tombouctou, Mali N18+168 80
Tome, Chile S78-366 103
Tomiko, Ontario T27+466 91
Tomini, G. of, Celebes, D86-004 65
Tomintoul, Scotland N20+572 40
Tomkinson Ra., Australia D38-260 110
Tommot, U.S.S.R. D51+590 63
Tomsk, U.S.S.R. G30+563 62
Tom's River, New Jersey S85+399 91
Tonala, Mexico U22+158 100
Tonate, French Guiana R44+049 105
Tonawanda, New York T23+430 96
Tonbridge, England M88+512 39
Tønder, Denmark M37+549 47
Tondi, India G66+098 70
Tonga, Sudan K84+094 81
Tonga, Is., Pacific Ocean Z60-220 106
Tongala, Victoria C31-363 109
Tongareva, I., Pacific Ocean Y50-092 107
Tongeren, Belgium M57+508 44
Tongobory, Madagascar K04-236 83
Tongoy, Chile S69-304 103
Tongres. See Tongeren.
Tongue & Kyle of, Scotland N26+585 40
Tongue R., Montana V08+454 98
Tonichi, Mexico V25+288 100
Tonk, India G85+262 70
Tonkin, Vietnam F00+214 69
Tongking, G. of, S.E. Asia E70+204 69
Tonkhil, Mongolia F68+464 64
Tonkova, U.S.S.R. G00+607 62
Tonle Sap, Cambodia F06+129 69
Tonneins, France M88+444 55
Tonnerre, France M66+478 54
Tonopah, Nevada V73+382 92
Tønsberg, Norway M27+593 47
Tooele, Utah V44+405 92
Toowoomba, Queensland B78-274 111
Top Oz., Karelskaya K80+657 62
Topeka, Kansas U34+390 95
Topolčany, Czechoslovakia L71+486 49
Torez, Ukraine K40+480 61
Torhout (Thourout), Belg. M71+511 44
Tori, India G31+237 73
Toriñana, C., Spain N56+430 52
Torino, Italy M44+451 56
Torit, Sudan K74+044 81
Torma, Estonia L19+588 47
Torne Trask, Sweden L66+684 46
Tornetråsk, Sweden L62+682 46
Tornio, Finland L35+659 46
Tornionjoki, Sweden L48+676 46
Tornquist, Argentina S13-382 103
Törökszentmiklós, Hungary L58+472 49
Toroni, G. of, Greece L38+401 59
Toronto, New South Wales B81-330 109
Toronto, Ontario T26+437 91
Toronto, S. Dakota U40+446 93
Tororo, Uganda K64+006 83
Toros Dağlari, Turkey K80+370 74
Torquay, England N21+505 38
Torre Annunziata, Italy M03+408 57
Torreblanca, Spain M89+402 53
Torre del Greco, Italy M04+408 57
Torrelaguna, Spain N21+408 52
Torrelapaja, Spain N12+415 53
Torrelavega, Spain N24+433 52
Torrens, L., S. Australia C74-310 109
Torrente, Spain N03+394 53
Torreon, Mexico U80+255 100
Torres, Mexico V34+287 100
Torres Is., Pacific Ocean A80-140 106
Torres Str., Queensland C50-104 111
Torres Novas, Portugal N51+395 52
Torres Vedras, Portugal N55+391 52
Torrevieja, Spain N04+380 53
Torridon, L., Scotland N34+576 40
Torrijos, Spain N28+400 52
Torrington, Connecticut S79+418 96
Torrington, Wyoming U86+421 93
Torrowangee, New S. Wales C51-314 109
Torrox, Spain N24+367 52
Torsby, Sweden M12+602 47
Tortola, I., Virgin Is. S28+185 101
Tortorici, Sicily M01+380 57
Tortosa, Spain M87+407 53
Tortue, I., Haiti S76+201 101
Tortuga I., Mexico V42+274 100
Torun, Poland L68+531 49
Tory, I. Ireland, Rep. N49+552 42
Torzhok, U.S.S.R. K61+571 60
Tosa B., Japan D08+334 68
Toscana, dep., Italy M23+434 56
Tosco-Emiliano, Appinnino, mts., Italy M26+444 56
Tossa, Spain M73+417 53
Tostado, Argentina S11-292 103
Totana, Spain N15+378 53
Totling, Tibet G61+314 70
Totma, U.S.S.R. K14+600 62
Totnes, England N22+504 38
Totonicapam, Guatemala U08+150 100
Totskoye, U.S.S.R. J43+525 61
Tottenham, New S. Wales C16-322 109
Tottori, Japan D05+355 68
Touba, Ivory Coast N46+084 80
Toubkal, mt., Morocco N48+310 80
Touggourt, Algeria M54+328 80
Toul, France M55+487 54
Toulon, France M55+431 55
Toulouse, France M82+436 55
Toungoo, Burma F51+190 71
Touquet, le, France M80+505 54
Touraine, prov., France M86+471 54
Tourane (Da Nang), Vietnam E71+161 69
Tourbis, L., Quebec S85+473 91
Tourcoing, France M71+507 54
Tour-du-Pin, la, France M58+456 54
Tournai, Belgium M70+506 44
Tournon, France M61+451 55
Tournus, France M61+465 54
Tours, France M86+474 54
Touws River, Cape Province L58-334 84
Towamba, New South Wales C02-371 109
Towanda, Pennsylvania T09+417 96
Towari, Celebes D81-046 65
Towcester, England N06+521 39
Tower City, N. Dakota U46+469 93
Townsend, Montana V39+463 93
Townsend, Mt., N.S.W. C10-364 109
Townsville, Queensland C19-193 111
Towoeti Danau, Celebes, D82-028 65
Towson, Maryland T09+394 96
Towy, R., Wales N25+519 38
Toyah L., Texas U81+313 94
Toyama & B., Japan C76+367 68
Tozeur, Tunisia M42+338 81
Trabzon, Turkey K33+410 74
Tracadie, New Brunswick S30+475 90
Tracy, Minnesota U34+442 93
Tradom, Tibet G36+303 71
Traer, Iowa U14+422 95
Trahiry, Brazil Q56-033 105
Trahynas, Brazil R22-144 105
Traiguen, Chile S76-382 103
Traiguen, I., Chile S83-455 103
Trail, British Columbia V76+493 88
Tralee & B., Ireland, Rep. N58+523 43
Tramore, Ireland, Rep. N43+522 43
Tranas, Sweden M00+581 47
Trancas, Argentina S32-263 103
Trancoso, Portugal N44+408 52
Trang, Thailand F33+076 69
Trangan, I., Indonesia D04-067 65
Trangie, New South Wales C12-321 109
Tranquebar, India G61+111 70
Tranqueira, Brazil Q82-082 105
Transcona, Manitoba U42+500 88
Transilvania, Romania L32+465 58
Transvaal, S. Africa L00-250 84
Transylvanian Alps, Romania L42+450 58
Trapani, Sicily M15+380 57
Traralgon, Victoria C21-382 109
Trasimeno, L., Italy M17+431 56
Trasparga, Spain N47+431 52
Traunstein, W. Germany M14+478 48
Travancore, India G80+090 70
Travellers L., New S. Wales C47-333 109
Traverse B., Michigan T63+451 91
Traversay Is., Atlantic Ocean P85-560 27
Traverse City, Michigan T64+448 91
Travis, L., Texas U48+304 95
Trawbreaga B., Ireland, Rep. N44+553 42
Třevič, Czechoslovakia L85+492 49
Trebinje, Yugoslavia L70+427 58
Trebizond. See Trabzon
Tree River Post, N.-W. Terr. V47+672 88
Tregaron, Wales N24+522 38
Treig, L., Scotland N28+568 41
Treinta-y-Tres, Uruguay R57-332 103
Trelew, Argentina S32-432 103
Trelleborg, Sweden M11+554 47
Tremadoc B., Wales N26+528 38
Tremblant, Mt., Quebec S87+463 91
Tremiti Is., Italy L87+420 56
Tremont, Maine S50+443 90
Tremp, Spain M85+422 53
Trencin, Czechoslovakia L72+489 49
Trenel, Argentina S26-355 103
Trenque Lauquen, Argentina S17-359 103
Trent. See Trento
Trent Canal, Ontario T24+445 91
Trent, R., England N04+530 37
Trentino-Alto Adige, reg., Italy M22+465 56
Trento, Italy M23+461 56
Trenton, Georgia T63+348 97
Trenton, Michigan T49+422 91
Trenton, Missouri U22+401 95
Trenton, New Jersey S89+402 96
Trenton, Ontario T16+442 91
Trenton, Tennessee T84+360 97
Tréport, le, France M82+501 54
Tres Arroyos, Argentina S02-384 103
Tres Lomas, Argentina S17-364 103
Tres Marias, Is., Mexico V10+215 100
Tres Montes, Pen., Chile T02-469 103
Tres Virgenes, Las, Mexico V46+274 100
Treves. See Trier
Trevino, Mexico U68+260 100
Treviso, Italy M17+457 56
Trevna, Bulgaria L27+428 58
Triabunna, Tasmania C13-425 109
Triana, Spain N36+374 52
Tricase, Italy L70+399 57
Trichinopoly. See Tiruchirapalli
Trichur, India G82+106 70
Trida, New South Wales C30-330 109

Trier, *W. Germany* M50+497 **48**
Trieste, *Italy* M07+457 **56**
Trikeri Str., *Greece* L41+390 **59**
Trikkala, *Greece* L50+396 **59**
Trikomo, *Cyprus* K67+353 **76**
Trim, *Ireland, Rep.* N41+536 **43**
Trincomalee, *Sri Lanka* G53+086 **70**
Trinidad, *Bolivia* S28–148 **104**
Trinidad, *Colorado* U87+372 **94**
Trinidad, *Cuba* T29+218 **97**
Trinidad, *Uruguay* R72–336 **103**
Trinidad, I., *Argentina* S12–392 **103**
Trinidad, I., *Atlantic Ocean* P87–203 **85**
Trinidad I., *West Indies* S07+105 **104**
Trinity & B., *Newfoundland* R50+482 **90**
Trinity, *Texas* U32+310 **95**
Trinity Pen, *Antarctica* R75–640 **27**
Trinity R., *Texas* U30+312 **95**
Trionto C., *Italy* L78+396 **57**
Tripoli, *Lebanon* K55+345 **76**
Tripoli (Tarabulus), *Libya* M10+328 **81**
Tripolis, *Greece* L46+375 **59**
Tripolitania, *Libya* M00+300 **81**
Tripura, *India* F80+240 **71**
Tristan da Cunha, *Atlantic Oc.* N76–372 **85**
Triunfo, *Mexico* V31+239 **100**
Trivandrum, *India* G79+085 **70**
Trmbesh, *Bulgaria* L27+434 **58**
Trn, *Bulgaria* L44+428 **58**
Trnava, *Czechoslovakia* L75+484 **49**
Trobriand Is., *Papua New Guinea* B84–086 **111**
Trogir, *Yugoslavia* L82+435 **56**
Trios Pistoles, *Quebec* S55+481 **90**
Trois Ponts, *Belgium* M55+504 **44**
Trois Rivières, *Quebec* S76+464 **91**
Troitsk, *U.S.S.R.* H81+540 **61**
Troitsk, *U.S.S.R.* K07+541 **61**
Troitsko Pechorsk, *U.S.S.R.* J23+629 **62**
Trollhättan, *Sweden* M16+583 **47**
Trollheimen, *Norway* M36+629 **46**
Tromen, mt., *Argentina* S60–371 **103**
Tromsø, *Norway* L66+697 **46**
Trondheim & Fd., *Norway* M28+635 **46**
Troödos, *Cyprus* K73+349 **76**
Troon, *Scotland* N28+555 **41**
Tropea, *Italy* L85+387 **57**
Troppau. *See* Opava
Trosa, *Sweden* L75+589 **47**
Trossachs, *Scotland* N26+562 **41**
Trout Lake, *Michigan* T60+462 **91**
Trowbridge, *England* N13+513 **39**
Troy, *New York* S82+427 **91**
Troy, *Turkey* L22+400 **74**
Troyes, *France* M66+483 **54**
Truba, *Saudi Arabia* K11+283 **74**
Truer Ra., *Northern Territory, Australia* D21–222 **110**
Trujillo, *Honduras* T66+158 **101**
Trujillo, *Peru* T24–082 **104**
Trujillo, *Spain* N35+395 **52**
Trujillo, *Venezuela* S62+093 **104**
Truk, I., *Caroline Is.* B82+070 **106**
Truksum, *Tibet* G40+300 **71**
Trumbull, *Mt., Arizona* V50+364 **92**
Trundle, *New South Wales* C15–329 **109**
Truns, *Switzerland* M36+467 **45**
Truro, *England* N30+502 **38**
Truro, *Nova Scotia* S19+454 **90**
Truro, *S. Australia* C65–344 **109**
Truskmore, *Ireland, Rep.* N50+544 **42**
Trutnov, *Czechoslovakia* L85+506 **49**
Trzebnica, *Poland* L78+514 **49**
Tržič, *Yugoslavia* M04+464 **56**
Tsabong, *Botswana* L46–262 **84**
Tsagan Olom, *Mongolia* F50+467 **64**
Tsahura, *Yemen, South* J70+148 **74**
Tsangbe, *Bhutan* G05+271 **73**
Tsanghsien. *See* Wuchow
Tsangwu, *China* E51+235 **67**
Tsaochow. *See* Hotseh
Tsaokiang, *China* E28+376 **66**
Tsaritsyn. *See* Volgograd
Tsavo Nat. Park, *Kenya* K40–028 **83**
Tschenstochau. *See* Czestochowa
Tschiertschen, *Switzerland* M32+468 **45**
Tseelim, *Israel* K63+313 **76**
Tsehchow. *See* Tsincheng
Tselinograd, *Kazakh* H21+512 **52**
Tsemah, *Israel* K56+327 **76**
Tsengshing, *China* E37+233 **67**
Tses, *Namibia* L70–260 **84**
Tshikapa, *Zaire* L56–064 **82**
Tsho Mirari L., *Kashmir* G70+329 **72**
Tsimlyanskoye Vdkhr., *U.S.S.R.* K12+470 **61**
Tsinan, *China* E17+367 **66**
Tsincheng, *China* E43+353 **66**
Tsinchow. *See* Tienshui
Tsing-chow, *China* E29+381 **66**
Tsingchow. *See* Yitu
Tsing Hai *See* Ching Hai
Tsingkiang, *China* 27+280 **67**
Tsingkiang, *China* E06+336 **66**
Tsingkow, *China* E05+348 **66**
Tsingtao, *China* D88+361 **66**
Tsingtze (Singtze), *China* E23+294 **67**
Tsingyüan, *See* Paoting
Tsingyün, *China* E42+237 **67**
Tsining, *China* E20+354 **64**
Tsinkiang, *China* E09+249 **67**
Tsinsien, *China* E22+284 **67**
Tsinyang, *China* E42+351 **66**
Tsitsihar, *China* D66+474 **64**
Tsivilsk, *U.S.S.R.* J71+558 **61**
Tsivory, *Madagascar* J84–242 **83**
Tskhinvali, *Gruzinskaya* K07+425 **62**
Tso-motre-tung, L., *Tibet* G10+284 **71**
Tsu, *Japan* C81+347 **68**
Tsugaru Str., *Japan* C54+416 **68**
Tsugitaka, mt., *Taiwan* D82+248 **64**
Tsungfa, *China* E38+236 **67**
Tsungming, *China* D81+316 **66**
Tsungtso, *China* E76+224 **64**
Tsunhwa, *China* E12+403 **66**
Tsunyi, *China* E79+277 **67**
Tsuruga, *Japan* C83+356 **68**
Tsuruoka, *Japan* C61+387 **68**
Tsuyama, *Japan* D06+350 **68**
Tsuyung, *China* F20+250 **64**
Tua, *Portugal* N45+412 **52**
Tua, *Zaire* L80–036 **82**
Tuakau, *New Zealand* A30–373 **112**
Tuam, *Ireland, Rep.* N53+535 **43**
Tuamarina, *New Zealand* A36–414 **112**
Tuamotu Arch., *Pacific Oc.* X30–200 **107**
Tuao, *Philippines* D82+178 **65**
Tuapse, *U.S.S.R.* K36+441 **62**
Tuatapere, *New Zealand* A74–461 **112**
Tubai, I., *Society Islands* Y10–160 **107**
Tubarão, *Brazil* R24–285 **103**
Tubas, *Jordan* K58+323 **76**
Tubbercurry, *Ireland, Rep.* N52+540 **42**
Tubingen, *W. Germany* M36+485 **48**
Tubize, *Belgium* M65+507 **44**
Tubuai, I., *Austral Islands* X88–210 **107**
Tubutama, *Mexico* V39+308 **100**
Tucacas, *Venezuela* S49+108 **104**
Tuckernuck I., *Massachusetts* S61+413 **96**
Tuckerton, *New Jersey* S86+396 **91**
Tucson, *Arizona* V36+322 **94**
Tucson Ra., *Arizona* V37+324 **94**
Tucumcari, *New Mexico* U82+352 **94**
Tucunare, *Brazil* R63–051 **105**
Tucupita, *Venezuela* S12+090 **104**
Tucurui, *Brazil* R26–038 **105**
Tudela, *Spain* N10+421 **53**
Tufi, *Papua New Guinea* C04–092 **111**
Tug, *Turkey* K16+385 **74**
Tuguegarao, *Philippines* D80+176 **65**
Tugur, *U.S.S.R.* C79+537 **63**
Tukums, *Latvia* L41+569 **47**
Tula, *Mexico* U55+200 **100**
Tula, *Mexico* U58+230 **100**
Tula, *U.S.S.R.* K44+542 **60**
Tulan, *China* F38+369 **64**
Tulancingo, *Mexico* U50+201 **100**
Tularosa, *New Mexico* V06+330 **94**
Tularosa Basin, *New Mexico* V09+329 **94**
Tulcan, *Ecuador* T16+008 **104**
Tulcea, *Romania* L07+452 **58**
Tulchin, *Ukraine* L07+487 **60**
Tulear, *Madagascar* K08–234 **83**
Tuli, *Zimbabwe* L04–220 **84**
Tulkarm, *Jordan* K60+323 **76**
Tullahoma, *Tennessee* T68+353 **97**
Tullamore, *Ireland, Rep.* N45+533 **43**
Tullamore, *New S. Wales* C15–327 **109**
Tulle, *France* M79+453 **55**
Tullow, *Ireland, Rep.* N40+528 **43**
Tulsa, *Oklahoma* U36+362 **95**
Tulsk, *Ireland, Rep.* N49+538 **43**
Tulu, *Ethiopia* K22+072 **83**
Tulua, *Colombia* T08+041 **104**
Tulun, *U.S.S.R.* F27+545 **63**
Tumaco & Rado de, *Colombia* T22+017 **104**
Tumany, *U.S.S.R.* B55+611 **63**
Tumbarumba, *N.S.W.* C12–358 **109**
Tumbes, *Peru* T33–035 **104**
Tumit-Guna, *China* E55+414 **66**
Tumkur, *India* G77+132 **70**
Tumlong, *India* G08+274 **73**
Tummel, R., *Scotland* N24+567 **41**
Tummo, *Libya* M06+224 **81**
Tump, *Pakistan* H76+260 **70**
Tumu, *Ghana* N12+108 **80**
Tumucumaque, Sa., *Brazil* R52+018 **105**
Tumupasa, *Bolivia* S48–142 **104**
Tumut & R., *New S. Wales* C11–354 **109**
Tunas de Zaza, *Cuba* T28+216 **101**
Tunbridge Wells, *England* M88+511 **39**
Tuncurry, *New South Wales* B76–321 **109**
Tundla, *India* G72+272 **70**
Tundubai, *Sudan* L44+146 **81**
Tunduru, *Tanzania* K46–112 **83**
Tüngan, *China* E53+264 **67**
Tungchang. *See* Liaocheng
Tungchow. *See* Tali
Tungchwan. *See* Hweitseh
Tungchwan. *See* Santai
Tunghai, *China* E04+346 **66**
Tungho, *China* D38+460 **64**
Tunghsien, *China* E20+398 **66**
Tunghwa, *China* D56+416 **64**
Tungjen, *China* E65+277 **67**
Tungkun, *China* E37+230 **67**
Tungkwan, *China* E59+346 **66**
Tungkwan, *China* E65+350 **66**
Tungliao, *China* D76+436 **64**
Tungshan. *See* Suchow
Tungtai, *China* D87+329 **66**
Tung Ting Hu, *China* E45+290 **67**
Tunguska, R., *U.S.S.R.* F30+640 **63**
Tunhwang, *China* F61+402 **64**
Tuni, *India* G44+173 **71**
Tunica, *Mississippi* U02+347 **97**
Tunis, *Tunisia* M30+368 **81**
Tunisia, *N. Africa* M30+350 **81**
Tunja, *Colombia* S81+056 **104**
Tunnsjø, *Norway* M10+647 **46**
Tunuyan & R., *Argentina* S55–335 **103**
Tuoy Khaya, *U.S.S.R.* E51+622 **63**
Tuparoa, *New Zealand* A10–379 **112**
Tupelo, *Mississippi* T82+343 **97**
Tupilco, *Mexico* U20+184 **100**
Tupinambaranas, I., *Brazil* R80–034 **104**
Tupiza, *Bolivia* S34–213 **104**
Tupper Lake, *New York* S87+442 **91**
Tuquarussu, *Brazil* R20–102 **105**
Tuquerres, *Colombia* T15+010 **104**
Tura, *India* F89+255 **71**
Tura, *U.S.S.R.* F30+641 **63**
Turaba, *Saudi Arabia* K20+208 **74**
Turakom, *Laos* F15+184 **69**
Turbat-i-Heideri, *Iran* J06+353 **75**
Turbat-i-Jam, *Iran* H86+353 **75**
Turbo, *Colombia* T10+081 **104**
Turda, *Romania* L37+466 **58**
Tureia I., *Tuamotu Arch.* X20–208 **107**
Turfan, *Sinkiang, China* G02+429 **64**
Turgay, *Kazakh* H69+499 **62**
Turgutlu, *Turkey* L14+385 **74**
Türi, *Estonia* L27+588 **47**
Turiaçu, *Brazil* R02–018 **105**
Turiamo, *Venezuela* S46+105 **104**
Turin. *See* Torino
Turkestan, *Kazakh, etc.* H40+432 **62**
Turkey, rep., *Europe-Asia* K78+390 **51**
Turkmenskaya, rep., *U.S.S.R.* J10+405 **62**
Turks Is., *Bahamas, The* S67+214 **101**
Turku, *Finland* L47+604 **47**
Turneffe Is., *Belize* T77+174 **101**
Turnhout, *Belgium* M60+513 **44**
Tûrnoovo, *Bulgaria* L27+430 **58**
Turnu Severin, *Romania* L44+446 **58**
Turquino, Pico de, *Cuba* T10+200 **101**
Turr, *Ethiopia* K08+064 **83**
Turrialba, *Costa Rica* T52+100 **101**
Turshiz, *Iran* J10+352 **75**
Turtkul, *Uzbek.* H84+415 **62**
Turtle Mts., *N. Dakota* U61+490 **93**
Turukta, *U.S.S.R.* E30+610 **63**
Turukhansk, *U.S.S.R.* G11+657 **62**
Turun, *Iran* J20+355 **75**
Turut, *Iran* J29+355 **75**
Turzovka, *Czechoslovakia* L68+494 **49**
Tus, *Iran* J03+366 **75**
Tuscaloosa, *Alabama* T76+332 **97**
Tuscarora Mts., *Pa.* T17+402 **96**
Tuscola, *Illinois* T80+398 **91**
Tuscumbia, *Alabama* T76+347 **97**
Tuscumbia, *Missouri* U15+383 **97**
Tuticorin, *India* G71+090 **70**
Tuttlingen, *W. Germany* M37+479 **48**
Tutuila, I., *Samoa* Z33–150 **106**
Tuvalu, *Pacific Ocean* A15–090 **106**
Tuwairifa, *Saudi Arabia* J62+216 **74**
Tuweiq, Jeb. el, *Jordan* K46+295 **76**
Tuxpan, *Mexico* U44+210 **100**
Tuxpan, *Mexico* V01+218 **100**
Tuxtepec, *Mexico* U37+181 **100**
Tuxtla & Vol. de, *Mexico* U31+185 **100**
Tuxtla Gutierrez, *Mexico* U18+168 **100**
Tuy, *Spain* N52+421 **52**
Tuyen-Quang, *Vietnam* E89+217 **69**
Tuy-hoa, *Vietnam* E64+131 **69**
Tuyun, *China* E75+263 **67**
Tuz Gölu, *Turkey* K70+386 **74**
Tuzla, *Yugoslavia* L68+446 **58**
Tvärån, *Sweden* L54+656 **46**
Tvurditsa, *Bulgaria* L26+427 **58**
Twante, *Burma* F54+166 **71**
Tweed, *Ontario* T14+445 **91**
Tweed, R., *Scotland* N13+557 **41**
Tweedsmuir Hills, *Scotland* N20+554 **41**
Tweedsmuir Park, *B.C.* W35+534 **88**
Twelve Pins, *Ireland, Rep.* N59+535 **43**
Twenty-five de Mayo, *Argent.* S46–380 **103**
Twenty-five de Mayo, *Argent.* S01–354 **103**
Twin Buttes, *Montana* V02+486 **93**
Twin Falls, *Idaho* V57+425 **92**
Twofold B., *New S. Wales* C00–370 **109**
Two Harbors, *Minnesota* U10+470 **93**
Two Mountains, L. of, *Que* S86+455 **91**
Two Rivers, *Wisconsin* T76+442 **91**
Tyler, *Texas* U31+322 **98**
Tygda, *U.S.S.R.* D52+532 **63**
Tyler, *Texas* U32+324 **95**
Tyndinski, *U.S.S.R.* D61+553 **63**
Tyndall, Mt., *New Zealand* A55–433 **112**
Tyne & Wear, co., *England* N09+550 **37**
Tynemouth, *England* N08+550 **37**
Tynset, *Norway* M25+623 **46**
Tyr (Sour), *Lebanon* K59+330 **76**
Tyrone, *Pennsylvania* T19+407 **96**
Tyrone, co., *N. Ireland* N43+546 **42**
Tyrrell, L., *Victoria* C43+354 **109**
Tyrrhenian Sea, *Italy* M18+400 **57**
Tyumen, *U.S.S.R.* H57+572 **62**
Tywyn, *Wales* N24+526 **38**
Tzechung, *China* E33+364 **66**
Tzeya Ho, *China* E26+380 **66**
Tzeyang, *China* E18+356 **66**
Tzeyun, *China* E82+256 **67**
Uani, *Nicaragua* T58+138 **101**
Uau el Chebir, *Libya* L78+252 **81**
Uaupés & R., *Brazil* S42–001 **104**
Uba, *Brazil* Q78–211 **105**
Ubait, *Saudi Arabia* K33+285 **74**
Ubari, *Libya* M14+266 **81**
Uberaba, *Brazil* R18–197 **105**
Uberlandia, *Brazil* R20–190 **105**
Überlingen, *W. Germany* M35+477 **48**
Ubon Muang, *Thailand* F01+153 **69**
Ubsa Nor, *Mongolia* F73+503 **63**
Ucayali, R., *Peru* S88–060 **104**
Uch, *Pakistan* H23+293 **72**
Uchiza, *Peru* T08–084 **104**
Uckfield, *England* M89+510 **39**
Udain, *Yemen* K06+141 **74**
Udaipur, *India* H07+246 **70**
Uddevalla, *Sweden* M19+584 **47**
Udd Jaur, *Sweden* L73+660 **46**
Uden, *Netherlands* M56+517 **44**
Udine, *Italy* M11+461 **56**
Udong, *Cambodia* F01+117 **69**
Udon Thani, *Thailand* F13+175 **69**
Udskaya Guba, *U.S.S.R.* C85+550 **63**
Udzha, *U.S.S.R.* E19+717 **63**
Uelen, *U.S.S.R.* Z30+660 **63**
Ueno, *Japan* C82+348 **68**
Ufa, *U.S.S.R.* J24+547 **61**
Uganda, *E. Africa* K70+010 **83**
Ugwashi-Uku, *Nigeria* M50+062 **82**
Uherske Hradiště, *Czech.* L75+491 **49**
Ui Failghe. *See* Offaly
Uinta Mts., *Utah* V36+408 **98**
Uist, North, I., *Scotland* N43+576 **40**
Uist, South, I., *Scotland* N43+573 **40**
Uitenhage, *Cape Province* L28–338 **84**
Uitgeest, *Netherlands* M62+525 **44**
Ujhani, *India* G66+280 **73**
Ujjain, *India* G85+230 **70**
Ujpest, *Hungary* L65+476 **49**
Ujung Pandang, *Celebes* E03–052 **65**
Ukermark (Uckermark), *E. Germany* M08+532 **48**
Ukhta, *Karelskaya* K85+652 **62**
Ukiah, *California* W20+391 **92**
Ukmerge, *Lithuania* L31+553 **47**
Ukraine, rep., *U.S.S.R.* L00+490 **60**
Ulaanbaatar, *Mongolia* E79+479 **64**
Ulangom, *Mongolia* F77+500 **63**
Ulan Ude, *U.S.S.R.* E74+520 **63**
Ulcinj, *Yugoslavia* L65+419 **58**
Ulithi, I., *Pacific Ocean* C60+100 **106**
Ulladulla, *New S. Wales* B87–354 **109**
Ullapool, *Scotland* N31+579 **40**
Ullared, *Sweden* M14+571 **47**
Ulldecona, *Spain* M87+406 **53**
Ullswater, L., *England* N18+546 **37**
Ullung Do, *Sea of Japan* D25+376 **68**
Ulm, *W. Germany* M30+484 **48**
Ulmarra, *New South Wales* B72–296 **109**
Ulster, prov., *Ireland, Rep.-N. Ire.* N48+548 **42**
Ulster Canal, *Ireland, Rep.-N. Ire.* N42+542 **42**
Ultima, *Victoria* C41–355 **109**
Ulua, *Honduras* T76+158 **101**
Ulukişla, *Turkey* K63+376 **74**
Ulva, I., *Scotland* N37+565 **41**
Ulverston, *England* N19+542 **37**
Ulverstone, *Tasmania* C23–412 **109**
Ulyanovsk, *U.S.S.R.* J70+544 **61**
Ülzen, *W. Germany* M27+530 **48**
Uman, *Ukraine* K88+488 **60**
Umanak Fd., *Greenland* R35+710 **26**
Umarkot, *Pakistan* H31+253 **70**
Umbria, reg., *Italy* M15+429 **56**
Umea, *Sweden* L58+638 **46**
Umm Ar Rusays, *Oman* J07+205 **75**
Umm el Qulban, *Saudi Arabia* K20+279 **74**
Umm Kuteira, *Sudan* L30+146 **81**
Umm Lej, *Saudi Arabia* K46+250 **74**
Umm Qasr, *Iraq* J73+300 **74**
Umm Ruwaba, *Sudan* K84+128 **81**
Umnak I., *Aleutian Is.* Z20+529 **99**
Umtali, *Zimbabwe* K74–188 **84**
Umtata, *Cape Province* L08–318 **84**
Umvuma, *Zimbabwe* K86–194 **84**
Una, *India* G82+315 **72**
Una R., *Yugoslavia* L80+452 **56**
Unadilla, *New York* T02+423 **96**
Unalakleet, *Alaska* Y65+637 **99**
Unalaska, *Aleutian Is.* Z10+535 **99**
Uncastillo, *Spain* N06+424 **53**
Uncia, *Bolivia* S39–185 **104**
Uncompahgre Plat., *Colorado* V20+385 **94**
Underbool, *Victoria* C49–352 **109**
Undur Khan, *Mongolia* E57+474 **64**
Ungarie, *New South Wales* C18–336 **109**
Ungava B., *Quebec* S45+594 **89**
União, *Brazil* Q77–045 **105**
União, *Brazil* S69–096 **104**
União da Victoria, *Brazil* R36–262 **103**
União Marara, *Brazil* S11–008 **104**
Uniejów, *Poland* L67+520 **49**
Unimak I., *Aleutian Is.* Y85+544 **99**
Unini, *Peru* S84–106 **104**
Union, *Argentina* S35–352 **103**
Union, *Argentina* S50–292 **103**
Union, *Missouri* U06+384 **97**
Union, *S. Carolina* T40+347 **97**
Union City, *Tennessee* T85+364 **97**
Union of Soviet Socialist Republics, (U.S.S.R.), *Europe-Asia* **30-31**
Uniontown, *Kentucky* T77+378 **97**
Uniontown, *Pennsylvania* T29+396 **96**
Unionville, *Missouri* U18+405 **95**
Unionville, *Nevada* V80+404 **92**
United Arab Emirates, *S.-W. Asia* J35+240 **75**
United Kingdom of Gt. Britain & N. Ire., *N.-W. Europe* **34**
United States of America (U.S.A.) **98-99**
United States Ra. *N.-W. Terr.* T30+810 **26**
Unnao, *India* G57+265 **73**
Unst, I., *Scotland* N05+607 **40**
Unterwalden, canton, *Switz.* M41+469 **45**
Unzha, *U.S.S.R.* K06+580 **61**
Uozu, *Japan* C75+368 **68**
Upata, *Venezuela* S15+081 **104**
Upemba L., *Zaire* L22–086 **82**
Upernivik, *Greenland* R40+730 **26**
Upington, *Cape Province* L52–284 **84**
Upolu, I., *Samoa* Z40–140 **106**
Upper Marlboro, *Maryland* T10+388 **96**
Upper Sandusky, *Ohio* T50+408 **91**
Upper Seal L., *Quebec* S84+558 **89**
Upper Volta, rep., *W. Afr.* N15+130 **80**
Uppsala, *Sweden* L74+599 **47**
Ur, *Iraq* J85+310 **74**
Uracoa, *Venezuela* S14+091 **104**
Urakawa, *Japan* C43+422 **68**
Ural, R., *U.S.S.R.* J54+508 **62**
Uralla, *New South Wales* B82–306 **109**
Uralsk, *U.S.S.R.* J52+513 **62**
Uralskiye Khrebet, *U.S.S.R.* J10+535 **62**
Urana, *New South Wales* C23–354 **109**
Uranium City, *Saskatchewan* V20+598 **88**
Urapunga, *N. Terr., Aust.* D03–147 **110**
Ura Tyube, *U.S.S.R.* H36+400 **62**
Urawa, *Japan* C62+358 **68**
Urbakh, *U.S.S.R.* J78+512 **61**
Urcos, *Peru* S70–137 **104**
Urda, *U.S.S.R.* J75+488 **62**
Urdzhar, *U.S.S.R.* G50+470 **62**
Ure R., *England* N11+543 **37**
Ures, *Mexico* V32+292 **100**
Urfa, *Turkey* K37+372 **74**
Urgun, *Afghanistan* H35+329 **75**
Uri, canton, *Switzerland* M38+468 **45**
Uribe, *Colombia* S85+031 **104**
Uribia, *Colombia* S73+116 **104**
Urisino, *New South Wales* C38–297 **109**
Urnasch, *Switzerland* M34+473 **45**
Urtazymsk, *U.S.S.R.* J07+520 **61**
Urtuin, *Mongolia* E26+462 **64**
Uruapan, *Mexico* U72+194 **100**
Urubamba & R., *Peru* S74–134 **104**
Urucará, *Brazil* R76–024 **105**
Urucu, *Brazil* Q64–177 **105**
Uruçui, *Brazil* Q87–072 **105**
Uruguaiana, *Brazil* R72–297 **103**
Uruguay, rep., *S. America* **103**
Uruguay, R., *Uruguay, etc.* R81–334 **103**
Urumchi, *Sinkiang, China* G14+437 **62**
Urumes Surhra, *Syria* K48+361 **76**
Urussanga, *Brazil* R26–286 **103**
Urville, Tg. d', *New Guinea* C73–015 **65**
Uryupinsk, *U.S.S.R.* K18+508 **61**
Urzhum, *U.S.S.R.* J60+571 **61**
Urziceni, *Romania* L20+446 **58**
Usak, *Turkey* L04+387 **74**
Usakos, *Namibia* L86–220 **84**
Usborne, mt., *Falkland Is.* R84–516 **103**
Usedom, *E. Germany* M06+540 **48**
Ushant I. *See* Quessant, I. d'
Ushirombo, *Tanzania* K78–034 **83**
Ush Tobe, *U.S.R.R.* G69+455 **62**
Ushuaia, *Argentina* S50–548 **103**
Usk, *Wales* N17+517 **38**
Usk, R., *Wales* N19+518 **38**
Uska, *India* G41+272 **73**

Uskedal, Norway M55+599 47
Uskudar, Turkey L06+411 74
Usole, Siberskoye, U.S.S.R. F09+528 63
Uspenskiy, U.S.S.R. H13+488 62
Usquil, Peru T21–079 104
Ussel, France M76+456 54
Ussuri, R., U.S.S.R. D08+465 63
Ussuriysk, U.S.S.R. D18+437 63
Ust Aldan, U.S.S.R. D35+635 63
Ust Amginskoye, U.S.S.R. D01+628 63
Ust Apuka, U.S.S.R. A61+605 63
Ust Belaya, U.S.S.R. A40+652 63
Ust' Bolsheretsk, U.S.S.R. B52+527 63
Ust' Chaun, U.S.S.R. A57+688 63
Uster, Switzerland M38+473 45
Usti nad Labem, Czech. M05+507 48
Ust Ishim, U.S.S.R. H25+575 62
Ust Kamenogorsk, Kazakh. G45+500 62
Ust Khayryuzovo, U.S.S.R. B49+570 63
Ust Kut, U.S.S.R. E85+570 63
Ust Maya, U.S.S.R. D02+604 63
Ust' Nera, U.S.S.R. C31+644 63
Ust Sopochnoye, U.S.S.R. B55+560 63
Ust Tsilma, U.S.S.R. J48+654 62
Ust Uda, U.S.S.R. F10+543 63
Ust Urt, plat., U.S.S.R. J30+440 62
Ust Usa, U.S.S.R. J18+660 62
Ust Uskoye, U.S.S.R. H66+543 61
Ust Yenisei Port, U.S.S.R. G34+698 62
Ustyuzhna, U.S.S.R. K52+588 60
Usumacinta, R., Mexico U08+168 100
Usumbura (Bujumbura), Burma L04–034 83
Utah, state, U.S.A. V45+391 98
Utah L., Utah V41+402 92
Utajarvi, Finland L22+647 46
Utena, U.S.S.R. L27+555 47
Utete, Tanzania K38–080 83
Uthal, Pakistan H50+257 70
Utiarity, Brazil R80–131 104
Utica, New York T01+431 91
Utiel, Spain N07+396 53
Utikuma L., Alberta V63+557 88
Utraula, India G46+273 73
Utrecht, Natal K88–276 84
Utrecht & prov., Netherlands M59+521 44
Utrera, Spain N35+372 52
Utsjoki, Finland L18+699 46
Utsunomiya, Japan C60+366 68
Uttar Pradesh, India G65+280 70
Uttaradit, Thailand F30+176 69
Uusikaarlepyy, Finland L45+635 46
Uusikaupunki, Finland L51+608 47
Uvac, Yugoslavia L63+436 58
Uvat, U.S.S.R. H38+591 62
Uvéa, I., Loyalty Islands A78–205 106
Uvira, Zaire L06–034 83
Uvs Nuur, lake, Mongolia F73+503 63
Uxbridge, Massachusetts S70+421 96
Uxbridge, Ontario T25+441 91
Uxmal, Mexico T89+204 100
Uyu Chaung R., Burma F55+252 71
Uyuni, Bolivia S41–205 104
Uzbekskaya, rep., U.S.S.R. H60+400 62
Uzdin, Yugoslavia L56+452 58
Uzgen, U.S.S.R. H10+406 62
Uzhgorod, U.S.S.R. L46+486 60
Uzyansk, U.S.S.R. J12+536 61
Vaal R., S. Africa L30–282 84
Vaalwater, Transvaal L10–242 84
Vaasä, Finland L50+631 46
Vac, Hungary L65+478 49
Vache, I. La, Haiti S82+181 101
Vadsø, Norway L02+701 46
Vadüz, Liechtenstein M33+471 45
Værøy, Norway M14+677 46
Vags Fd., Norway L78+690 46
Vah, R., Czechoslovakia L73+485 49
Vaila, I., Scotland N09+602 40
Vairowal, India G89+314 72
Valais, canton, Switzerland M47+462 45
Val Brillant, Quebec S45+485 90
Valcheta, Argentina S37–407 103
Valday, U.S.S.R. K69+579 60
Valday Hills, U.S.S.R. K72+576 60
Valdepeñas, Spain N21+388 52
Valderredible, Spain N24+428 52
Valderrobres, Spain M89+409 53
Valdez, Alaska X70+610 99
Valdez, Pen., Argentina S24–422 103
Valdivia, Chile S80–398 103
Valdosta, Georgia T50+308 97
Valea-lui-Mihai, Romania L47+475 49
Valença, Brazil Q71–066 105
Valençay, France M81+471 54
Valence, France M61+450 55
Valencia, Spain N02+395 53
Valencia, Venezuela S48+102 104
Valencia, Gulf of, Spain N87+394 53
Valencia de Alcantara, Spain N43+394 52
Valencia de Don Juan, Spain N33+423 52
Valenciennes, France M69+503 54
Văleni de Munte, Romania L24+452 58
Valencia I., Ireland, Rep. N62+519 43
Valentin, mt., Chile S80–465 103
Valentine, Nebraska U64+428 94
Valera, Venezuela S63+093 104
Valga, U.S.S.R. L24+578 47
Valjala, U.S.S.R. L43+584 47
Valjevo, Yugoslavia L61+443 58
Valkeakoski, Finland L35+612 47
Valkenburg, Netherlands M55+509 44
Valladolid, Mexico T77+205 100
Valladolid, Spain N28+416 52
Valldemosa, Balearic Is. M74+397 53
Valle-D'Aosta, reg., Italy M47+457 58
Valle de La Pascua, Venez. S36+092 104
Valle de Santiago, Mexico U68+203 100
Valledupar, Colombia S79+104 104
Vallejo, California W13+381 92
Vallenar, Chile S65–284 103
Valletta, Malta M03+359 57
Valley City, N. Dakota U48+469 93
Valleyfield, Quebec S85+453 91
Vallgrund, Finland L52+632 46
Vallorbe, Switzerland M52+467 45
Valmaseda, Spain N19+432 52
Valmiera, U.S.S.R. L27+575 47
Valognes, France N09+495 54
Valona. See Vlone
Valona B., Albania L63+404 59
Valoria la Buena, Spain L63+418 52
Valparaiso, Chile S70–330 103
Valparaiso, Indiana T72+414 95
Valparaiso, Mexico U81+228 100
Vals Platz, Switzerland M35+466 45
Valtimo, Finland L07+637 46
Valverde de Jucar, Spain N14+397 53
Valverde del Caming, Spain N40+376 52
Van & Gölu, Turkey K10+385 74
Vana Vändra, Estonia L30+587 47
Van Buren, Arkansas U26+354 99
Van Buren, Maine S48+471 90
Van Buren, Missouri U06+370 97
Vanceboro, Maine S45+455 90
Vancouver, Brit. Columbia W19+493 88
Vancouver, Washington W16+456 92
Vancouver I., Brit. Columbia W34+500 88
Vancouver, Mt., Yukon X26+605 88
Vandalia, Illinois T85+389 95
Van Diemen, C., N.T., Aust. D27–111 110
Van Diemen G.;
N. Territory, Australia D18–119 110
Vanegas, Mexico U66+239 100
Vänern, L., Sweden M12+589 47
Vänersborg, Sweden M16+584 47
Vangaindrano, Madagascar J74–234 83
Van Horn Mts., Texas V00+308 94
Vankarem, U.S.S.R. Z66+678 63
Vanndale, Arkansas U05+353 97
Vannes, France N17+477 54
Vannøy, Norway L60+701 46
Vanovara, U.S.S.R. F15+604 63
Vanrhynsdorp, South Africa L68–316 84
Vanuatu, Pac. Oc. A70–170 106
Vanua Levu, I., Fiji A04–170 106
Var, dep., France M52+435 55
Varanasi, India G42+254 73
Varanger-halvøya, Norway L00+700 46
Varanger Halvøy, Norway L06+704 46
Varaždin, Yugoslavia L82+463 56
Varberg, Sweden M16+571 47
Vardar R., Greece, etc. L46+414 58
Vardø, Norway K84+703 46
Vares, C. de, Spain N46+435 52
Varese, Italy M38+458 56
Varkaus, Finland L13+623 46
Varna, Bulgaria L12+432 58
Varnavin, U.S.S.R. K00+574 61
Värtsilä, Finland K86+622 46
Vasht, Iran H83+282 75
Vasknarva, U.S.S.R. L14+590 47
Vassar, Michigan T51+434 91
Vastanfors, Sweden L85+600 47
Västerås, Sweden L81+597 47
Väster Dal Älv, Sweden M10+611 47
Västervik, Sweden L80+578 47
Vasvar, Hungary L78+471 49
Vatican City (Citta del
Vaticano), Italy M15+417 57
Vaticano C., Italy L85+387 57
Vatna Jökull, Iceland P12+645 46
Vatomandry, Madagascar J66–194 83
Vättern, L., Sweden M04+580 47
Vättis, Switzerland M33+469 45
Vaucluse, dep., France M59+440 55
Vaud, canton, Switzerland M51+466 45
Vaughn, New Mexico V00+348 94
Vaxjö, Sweden M01+569 47
Vaygach, Ostrov, U.S.S.R. J00+700 62
Vechel, Netherlands M55+516 44
Vedia, Argentina S10–344 103
Vedrin, Belgium M61+505 44
Veere, Netherlands M68+516 44
Vega & Fd., Norway M18+656 46
Vegornitis, L., Greece L49+407 59
Vegreville, Alberta V43+536 88
Vejle, Denmark M33+557 47
Vela, Argentina R88–374 103
Velaines, Belgium M69+507 44
Velebit Planina, Yugoslavia L88+445 56
Veles, Yugoslavia L49+417 58
Velestinon, Greece L43+394 59
Velez Rubio, Spain N12+377 53
Veliki Ustyug, U.S.S.R. J83+609 62
Velikiye Luki, U.S.S.R. K87+564 60
Velizh, U.S.S.R. K83+556 60
Velletri, Italy M13+417 57
Vellore, India G66+129 70
Velp, Netherlands M54+520 44
Velsen, Netherlands M62+525 44
Velsk, U.S.S.R. K17+611 60
Venado, Mexico U66+230 100
Venado Tuerto, Argentina S12–337 103
Vendee, dep., France N10+467 54
Vendôme, France M84+478 54
Venendaal, Netherlands M57+520 44
Veneto, reg., Italy M16+454 56
Venezia, & G. di, Italy M16+454 56
Venezuela, rep., S. America 104
Venezuela, G. de, Venezuela S66+115 104
Vengurla, India H08+159 70
Venice. See Venezia
Venlo, Netherlands M53+514 44
Vennacher, L., Scotland N26+562 41
Venraij, Netherlands M54+515 44
Ventotene, I., Italy M10+408 57
Ventspils, U.S.S.R. L50+574 47
Ventura, California V86+343 92
Venus B., Australia C26–388 109
Vera, Argentina S02–294 103
Vera, Spain N11+372 53
Veracuz and state, Mexico U37+191 100
Veramin, Iran J49+354 75
Veraval, India H28+209 70
Verbania, Switzerland M39+460 45
Vercelli, Italy M39+453 56
Verde, C., See Vert, C.
Verde R., Arizona V40+338 94
Verdun, France M58+491 54
Verdun, Quebec S82+455 91
Vereshchagino, U.S.S.R. G15+641 62
Vereshchagino, U.S.S.R. J31+581 61
Vereya, U.S.S.R. K54+553 61
Verga C., Guinea N88+104 80
Vergara, Uruguay R53–329 103
Vergennes, Vermont S79+441 91
Verin, Spain N44+419 52
Verkhne Imbatskoe, U.S.S.R. G12+632 62
Verkhne Ulkhne, U.S.S.R. J06+538 61
Verkhne Vilyuysk, U.S.S.R. D88+633 63
Verkhoturye, U.S.S.R. H67+589 62
Verkhoyansk, U.S.S.R. D09+672 63
Verkhoyanskiy Khr., U.S.S.R. D30+650 63
Vermilion, S. Dakota U42+428 93
Vermilion B., Louisiana U12+296 95
Vermont, state, U.S.A. S80+437 99
Vernal, Utah V28+404 94
Verneuil, France M86+487 54
Vernon, British Columbia V85+503 88
Veroia, Greece L47+405 59
Verona, Italy M24+454 56
Vernon, Texas U55+342 95
Verrieres, les, Switzerland M51+469 45
Versailles, France M77+488 54
Versailles, Kentucky T59+381 97
Versam, Switzerland M34+468 45
Vert, C., Senegal P16+148 80
Verte, I., Quebec S57+480 90
Vertrijk, Belgium M61+508 44
Verviers, Belgium M55+506 44
Vervins, France M66+498 54
Vesanto, Finland L21+629 46
Vesoul, France M53+476 54
Vessem, Netherlands M58+514 44
Vest Fd., Norway M06+678 46
Vesta, Costa Rica T48+097 101
Vesterålen, Is., Norway M00+693 46
Vest Vägöy, Norway M06+682 46
Vesyegonsk, U.S.S.R. K47+587 60
Veszprem, Hungary L73+471 49
Vetluga, U.S.S.R. J85+579 61
Vetluga, R., U.S.S.R. J89+573 62
Veurne, Belgium M74+511 44
Vevey, Switzerland M49+465 45
Vex, Switzerland M46+462 45
Viacha, Bolivia S50–166 104
Viana, Brazil Q88–031 105
Viborg, Denmark M34+564 47
Vibo Valentia, Italy L83+387 57
Vicente de la Barquera, S.,
Spain N26+434 52
Vicenza, Italy M21+455 56
Vich, Spain M76+419 53
Vichuquen, Chile S72–348 103
Vichy, France M69+461 54
Vicksburg, Mississippi U06+324 97
Vicosa, Brazil Q66–036 105
Victor Harbour, S. Australia C69–356 109
Victoria, Argentina S01–325 103
Victoria, British Columbia W20+485 88
Victoria, Hong Kong E34+220 64
Victoria, Texas U42+288 94
Victoria, state, Australia — 111
Victoria Falls, Zimbabwe L24–178 84
Victoria I., N.-W. Territories V30+710 88
Victoria L., New S. Wales C52–340 109
Victoria L., Uganda, etc. K70–010 83
Victoria Ld., Antarctica B30–740 27
Victoria Mt., Burma F67+214 71
Victoria, Mt.,
Papua New Guinea C17–088 111
Victoria, R., N.Terr., Aust. D26–154 110
Victoria do Mearim, Brazil Q87–034 105
Victoria Point, Burma F39+100 71
Victoria River Downs
N. Territory, Australia D14–162 110
Victoriaville, Quebec S72+461 91
Victoria West, South Africa L42–314 84
Victorica, Argentina S32–361 103
Vicuna, Chile S64–300 103
Vidago, Portugal N45+417 52
Vidin, Bulgaria L43+440 58
Viedma, Argentina S18–407 103
Viedma, L., Argentina S74–496 103
Vienna (Wien), Austria L82+482 49
Vienne, France M61+455 54
Vienne, dep., France M88+465 54
Vienne R., France M87+471 54
Vientiane, Laos F15+180 69
Vieques, I. de, West Indies S32+182 101
Vierlingsbeek, Netherlands M54+516 44
Vierwaldstatter See, Switz. M39+470 45
Vierzon Ville, France M78+472 54
Vietnam S.E.Asia E70+195 69
Vigan, Philippines D87+176 65
Vigan, le, France M68+440 55
Vigia, Brazil R19–008 105
Vigia Chico, Mexico T74+197 100
Vigo & R., Spain N52+422 52
Vigrestad, Norway M56+585 47
Vihanti, Finland L30+645 46
Vijayanagar, India G80+154 70
Vijayavada, India G56+165 70
Vijosë R., Albania L62+406 59
Vikaviskis, U.S.S.R. L42+546 47
Vikna, Norway M24+649 46
Vila Arriage, Angola M10–146 82
Vila de Cangombe, Angola L60–144 82
Vila de João Belo, Mozamb. K68-252 84
Vila Lugela, Mozambique K48-170 84
Vila Luso, Angola L60-120 82
Vila Machado, Mozambique K64-194 84
Vila Manica, Mozambique K72-190 84
Vilanculos, Mozambique K58-220 84
Vilani, U.S.S.R. L18+566 47
Vila Nova de Famalicão,
Portugal N51+414 52
Vila Nova de Gerveira, Port. N52+419 52
Vila Pereira de Eça, Angola L86–172 84
Vila Pery, Mozambique K70–194 84
Vila Real, Portugal N47+413 52
Vilar Formoso, Portugal N41+406 52
Vila Serpa Pinto, Angola L80–146 82
Vila Velha de Rodao, Port. N46+397 52
Vila Verissimo, Angola L56–082 82
Vila Viçosa, Portugal N44+388 52
Vilcheka, Os., Arctic Ocean H85+807 62
Vilhelmina, Sweden L80+646 46
Vilhena, Brazil S01–126 104
Viljandi, U.S.S.R. L26+584 47
Villa Angela, Argentina S04–275 103
Villa Bella, Bolivia S32–105 104
Villa Bens, Morocco N81 + 274 80
Villa Bittencourt, Brazil S56–015 104
Villablino, Spain N38+430 52
Villacañas, Spain N20+396 52
Villacarriedo, Spain N22+432 52
Villach, Austria M07+465 48
Villa Cisneros, See Dakhla
Villa Constitucion, Argentina S02–332 103
Villa del Rosario, Paraguay R73–245 103
Villa de Rosario, Argentina S22–316 103
Villa Dolores, Argentina S31–319 103
Villafranca, Spain N41+426 52
Villafranca del Cid, Spain N02+404 53
Villafranca del Panadés, Sp. M80+413 53
Villaguay, Argentina R84–319 103
Villa Guillermina, Argentina R87–282 103
Villa Hermosa, Mexico U18+179 100
Villa Hidalgo, Mexico U87+261 100
Villa Iris, Argentina S20–382 103
Villa Jordão, Brazil S73–095 104
Villajoyosa, Spain N01+385 53
Villalba, Spain N46+432 52
Villaldama, Mexico U62+264 100
Villalón de Campos, Spain N30+421 52
Villalonga, Argentina S16–400 103
Villalpando, Spain N33+419 52
Villa Maria, Argentina S20–324 103
Villa Mercedes, Argentina S33–336 103
Villa Montes, Bolivia S21–212 104
Villa Murtinho, Brazil S32–104 104
Villaneuva de Cordoba, Sp. N28+383 52
Villa Nova, Brazil R77–068 105
Villa Nova, Brazil Q39–104 105
Villanova, Greece L11+364 59
Villa Novo, Brazil R41–012 105
Villanueva-de-la-Serena, Sp. N35+390 52
Villanueva-y Geltrú, Spain M81+413 53
Villaodrid, Spain N43+433 52
Villaputzu, Sardinia M33+395 57
Villarcayo, Spain N21+429 52
Villareal, Spain N01+399 53
Villarrica, Chile S74–392 103
Villarrica, Paraguay R68–257 103
Villarrobledo, Spain N16+393 53
Villa Sanjurjo, Morocco N24+352 80
Villavicencio, Colombia S76+040 104
Villaviciosa, Spain N32+435 52
Villa Viejo, Colombia T02+030 104
Villazon, Bolivia S34–220 104
Villefort, France M67+444 55
Villefranche-de-Rouergue,
France M78+443 55
Ville Marie, Quebec T27+473 91
Villena, Spain N05+386 53
Villeneuve-sur-Lot, France M86+444 55
Villeurbanne, France M61+458 54
Villingen, W. Germany M39+481 48
Villisca, Iowa U30+409 95
Villo-Duca-Abruzzi, Somalia J86+026 83
Villupuram, India G62+121 70
Vilnyus (Vilna), Lithuania L28+546 47
Vilvoorde, Belgium M63+509 44
Vilyui, R., U.S.S.R. E30+670 63
Vilyuysk, U.S.S.R. D80+637 63
Vimioso, Portugal N39+417 52
Vimperk, Czechoslovakia M08+490 48
Viña del Mar, Chile S70–330 103
Vinai Haven I., Maine S53+441 90
Vinaroz, Spain M87+405 53
Vincennes, Indiana T75+386 95
Vinchiaturo, Italy M02+415 57
Vindel Alv, Sweden L70+651 46
Vindhya Ra., India G80+222 70
Vineland, New Jersey T00+395 96
Vineyard Sd., Massachusetts S64+414 96
Vinh, Vietnam E86 + 187 69
Vinh Loi, Vietnam E85 + 093 69
Vinita, Oklahoma U32+366 95
Vinkovci, Yugoslavia L67+453 58
Vinnitsa, Ukraine L10+492 60
Vintes, Ecuador T28–015 104
Vinton, Iowa U12+422 95
Viransehir, Turkey K31+374 74
Virden, Manitoba U65+498 88
Virgin Is., West Indies S28+185 101
Virginia, Ireland, Rep. N42+538 42
Virginia, Minnesota U15+475 93
Virginia, state, U.S.A. T27+374 99
Virginia City, Montana V42+452 93
Virginia Falls, N.-W. Terr. W32+616 88
Viroqua, Wisconsin U05+436 91
Virovitica, Yugoslavia L76+458 58
Virpazar, Yugoslavia L65+423 58
Virtasalmi, Finland L15+621 46
Virton, Belgium M57+496 44
Virtsu, Estonia L39+586 47
Viru, Peru T22–084 104
Vis, I., Yugoslavia L83+430 56
Visalia, California V86+363 92
Visby, Gotland, Sweden L70+577 47
Viscount Melville Sd.,
N.-W. Territories V30+732 88
Visé, Belgium M56+507 44
Viseu, Portugal N47+407 52
Vishakhapatnam, India G40+177 71
Viški, Latvia L19+561 47
Viso, Mte., Italy M48+447 56
Visoko, Yugoslavia L71+440 58
Visp, Switzerland M43+463 45
Vista Alegre, Brazil S06+017 104
Vistula (Wisla), R., Poland L50+515 49
Vitebsk, Byelorussia K89+551 60
Viterbo, Italy M17+424 56
Vitigudino, Spain N38+410 52
Viti Levu, I., Fiji A10–177 106
Vitim, R., U.S.S.R. E40+590 63
Vitoria, Brazil Q62–203 105
Vitoria, Spain N16+429 53
Vitry-le-François, France M62+487 54
Vitteaux, France M63+474 54
Vittoria, Sicily M03+369 57
Viver, Spain N04+399 53
Vivero, Spain N45+434 52
Vivi, U.S.S.R. F41+640 63
Vivonne & B., S. Australia C77–359 109
Vivorata, Argentina R76–378 103
Vizeu, Brazil R07–012 105
Vizianagram, India G39+181 71
Vizirul Romania L14+449 58
Vizovice, Czechoslovakia L73+492 49
Vizzini, Sicily M02+372 57
Vlaanderen, Oost, Belgium M68+509 44
Vlaanderen, West, Belgium M72+510 44
Vlaardingen, Netherlands M64+519 44
Vladimir, U.S.S.R. K28+561 60
Vladimirovka, U.S.S.R. J83+484 61
Vladivostok, U.S.S.R. D18+430 63
Vlieland I., Netherlands M60+533 44
Vlissingen, Netherlands M69+514 44
Vlone, Albania L63+405 59
Vltava R., Czechoslovakia M03+504 48
Voghera, Italy M36+450 56
Vohemar, Madagascar J60–134 83
Võhma, Estonia L27+586 47
Voi, Kenya K38–034 83

Voiotia, Greece L39+382 59
Voiron, France M57+452 54
Voitsberg, Austria L89+470 48
Voiviis, L., Greece L43+395 59
Vojvodina, Yugoslavia L60+454 58
Volcano B., Japan C56+424 68
Volga, R., U.S.S.R. J85+477 62
Volgograd, U.S.S.R. K04+487 61
Volissos, Greece L24+385 59
Volkhov, R., U.S.S.R. K78+596 60
Vollenhove, Netherlands M54+527 44
Volochanka, U.S.S.R. F64+710 63
Volochisk, Ukraine L23+495 60
Vologda, U.S.S.R. K32+592 60
Volokolamsk, U.S.S.R. K54+561 60
Vólos, Greece L42+394 59
Volosinov, Yugoslavia L59+456 58
Volovets, Ukraine L40+488 60
Volozhin, Byelorussia L22+541 60
Volsk, U.S.S.R. K60+595 60
Volsk, U.S.S.R. J75+521 61
Volta R., Ghana M88+060 80
Voltveti, Estonia L30+582 47
Voneche, Belgium M60+501 44
Voorburg, Netherlands M64+521 44
Voorschoten, Netherlands M63+521 44
Voorst, Netherlands M53+522 44
Voorthuizen, Netherlands M56+522 44
Vopnafjordhur, Iceland N88+658 46
Vorab, mt., Switzerland M35+469 45
Vorarlberg, Austria M31+472 48
Vorauen, Switzerland M36+470 45
Vorkuta, U.S.S.R. H67+674 62
Vormsi, I., Estonia L40+590 47
Voronezh, U.S.S.R. K35+517 60
Voroshilovgrad, Ukraine K34+486 60
Vosges, dep. & mts., France M50+482 54
Voss, Norway M51+606 47
Vostock I., Pacific Ocean Y15–100 107
Votkinsk, U.S.S.R. J36+570 61
Voulijoki, Finland L18+642 46
Vouvry, Switzerland M49+463 45
Vouziers, France M62+493 54
Voxna, Sweden L86+613 47
Voyampolka, U.S.S.R. B33+584 63
Voznesensk U.S.S.R. K82+475 60
Vrancv, Czechoslovakia L50+489 49
Vrangelya, Ostrov, I., U.S.S.R. A00+718 63
Vranje, Yugoslavia L49+425 58
Vratsa, Bulgaria L39+432 58
Vrbitsa, Bulgaria L20+430 58
Vrchovina Ceskomoravska,
Czechoslovakia L84+495 49
Vredefort, O.F.S. L16–270 84
Vrin, Switzerland M36+467 45
Vrindaban, India G73+276 73
Vroomshoop, Netherlands M51+524 44
Vršac, Yugoslavia L52+451 58
Vrútky, Czechoslovakia L67+491 49
Vryburg, Cape Province L32–270 84
Vučitrn, Yugoslavia L54+428 58
Vukovar, Yugoslavia L66+454 58
Vulcan, Missouri U04+374 97
Vulcano, I., Italy M00+384 57
Vulpera, Switzerland M28+468 45
Vyatka (Kirov), U.S.S.R. J62+586 61
Vyatka, R., U.S.S.R. J65+577 62
Vyazemski, U.S.S.R. D01+475 63
Vyazma, U.S.S.R. K63+551 60
Vyazniki, U.S.S.R. K17+563 61
Vyborg, U.S.S.R. L07+606 60
Vyrnwy, L., Wales N21+528 38
Vyrtsyarv Oz., Estonia L24+583 47
Vyru, Estonia L18+578 47
Vyshniy Volochek, U.S.S.R. K63+576 60
Vyskov, Czechoslovakia L78+493 49
Vytegra, U.S.S.R. K52+610 60
Wa, Ghana N14+102 80
Waalwijk, Netherlands M60+517 44
Wabash R., Indiana T76+392 95
Wabiskaw R., Alberta V55+568 88
Waboose Dam, Ontario T78+506 89
Wabos, Ontario T55+468 91
Wabra, Saudi Arabia J56+274 74
Wabuda, I.,
Papua New Guinea C38–084 111
Waco, Texas U43+315 95
Wad, Pakistan H51+272 70
Waddamana, Tasmania C20–421 109
Wadden Zee, Netherlands M57+533 44
Waddington Mt., B.C. W33+513 88
Wadebridge, England N29+505 38
Wadena, Minnesota U31+464 93
Wadesboro, N. Carolina T31+350 97
Wad Hamid, Sudan K74+166 81
Wadi-es-Sir, Jordan K55+320 76
Wadi Gemal I., Egypt K60+246 81
Wadi Halfa, Sudan K82+216 81
Wadi Musa, Jordan K57+303 76
Wadi Medani, Sudan K70+144 81
Wafi, Saudi Arabia K07+249 74
Wageningen, Netherlands M56+520 44
Wager B., N.-W. Territories U00+654 89
Wagga Wagga, N.S.W. C16–351 109
Wagin, W. Australia E15–332 110
Wagoner, Oklahoma U34+360 95
Wahabis, Saudi Arabia K20+243 74
Wahla, Saudi Arabia K20+180 74
Wahoo, Nebraska U40+412 95
Waiau, New Zealand A41–426 112
Waichow. See Waiyeung
Waigeo, I., New Guinea D26–002 65
Waiheke I., New Zealand A29–368 112
Waihi, New Zealand A25+374 112
Waikaia, New Zealand A67–457 112
Waikare Moana, N.Z. A17–387 112
Waikari, New Zealand A44–429 112
Waikato, R., New Zealand A25–382 112
Waikerie, S. Australia C60–342 109
Waikouaiti, New Zealand A55–456 112
Waimakariri, R., N.Z. A46–434 112
Waimate, New Zealand A54–447 112
Waimes, Belgium M53+504 44
Wainfleet, England M89+531 37
Wainganga R., India G61+212 70
Waingapu, Sumba I., Indon. D89–096 65
Wainwright, Alaska Y60+705 99
Waipara, New Zealand A41–430 112
Waipawa, New Zealand A20–399 112
Waipukurau, New Zealand A20–400 112
Wairarapa, L., New Zealand A28–412 112
Wairau, R., New Zealand A40–416 112
Wairio, New Zealand A72–458 112
Wairoa, New Zealand A16–391 112
Wais, Iran J66+315 74
Waitara, New Zealand A34–390 112
Waitomo, New Zealand A29–383 112
Waiuku, New Zealand A32–372 112
Waiyeung, China E33+231 67
Wajir, Kenya K30+016 83
Wakamatsu, Japan C60+375 68
Wakasa B., Japan C86+357 68
Wakatipu, L., N.Z. A68–451 112
Wakayama, Japan C89+342 68
Wakba, Jordan K54+303 74
Wake I., Pacific Ocean A80+192 106
Wakefield, England N09+537 37
Wakonichi L., Quebec S84+501 90
Wakrah, Qatar, Arabia J51+252 75
Waksa, Iraq K07+308 74
Wakuan Hu, China E18+324 66
Walachia, Romania L24+448 58
Walbrzych, Poland L82+508 49
Walcha, New South Wales B81–310 109
Walcheren I., Netherlands M69+515 44
Wald, Switzerland M37+473 45
Waldia, Ethiopia K32+118 83
Waldoboro, Maine S56+441 90
Waldport, Oregon W24+444 92
Walen See, Switzerland M35+471 45
Walenstadt, Switzerland M34+471 45
Wales, Great Britain N20+524 34
Walgett, New South Wales C11–300 109
Walgreen Coast, Antarctica U50–720 27
Walhalla, S. Carolina T48+347 97
Walhalla, Victoria C21–379 109
Walker, Minnesota U28+471 93
Walker, L., Nevada V82+388 92
Walker's Ra., Oregon W10+434 92
Walkerton, Ontario T37+441 91
Walkerville, Ontario T48+424 91
Wallace, Idaho V65+475 92
Wallaceburg, Ontario T43+426 91
Wallal, Western Australia D85–198 110
Wallaroo, S. Australia C75–340 109
Wallasey, England N18+534 37
Wallaston, Mt.,
N. Territory, Australia D15–166 110
Walla Walla, New S. Wales C19–358 109
Walla-Walla, Washington V80+461 92
Wallenpaupack, L., Pa. T01+414 96
Wallingford, England N07+516 39
Wallis L., New South Wales B76–322 109
Wallowa Mts., Oregon V74+452 92
Wallsend, New S. Wales B81–329 109
Walney I., England N20+541 37
Walnut Cove, N. Carolina T31+363 97
Walsall, England N12+526 37
Walsenburg, Colorado U88+376 94
Walsoorden, Netherlands M66+514 44
Walterboro, S. Carolina T34+329 97
Waltham, England M87+518 39
Waltham, Massachusetts S67+424 96
Waltham, Quebec T12+459 91
Walton, New York T01+422 96
Walvis Bay, Namibia M02-230 84
Walwale, Ghana N04+104 80
Wamba, Zaire L12+020 83
Wamel, Netherlands M57+519 44
Wampsville, New York T04+430 91
Wana, Pakistan H33+323 72
Wanaaring, New S. Wales C35–297 109
Wanaka & L., New Zealand A65–445 112
Wanbi, S. Australia C58–348 109
Wandiwash, India G62+126 70
Wandre, Belgium M56+507 44
Wandsbek, W. Germany M30+536 48
Wan Fou Shan, China E32+292 67
Wanganella, New S. Wales C31–352 109
Wanganui & R., N.Z. A30–399 112
Wangaratta, Victoria C22–364 109
Wangyehmiao, China D77+460 64
Wanhsien, China E70+308 66
Wankie, Zimbabwe L20–184 84
Wanping, China E21+398 66
Wantage, England N08+516 39
Wanyuan, China E70+321 66
Wapeelo, Iowa U08+412 95
Wappapello Res., Missouri U02+370 95
Wapheton, N. Dakota U40+462 98
Wapiti R., Alberta V87+548 88
Warandab, Ethiopia K06+070 83
Warangal, India G62+180 70
Waratah, Tasmania C27–415 109
Waratah B., Victoria C24–388 109
Warburton, Victoria C26–378 109
Wardair, Ethiopia J89+068 83
Wardha & R., India G68+208 70
Ware, England N00+518 39
Waremme, Belgium M58+507 44
Warialda, New South Wales B86–296 109
Warka, Poland L53+518 49
Warmbad, Namibia L66-284 84
Warmbaths, Transvaal L10–250 84
Warm Springs, Virginia T28+380 97
Warnemünde, E. Germany M17+542 48
Warner L., Oregon V89+423 92
Warneton, Belgium M72+507 44
Warora, India G65+203 70
Warracknabeal, Victoira C45–363 109
Warragul, Victoria C25–382 109
Warrego, R., New S. Wales C28–296 109
Warren, Arkansas U13+336 97
Warren, Illinois U00+425 91
Warren, Minnesota U40+482 93
Warren, New South Wales C13–318 109
Warren, Ohio T35+413 91
Warren, Pennsylvania T25+418 96
Warrenpoint, N. Ireland N37+541 42
Warrensburg, Missouri U22+388 95
Wellington, I, Chile T00–495 103
Warrenton, Virginia T17+387 96
Warri, Nigeria M56+056 80
Warrington, England N16+534 37
Warrnambool, Victoria C45–384 109
Warroad, Minnesota U32+489 93
Warroh, Ethiopia K12+086 83
Warrumbungle Ra., N.S.W. C03–313 109
Warsaw, Indiana T65+412 91
Warsaw, New York T19+427 96
Warsaw, N. Carolina T19+350 97
Warsaw. See Warszawa
Warszawa, Poland L54+523 49
Warta, Poland L68+517 49
Warta R., Poland L71+524 49
Wartburg, Tennessee T57+361 97
Warwick, Queensland B78–280 111
Warwick, Rhode Island S68+417 96
Warwick & co., England N09+524 37
Wasatch Mts., Utah V36+400 94
Waseca, Minnesota U20+440 93
Wasen, Switzerland M43+471 45
Wash, The, England M88+530 37
Washakie Needle, Wyoming V27+438 93
Washburn, Wisconsin U06+467 93
Washington,
District of Columbia T12+389 91
Washington, Indiana T72+386 95
Washington, Iowa U10+413 95
Washington, Missouri U07+386 97
Washington, New Jersey T00+407 96
Washington, N. Carolina T12+355 97
Washington, Ohio T51+396 91
Washington, Pennsylvania T32+402 91
Washington, Virginia T19+387 96
Washington, state, U.S.A. V12+475 98
Washington I., Pacific Ocean Y60+048 106
Washington Ld., Greenland S00+800 26
Washington, Mt., N.H. S67+443 91
Washir, Afghanistan H66+321 75
Washuk, Pakistan H61+277 70
Wasmes, Belgium M67+504 44
Wassen, Switzerland M38+467 45
Wataroa, New Zealand A58–433 112
Watchet, England N20+512 38
Waterbury, Connecticut S78+415 96
Waterford, New Brunswick S32+457 90
Waterford (Port Láirge),
Ireland, Rep. N43+522 43
Waterford Harb., Ireland, Rep. N42+522 43
Waterloo, Belgium M64+507 44
Waterloo, Illinois U01+384 97
Waterloo, Iowa U14+425 95
Waterloo, Ontario T33+435 91
Waterloo, Quebec S75+454 91
Watertown, New York T06+440 91
Watertown, S. Dakota U43+449 93
Watertown, Wisconsin T82+432 91
Waterville, Maine S58+446 90
Watervliet, New York S82+428 96
Waterways, Alberta V38+564 88
Watford, England N03+517 39
Watford City, N. Dakota U80+479 93
Watkins Glen, New York T12+424 96
Watlings I., Bahamas, The S88 + 240 101
Watonga, Oklahoma U51+358 95
Watou, Belgium M74+508 44
Watrous, Saskatchewan V02+513 88
Watsa, Zaire L02+028 83
Watseka, Illinois T76+408 95
Watson, Utah V24+398 94
Watsonville, California W11+369 92
Watt, New Brunswick S43+454 90
Watts Bar L., Tennessee T58+355 97
Wattsville, Alabama T67+336 97
Wau, Papua New Guinea C20–074 111
Wau, Sudan L12+078 81
Wauchope, New South Wales B74–315 109
Wauchula, Florida T41+276 97
Waukaringa, S. Australia C64–323 109
Waukegan, Illinois T77+424 95
Waukesha, Wisconsin T78+430 95
Waupaca, Wisconsin T85+444 91
Waupun, Wisconsin T82+436 91
Waurika, Oklahoma U48+342 95
Wausau, Wisconsin T88+450 91
Wautoma, Wisconsin T86+442 91
Wauwatosa, Wisconsin T79+431 91
Wave Hill, N. Terr., Aust. D24–175 110
Waveney, R., England M81+525 39
Waverley, Iowa U14+428 95
Waverly, New York T09+420 96
Waverly, Ohio T48+392 91
Wavre, Belgium M62+507 44
Waxahachie, Texas U41+324 95
Waycross, Georgia T44+312 97
Wayland, Ontario T53+480 91
Wayne, W. Virginia 145+382 97
Waynesboro, Georgia T42+330 97
Waynesboro, Pennsylvania T16+398 96
Waynesville, N. Carolina T48+355 97
Waynoka, Oklahoma U54+366 95
Wazirabad, Pakistan H05+324 72
Weald, The, England M89+511 39
Wear, R., England N10+548 37
Weatherford, Texas U46+328 95
Weatherly, Pennsylvania T06+410 96
Weaver, R., England N16+532 37
Webb City, Missouri U26+372 95
Webbwood, Ontario T41+463 91
Webster, S. Dakota U45+453 93
Webster City, Iowa U22+425 95
Webster Springs, W. Virginia T33+385 97
Wechelderzande, Belgium M61+513 44
Weda B., Halmahera, Indon. D40+002 65
Weddell I., Falkland Islands S06–518 103
Weddell Sea, Antarctica Q00–700 27
Wedderburn, Victoria C39–364 109
Wedgeport, Nova Scotia S36+437 90
Wednesbury, England V12+526 37
Weed, California W14+414 92
Weedon, Quebec S68+458 91
Weedsport, New York T09+430 96
Weeping Water, Nebraska U37+408 95
Weert, Netherlands M56+512 44
Weesen, Switzerland M35+471 45
Weesp, Netherlands M60+523 44
Wee Waa, New S. Wales C04–302 109
Weichang, China E11+418 66
Weiden, W. Germany M17+496 48
Weifang, China E06+367 66
Wei-hai, China D78+374 66
Wei Ho, R., China E76+342 64
Weihwei. See Chihsien
Weilmoringle, New S. Wales C19–292 109
Weimar, E. Germany M22+509 48
Weipa, Queensland C48–130 111
Weinfelden, Switzerland M35+476 45
Weiser, Idaho V72+442 92
Wei Shan Hu, China E18+350 66
Weissenfels, E. Germany M18+512 48
Weisshorn, mt., Switzerland M44+461 45
Weissmies, mt., Switzerland M42+461 45
Weisstannen, Switzerland M34+470 45
Wejh, Saudi Arabia K51+263 74
Welch, W. Virginia T38+375 97
Weldon, N. Carolina T16+364 97
Welford, Queensland C38–251 111
Welland, Ontario T25+430 91
Welland, R., England N03+527 37
Wellesley Is., Queensland C63–164 111
Wellin, Belgium M59+501 44
Wellingborough, England N04+523 37
Wellington, Kansas U42+372 95
Wellington, New S. Wales C06–326 109
Wellington, New Zealand A31–413 112
Wellington, S. Australia C64–354 109
Wellington, I., Chile T00–495 103
Wellington L., Victoria C16–380 109
Wells, Norfolk, England M85+530 39
Wells, Somerset, England N16+512 38
Wells, Nevada V60+411 92
Wellsboro, Pennsylvania T14+418 96
Wellsville, Missouri U10+390 95
Wellsville, New York T18+421 96
Wels, Austria M06+482 48
Welsford, New Brunswick S38+455 90
Welshpool, Wales N19+526 38
Welwyn Garden City, Eng. N01+518 39
Wema, Zaire L50–006 82
Wembo Niama, Zaire L32–042 82
Wemyss Bay, Scotland N29+559 41
Wenatchee, Washington W02+474 92
Wenchow, China D86+280 67
Wenshan, China F04+236 67
Wensi, China E53+353 66
Wentworth, New S. Wales C48–341 109
Weobley, England N17+522 38
Wernhout, Netherlands M62+514 44
Werribee, Victoria C32–379 109
Werris Creek, New S. Wales B86–313 109
Wervershoof, Netherlands M59+527 44
Wervik, Belgium M72+508 44
Wesel, W. Germany M50+517 48
Wesenberg, E. Germany M12+532 48
Weser, R., W. Germany M36+526 48
Wessel Is., N. Terr., Aust. C81–112 111
Wesson, Mississippi U02+317 97
West B., Louisiana T75+291 95
West Allis, Wisconsin T79+431 91
West Barra, Scotland N08+601 40
West Bay City, Michigan T54+436 91
West Bend, Wisconsin T79+435 91
West Bengal, India G15+224 71
West Branch, Michigan T55+443 91
West Bromwich, England N12+525 37
Westbrook, Maine S62+437 90
Westbury, Tasmania C19–415 109
Westby, New South Wales C16–355 109
West Calder, Scotland N21+559 41
West Chester, Pennsylvania T04+399 96
Westerly, Rhode Island S71+413 96
Westende, Belgium M73+512 44
Western Australia, state, Aust. 110
Western Samoa, Samoa Z60–150 10
Wester Schelde, Netherlands M67+514 44
Westfalen, W. Germany M42+518 48
Westfield, Massachusetts S76+421 91
Westfield, New Brunswick S38+454 90
Westfield, New York T28+423 96
Westfield, Pennsylvania T16+419 96
West Frankfort, Illinois T84+379 95
West Hartlepool, England N07+547 37
West Indies, Caribbean Sea S70+200 85
West Irian (Irian Barat), See Irian Jaya
West Linton, Scotland N20+557 41
West Lothian, co., See Lothian
Westmeath, co., Ireland, Rep. N45+535 43
Westminster, Maryland T12+396 96
Westmorland, co., See Cumbria
West Nicholson, Zimbabwe L04–212 84
Weston, Sabah E26+053 65
Weston, West Virginia T33+390 91
Weston-super-Mare, England N18+513 38
Westplains, Missouri U12+368 95
West Point, Arkansas U10+352 97
West Point, Georgia T61+329 97
West Point, Mississippi T82+336 95
Westpoint, Nebraska U40+418 95
West Point, New York S84+413 96
West Point, Virginia T11+375 97
Westport, Ireland, Rep. N57+538 42
Westport, New Zealand A50–417 112
Westport, Ontario T09+447 91
Westray I. & Firth, Scot. N18+593 40
West Riding, See West Yorkshire
West Union, Iowa U12+430 95
West Virginia, state, U.S.A. T40+384 99
Westwoud, Netherlands M59+527 44
West Yorkshire, Eng. N10+537 37
Wetar, I. & Str., Indonesia D52–080 65
Wetaskiwin, Alberta V50+532 88
Wetterhorn, mt., Switzerland M41+466 45
Wetumpka, Alabama T67+326 97
Wewoka, Oklahoma U40+352 95
Wexford & co., Ireland, Rep. N39+523 43
Wexford B. & Harb., Ireland, Rep.
N37+523 43
Wey, R., England N03+514 39
Weybridge, England N03+514 39
Weyburn, Saskatchewan U83+497 88
Weymont, Quebec S83+479 91
Weymouth, England N15+506 38
Weymouth, Nova Scotia S36+444 90
Whakataki, New Zealand A22–408 112
Whakatane, New Zealand A18–380 112
Whale R., Quebec S44+574 89
Whale, R., Gt., Quebec T15+551 89
Whale, R., Lit., Quebec T08+555 89
Whales, B. of, Antarctica Z00–790 27
Whalsay, I., Scotland N06+604 40
Whangarei, New Zealand A34–358 112
Wharanui, New Zealand A35–419 112
Wharfe, R., England N09+539 37
Wharton, Texas U36+293 95
Wheatland, Wyoming V00+420 93
Wheatland Res., Wyoming V04+418 93
Wheaton, Minnesota U39+458 93
Wheeler Dam & L., Alabama T73+348 97
Wheeler Pk., Nevada V56+391 92
Wheeling, W. Virginia T34+401 91
Whetstone Buttes, N. Dakota U77+462 93
Whitbourne, Newfoundland R51+474 90
Whitby, England N04+545 37
Whitby, Ontario T24+439 91
Whitchurch, Salop, Eng. N16+530 37
Whitchurch, Hants, Eng. N08+512 39

White B., *Newfoundland* R68+500 **90**
White L., *Louisiana* U14+298 **95**
White Mts., *New Hampshire* S68+443 **91**
White R., *Arkansas* U12+360 **95**
White R., *Indiana* T74+385 **97**
White R., *S. Dakota* U73+439 **98**
White R., *Utah, etc.* V24+400 **94**
White R., *Yukon* X32+632 **88**
White Cliffs, *New S. Wales* C42-309 **109**
White Earth, *N. Dakota* U77+484 **93**
Whitefish, *Montana* V58+483 **98**
Whitefish B., *Michigan* T59+469 **91**
Whitehall, *Michigan* T68+434 **91**
Whitehall, *New York* S80+435 **91**
Whitehaven, *England* N21+545 **37**
Whitehorse, *Yukon* X00+606 **88**
White Horse Hills, *England* N10+515 **39**
White Mark, *Tasmania* C13-401 **109**
White Pass, *Brit. Columbia* W88+596 **88**
White Plains, *New York* S83+410 **96**
White River, *Ontario* T61+488 **89**
White River, *S. Dakota* U65+435 **93**
White River Junction, *Vermont* S74+434 **99**
White Russia (Byelorussia) rep., *U.S.S.R.* L12+536 **60**
White Sulphur Springs, *Montana* V36+465 **93**
White Volta, R., *Ghana* N06+088 **80**
Whitfield, *Victoria* C22-368 **109**
Whiting, *New Jersey* S86+399 **91**
Whitley Bay, *England* N09+551 **37**
Whitney, *Ontario* T19+455 **91**
Whitney, Mt., *California* V80+366 **92**
Whittier, *California* V78+339 **92**
Whittlesea, *Victoria* C29-375 **109**
Whitton, *New South Wales* C23-345 **109**
Wholdaia L., *N.-W. Terr.* U86+604 **88**
Whyalla, *S. Australia* C75-330 **109**
Wiarton, *Ontario* T37+447 **91**
Wichita, *Kansas* U44+377 **95**
Wichita Falls & R., *Texas* U50+338 **95**
Wichita Mts., *Oklahoma* U54+347 **95**
Wick, *Scotland* N19+584 **40**
Wickliffe, *Missouri* T86+370 **95**
Wicklow & co., *Ireland, Rep.* N36+530 **43**
Wicklow Hd., *Ireland, Rep.* N36+530 **43**
Wicklow Mts., *Ireland, Rep.* N39+530 **43**
Widnes, *England* N16+534 **37**
Wielbark, *Poland* L54+534 **49**
Wielen, *Poland* L83+528 **49**
Wieliczka, *Poland* L60+500 **49**
Wielun, *Poland* L69+512 **49**
Wien, *Austria* L82+482 **49**
Wiener Neustadt, *Austria* L83+478 **49**
Wierzbnik, *Poland* L53+511 **49**
Wiesbaden, *W. Germany* M41+501 **48**
Wiesen, *Switzerland* M32+467 **45**
Wigan, *England* N16+536 **37**
Wight, I. of, *England* N08+507 **39**
Wigton, *England* N19+548 **37**
Wigtown, *Scotland* N27+549 41
Wigtown B., *Scotland* N25+548 **41**
Wijhe, *Netherlands* M53+524 **44**
Wijk, *Netherlands* M56+508 **44**
Wijk, *Netherlands* M58+520 **44**
Wil, *Switzerland* M36+475 **45**
Wilcannia, *New S. Wales* C41-316 **109**
Wildhorn, mt., *Switzerland* M46+464 **45**
Wildstrubel, mt., Switzerland M45+464 **45**
Wildwood, *Florida* T42+288 **97**
Wildwood, *New Jersey* S89+390 **91**
Wilhelmshaven, *W. Germany* M41+535 **48**
Wilkes Ld., *Antarctica* E20-690 **27**
Wilkes Barre, *Pennsylvania* T05+412 **96**
Wilkesboro, *N. Carolina* T37+362 **97**
Wilkin's Str., *Antarctica* S80-710 **27**
Wilkolaz, *Poland* L46+510 **49**
Willamette R., *Oregon* W19+449 **92**
Willcox, *Arizona* V29+323 **94**
Willemsdorp, *Netherlands* M62+517 **44**
Willemstad, *Curaçao I.* S53+121 **104**
Willemstad, *Netherlands* M63+517 **44**
William, Mt., *Victoria* C44-374 **109**
Williams, *Arizona* V43+352 **94**
Williams Pt., *North-West Territories* V68+688 **88**
Williamsburg, *Kentucky* T55+368 **97**
Williamsburg, *Virginia* T10+372 **97**
Williamsport, *Indiana* T74+403 **95**
Williamsport, *Pennsylvania* T13+413 **96**
Williamston, *N. Carolina* T13+358 **97**
Williamsville, *Missouri* U03+370 **97**
Willimantic, *Connecticut* S73+417 **96**
Williston, *Cape Province* L54-314 **84**
Williston, *N. Dakota* U82+481 **93**
Willmar, *Minnesota* U30+451 **93**
Willochra, *S. Australia* C71-322 **109**
Willow L., *N.-W. Territories* W07+620 **88**
Willow Creek, *Montana* V40+458 **93**
Willow Lake R., *N.-W. Terr.* W15+620 **88**
Willowmore, *Cape Province* L38-332 **84**
Willow Springs, *Missouri* U12+370 **95**
Wills Mt., *Pennsylvania* T22+399 **96**
Wilmette, *Illinois* T77+422 **91**
Wilmington, *California* V80+338 **92**
Wilmington, *Delaware* T03+397 **96**
Wilmington, *N. Carolina* T18+342 **97**
Wilmington, *S. Australia* C72-326 **109**
Wilnis, *Netherlands* M61+522 **44**
Wilno, *Ontario* T15+455 **91**
Wilson, *N. Carolina* T18+357 **97**
Wilson's Prom., *Victoria* C22-388 **109**
Wilsonville, *Alabama* T69+332 **97**
Willunga, *S. Australia* C69-353 **109**
Wiltshire (Wilts), co., *Eng.* N11+514 **39**
Wiluna, *W. Australia* D88-266 **110**
Wimbledon, *N. Dakota* U51+472 **93**
Wimmera, R., *Victoria* C47-368 **109**
Winburg, *Orange Free State* L18-286 **84**
Winchendon, *Massachusetts* S72+427 **91**
Winchester, *England* N08+511 **39**
Winchester, *Kentucky* T55+380 **97**
Winchester, *Ontario* T02+451 **91**
Winchester, *Tennessee* T69+352 **97**
Winchester, *Virginia* T19+392 **96**
Wind R., *Yukon* X00+654 **88**
Wind Cave Nat. Pk., *S. Dak.* U82+434 **93**
Windermere & L., *England* N18+544 **37**
Windhoek, *Namibia* L78-226 **84**
Windom, *Minnesota* U31+439 **93**
Wind River Pk. & Mts., *Wyoming* V25+424 **98**
Windsor, *Colorado* V00+405 **94**
Windsor, *Connecticut* S76+419 **96**
Windsor, *England* N04+515 **39**
Windsor, *Missouri* U21+386 **95**
Windsor, *N. Carolina* T12+361 **97**
Windsor, *New South Wales* B86-337 **109**
Windsor, *Nova Scotia* S25+450 **90**
Windsor, *Ontario* T48+423 **91**
Windsor, *Quebec* S72+456 **91**
Windsor, *Vermont* S75+435 **91**
Windward Is., *West Indies* S06+138 **101**
Windward Pass., *West Indies* S84+200 **101**
Winfield, *Kansas* U42+372 **95**
Winfield, *W. Virginia* T41+385 **97**
Wingen, *New South Wales* B85-319 **109**
Wingene, *Belgium* M70+510 **44**
Wingham, *New South Wales* B77-319 **109**
Wingham, *Ontario* T38+439 **91**
Winisk R., *Ontario* T70+548 **89**
Winnebago, *Minnesota* U25+438 **93**
Winnebago L., *Wisconsin* T81+440 **91**
Winnemucca, *Nevada* V76+410 **92**
Winnemucca L., *Nevada* V86+400 **92**
Winner, *S. Dakota* U42+434 **93**
Winnett, *Montana* V20+470 **93**
Winnfield, *Louisiana* U16+319 **97**
Winnipeg, *Manitoba* U43+499 **88**
Winnipeg, L., *Manitoba* U45+526 **88**
Winnipegosis, *Manitoba* U60+514 **88**
Winnipegosis, L., *Manitoba* U60+530 **88**
Winnipesaukee, L., *N.H.* S68+436 **91**
Winnsboro, *S. Carolina* T37+344 **97**
Winona, *Minnesota* U10+441 **93**
Winscale, *England* N21+544 **37**
Winschoten, *Netherlands* M48+533 **44**
Winslow, *Arizona* V34+350 **94**
Winsted, *Connecticut* S78+419 **96**
Winston Salem, *N. Carolina* T32+361 **97**
Winter Ra., *Oregon* W09+430 **92**
Winterhaven, *California* V58+327 **92**
Winter Haven, *Florida* T39+281 **97**
Winterport, *Maine* S53+446 **90**
Winterset, *Iowa* U24+413 **95**
Winterswijk, *Netherlands* M49+520 **44**
Winterthur, *Switzerland* M38+475 **45**
Winton, *New Zealand* A69-462 **112**
Winton, *Queensland* C41-222 **111**
Wirksworth, *England* N09+531 **37**
Wirrabara, *S. Australia* C71-330 **109**
Wirral Pen., *England* N18+533 **37**
Wirrega, *S. Australia* C56-362 **109**
Wirt, *Minnesota* U23+478 **93**
Wisbech, *England* M89+527 **37**
Wisconsin, state, *U.S.A.* U07+447 **99**
Wisconsin R., *Wisconsin* T89+452 **91**
Wisconsin Rapids, *Wisconsin* T89+444 **91**
Wise, *Virginia* T46+370 **97**
Wishaw, *Scotland* N23+558 **41**
Wishek, *N. Dakota* U58+462 **93**
Wisla (Vistula), R., *Poland* L51+517 **49**
Wismar, *E. Germany* M22+539 **48**
Witham, R., *England* N02+532 **37**
Withlacoochee B., *Florida* T57+290 **99**
Witputs, *Namibia* L80-276 **84**
Witry, *Belgium* M56+498 **44**
Witten, *W. Germany* M46+515 **48**
Wittenberg, *E. Germany* M14+519 **48**
Wittenberge, *E. Germany* M19+530 **48**
Wittenoon, *Western Aust.* E09-213 **110**
Wittingen, *W. Germany* M26+527 **48**
Wittstock, *E. Germany* M15+532 **48**
Wivenhoe, *England* M84+518 **39**
Wloclawek, *Poland* L66+526 **49**
Wodonga, *Victoria* C19-361 **109**
Woerden, *Netherlands* M61+521 **44**
Wognum, *Netherlands* M60+527 **44**
Wohlen, *Switzerland* M40+473 **45**
Wokam, I., *Indonesia* D03-058 **65**
Wolbrom, *Poland* L61+504 **69**
Woleai, I., *Caroline Islands* C40+065 **106**
Wolfe I., *Ontario* T08+442 **91**
Wolfeboro, *New Hampshire* S67+436 **91**
Wolfe City, *Texas* U36+332 **95**
Wolf Point, *Montana* V04+481 **93**
Wolfsberg, *Austria* M01+468 **48**
Wolfville, *Nova Scotia* S26+450 **90**
Wolgast, *E. Germany* M08+540 **48**
Wolhusen, *Switzerland* M42+471 **45**
Wollaston, *England* N04+522 **39**
Wollaston Foreland, *Greenland* P28+740 **26**
Wollaston, Is., *Chile* S44-557 **103**
Wollaston L., *Saskatchewan* U80+584 **88**
Wollongong, *New S. Wales* B85-344 **109**
Wolseley, *S. Australia* C54-364 **109**
Wolstenholme, C., *Quebec* T15+621 **89**
Wolvega, *Netherlands* M54+529 **44**
Wolverhampton, *England* N13+526 **37**
Wolvertem, *Belgium* M64+509 **44**
Wolverton, *England* N05+521 **39**
Woman River, *Ontario* T46+475 **91**
Wonoka, *S. Australia* C70-317 **109**
Wonsan, *Korea* D45+391 **64**
Wonthaggi, *Victoria* C27-386 **109**
Wood R., *Saskatchewan* V12+500 **88**
Woodbridge, *England* M82+521 **39**
Wood Buffalo Park, *Alberta* V50+594 **88**
Woodburn, *New South Wales* B70-290 **109**
Woodbury, *New Jersey* T01+398 **96**
Woodford, *Newfoundland* R49+474 **90**
Woodlark I., *Papua New Guinea* B74+093 **111**
Woodroffe, Mt., *S. Australia* D23-264 **110**
Woods, L., *N. Terr., Aust.* D10-179 **110**
Woods, L. of the, *Ontario* U30+494 **88**
Woods Hole, *Massachusetts* S64+415 **96**
Woodside, *Utah* V32+392 **94**
Woodside, *Victoria* C19-385 **109**
Woodstock, *Illinois* T80+424 **95**
Woodstock, *New Brunswick* S45+461 **90**
Woodstock, *Ontario* T35+432 **91**
Woodstock, *Vermont* S75+436 **96**
Woodstock, *Virginia* T21+388 **96**
Woodsville, *New Hampshire* S72+441 **91**
Woodville, *New Zealand* A24-403 **112**
Woodward, *Oklahoma* U57+364 **95**
Wooler, *England* N12+555 **37**
Wooltana, *S. Australia* C64-305 **109**
Woolwich, *England* N00+515 **39**
Woomera, *S. Australia* C82-312 **111**
Woonsocket, *Rhode Island* S69+420 **96**
Woonsocket, *S. Dakota* U50+441 **93**
Worcester, *Cape Province* L64-338 **84**
Worcester, *England* N13+522 **37**
Worcester, *Massachusetts* S71+423 **91**
Worcester, co., *See* Hereford & Worcs.
Workington, *England* N21+546 **37**
Worksop, *England* N07+533 **37**
Workum, *Netherlands* M57+530 **44**
Worland, *Wyoming* V18+440 **93**
Worms, *W. Germany* M40+496 **48**
Worthing, *England* N02+508 **39**
Worthington, *Minnesota* U32+436 **93**
Worthington, *Ontario* T39+464 **91**
Wotho, I., *Marshall Islands* A85+100 **106**
Woudenberg, *Netherlands* M57+521 **44**
Woudrichem, *Netherlands* M60+518 **44**
Wounta, *Nicaragua* T51+135 **101**
Wour, *Chad* L86+212 **81**
Wouw, *Netherlands* M64+515 **44**
Wowoni, I., *Indonesia* D72-041 **65**
Wrangel I. *See* Vrangelya, Ostrov
Wrangell, *Alaska* W70+564 **99**
Wrangell, Mt., *Alaska* X62+616 **99**
Wrath C., *Scotland* N30+586 **40**
Wray, *Colorado* U74+400 **94**
Wrexham, *Wales* N18+530 **38**
Wright, Mt., *New S. Wales* C46-312 **109**
Wrightsville, *Georgia* T46+327 **97**
Wrightsville Beach, *North Carolina* T17+342 **97**
Wrigley, *N.-W. Territories* W25+637 **88**
Wroclaw, *Poland* L78+511 **49**
Wroxham, *England* M82+527 **39**
Wuchang, *China* D46+449 **64**
Wuchang, *China* E34+305 **67**
Wuchow (Tsangwu), *China* E51+235 **67**
Wuchwan, *China* E51+411 **66**
Wudam, *Saudi Arabia* J15+238 **75**
Wuhan, *China* E32+304 **66**
Wuhing. *See* Huchow
Wuhsien. *See* Soochow
Wuhu, *China* E09+314 **66**
Wukang, *China* E56+268 **67**
Wukari, *Nigeria* M32+078 **81**
Wukiang, *China* E25+380 **66**
Wu Kiang, R., *China* E72+280 **64**
Wular L., *Kashmir* H02+344 **72**
Wuntho, *Burma* F55+239 **71**
Wuppertal, *W. Germany* M47+513 **48**
Wurttemberg, *W. Germany* M36+485 **48**
Wurzburg, *W. Germany* M30+498 **48**
Wurzen, *E. Germany* M14+514 **48**
Wushih, *Hainan Island* E62+192 **64**
Wusiang, *China* E42+368 **66**
Wusih, *China* D88+316 **66**
Wuti, *China* E14+377 **66**
Wutsin, *China* E00+318 **66**
Wuustwezel, *Belgium* M63+514 **44**
Wuwei, *China* F14+379 **66**
Wu Yi Shan, *China* E21+270 **67**
Wuyüan, *China* E70+411 **66**
Wuyuon, *China* D32+490 **64**
Wyalong, West, *New S. Wales* C17-339 109
Wyandotte, *Michigan* L49+422 **91**
Wyangala Res., *New South Wales* C06-339 **109**
Wye, R., *England-Wales* N16+520 **38**
Wyk, *W. Germany* M39+547 **48**
Wymondham, *England* M83+526 **39**
Wyndham, *New Zealand* A66-463 **112**
Wyndham, *W. Australia* D41-154 **110**
Wynne, *Arkansas* U05+352 **95**
Wynyard, *Tasmania* C26-410 **109**
Wyoming, state, *U.S.A.* V26+436 **98**
Wyoming Pk., *Wyoming* V34+426 **93**
Wyong, *New South Wales* B82-333 **109**
Wysokie Mazowieckie, *Poland* L45+529 **49**
Wyszkow, *Poland* L51+526 **49**
Wytheville, *Virginia* T37+369 **97**
Xanthi, *Greece* L31+412 **58**
Xanxere, *Brazil* R45-268 **103**
Xapuri, *Brazil* S52-107 **104**
Xenia, *Montana* V31+486 **93**
Xeró, *See* Peristera I.
Xibury, *Brazil* S43-053 **104**
Xilokastron, *Greece* L44+381 **59**
Xingu, *Brazil* S55-082 **104**
Yaan, *China* F11+300 **64**
Yaapeet, *Victoria* C48-358 **109**
Yaate, *Lebanon* K53+340 **76**
Yablonovy Khrebet Mts., *U.S.S.R.* E50+510 **63**
Yabrud, *Syria* K50+339 **76**
Yackandandah, *Victoria* C17-362 **109**
Yacuiba, *Bolivia* S22-218 **104**
Yagvildino, *U.S.S.R.* J21+558 **61**
Yakhtul, *Yemen* K10+135 **74**
Yakima, *Washington* W03+466 **92**
Yako, *Volta* N14+128 **80**
Yakoma, *Zaire* L46+038 **82**
Yaku Kaikyo, *Japan* D25+303 **68**
Yaku Shima, *Japan* D27+303 **68**
Yakutsk, *U.S.S.R.* D31+621 **63**
Yale, *British Columbia* W08+496 **88**
Yale, *Michigan* T47+432 **91**
Yalgoo, *W. Australia* E20-282 **110**
Yalinga, *Cent. Afr. Rep.* L40+065 **81**
Yallourn, *Victoria* C22-381 **109**
Yalouke, *Cent. Afr. Rep.* L78+054 **81**
Yalpunga, *New S. Wales* C48-289 **109**
Yalta, *U.S.S.R.* K64+446 **60**
Yalu, *China* D77+483 **64**
Yalu R., *China, etc.* D60+407 **64**
Yalung R., *China* F28+314 **64**
Yalutorovsk, *U.S.S.R.* H53+568 **62**
Yamada, *Japan* C79+345 **68**
Yamagata, *Japan* C58+382 **68**
Yamaguchi, *Japan* D21+342 **68**
Yamal, Pol., *U.S.S.R.* H30+715 **62**
Yamba, *New South Wales* B70-294 **109**
Yambol, *Bulgaria* L21+425 **58**
Yamdena I., *Indonesia* D22+077 65
Yamdok Tso, *Tibet* F85+290 **71**
Yamethin, *Burma* F52+204 **71**
Yampol, *U.S.S.R.* L10+483 **60**
Yampol, *U.S.S.R.* L23+499 **60**
Yamsk, *U.S.S.R.* B66+593 **63**
Yamuna R., *India* G58+260 **73**
Yanac, *Victoria* C51-361 **109**
Yanam, *India* G47+168 **71**
Yanaoca, *Peru* S69-143 **104**
Yancannia, *New S. Wales* C44-303 **109**
Yanco, *New South Wales* C22-346 **109**
Yanda, R., *New South Wales* C25-310 **109**
Yandoon, *Burma* F56+170 **71**
Yangchow, *China* E04+323 **66**
Yangihissar, *Sinkiang, China* G83+389 **72**
Yang-kao, *China* E38+404 **66**
Yangku. *See* Taiyuan
Yangtze Kiang, R., *China* E70+308 **66**
Yangyuan, *China* E34+401 **66**
Yankton, *S. Dakota* U44+429 **93**
Yannina. *See* Ioannina
Yantabulla, *New S. Wales* C30-294 **109**
Yaoundé, *Cameroon* M20+038 **81**
Yap, I., *Pacific Ocean* C70+093 **106**
Yapen I., *Irian Jaya, Indon.* C82+018 65
Yaraka, *Queensland* C36-248 **111**
Yarda, *Chad* L66+184 **81**
Yare R., *England* M81+526 **39**
Yarensk, *U.S.S.R.* J65+623 **62**
Yarim, *Yemen* K04+145 **74**
Yarkand, *Sinkiang, China* G77+384 **72**
Yarmouth, *I. of Wight, Eng.* N09+507 **39**
Yarmouth, *Maine* S61+438 **90**
Yarmouth, *Nova Scotia* S37+438 **90**
Yarmouth, Great, *England* M80+526 **39**
Yaroslavl, *U.S.S.R.* K30+576 **60**
Yarram, *Victoria* C20-385 **109**
Yarrawonga, *Victoria* C24-360 **109**
Yarrow, R., *Scotland* N18+555 **41**
Yartsevo, *U.S.S.R.* G00+602 **63**
Yarumal, *Colombia* T03+070 **104**
Yarylgach, *U.S.S.R.* K73+456 **60**
Yasanyama, *Zaire* L53+042 81
Yasin, *Kashmir* H10+364 **72**
Yasothon, *Thailand* F04+158 **65**
Yass & R., *New S. Wales* C07-348 **109**
Yatakala, *Niger* M88+146 **80**
Yathkyed L., *N.-W. Terr.* U35+630 **88**
Yatsushiro, *Japan* D26+325 **68**
Yatta, *Jordan* K59+314 **76**
Yatung, *Tibet* G06+274 **71**
Yauca, *Peru* S87-157 **104**
Yauri, *Peru* S69-148 **104**
Yautepec, *Mexico* U54+188 **100**
Yavarete, *Colombia* S54-002 **104**
Yawata, *Japan* D25+338 **68**
Yazd, *Iran* J33+319 **75**
Yazdan, *Iran* H85+337 **75**
Yazoo City, *Mississippi* U02+328 **95**
Ybbs, *Austria* M00+482 **48**
Ye, *Burma* F43+153 **71**
Yea, *Victoria* C27-372 **109**
Yecla, *Spain* N07+386 **53**
Yecora, *Mexico* V22+288 **100**
Yéfira, *Greece* L44+407 **59**
Yefremov, *U.S.S.R.* K42+532 **60**
Yegros, *Paraguay* R68-265 **103**
Yehcheng. *See* Karghalik
Yehkiatsi, *China* E24+318 **64**
Yehpaishow, *China* E01+413 **66**
Yehsien, *China* E00+372 **66**
Yelabuga, *U.S.S.R.* J47+558 **61**
Yelan, *U.S.S.R.* K08+509 **61**
Yelatma, *U.S.S.R.* K20+550 **61**
Yeldyak, *U.S.S.R.* J20+556 **61**
Yelets, *U.S.S.R.* K39+526 **60**
Yelizarovo, *U.S.S.R.* H45+615 **62**
Yell, I. & Sd., *Scotland* N07+606 **40**
Yellandu, *India* G59+177 **70**
Yellow Mt., *New S. Wales* C19-327 **109**
Yellow R. *See* Hwang Ho
Yellow Sea, *China* D78+350 **66**
Yellowhead Pass, *Alberta* V80+532 **88**
Yellowstone L., *Wyoming* V32+440 **98**
Yellowstone Nat. Pk., *Wyo.* V34+447 **93**
Yellowstone R., *Montana, etc.* U86+473 **93**
Yellowtail Res., *Montana* V20+450 **93**
Yemanzhelinka, *U.S.S.R.* H82+548 **61**
Yemen, *Asia* K10+173 **74**
Yemen, South *Asia* J80+150 **74**
Yenakiyevo, *Ukraine* K41+482 **60**
Yenan (Fushih), *China* E63+366 **66**
Yenangyaung, *Burma* F60+204 **71**
Yen-Bay, *Vietnam* F02+216 **69**
Yenbo, *Saudi Arabia* K42+242 **74**
Yencheng, *China* D89+333 **66**
Yenchih, *China* F50+420 **64**
Yenchow. *See* Kienteh
Yenchow. *See* Tzeyang
Yenda, *New South Wales* C23-343 **109**
Yenise, R., *U.S.S.R.* G20+680 **62**
Yeniseysk, *U.S.S.R.* F78+583 **63**
Yeniseyskiy Zaliv, *U.S.S.R.* G60+724 **62**
Yenki, *China* D32+428 **64**
Yenki (Kara Shahr), *China* G22+421 **62**
Yenping. *See* Nanping
Yentai, *China* D82+375 **66**
Yeoval, *New South Wales* C08-328 **109**
Yeovil, *England* N16+510 **38**
Yeper, *Belgium* M73+508 **44**
Yeráki, *Greece* L44+370 **59**
Yerbogachen, *U.S.S.R.* E73+614 **63**
Yerevan, *Armyanskaya, U.S.S.R.* K03+402 **62**
Yerofei Pavlovich, *U.S.S.R.* D78+540 **63**
Yeropol, *U.S.S.R.* A66+651 **63**
Yeshbum, *Yemen, South* J79+145 **74**
Yessei, *U.S.S.R.* F17+683 **63**
Yeste, *Spain* N14+384 **53**
Yesud ha Ma'ala, *Israel* K56+331 **76**
Yetman, *New South Wales* B86-289 **109**
Yeu, *Burma* F57+228 **71**
Yeu, I. d', *France* N14+467 **54**
Yeungkong, *China* E48+217 **64**
Yevsyeevo, *U.S.S.R.* B69+673 **63**
Yeysk, *U.S.S.R.* K40+465 **62**
Yezd-i-Khast, *Iran* J47+316 **75**
Yhu, *Paraguay* R66-250 **103**
Yi, R., *Uruguay* R71-333 **103**
Yianisadhes Is., *Crete* L22+354 **59**
Yiannitsá, *Greece* L46+407 **59**
Yibna, *Israel* K62+319 **76**
Yidha, *Greece* L45+406 **59**
Yihsien, *China* E26+394 **66**
Yingchisa. *See* Yangihissar
Yingchow. *See* Fowyang
Yingchwan, *China* E82+385 **66**
Yinghsien, *China* E41+395 **66**
Yingkow, *China* D77+407 **66**
Yingtak, *China* E40+242 **67**
Yinkanie, *S. Australia* C58-343 **109**
Yioura, I., *Greece* L32+376 **59**

Yithion, *Greece* L45+368 **59**
Yitu, *China* E09+367 **66**
Yiyang, *China* E46+287 **67**
Yocalla, *Bolivia* S36–192 **104**
Yochow. *See* Yoyang
Yogovsk, *U.S.S.R.* J22+576 **61**
Yogyakarta, *Java* E58+079 **65**
Yoho Park, *Brit. Columbia* V70+512 **88**
Yokkaichi, *Japan* C80+350 **68**
Yoko, *Cameroon* M16+056 **81**
Yokohama, *Japan* C62+354 **68**
Yokosuku, *Japan* C62+352 **68**
Yokote, *Japan* C57+393 **68**
Yola, *Nigeria* M16+092 **81**
Yonago, *Japan* D10+354 **68**
Yone Zawa, *Japan* C59+379 **68**
Yonkers, *New York* S83+409 **96**
Yonne, dep., *France* M69+478 **54**
York, *Alabama* T80+325 **97**
York, *England* N07+539 **37**
York, *Nebraska* U46+408 **95**
York, *Pennsylvania* T11+400 **96**
York, *W. Australia* E19–319 **110**
York C., *Greenland* S50+760 **26**
York, C., *Queensland* C45–108 **111**
York R., *Virginia* T10+374 **97**
York Sd., *W. Australia* D58–150 **110**
Yorke Pen., *S. Australia* C74–346 **109**
Yorketown, *S. Australia* C75–350 **109**
York Factory, *Manitoba* U16+567 **89**
Yorkshire, North, co., *Eng.* N08+542 **37**
Yorkshire Moors, *England* N05+544 **37**
Yorkshire Wolds, *England* N03+540 **37**
Yorkton, *Saskatchewan* U75+511 **88**
Yorktown, *Virginia* T09+372 **97**
York Village, *Maine* S64+432 **90**
Yoro, *Honduras* T71+150 **101**
Yosemite Nat. Park, *Cal.* V88+379 **92**
Yoshkar Ola, *U.S.S.R.* J72+568 **61**
Youghal & Harb., *Ireland, Rep.* N47+519 **43**
Youghiogheny River Res., *Penn. etc.* T27+397 **96**
Youkadouma, *Cameroon* M00+036 **81**
Young, *New South Wales* C10+343 **109**
Younghusband Pen., *S. Aust.* C64–360 **109**
Youngstown, *Ohio* T34+411 **91**
Yount Pk., *Wyoming* V30+440 **93**
Yoyang, *China* E40+294 **67**
Yozgat, *Turkey* K62+398 **74**
Ypres (Yeper), *Belgium* M73+508 **44**
Ypsilanti, *Michigan* T52+423 **91**
Yreka, *California* W16+417 **92**
Ysabel, I., *Solomon Islands* B35–080 **106**
Yssingeaux, *France* M65+451 **55**
Ystad, *Sweden* M07+555 **47**
Ytterhogdal, *Sweden* M01+622 **46**
Yüanchow. *See* Chihkiang
Yüanchow. *See* Ichun
Yüanling, *China* E58+285 **67**
Yubalia, *S. Australia* C58–336 **109**
Yubi C., *Morocco* N78+280 **80**
Yucamani, mt., *Peru* S60–170 **104**
Yucatan, state, *Mexico* T84+208 **100**
Yucatan Chan., *Mex.-Cuba* T66+216 **101**
Yugoslavia (Jugoslavia), *Cent. Europe* L70+440 **51**
Yuhsien, *China* E32+398 **66**
Yuhwan, *China* D82+282 **67**
Yukhnov, *U.S.S.R.* K59+548 **60**
Yukon Terr., *Canada* W80+610 **88**
Yukon, R., *Alaska* Y60+626 **99**
Yulin, *China* E62+383 **66**
Yuma, *Arizona* V58+329 **98**
Yuma, *Colorado* U76+401 **94**
Yumen, *China* F50+410 **63**
Yungchow. *See* Lingling
Yungera, *Victoria* C41–348 **109**
Yungfu, *China* E60+250 **67**
Yungki. *See* Kirin
Yungkia. *See* Wenchow
Yungnien, *China* E31+368 **66**
Yungning (Nanning), *China* E70+228 **67**
Yungning, *China* F25+277 **64**
Yungping. *See* Lulung
Yungshun, *China* E61+290 **67**
Yungsin, *China* E33+270 **67**
Yungsui, *China* E63+286 **67**
Yungtsi, *China* E59+349 **66**
Yunhsien, *China* E54+329 **66**
Yunsi, *China* E57+331 **66**
Yunta, *S. Australia* C63–326 **109**
Yurievets, *U.S.S.R.* K11+574 **61**
Yurimaguas, *Peru* T07–059 **104**
Yurlovka, *U.S.S.R.* J79+536 **61**
Yurmysh, *U.S.S.R.* H70+572 **61**
Yushu, *China* F50+332 **64**
Yütze, *China* E44+377 **66**
Yuyang, *China* E67+288 **67**
Yuyu, *China* E46+402 **66**
Yverdon, *Switzerland* M50+468 **45**
Ywathit, *Burma* F45+192 **71**
Zaachila, *Mexico* U41+168 **100**
Zaandam, *Netherlands* M61+524 **44**
Zabid, *Yemen* K11+141 **74**
Zabrze, *Poland* L67+504 **49**
Zacapa, *Guatemala* T88+149 **100**
Zacapoaxtla, *Mexico* U46+198 **100**
Zacatecas & state, *Mexico* U76+228 **100**
Zadar, *Yugoslavia* L89+441 **56**
Zadonsk, *U.S.S.R.* K36+524 **60**
Zafarabad, *Iran* J75+390 **74**
Zafarwal, *Pakistan* H01+323 **72**
Zafra, *Spain* N38+384 **52**
Zagazig, *Egypt* K80+306 **81**
Zagreb, *Yugoslavia* L84+458 **56**
Zahedan, *Iran* H84+295 **75**
Zahle, *Lebanon* K55+338 **76**
Zahran, *Saudi Arabia* K06+174 **74**
Zaidiya, *Yemen* K12+152 **74**
Zainsk, *U.S.S.R.* J47+553 **61**
Zaire, rep., *Cent. Africa* L50–050 **82**
Zaisan, *Kazakh.* G30+474 **62**
Zaječar, *Yugoslavia* L46+439 **58**
Zakho, *Iraq* K13+373 **74**
Zakin, *Afghanistan* H81+326 **75**
Zakinthos, I., *Greece* L56+378 **59**
Zakroczyn, *Poland* L55+498 **49**
Zákros, *Crete* L22+351 **59**
Zalău, *Romania* L42+472 **49**
Zalew Wiślany, *Poland* L62+544 **49**
Zalma, *Missouri* U01+370 **97**
Zambia, *Africa* L30–150 **84**
Zambezi R., *S.-E. Africa* K52–186 **84**
Zamboanga, *Philippines* D77+070 **65**
Zamora, *Ecuador* T22–042 **104**
Zamora de Hadalgo, *Mex.* U74+199 **100**
Zamora, *Spain* N34+415 **52**
Zandberg, *Netherlands* M48+529 **44**
Zandvoort, *Netherlands* M63+524 **44**
Zanesville, *Ohio* T42+399 **91**
Zangla, *Kashmir* G78+336 **72**
Zanjan, *Iran* J69+367 **74**
Zante. *See* Zakinthos I.
Zanzibar & I., *E. Africa* K34–062 **83**
Zapala, *Argentina* S61–388 **103**
Zapallar, *Argentina* R87–265 **103**
Zapata Pen., *Cuba* T40+223 **101**
Zaporozhye, *Ukraine* K59+479 **60**
Zara, *Turkey* K44+399 **74**
Zara. *See* Zadar
Zaragoza, *Colombia* S89+074 **104**
Zaragoza, *Mexico* U57+241 **100**
Zaragoza, *Spain* N05+416 **53**
Zaragozo, *Mexico* U81+260 **100**
Zaraguro, *Ecuador* T25–036 **104**
Zarand, *Iran* J20+308 **75**
Zarasai, *Lithuania* L22+558 **47**
Zarauz, *Spain* N13+433 **53**
Zaraza, *Venezuela* S32+094 **104**
Zaria, *Nigeria* M44+110 **80**
Zarki, *Poland* L64+507 **49**
Zarnūqa, *Saudi Arabia* J61+250 **74**
Zarqa, *Jordan* K53+321 **76**
Zaruma, *Ecuador* T28–038 **104**
Zarzis, *Tunisia* M35+335 **81**
Zatec, *Czechoslovakia* M09+503 **48**
Zavitinsk, *U.S.S.R.* D33+500 **63**
Zawiercie, *Poland* L63+505 **49**
Zaysan, Oz., *Kazakh* G35+480 **62**
Zbaszyn, *Poland* L84+522 **49**
Zdunska Wola, *Poland* L66+516 **49**
Zealand, *New Brunswick* S41+461 **90**
Zealand. *See* Sjaelland
Zebak, *Afghanistan* H21+364 **75**
Zebdani, *Syria* K53+337 **76**
Zebid Qadhima, *Saudi Arabia* K35+224 **74**
Zeebrugge, *Belgium* M71+513 **44**
Zeehan, *Tasmania* C28–419 **109**
Zeeland, prov., *Netherlands* M67+515 **44**
Zeerust, *Transvaal* L24–256 **84**
Zegharta, *Lebanon* K55+344 **76**
Zeila, *Somalia* K10+112 **83**
Zeist, *Netherlands* M58+521 **44**
Zeitz, *E. Germany* M17+510 **48**
Zelaf, *Syria* K46+329 **76**
Zele, *Belgium* M66+511 **44**
Železná Ruda, *Czech.* M11+491 **48**
Zella, *Libya* L76+284 **81**
Zelman, *U.S.S.R.* J84+507 **61**
Zemio, *Cent. Afr. Rep.* L30+050 **81**
Zemun, *Yugoslavia* L57+448 **58**
Zenica, *Yugoslavia* L73+442 **58**
Zepce, *Yugoslavia* L72+445 **58**
Zermatt, *Switzerland* M43+460 **45**
Zernez, *Switzerland* M29+467 **45**
Zetland (Shetland), *Scot.* N07+604 **40**
Zevenbergen, *Netherlands* M62+516 **44**
Zeya, *U.S.S.R.* D47+537 **63**
Zeyma, *Saudi Arabia* K29+217 **74**
Zgierz, *Poland* L63+519 **49**
Zgorzelec. *See* Görlitz.
Zhdanov, *Ukraine* K44+471 **60**
Zhigansk, *U.S.S.R.* D70+667 **63**
Zhitomir, *Ukraine* L08+504 **60**
Zhmerinka, *Ukraine* L10+490 **60**
Ziarat, *Pakistan* H43+304 **70**
Ziba. *See Dhaba.*
Zidani Most, *Yugoslavia* L89+461 **56**
Ziemupe, *Latvia* L53+568 **47**
Zierikzee, *Netherlands* M66+516 **44**
Zijpe, *Netherlands* M66+517 **44**
Zikhron Ya'aqoy, *Israel* K60+325 **76**
Zile, *Turkey* K54+402 **74**
Zilfi, *Saudi Arabia* K02+262 **74**
Zilina, *Czechoslovakia* L67+492 **49**
Zima, *U.S.S.R.* F18+540 **63**
Zimapan, *Mexico* U56+207 **100**
Zimbabwe, *S.E. Africa* L00–200 **84**
Zinder, *Niger* M36+138 **81**
Zingst, pen., *E. Germany* M14+544 **48**
Zion Nat. Park, *Utah* V48+374 **92**
Zira, *India* H00+310 **72**
Ziraquira, *Colombia* S84+050 **104**
Zirc, *Hungary* L73+473 **49**
Zitacuaro, *Mexico* U63+193 **100**
Zittau, *E. Germany* M01+509 **48**
Zizers, *Switzerland* M32+469 **45**
Zlatoust, *U.S.S.R.* J02+551 **61**
Zmeinogorsk, *U.S.S.R.* G47+511 **62**
Znin, *Poland* L74+528 **49**
Znojmo, *Czechoslovakia* L84+489 **49**
Zoar, *Labrador* S19+558 **89**
Zofingen, *Switzerland* M42+473 **45**
Zoisa, *Tanzania* K50–058 **83**
Zolder, *Belgium* M58+510 **44**
Zollino, *Italy* L71+402 **57**
Zolotoye, *U.S.S.R.* J85+508 **61**
Zomba, *Malawi* K58–154 **83**
Zonguldak, *Turkey* K78+416 **74**
Zorita, *Spain* N34+393 **52**
Zoute, Het, *Belgium* M70+514 **44**
Zoutkamp, *Netherlands* M52+533 **44**
Zrenjanin, *Yugoslavia* L58+454 **58**
Zuara, *Libya* M18+328 **81**
Zuevka, *U.S.S.R.* J55+585 **61**
Zug & canton, *Switzerland* M39+472 **45**
Zuger See, *Switzerland* M39+471 **45**
Zuhab, *Iran* J85+347 **74**
Zuid Beijerland, *Netherlands* M64+518 **44**
Zuider Zee. *See* IJsselmeer
Zuidland, *Netherlands* M65+518 **44**
Zuid Natoena Eiln., *Indon.* E66+028 **65**
Zuidwolde, *Netherlands* M51+527 **44**
Zuila, *Libya* L88+262 **81**
Zukur, Jab., *Yemen* K13+140 **74**
Zula, *Ethiopia* K32+152 **83**
Zulfikar, *Afghanistan* H82+356 **75**
Zumbo, *Mozambique* K88–156 **84**
Zumpango, *Mexico* U54+198 **100**
Zundert, *Netherlands* M62+515 **44**
Zungeru, *Nigeria* M54+098 **80**
Zuni, Mt., *New Mexico* V18+352 **94**
Zürich & canton, *Switz.* M39+474 **45**
Zürich See, *Switzerland* M38+472 **45**
Zurzach, *Switzerland* M40+476 **45**
Zutphen, *Netherlands* M53+522 **44**
Zwai L., *Ethiopia* K38+078 **83**
Zwartsluis, *Netherlands* M54+526 **44**
Zweelo, *Netherlands* M50+528 **44**
Zweibrucken, *W. Germany* M47+493 **48**
Zweisimmen, *Switzerland* M46+466 **45**
Zwickau, *E. Germany* M15+507 **48**
Zwoleń, *Poland* L51+513 **49**
Zwolle, *Netherlands* M53+525 **44**
Żyrardów, *Poland* L57+521 **49**
Zyryanka, *U.S.S.R.* B85+645 **63**
Zyryanovsk, *Kazakh.* G35+498 **62**
Zyyi, *Cyprus* K70+347 **76**

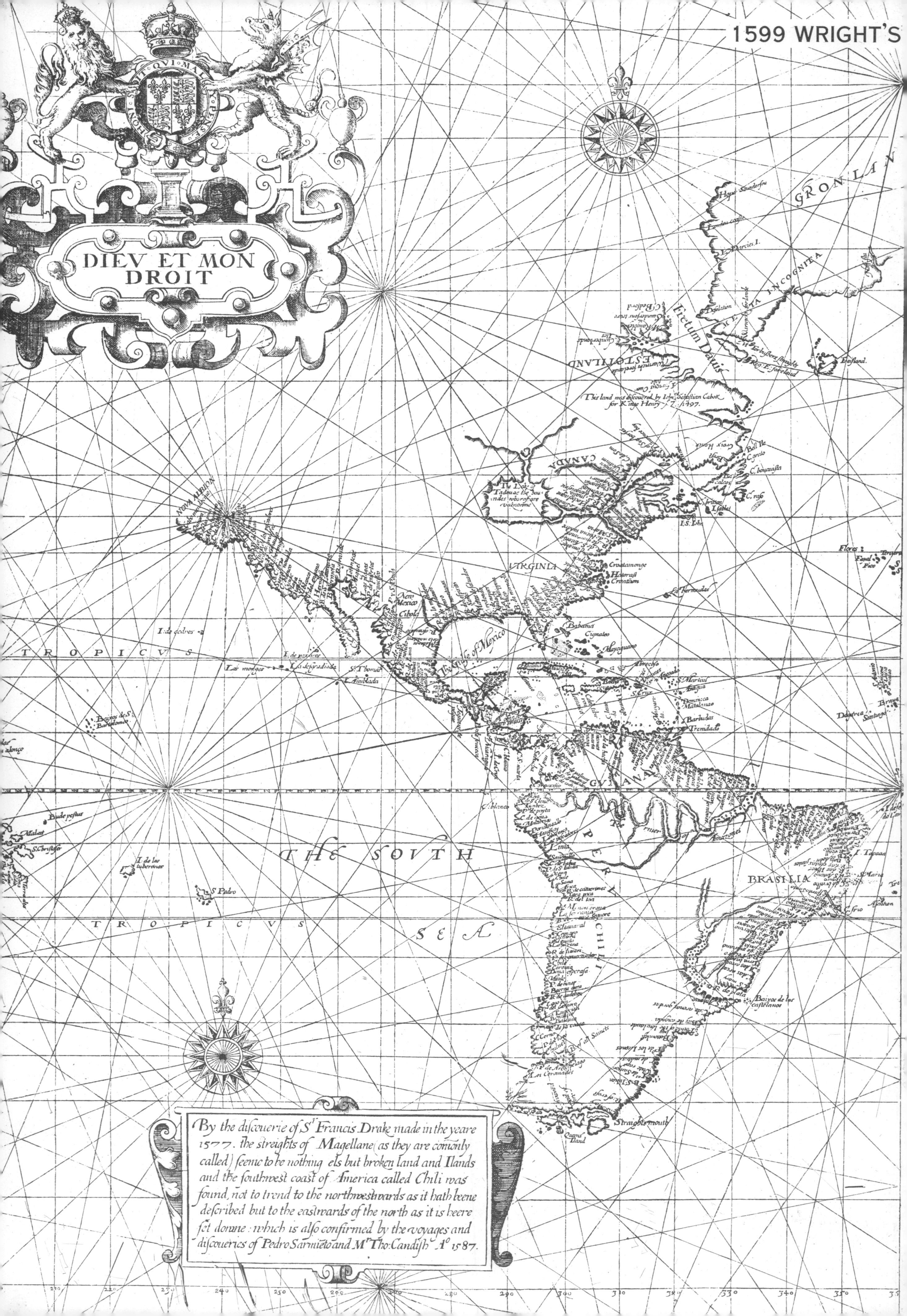
1599 WRIGHT'S
DIEV ET MON DROIT
GRON LAN
TERRA INCOGNITA
Fretum Dauis
ESTOTILAND
This land was discouered by Iohn Sebastian Cabot for Kinge Henry 7. 1497.
CANADA
NOVA ALBION
VIRGINIA
New Mexico
The Gulfe of Mexico
Bermudas
TROPICVS
GVIANA
PERV
THE SOVTH SEA
BRASILIA
CHILI
Straights mouth
By the discouerie of Sr Francis Drake made in the yeare 1577. the streights of Magellane (as they are comonly called) seeme to be nothing els but broken land and Ilands and the southwest coast of America called Chili was found, not to trend to the northwestwards as it hath beene described but to the eastwards of the north as it is heere set downe: which is also confirmed by the voyages and discoueries of Pedro Sarmieto and Mr Tho: Candish Ao 1587.